Practices in Children's Nursing

Guidelines for Hospital and Community

SECOND EDITION

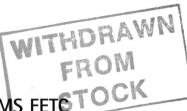

Edited by

Ethel Trigg MBA RN RSCN DMS FETC

General Manager and Children's Lead, Sussex Downs and Weald Primary Care Trust, Sussex, UK

Toby A. Mohammed MN (Specialty in Education) PGCE RGN RSCN RNT

Senior Nurse (Practice Development), Yorkhill Operating Division of NHS Greater Glasgow, Glasgow, UK

Foreword by

Sally Huband

Formerly Senior Lecturer, Paediatrics, Sussex and Kent Institute, Brighton, UK

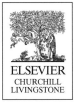

ELSEVIER
CHURCHILL
LIVINGSTONE

EDINBURGH LONDON NEW YORK OXFORD PHILADELPHIA ST LOUIS SYDNEY TORONTO 2006

ELSEVIER
CHURCHILL
LIVINGSTONE

First edition 2000
Second edition 2006

ISBN 0 443 10022 5

British Library Cataloguing in Publication Data
A catalogue record for this book is available from the British Library

Library of Congress Cataloging in Publication Data
A catalog record for this book is available from the Library of Congress

Note
Knowledge and best practice in this field are constantly changing. As new research
and experience broaden our knowledge, changes in practice, treatment and drug
therapy may become necessary or appropriate. Readers are advised to check the most
current information provided (i) on procedures featured or (ii) by the manufacturer of
each product to be administered, to verify the recommended dose or formula, the
method and duration of administration, and contraindications. It is the responsibility
of the practitioner, relying on their own experience and knowledge of the patient, to
make diagnoses, to determine dosages and the best treatment for each individual
patient, and to take all appropriate safety precautions. To the fullest extent of the law,
neither the publisher nor the editors assume any liability for any injury and/or
damage to persons or property arising out of or related to any use of the material
contained in this book.

The Publisher

Working together to grow
libraries in developing countries

www.elsevier.com | www.bookaid.org | www.sabre.org

ELSEVIER   BOOK AID International   Sabre Foundation

ELSEVIER your source for books,
journals and multimedia
in the health sciences

www.elsevierhealth.com

The
Publisher's
policy is to use
**paper manufactured
from sustainable forests**

Printed in China

Contents

Clinical Coordinators

BIRMINGHAM

Julia Fearon RGN RSCN BSc (Complementary Therapy)
Independent Children's Nurse and
Complementary Practitioner; formerly Laser
Nurse Specialist, Birmingham Children's
Hospital, Birmingham, UK

*Appendix 2 Complementary therapies, Practices 3, 10,
15, 16, 17, 21, 27*

BRISTOL

Louise Dyer MSc BSc (Hons) RNT (Cert Ed) RCNT RSCN
RN
Senior Lecturer, School of Maternal and Child
Health, University of the West of England,
Bristol, UK

Practices 1, 6, 9, 11, 14, 24, 29, 31

GLASGOW

Toby A. Mohammed MN (Specialty in Education) PGCE
RGN RSCN RNT
Senior Nurse (Practice Development), Yorkhill
Operating Division of NHS Greater Glasgow,
Glasgow, UK

*Practices 4, 7, 12, 13, 18 (joint with Sheffield), 19, 32,
35, 36, 37*

SHEFFIELD

Pat Wilson RSCN RN
Modern Matron, Sheffield Children's Hospital,
Sheffield, UK

*Practices 5, 8, 18 (joint with Glasgow), 20, 22, 23, 26,
33, 34*

SUSSEX

Ethel Trigg MBA RN RSCN DMS FETC
General Manager and Children's Lead, Sussex
Downs and Weald Primary Care Trust, Sussex,
UK

*Appendix 1 Play, Practices 2, 25, 28, 30, Community
perspective boxes*

Contributors

Susan Aitkenhead MSc PGDip Palliative Care RSCN
Professional Advisor (Children's Nursing),
Nursing and Midwifery Council; formerly
Consultant Nurse (Paediatric Pain
Management), Glasgow, UK

Susan Alexander MN BA RGN RM ENB 405
Clinical Educator, Paediatric Department, The
Queen Mother's Hospital, Yorkhill Operating
Division of NHS Greater Glasgow, Glasgow, UK

Christopher Bunford RGN RSCN
Nutritional Care Charge Nurse, Birmingham
Children's Hospital, Birmingham, UK

Lynne Chadburn EN RSCN BOA Orth Tech Cert
Paediatric Casting Practitioner, A&E
Department, Sheffield Children's Hospital,
Sheffield, UK

Fiona Clements BSc (Hons) RGN
Resuscitation Officer, Yorkhill Operating
Division of NHS Greater Glasgow, Glasgow,
UK

Janice Colson MA RSCN RGN Dip Nursing Education RNT
Principal Lecturer Child Health, Faculty of
Health Care & Social Sciences, University of
Luton, Stoke Mandeville Hospital, Aylesbury,
UK

Kerry Cook RGN RN(Child) BA (Hons) ITEC Dip ENB 160
PGDip
Senior Lecturer, Children's Nursing Team,
School of Health and Social Sciences, Coventry
University, Coventry; formerly Clinical Practice
Development Facilitator, Professional

Development Team, Birmingham Children's
Hospital, Birmingham, UK

Mark Denial EN(G) RGN RSCN
Paediatric Diabetes Nurse Specialist, Sheffield
Children's Hospital, Sheffield, UK

Jacqueline Denyer RGN RSCN RHV
Clinical Nurse Specialist for Epidermolysis
Bullosa (Paediatric), DebRA UK and Great
Ormond Street Hospital for Sick Children,
London, UK

Michaela Dixon PGCE (HE) BSc (Hons) ENB 415 RSCN RGN
Senior Lecturer, School of Maternal and Child
Health, University of the West of England,
Bristol; Clinical Development Nurse, Paediatric
Intensive Care Unit, Bristol Royal Hospital for
Children, Bristol, UK

Barbara Doyle MSc RGN RSCN

Senior Sister/Ward Manager, Sheffield
Children's Hospital, Sheffield, UK

Louise Dyer MSc BSc (Hons) RNT (Cert Ed) RCNT RSCN RN
Senior Lecturer, School of Maternal and Child
Health, University of the West of England,
Bristol, UK

Bev Embling BSc (Hons) ENB 640 RN (Child) Dip HE RGN
Senior Staff Nurse, Barbara Russell Children's
Unit, Frenchay Hospital, Bristol, UK

Julia Fearon RGN RSCN BSc (Complementary Therapy)
Independent Therapist, formerly Laser Nurse
Specialist, Birmingham Children's Hospital,
Birmingham, UK

Teresa Figari Bsc (Hons) RSCN
Junior Sister, Infants Cardiology, Birmingham
Children's Hospital, Birmingham, UK

Catherine Furze PGCE (HE) BSc (Hons) RN (Child) ENB
405 RGN
Senior Lecturer in Children's Nursing, School of
Maternal and Child Health, University of the
West of England, Bristol, UK

Vikki Garrick BSc RGN RSCN
Tissue Viability Nurse Specialist, Yorkhill
Operating Division of NHS Greater Glasgow,
Glasgow, UK

Rebecca Giles RN (Child) BSc (Hons) Clinical Nursing
Studies ENB 415
Junior Sister, Paediatric Intensive Care Unit,
Birmingham Children's Hospital, Birmingham,
UK

Liz Gough BSc (Hons) Nursing RGN RSCN Intensive Care
Nursing of Children Pathway
Research and Audit Junior Sister, PICU,
Birmingham Children's Hospital, Birmingham,
UK

Margaret Henderson RSCN RGN RM
UTI Sister, Yorkhill Operating Division of NHS
Greater Glasgow, Glasgow, UK

Sandi Hillery RGN RSCN BSc (Hons) Community
Specialist Practice in Community Health Care, Community
Children's Nursing FETC ENB 923
Outreach Team Leader, Shooting Star House,
Children's Hospice, Hampton, UK
(*Community perspective boxes*)

Jane Hutchins BSc(Hons) Health Care RGN RSCN DPSN 2
Sister/Ward Manager, Sheffield Children's
Hospital, Sheffield, UK

Tricia Kleidon BSc (Nursing)
Clinical Nurse Specialist, Great Ormond Street
Hospital for Sick Children, Department of
Radiology, London, UK

Heather Laird RN BSc

Research Nurse, UCLH NHS Hospital Trust,
London, UK

Karen Leitch RSCN Dip Nursing Studies
UTI Sister, Yorkhill Operating Division of NHS
Greater Glasgow, Glasgow, UK

Maureen Lilley MSc BSc (Hons) Adv Pract Dip
(Independent/supplementary nurse prescribing) RGN RSCN
Paediatric Nurse Practitioner, Ambulatory Care
Unit, Yorkhill Operating Division of NHS
Greater Glasgow, Glasgow, UK

Fiona Lynch RSCN
Staff Nurse, Sheffield Children's Hospital,
Sheffield, UK

Bernadette McGarry BSc RSCN
Practice Education Facilitator, Yorkhill Nursing
and Midwifery Research and Practice
Development Unit, Yorkhill Operating
Division of NHS Greater Glasgow, Glasgow,
UK

Nan McIntosh BSc (Hons), Adv Pract Dip RSCN RGN
Nurse Practitioner, Haematology/Oncology,
Yorkhill Operating Division of NHS Greater
Glasgow, Glasgow, UK

Susan Macqueen MSc RGN RSCN
Senior Nurse Specialist and Head Clinician
Infection Control, Department of Microbiology,
Great Ormond Street Hospital for Sick Children,
London, UK

Christina Maddox PG Cert Dip HE (Part 15) RGN
Lecturer in Children's Nursing, School of
Maternal and Child Health, University of the
West of England, Bristol, UK

Toby A. Mohammed MN (Specialty in Education) PGCE
RGN RSCN RNT
Senior Nurse (Practice Development), Yorkhill
Operating Division of NHS Greater Glasgow,
Glasgow, UK

Hermione Montgomery RGN RSCN RM BSc (Hons)
LTHE
Lead Nurse, Quality of Care, Birmingham
Children's Hospital NHS Trust, Birmingham,
UK

Dawn Moss RGN RSCN CCN (SPQ) HV BSc (Hons)
Nurse Consultant in Child Health, NHS
Borders, Melrose, and Napier Unversity,
Edinburgh, UK

Beryl Pearson RN RSCN RCNT CertEd (FE/HE) Med
(FE/HE)
Staff Tutor Nursing, Open University, Bristol,
UK

Sue Pickup MMedSci (Clinical Nursing) RGN RSCN
CNS Pain Management, Sheffield Children's
NHS Trust, Sheffield, UK

Susan Rideout MSc (Oxon) BSc (Hons) Grad Dip Phys
MCSP SRP
Clinical Specialist, Physiotherapist,
Paediatric Neurosciences, Birmingham
Children's Hospital, Birmingham, UK

Stephen Rowley RSCN MSc BSc (Hons)
Clinical Lead and Senior Nurse Haematology,
UCLH NHS Hospital Trust, London, UK

Rachel Sales RN PG Dip HE BSc (Hons) Dip HE Nursing
Senior Lecturer, School of Maternal and Child
Health, University of the West of England,
Bristol, UK

Brian Silverwood RGN RSCN ENB 998 N49, 870
Former Ward Manager (Orthopaedics), Sheffield
Children's Hospital, Sheffield, UK

Louise Simmons RN (Child) ENB 970
Liaison Sister, Inherited Metabolic Disorders,
Birmingham Children's Hospital, Birmingham,
UK

Stella Snell RGN RSCN ENB 998, 923, R92
Clinical Nurse Specialist – Paediatric
Continence, St George's Healthcare NHS Trust,
London, UK

Joyce Stebbings NNEB HPS
Play Service Manager, Royal Alexandra
Children's Hospital, Brighton, UK

Sue Tulp Adv Dip Nursing Studies, RN (Child)
Staff Nurse, Sheffield Children's Hospital,
Sheffield, UK

Rosemary Turnbull RSCN BSc (Hons) Child Health ENB
N25, 998
Paediatric Dermatology Specialist Nurse,
Chelsea & Westminster Hospital, London, UK

Alison Warren RGN RSCN ENB 415, 998 APLS/EPLS
Instructor
Senior Nursing Sister, Paediatric Intensive Care
Unit, Birmingham Children's Hospital,
Birmingham, UK

Melanie Wilson RN (Child) Dip Health Studies
Sister, Sheffield Children's Hospital, Sheffield, UK

Foreword

I am delighted to be asked to write a foreword to the second edition of this book. The first edition was welcomed by children's nurses throughout the UK as no previous text had addressed the practical skills required by children's nurses in both hospital and the community. However, children's nursing progresses and as more nursing research is undertaken and medical knowledge increases, books quickly become dated and need to be rewritten and brought up to date. Ethel Trigg, one of the original editors, and Toby Mohammed, a clinical coordinator of the first edition, have done an excellent job in maintaining the original format but ensuring the information is relevant to the children's nurses of today. The first edition was translated into Italian and was also chosen by the International Council of Nurses to be one of the books in mobile libraries, sent to several African countries. I am sure that this second edition will be equally successful. Many congratulations to all who have been involved.

Brighton 2005   Sally Huband

Preface

When we were approached by the publishers and asked if we were willing to undertake a second edition, both Sally and I were delighted that the first edition had done so well, warranting an update. Sally and my wish was to see this as a well-thumbed book in as many children's units as possible, so imagine my feelings when I walked onto a children's unit as a visitor to see the first edition in use and far from new.

As Sally decided not to proceed with the second edition due to a rewarding and full retirement, Toby Mohammed – one of the original contributors – agreed to join me. Toby has been a brilliant co-editor, bringing new thoughts and approaches to this edition.

Ethel Trigg 2005

About the second edition

Following a positive review, we decided to maintain the original structure for the practices. Where possible, we approached the original five children's centres and authors. Many were delighted to be asked to contribute and have updated their original practices. However, there is a range of new names, adding different dimensions from the first edition. Our aim was to keep as near to the original format as possible and to continue to ensure that this manual is easy to read and gives good practice guidelines in the delivery of care to sick and vulnerable children. The authors were asked to add new material and references where appropriate and in many areas this was overwhelming. This was particularly noticeable in the Concepts chapter, which has attempted to incorporate and make comments on the differences between the countries of the UK, while addressing the many national documents and directives that have been issued since the publication of the first edition. It was interesting to see how children's nurses have developed and embraced many new areas that would have originally been thought of as 'no man's land'. This was proven on many occasions when authors indicated that it was easier to rewrite the practice than to try to update around the original text. As before, all practices have been read by two community nurses and updates to these sections have been made. All practices have been peer reviewed by an author from another centre.

We do hope you will find this updated and revised edition as useful as the first, and that again it will become a well-thumbed book to guide good practice and safe care.

Ethel Trigg
Toby A. Mohammed

Sussex and Scotland 2005

Acknowledgements

The clinical coordinators would like to acknowledge the support and contribution of the following people during the update of the specific practices.

Birmingham
All of the contributors who updated practices and also Liz Morgan (Director of Nursing) and Kim Fowler (Liaison Health Visitor) for their support.

Glasgow
All of the contributors who updated practices and Elaine Harrison (Transfusion Practitioner), Julie Smith (Project Nurse/GRASP Coordinator), Theresa Tchehrasi (Clinical Educator), Alison McGuire (IV Coordinator), Pamela Joanidis (Senior Infection Control Nurse) and Linda Wolfson (Breast Feeding Coordinator) for their involvement in the peer review process. A special thanks to Mhairi and Eilidh Thomson for allowing us to use their photographs in Figures 18.2 and 18.3 (Practice 18 Pain Management).

Sheffield
All of the contributors who updated practices and those involved in the peer review process. We are also grateful to Hussein Khatib who offered the services of the Sheffield staff for the first edition, to Lorraine Fitter, Support Manager (Nursing), and to Nicola Rogers, Paediatric Diabetes Nurse Specialist.

Bristol
Colleagues in the School of Maternal and Child Health at the Faculty of Health and Social Care, University of the West of England.

The support and contribution of the following are also acknowledged: Patsy Campbell and David Fulton, staff at the nursing libraries at the University of Luton; Caroline Rudoni, Clinical Nurse Specialist (Stoma Care) and Rachael Bolland, Lecturer Practitioner (Paediatrics), St George's Healthcare NHS Trust, London; and Emma Potter (Epsom Children's Home Care Team) for assistance with the Community Perspective boxes.

Concepts

Janice Colson

INTRODUCTION

The health of children today has been the subject of wide-ranging investigation and changes in approach due to failures in old and outdated systems. The publication of a number of key documents has already made and will continue to make considerable impact and will underpin the developments and implementation of child health for the next 10 years or more. These include *Learning from Bristol* (Kennedy 2001), the *Victoria Climbie Inquiry* (DoH 2003a), the *National Service Framework for Children and Young People* (DoH 2004a) and *Every Child Matters* (DoH 2004b), all of which have been used to inform the NHS service reviews being undertaken across the United Kingdom (UK). Each of these documents makes its own unique contribution and provides the fundamental principles to this chapter. However, it is important to remember that the differing countries of the UK have their own particular nuances related to legislation and child care provision. Therefore, practitioners must be aware of relevant legislation that applies to the country in which they practise.

Every Child Matters (DoH 2004b) is about radical change for the delivery of children's services to improve the outcomes for the child. It is about making children's services more child-centred, and integrating them around the needs of children and young people by listening to children and their families. The emphasis is about early intervention and not crisis-driven action. 'Follow the child' is the key theme. In order to follow this approach, the boundaries and traditions that nurses have had imposed on and by themselves will need to be broken down and care and safety located as close to the child as possible. This work will change the way children's services are delivered, with emphasis that this will be managed by frontline staff who understand the changing face of children's services.

There are five themed outcomes that set the scene for delivering improved services for children:

- Be healthy
- Stay safe
- Enjoy and achieve
- Make a positive contribution
- Achieve economic well-being.

Every Child Matters is an essential for all professionals working with children and young people.

A recommendation from *Every Child Matters* suggested that the Chief Nursing Officer (CNO) of England look at the role of nursing and midwifery in the health and well-being of vulnerable children and young people. The CNO's review made a number of recommendations which included increasing the number of school nurses, strengthening the public health role of nurses, the integration and co-location of practitioners, strengthening the role of nurses who work in general practice and improving leadership on child protection (DoH 2004c). These will have an impact on the role of any nurse who works with children and young people.

Nurses are responding to these changes by enhancing and broadening their roles and looking at how roles and care can be integrated, thus allowing improvement in the overall quality of care which children and their families receive. This involves moving away from the traditional nursing image and undertaking tasks which previously were performed only by doctors and other professionals.

The nurse must continue to develop and be recognised as a professional practitioner, with an ever-extending repertoire of skills. The new practitioner is one who is educated to practise from a sound, research-based knowledge. Current practitioners in children's nursing sometimes feel that they do not have the opportunity to provide much 'hands-on care'. This feeling has to be considered in the context of changes in care. One such change is the philosophy of family-centred care and partnership being central to the service provided in children's nursing (Kenny 2003). Family-centred care is a concept that has been familiar to children's nurses for a number of years. More recently, the National Service Framework's standard for hospital services states that child-centred services are those that 'treat children, young people and parents as partners in care' (DoH 2004a, p. 9). Therefore, whilst parents and other family members are doing what were previously considered 'nursing duties', nurses have to develop a very special set of skills that enable them to care for vulnerable children and families. These skills include the responsibility for teaching families, providing support and helping families to make decisions in the best interests of their infant or child, whether sick or healthy, and may present nurses with situations in which they have to make some difficult decisions. Nurses must feel confident about the delivery of their practical skills and that they can think in a clear and rational manner about the emotional and social care they provide. Kitson (2004) emphasises the need for nurses of the future to be able to deliver integrated care across a range of settings, undertaking a range of activities on their own initiative such as independent prescribing, referral, admission and discharge within the co-located care setting.

ACCOUNTABILITY

Practice for the children's nurse is broad and varied. It ranges from delivery of care within the intensive care setting, to the provision of home support to children with long-term and chronic healthcare needs. Their role involves not only dealing with the individual child, but also working very closely with their families (Dearmun et al 1995).

Whatever the practice, the qualified nurse is accountable for personal decisions and actions. This fact is emphasised in the *Code of Professional Conduct* (NMC 2004) and is the practitioner's need to maintain and develop knowledge and competence (Donaldson 1997). To be able to deliver care within acute and community settings is of equal importance for children's nurses as their roles are increasingly becoming community focused. In both of these situations the responsibility to practise intelligently is with the individual nurse. Accountability may be defined as 'the obligation of being answerable for one's own judgements and actions' (Martin 2004, p. 3). This definition provides evidence of an abstract concept which nurses should explore further. Accountability is a term frequently used by and about nurses and so each nurse should be able to define this in the context of personal practice. Student nurses often ask questions such as: 'If we give a wrong drug, who is accountable?' or 'Supposing a child injures himself whilst he is playing with me in the playroom, am I accountable?' Students may challenge registered nurses by posing such questions; however, it is important for them to explore the issues whilst they are still students. Although it is impossible to explore every conceivable situation, students should be provided with guiding principles which will help in their decision-making. The Nursing and Midwifery Council's guide for students (NMC 2002b) stresses that, although not professionally accountable, students must act at all times in the interests of the patients with whom they come into contact during their practice experience. Therefore, when playing with a child in the playroom, the student nurse should make every effort to ensure that the child is supervised within a safe environment appropriate to the child's age and stage of development.

Qualified nurses also have unanswered questions about accountability and their extending scope of professional practice. Qualified practitioners are, on the whole, very aware of the implications of ever-expanding boundaries of practice and thus realise that there is no room for complacency. Therefore, it would seem pertinent to explore what it does mean for a nurse to be accountable.

The Department of Health, in the response to the Report of the Public Inquiry into children's heart surgery at the Bristol Royal Infirmary 1984–1995, calls for the need to improve lines of accountability at local and national levels (DoH 2002). Therefore, it would seem that accountability has now been recognised as the high-profile concept it is in relation to the caring professions.

The revised *Code of Professional Conduct* from the Nursing and Midwifery Council (2004) states that its purpose is to 'inform the professions . . . in the exercise of their professional accountability and practice' and refers to accountability on a number of occasions. The Code states quite clearly what a registered nurse is personally accountable for, and provides a set of guiding principles as an aid to

practitioners to understand and implement their accountability (Pyne 1998).

The Code also provides guidelines for the professions and, like all guidelines, may be open to interpretation by individuals. Nurses should avoid individual interpretations of their professional accountability since in so doing they may bring their careers into jeopardy, together with the reputations of their employing institutions and the profession.

Howard (1997) states that practice with accountability is a key concept in the effective delivery of health care in modern nursing. This suggests that nurses have not always been willing or able to be accountable for their practice. Nursing has changed and will continue to change for it to be a dynamic profession. The latter decades of the 20th century witnessed a greater diversity of career pathways for children's nurses (Cox et al 2003) and these have required breaking down the boundaries of practice and accountability.

Some nurses and health visitors have undertaken further academic programmes in order to support the development of their roles. One such programme, which has gained professional and media interest, is nurse prescribing. Nurses who have undertaken this educational programme are now prescribing medications from the *Nurses Prescribing Formulary*. In some specialist roles (e.g. the advanced neonatal nurse practitioners), nurses have developed knowledge and skills to enable them to assess, plan and deliver care that previously was considered the role of a doctor. These nurses are trained to undertake such procedures as resuscitation and intubations in critical situations where the wrong decision or action may jeopardise the life of the infant/child. The majority of nurses undertaking these specialist skills are now educated to degree level and, at times, masters degree level, with an increasing number achieving higher academic accolades at doctorate level. Nurses practising at these advanced levels are making judgements and taking actions which may involve life and death situations. Recent research (Ward Platt & Brown 2004) identifies that good-quality neonatal care can be provided by neonatal nurse practitioners without the support of junior paediatricians. The new role of nurse consultant enables more nurses to develop in-depth expertise in a particular area and to gain recognition of their specialist knowledge. These roles are in keeping with the recommendations made by the Department of Health in *Making a Difference* (DoH 1999) where it is stated that, by developing nurses' roles, services for patients will be improved and nurses' careers enhanced.

Today there is an increasing need to be able to recognise and deal with the mental health problems of children and young people. This is a specialist area where the lack of resources in both manpower and facilities often means that children with mental health problems are being admitted to general paediatric wards. In this environment they are cared for by nurses who do not always have the specialist knowledge and skills to deal with their particular problems. Thus staff and patients are in a vulnerable position. The National Service Framework (NSF) (DoH 2004a) stresses that child and adolescent mental health is an integral part of all children's services. It goes on to state that where a hospital is providing a service for children, then the staff should have an understanding of how to assess and address the emotional well-being of children. The CNO's review of nursing, midwifery and health visiting states that children in acute settings would greatly benefit from nurses who have more skills in mental health and improved access to Child and Adolescent Mental Health Services (CAMHS). Staff should also be able to identify any significant mental health problems. The need for a strong liaison with CAMHS, including psychiatry, psychology and family therapy, is also stressed. Section 4.27 of the NSF (DoH 2004a) calls for all hospitals treating children and young people to have policies and liaison arrangements in place to deal with child and adolescent mental health problems, ranging from overdoses and deliberate self-harm to child protection and long-term life-threatening diseases. In addition, nurses working with school-age children should have appropriate competencies for working with this age group.

In reality, the Royal College of Nursing (RCN) have recognised that there is an urgent need for short-term targeting of education and training to bridge this knowledge and skills gap and have responded with guidelines (RCN 2004).

The increasing move towards caring for sick children in their own homes (Whiting 1997, Hughes & Callery 2004) puts more pressure on the nurse in the community. The section on nursing practices in the community addresses the role of the community children's nurse. These nurses are often isolated from colleagues for long periods during their working day, making it difficult to discuss issues when uncertainty arises. They should not feel obligated to undertake practices for which they do not have appropriate skills. However, they are responsible for their own knowledge base and effective decision-making, since their level of accountability is no more or less than that of any other nurse.

Care for a sick child at home is mainly provided by the parents, but, when visiting the family, the community nurse will be expected to provide support, guidance and some care. Parents need to see evidence of a competent and confident practitioner. Such situations provide the ultimate opportunity for nurses to exercise their professional judgement. Carter and Campbell (1997) identify professional judgement as a complex concept and state that 'no single decision will be the same as another individual decision'.

Where individual nurses are working within a team of professionals, then update and professional dialogue are more likely to happen than when a nurse is working independently, for example in the long-term continuing care environment for a child dependent on technology at home. Children with long-term conditions are cared for by care assistants or nursery nurses/healthcare support workers who may only have had the technical training to provide the specific care needed by that child (Beale 2002) and are supervised and supported by one or two trained nurses. In these circumstances, where does the line of accountability lie? Although these carers are part of a larger team, they will be alone with the child at home. This form of care is a growing source of support to families in need of respite and, whilst Beale is emphatic that the most fragile children are still cared for by qualified children's nurses, there is no doubt that the use of support workers is on the increase in all care settings. Work is currently being undertaken by the Department of Health to explore the lines of accountability as part of a wider review of the role of support workers (Mullaly 2003). The qualified nurse is accountable at all times and, by delegating work to a person who is not registered with the NMC, is accountable to ensure that the person is suitably trained to undertake care at the appropriate level.

Isolation in practice should be avoided and to that end student nurses are not generally permitted to carry their own case load in the community. Although in the past vacant posts in the community were seldom taken as first posts for newly qualified nurses, skill mix into community teams is now more acceptable and more newly qualified staff are interested in community career pathways. Wherever newly qualified nurses seek work, they do require support and guidance from more experienced staff in order to make the transition from student to registered practitioner (NMC 2002a). To aid this process, the NMC (2002a) recommend a period of supported practice of no less than 4 months. This process is termed preceptorship and involves the newly qualified practitioner working alongside an experienced practitioner who provides help, support and advice. Clinical supervision is another means of support for nurses at all levels and can be of value to lone practitioners.

Clinical supervision can be undertaken on a one-to-one basis with another colleague or as part of a group meeting of the team discussing issues related to patient care that have given concern and can be used as a vehicle to explore accountability and practice issues.

Nurses working in the current environment of constant change need to develop coping skills to manage the changing environment. In circumstances where nurses are exposed to new areas of practice, whether students or reg-istered practitioners, they must indicate any knowledge deficit and request appropriate orientation, education and support. It is the responsibility of all nurses to question when unsure and for nurses to constantly strive to add to their personal knowledge and perfection of their professional skills. Nurses must recognise that they can learn from each other. In addition, nurses should be proactive in seeking out appropriate study days and courses to attend, demonstrating their commitment to education and sound practice.

ADVOCACY

The *Code of Professional Conduct* (NMC 2004) does not make direct reference to the term advocate, but states that the nurse must promote the interests of patients and clients, including the provision of help to individuals and groups to enable them to gain access to health care. Martin (2004) defines an advocate as a practitioner, usually a nurse, who will promote and safeguard the well-being and interests of their patients by ensuring they are aware of their rights and have access to information to enable them to make informed decisions. This definition adds more depth to what is expected of the nurse when acting in the role of an advocate.

Rushton and colleagues (1996) state that advocacy on behalf of patients and their families is central to the practice of nursing, whilst Gates (1995) reminds readers of the origins of the word advocate, from the Latin *advocatus*, meaning one who is summoned to give evidence. Woodrow (1997) states that the concept of advocacy comes from legal practice, thus producing visions of courtroom scenes with lawyers pleading the case of their client. This concept and the Latin origins of the word advocate would appear to have some significance for nurses since, according to Mallick (1997), much of the literature on advocacy is concerned with patients' complaints. In such circumstances, nurses may well be called to give evidence about the care they have provided. Whether the evidence is verbal or in the form of written statements, there are important implications for the nurse. If a patient or a member of the patient's family complains about the care received, nurses may be held accountable.

Changes at national level are requiring nurses to demonstrate the ability to think about patients' rights and advocacy. *The NHS Plan* (DoH 2000a) requires trusts to appoint advocacy services (known as PALS) so that patient concerns may be addressed at the time of concern and in a timely matter. This early intervention has been supported by patients as they feel they are having their issues addressed as soon as possible. Research has identified that effective management of complaints comes from dealing with concerns at an early stage. Using complaints as a learning framework, rather than in a negative frame, can contribute to improved patient care by acknowledging possible shortfalls and, if necessary, by instituting changes to policy and practice. Also, involving patients in the complaint process wherever possible has proven to be effective.

Frequently, circumstances in the day-to-day care given to children provide nurses with ethical dilemmas and difficult decisions. *The NHS Plan* (DoH 2000a) makes a clear statement about the need for partnership between patients and professionals, a concept embraced some years ago in the majority of environments where children are nursed. Where nurses are working in partnership with parents and the child, trust is an essential element. Nurses are allowed into a privileged position and it is therefore important that nurses are aware of their own values and principles in any given situation. Charles-Edwards (2001), in reviewing advocacy and the role of the nurse, states that children are not likely to make formal requests for representation.

Children's nurses often struggle when attempting to define their advocacy role (Rushton et al 1996). Anecdotal evidence would suggest that they do not view it in the terms described above; rather, they interpret it within their daily activities of caring for children, speaking out and acting on behalf of the child. Examples of good practice from nurses' reflections on their role as advocate are provided below.

- A student nurse recalled how she had prevented a doctor from inserting an intravenous cannula into Jack's arm because he had not had a topical anaesthetic cream applied for the prescribed time.

- In a similar situation, Stephanie was hysterical at the thought of yet another blood test. Initially, her parents and the nurse could do nothing to calm her. The doctor was anxious to get the blood samples and requested that she should be held tightly to gain cooperation (Collier & Robinson 1997). The nurse, sensing the tensions, asked the doctor to wait whilst she got the 'bubble tubes'. These brightly coloured objects provided perfect distraction and the test went ahead without further problems.

Nurses frequently feel uncomfortable about restraining children for procedures when alternative methods may be as effective (RCN 1999). This has been re-emphasised more recently as the body of legislation and guidance about restraint has grown and the overriding message is that restraint should only take place if the child is likely to cause self-harm. Furthermore, in a survey by Collier and Robinson (1997), the majority of nurses felt that restraint rather than pain was the more likely cause of distress. The scenarios above provide evidence of nurses acting in the child's best interests based on knowledge supported by research.

These scenarios also highlight the probable imbalance of power between healthcare professionals and patients, particularly between doctors and children. They indicate the vulnerability of sick children and their need for support when confronted by paternalistic medical professionals (Charles-Edwards 2003). Whilst it would be unjust to label all doctors as paternalistic, there has been a tradition within medicine that the doctor knows best and therefore patients and nurses will do as they are told.

In fairness to medical colleagues, nurses can also sometimes be too eager to exert power over children and parents in their care. Making judgemental statements about parenting skills, displaying negative attitudes and failing to provide opportunities for parents to participate in their child's care are just some examples of how nurses might demonstrate that they think they know best.

Phillips (1994) states that it takes less time to tell a child what to do than to consult with the child about their wishes. Ondrusek et al (1998) and Charles-Edwards (2003) suggest that children will say 'yes' because it is seen as what they should do. Although this refers to the involvement of children in a research study, it may readily be translated into a variety of other situations including treatments. Such behaviour may enable the busy nurse, working within a punishing timescale, to complete the dressing, administer the intravenous drugs or apply the skin care. Children may comply with this type of behaviour, but it does not reflect the spirit of advocacy and raises questions about whose best interests are being served.

There are times when nurses may think that they are acting in a child's best interests. For example, in another situation, a staff nurse returned from the operating theatre to the children's ward with a child before her operation had taken place, because the anaesthetist was not ready to receive her into the anaesthetic room. The staff nurse had decided that it was in the child's best interests to wait in the less stressful ward environment rather than in the busy corridor by the operating theatre; there is no evidence to suggest that the nurse had consulted with the child. Furthermore, the child may have been told that, by the time she returned to the ward, her operation would be over. Also, the nurse may have caused the child's parents to be unnecessarily alarmed by the action of returning their child to the ward. In this scenario the nurse may have created more tension. It would seem that, if the nurse had not consulted with the child or explained what was happening, the nurse had confused the role of advocate with that of exerting power.

In almost every situation when a child is sick, parents and immediate family are faced with uncertainty and ambiguity about the treatment and outcomes of the illness. Additionally, in accepting that the child is ill, parents have to accept that the child needs to be cared for by health professionals and thus as parents they may have to relinquish some of their former parenting roles (Altschuler 1997). It would seem that there is a strong argument for not asking parents to relinquish their parenting role, but rather enabling them to adapt. Adaptation would involve re-establishing the parenting role from being parents of a well child to being parents of a sick child (Rennick 1986) and developing strategies to allow this to occur. Such strategies provide ideal opportunities for nurses to act in the child's best interests. This may be done through negotiating what care parents wish to participate in and that which they prefer to hand over to nurses. The idea of nurses being told by parents what they may do for their child could be difficult for some nurses to accept, particularly if they have to embrace the concepts of family-centred care and partnership. If nurses view advocacy as a dimension of the nursing role, then it would seem essential that the other aspects have to be incorporated into the nursing strategy.

Changes at national level are requiring nurses to demonstrate the ability to think about patients' rights and advocacy. Within the concept of family-centred care, the child is seen as part of the family; therefore, when advocating for the child, the nurse should also be an advocate for the family – or should she? This raises questions of how nurses view their advocacy role, particularly when confronted with situations where there may be conflicts of interest.

Conflicts of interest may arise out of a variety of situations and can place the nurse in a difficult position. For example, when children express their views about care regimes (as discussed in the section on informed consent), those views may be negative. Simon, aged 13, has been started on another course of painful intravenous antibiotic therapy. He is still very ill and cannot see an end to or even improvement in this illness. He expresses his unhappiness to his nurse and asks that the drugs are stopped. Purssell (1995) suggests that children need a powerful advocate and parents or guardians are in an ideal position for the role. In Simon's case this is not so. Mary, the nurse, knows that Simon's prognosis is poor and feels that she should raise the issue at the forthcoming multidisciplinary team meeting. She is also aware that Simon's parents and the team members will oppose any suggestions to review the care regime; they want everything possible to be done.

Issues of power and control are raised from this scenario. Mary thinks she will be acting in Simon's best interests. She is the nurse who has most interactions with him; she knows how ill he feels, but that he tries to be cheerful for his parents. Mary also feels that colleagues will experience a sense of failure if they change the care regime. Therefore, they will exert power over Simon and her to continue the treatment.

A further example of where nurses feel that conflicts of interest arise concerns video surveillance of parents when they are suspected of child abuse. Nurses are expected to assume a partnership with parents, whilst at the same time they know that parents are being subjected to covert video surveillance when left alone to care for their child. In situations such as these, nurses and other providers of care for children have to justify carefully what is essentially an invasion of privacy when they take steps to override parental prerogatives (Kohrman et al 1995).

Whilst the above situation arises infrequently and usually in units specially designed for monitoring work with parents who are suspected of abuse, it may be an issue for nurses in other care environments.

Another dimension of the nurse's advocacy role may be seen in working with parents to gain their child's cooperation in a treatment regime, for example teaching the child newly diagnosed as having diabetes about diet and administration of insulin. Similarly, an older child with cystic fibrosis may find the frequent drugs and physiotherapy tedious. Negotiation with child and parents can enable a more positive approach, with everyone acting in the child's best interests.

When nurses claim to be advocates for children, they should be fighting for appropriate standards of care for all children (Casey 1997) and should ensure that recent valuable national documents, for example the NSF (DoH 2004a) and *Every Child Matters* (DoH 2004b), are implemented in the care settings in which they work and that these documents are regularly audited and evaluated.

CONSENT

Consent within child healthcare has raised much concern within children's nursing for some time (Lowden 2002). Legislation across all four countries of the United Kingdom, and indeed international treaties, have identified the rights of children to be involved in the decision-making process (Children's Act (England and Wales) 1989, United Nations 1989, Children (Scotland) Act 1995) and this can be applied to the right to be involved in decisions about health care.

It is the intention of this section to highlight some of the key issues surrounding consent. However, nurses need to remember that legislation across the four countries of the United Kingdom has some differences regarding children's rights. Consequently, each individual nurse must update themselves on children's rights if they move employment between countries.

Gaining consent

Consent is the provision of permission from one person to another to do something on their behalf. Within health care, this is usually an act of caring and may range from helping a child to dress to the changing of a complex dressing on a wound and gaining consent for an invasive procedure (e.g. surgery). Healthcare workers are required by law to obtain consent from their patients before they commence any type of care or treatment (DoH 2001a). In addition to this being a legal requirement, it is also a fundamental part of good practice.

The British Medical Association (BMA) state that from an ethical perspective any person who is competent and informed can give consent for a medical or nursing procedure and stress that age is not always a major factor (BMA 2001). However, judging the competence of a child poses ethical and practical dilemmas for practitioners, especially where there is conflict between what the child wants and what the parents want for the child.

Traditionally, it has been accepted that consent is being given for medical and nursing treatments by virtue of the child being in hospital. Frequently, consent was implied informally rather than stated in a formal manner. Formal consent, by the signing of a form, was only requested and given prior to surgery. These circumstances meant that parents returning to their child after a brief spell of absence might find some change in the treatment regime. A further test may have been carried out or a new intravenous line inserted; the list is endless. Such situations clearly did not provide opportunities for information to be exchanged and consent given.

Today, when children require medical and nursing care, consent should be obtained before treatment is given. The reasons for this are ethical, clinical and legal. The NMC (2004) clearly identify that nurses must gain consent from their patients prior to giving any care or treatment. Consent is an everyday practical issue for nurses working with children and their families.

In order for consent to be legally valid, the following areas need to be addressed:

- The person providing consent must be a competent person who has the capacity to understand the information that is being given. This may be the individual themselves or a person legally appointed to act on an individual's behalf (DoH 2001a, NMC 2004).
- The person who is providing the consent must have been given enough information in order to make an informed judgement (NMC 2004).
- Consent is given voluntarily and without coercion (Charles-Edward 1995, NMC 2004).

It goes without saying, therefore, that in order to gain consent from an individual the nurse must ensure that that person understands what it is that they are being told, that they have been given enough information to make an informed decision and that consent is given voluntarily.

However, how does this apply to children? Can they truly give their consent? Would they really understand what is to happen? Do nurses (as adults) have the capacity to make information understandable to children?

These are all questions that children's nurses may raise when considering gaining consent from children. At times it may be considered easier and more straightforward to seek consent from legal primary carers. However, legislation now challenges nurses to consider gaining consent from children.

Competence to consent

Confirming whether or not a child is competent is pivotal to obtaining or involving them in the consent process and is probably the most controversial aspect of obtaining consent. Two issues arise out of deeming a child competent or not: the child's ability to be rational according to their level of cognitive ability, and the recognition by others of the child's autonomy. Under Scottish law the young person over the age of 16 years has the same right to consent or refuse as adults do (Marshall 1998). The situation is slightly different within England and Wales. The DoH (2001a) identify that between the ages of 16–18 years the parents may sometimes become involved. When a young person consents positively to treatment there is no problem. However, if the young person refuses then parents may intervene to allow the treatment to take place. The DoH (2001a) suggests that situations seldom reach this stage, although in extreme cases a court may be asked to decide.

The child's chronological age and competence will naturally influence their ability to participate in the decision-making process (Orr 1999). However, age and level of competence are not necessarily synonymous. Children can have developed a level of competence which can be the result of skilled care that has encouraged them to participate in decision-making about what happens to them. The Children (Scotland) Act 1995 clearly identifies the need to involve children in decisions being made regarding their care within local authorities and this is reflected across the countries of the UK. Coyne (1998) clearly identifies that children have views and that these views can provide a rich source of information on how they feel in a given situation. Nonetheless, in the early years of a child's life, decisions about health and welfare are normally made by the child's parents.

The consent of children under the age of 16 years has been the subject of much debate since the late 1980s and early 1990s. Gillick v West Norfolk and Wisbech Area Health Authority (1986) heralded changes in English law that were to be reflected across the UK. The case was focussed on the teenage child's right to consent to medical treatment without the parents' knowledge. The judge on the case ruled that a parent's degree of control over such areas varied with the child's understanding and intelligence. The Age of Legal Capacity (Scotland) Act (1991) clearly states that:

> Children under the age of 16 years can give their own consent if the medical practitioner attending the child considers the child capable of understanding the nature and possible consequences of the procedure or treatment.

This is reflected in similar Acts across the UK.

Within Scotland, once a child has been deemed as competent and capable of giving their consent, the parents lose any right that they have to consent on the child's behalf (Marshall 1998). Gulam (2004) makes a similar comment when considering Australian legislation. However, the courts may influence and overrule a child's consent and indeed that of a parent and this at times has been the subject of much media attention (Orr 1999, Alderson 2000, Lowden 2002).

Gaining a child's consent can be further complicated by the perception of the adult who is trying to involve them (Lowden 2002). Lowden (2002) argues that how the adult conveys relevant information, the terminology that they use, their belief in the rights of the child and their general knowledge and perception of the child may inhibit competence being developed in a child.

A child's competence to consent must be reflected upon and considered by the nurses within the context and country in which they practise.

Parental responsibilities

Parents, as adults, are often considered to be the most appropriate people from whom to gain consent when considering children. The individual Children's Acts of the countries of the UK clearly identify the responsibilities of parents regarding the issue of consent. Parental responsibility is regarded as something of utmost importance and not to be taken lightly. Interestingly, however, this is an area that may not be fully understood by professionals working within health care (Russell-Johnson 2004).

The Children's Acts of the countries of the UK identify adults who have parental responsibilities:

- the mother (whether or not married to the father)
- the child's natural father (if married to the mother)
- a legal guardian nominated by the parents prior to their death.

It is interesting to note that unmarried fathers within Scotland must have a Parental Responsibilities and Parental Rights agreement with the mother entered and registered (Marshall 1998).

Russell-Johnston (2004) identifies changes to the current legislation within England and Wales brought about by the Adoption and Children Act (2002).

In light of the above, it is therefore essential for the children's nurse to be fully aware of the adults who are legally responsible for giving consent for a child's treatment.

CLINICAL GOVERNANCE AND RISK MANAGEMENT

> Risk is the potential for an unexpected or unwanted outcome.
>
> Russell (1995)

Clinical governance was introduced as being central to the strategy for reforms to create a modern, dependable service which can consistently provide a fast responsive quality service to all parts of the country (DoH 1999). *An Organisation with a Memory*, published in 2000 (DoH 2000b), was implemented through *Building a Safer NHS for Patients* (DoH 2001b). This was followed by the introduction of the National Patient Safety Agency (NPSA) in 2001, which published *Seven Steps to Patient Safety* in 2003.

Clinical governance is an organisational concept (Donaldson 2000) and provides a framework through which NHS organisations can work to improve the quality of clinical services for patients (DoH 1999, Stower 2000). The implementation of clinical governance will create the type of health service where the poor professional practice of the past should no longer be evident. Donaldson (2000) identifies what clinical governance will mean for the organisation and for the individual. Organisations must create sound programmes of professional development; this will help to develop the use of evidence-based practice which, according to Wilson and Tingle (1999), should be part of everyday practice. The implementation of effective systems of clinical audit and risk management to monitor and detect poor outcomes of care and to intervene where these are caused by poor practice is another essential component. In addition, each organisation will need to ensure appraisal systems are provided for all staff. Individual practitioners will be required to keep up to date with their knowledge and skills, participate to the full in their organisation's clinical governance programme, recognise problems in their own performance and seek help appropriately. Concerns about a colleague's standard of practice must be reported; failure to do so will be considered unprofessional behaviour (Donaldson 2000).

Clinical governance would appear to be synonymous with quality and therefore it could be a means by which the negativity previously attached to risk management might be eliminated. Lugon and Secker-Walker (1999) suggest that there might be two distinct components within the clinical governance structure: clinical policy setting and clinical policy monitoring. Any policy setting and

monitoring will require standards and the NSF (DoH 2004a) standard for hospital services is just the first of a series on which the future of children's healthcare can be based.

There would appear to be three categories of risk which might be identified as follows:

- the risks for the child and parents
- the risks for the nurse
- the risks arising from research, which include both the patient and nurse.

Within the NSF, the standard relating to quality and safety of care provided states that 'children and young people should receive high quality, evidence-based hospital care developed through clinical governance and delivered by staff who have the right set of skills' (DoH 2004a, p. 21).

Whilst clinical governance is an inherent part of service planning and delivery where children and young people are concerned, there are some aspects that will require trusts to make separate responses. The NSF (DoH 2004a) highlights the need for clinical governance systems to recognise that children and young people are vulnerable and need to be provided for as a discrete group. In particular it states that:

- the care of children is given a specific focus within clinical governance arrangements
- a board level children's lead is appointed within the trust
- clinical governance is approached on a multidisciplinary and a multiagency basis
- an action plan for additional clinical governance arrangements should be part of the process
- an annual report on children's services in the hospital should be presented to the board
- health and safety policies should make explicit reference to children and young people
- a risk register of actual and potential risks in the care of children and young people should be developed.

Whilst the above list is not intended to be exhaustive, it does highlight some of the key issues. However, the need for the reporting and monitoring of significant events in the delivery of care to children is also highlighted and where these occur they should be used as learning opportunities for staff at all levels. Trusts must ensure that the policies are in place to enable staff to deal with critical incidents. Guy et al (2003) identifies that drug errors in the care of children are higher than in the general population. Therefore, when a drug error has occurred, staff need to know how it should be investigated and what support to give to children and their families. Staff should be able to access policies that describe individual staff roles and lines of accountability for errors. Usually errors have to be recorded on an incident form and these individual forms are part of the organisational process of monitoring risk from drug errors. At a local level, the ward manager should use the incident in a non-threatening way to create a learning experience for staff (DoH 2003a). The NPSA (2003) identifies strong leadership as an important part of the process of increasing safety and reducing risk. The introduction of the modern matron is to bring leadership to professional and direct care staff. According to Mullaly (2003), this new role will provide a visible, accessible and authoritative presence in the ward setting.

Within the context of this book the aim is to facilitate nurses in minimising risk to the child, to the parents and to themselves through effective risk management. Risks arising from research are described elsewhere (Charles-Edwards 1995, Coyne 1998). However, all nurses should be cognisant of the ethical issues of being involved and involving patients in the research process. Using the NSF (DoH 2004a) and the *Seven Steps to Patient Safety* (NPSA 2003), the remainder of this section will aim to explore how nurses might address the issues of risk for the child and family.

The complex and diverse nature of health care creates a forum for risk activities which may lead to unexpected or unwanted risks and outcomes as evidenced through adverse incidents relating to healthcare issues in recent years. Bowden (1996) argues that doctors and nurses should not be prevented from taking risks in the development of treatments and care regimes for patients, providing that the risks are as a result of decisions based on sound research knowledge and an understanding of what might be the possible consequences. Conversely, the environment where children are cared for, the people and the equipment they come into contact with can be potentially dangerous. Wilson and Tingle (1999) identify the escalating costs of health care leading to the need for reforms which consequently bring with them a number of risks. These include organisational, clinical, business and financial risks, all of which require to be assessed and controlled to reduce unnecessary liability.

Liability has frequently come from complaints about care by patients or their relatives. Bowden (1996) believes these may have arisen from:

- a lack of clear policies
- deficient working practices
- poorly defined responsibilities
- inadequate communications
- staff working beyond their level of competence.

It has been reported that of all patients admitted to hospitals in the UK, approximately 10% will experience an adverse outcome (DoH 2000b). In discussing issues of adverse outcomes, Smallman (2003) states that these figures largely apply to hospital settings, but similar issues occur in the primary care arena and other settings. Wherever the situation occurs, the reason for the complaint should be explored, issues identified and acted upon to try to prevent recurrence. Possible outcomes of this investigation can be a change of policy, practice and delivery of care. Complaints need to be dealt with promptly within the timeframes set down by the Department of Health.

Tingle (1995) cites the failure of communication as being a central feature in an analysis of complaints about the National Health Service written to *The Times* between 1993 and 1994. Complaints have escalated since the launch of government reforms in the early 1990s due to patients and parents being more aware of their personal rights. Through legislation and government initiatives such as *The Patient's Charter* (DoH 1996), they are invited to complain – and of course they do. Many complaints arise from poor communication and records which lack clarity. The potential for this in children's nursing is possibly greater, owing to the tripartite relationship between child, parents and nurse. Where a system such as individualised nursing or named nursing does not exist and everyone contributes, channels of communication may become blurred and there may be no evidence of which nurse did what procedure for which child. The implementation of a clinical supervision programme which facilitates improvements in communication with children and parents and the inclusion of more detail in records could go some way towards effective risk management.

However, according to Symons (1995), for all the letters of criticism there are approximately 10 times more of commendations received by hospitals. This is an encouraging fact and nurses should be eager to record all comments so that good practice can be extended and poor practice changed. The plan for the future is to involve patients in risk reduction.

Lugon and Secker-Walker (1999) suggest that often trusts have no formal or have only weak mechanisms for setting trust-wide clinical policies. This may be one reason why children are susceptible to risk as they are treated most frequently in hospitals and in the community, where as a client group they are in the minority. The accident and emergency department or minor injury unit is one area where children are the minority population. Within most hospitals they form on average 25% of the clients seen. This means that they are not usually seen by a paediatrician and may only on occasion be cared for by a children's nurse since not all accident and emergency departments have the staff skill mix to enable a children's nurse to be part of the staff on every shift. In such situations, the risks include:

- missing the diagnosis of a serious illness, e.g. meningitis (Hill 2000)
- the failure to recognise a seriously ill child and refer on to a more experienced practitioner
- the prescription of an incorrect drug dose.

When children come into contact with the health services, parents and carers naturally expect that their child will be protected (Smallman 2003); however, the issues raised highlight the vulnerability of the child despite the fact that whilst the child is in the care of the hospital the trust has a duty of care towards the child (Stower 2000).

Risks for the child and family may stem from a variety of sources and by using the first of the seven steps to safety it might be appropriate to consider how to build a safety culture for the child and family. This section is about the promotion of an open and fair culture, one where underlying causes for errors are identified rather than a 'quick to blame the individual' approach. In order for the culture to be open and fair, services for the child should be child-centred. The NSF (DoH 2004a) states that care should be delivered in a safe, suitable and child-friendly environment. Kennedy (2001) found that services often treated children as 'mini-adults' and staff who were well qualified to care for adults had had no additional training to teach them how to care for children. Those caring for children within the health services should be cognisant of the child's age and stage of development so that they can interpret the child's needs. This would ensure that when admitting a child, the child is neither frightened, for example a 13-year-old being cared for in an adult ward of elderly and possibly very ill people or, conversely, annoyed by being placed next to a distressed toddler on the children's ward. In addition, when cared for in an area designated for children, the child is more likely to be cared for by a children's nurse who will have the specialist knowledge and skills to communicate, and to work in partnership, with the child and family. It would seem that if the child is in an age-appropriate environment, the margin for error in accidents is likely to be reduced.

With reference to treatment and care, risks are associated with benefits and considered in categories of high risk/low benefit and low risk/high benefit. An example of high risk/low benefit might be the child who is being offered a second heart–lung transplant following rejection of the first one. Conversely, the measles, mumps and rubella (MMR) vaccination may be considered as a low risk/high benefit treatment (Richardson & Webber 1995).

Family-centred care is a concept central to philosophies in the majority of areas where children are nursed. Nurses should be aware of the risks involved when they do not define clearly what they mean by family-centred care. They should be able to provide evidence of negotiation which has taken place to establish exactly who will undertake which elements of care for the child. There is too much evidence which suggests that parents may feel unsupported and neglected in the care of their sick child (Darbyshire 1994). The NSF (DoH 2004a) highlights the various types of support which parents need and includes effective personal and material support. Much of what is stated in this section of the NSF reiterates what has been said by others in the past, but now it is being set in standards that healthcare workers are required to show evidence of meeting.

Aspects of family-centred care provide many additional examples of risks for children, parents and nurses. Feeding, or the provision of food for children to feed themselves, is usually considered to be a normal 'parenting skill'. However, when that food is to be administered via a nasogastric tube or gastrostomy, questions may arise over who should give the feeds. If the parents wish to give the feeds, then nurses must ensure a low risk/high benefit situation by teaching the parents this 'new skill' and monitoring their ability until all parties feel equally confident that the parents can carry out the practice. The risk is in handing over to parents what has previously been conceived as nursing care; the benefit is that parents and child can share the closeness of a mealtime together. Principles from this scenario can be transferred to many other practices which may involve parents, student nurses or nurses previously unfamiliar with a particular practice.

Risks for nurses may originate from many sources. Some risks arise from complaints by parents as a result of nurses failing in their duty of care. Examples of such failure might include inadequate securing of a nasogastric tube, resulting in the infant removing the tube and necessitating the passage of another, causing the child further distress. In caring for a child who is receiving fluids via a peripheral venous line, the nurse may fail to notice a swelling on the child's arm. When the electronic pump continues to alarm, a second nurse discovers the child's arm is oedematous and hard, indicating the severity of the extravasation.

A lack of written instructions may also give rise to failure in duty of care. For example, at the changeover of shifts, Nurse Small tells Nurse Knight that Joe is having 20 ml of milk 2-hourly and that his bottles are ready in the refrigerator. Once the day staff have left, Nurse Knight checks the care plan only to realise that Nurse Small has not completed this for her shift.

As the nurse completing the shift has not provided details of the care given, the new nurse has only the verbal report to rely on. This may lead to inappropriate care, with both nurses implicated for failing in their duty of care. Accurate, well-written care plans provide clinical evidence for determining the delivery of care and minimising risk. The treatment needs of children are very different and special attention must be given to babies and small children when giving them medicines and in the interpretation of results from services such as pathology (DoH 2004a). The findings of a small study by Guy et al (2003) identified that nurses, together with pharmacists, have a key role to play in identifying and preventing errors of prescribing being translated into errors of medication administration in paediatric settings.

There are risks which the nurse accepts in exercising duty of care, for example looking after an infectious patient (Chadwick & Tadd 1992), dealing with an aggressive person in the accident and emergency department, or teaching children and parents in the administration of drugs. Chadwick and Tadd (1992) emphasise that members of the nursing and medical professions are expected to assume a certain level of personal risk as part of their professional obligation. Dimond (2002) states that each nurse should be able to carry out a risk assessment of health and safety hazards in relation to colleagues, clients and the general public. This is an essential part of the role of the nurse since the management of risks must become everybody's business.

All nurses should be aware of the potential risks each time they enter into a situation with a child and/or the parents.

Local risk management systems designed to help NHS organisations in the effective management of incidents should be supported by an organisational risk management strategy and a programme of proactive risk assessments, together with the compilation of an organisational risk register. This will require trust boards to receive reports periodically and to demonstrate how learning has occurred and what measures have been implemented to improve care.

The risk assessment process should enable the creation of a risk profile and action plan which highlights issues for the most urgent attention. Stower (2000) presents a simple and clear model of risk assessment in which hazard inspection is the first step and the simple hazards are dealt with. Risk reduction and control is the next stage. Where other hazards remain these are then categorised into low, medium and high risk and appropriate methods of resolution are identified. Stower (2000) promotes the idea of engaging a colleague from another area to review the environment as fresh eyes are alert to those things that regular team members may overlook. However, it should always be borne in mind that the ultimate responsibility lies with those who have been especially trained in the job.

The third stage in the process is risk transference in which Bowden (1996) discusses insurance by trusts to cover claims on their behalf. Although this may seem beyond the domain of the majority of readers, the fact that there are funds to cover claims should not be a cause for complacency.

In conclusion, risk management is about the prevention or minimisation of risks within the process of providing care. Benefits of a risk management programme are improvements in the quality of patient care, reductions in damage and injury to patients, increases in patient activity and a better environment for staff. Strategies identified to achieve this include improved communications and record keeping which involve the child and family as active participants. The child and family should be encouraged to voice their opinions of the care received through systematic channels. Finally, clinical supervision (as discussed in the section on accountability) may enable a more open and honest approach to the delivery of care, both in hospital and in the community. Utilising these strategies may enable a positive and proactive approach to risk management in the future.

CHILD PROTECTION

If society is to protect children, then it is essential that everyone accepts responsibility for the welfare of children (Protecting Children 2003). As healthcare professionals, children's nurses are in direct contact with children on a daily basis whether in hospital or in the community, and therefore it is essential that they are aware of their own responsibilities in child protection. However, it must be recognised that local authorities, through their Social Services Departments, under statute, are the body responsible for protecting children (Hall 2003, Protecting Children 2003).

Child abuse is at times difficult to define and is identified by Corby (2000) as a socially defined construct being a product of a particular time, culture and context. It is not an absolute and unchanging phenomenon. Therefore any figures which relate to child protection need to be analysed with care. Prior to 1988 there were no national statistics kept in Britain about child abuse despite the fact that there had been a number of major incidents of abuse prior to 1988. Figures have been available since that time and the Department of Health collates the number of children on the child protection register annually (Corby 2000). The figures recorded provide evidence that child protection concerns increased with the formalisation of the protection processes and then decreased as the category of grave concern was eliminated in 1991 (Corby 2000).

During the three decades prior to the 21st century, there were a number of cases of child abuse concerning individual children which were so severe that the inquiries into them were named after the children.

In light of the above, the Victoria Climbie inquiry made by Lord Laming (DoH 2003a) and issues of child protection arising from it will be considered. The recommendations of this report have been implemented throughout the UK. Although all aspects of this chapter have some relevance to child protection – for example, listening to the voice of the child, advocating on behalf of the child – perhaps health professionals can be most effective in their recognition of the child at risk. Lack of communication and documentation have been identified as key factors that influence child protection cases (DoH 2003a, Hall 2003, Protecting Children 2003) and indeed were viewed as being major contributing factors to the death of Victoria. The Climbie Report made 108 recommendations, all aimed at improving services for children. However, the words of Smith (2003), outlining the Royal College of Nursing (RCN) guidance following the publication of this report, carry the strongest message that 'child protection is every nurse's responsibility'. The National Society for the Prevention of Cruelty to Children goes one step further and says it is everyone's business (NSPCC 2003). Therefore everyone who has any interaction with children in a professional capacity should be cognisant of the major recommendations of the Laming report. The 108 recommendations may, according to the RCN (Smith 2003), be summarised under the headings shown in Box 1.

The RCN guidelines recommend that training and education in child protection should be provided to all nurses who come into contact with children; it should feature in pre- and post-registration programmes with specific provision for those at post-registration undertaking work focused on child protection. However, it is widely recognised that multiprofessional/multiagency education is beneficial such that all parties involved in the process have a fuller understanding of their individual responsibilities (Hall 2003).

The NHS across the UK is committed to child protection, with hospitals/trusts appointing lead nurses and medical staff to provide support for staff within their organisations.

When working with children in any care setting, all nurses should be aware of the need to be vigilant for the child who may be the victim of abuse. This can manifest itself in many ways, with some behaviours being more obvious indicators than others; for example, the frozen watchfulness of the toddler who has been subject to physical harm, and the over-friendliness of another who has been neglected and possibly harmed as well, since evidence of more than one type of abuse may be seen in a single child. Older children may be looking for a confidante and do on occasions ask nurses to keep their secret, perhaps in terms of, 'If I tell you something, do you promise not to tell anyone else?' This may be because the child has been groomed by an abuser that the sexual behaviours they are engaging in are secret and the child should not tell anyone else. Therefore the child has displayed a lot of courage to get to the point of asking the nurse to keep this secret. When a child does ask for a confidence to be kept, then the nurse must do so, providing that the child is competent (see section on informed consent). In addition, if the nurse has reasonable cause to suspect that the child is suffering or likely to suffer significant harm, then they can justify disclosure. However, the child must be alerted to the fact that the nurse will have to disclose.

Every nurse should be familiar with the procedure for what to do when concerned that a child may be at risk or has been abused in some way. The Laming report highlighted that there were many documents available relating to child protection procedures and therefore professionals might become confused or indeed be using out-of-date material. To this end, *What to do if you're worried a child is being abused* (DoH 2003b) was released in May 2003. This comprehensive document should eliminate the need for individual bodies to produce their own and provides staff with a practical guide to do their job.

Box 1   Major recommendations of the Laming report

Changes in services to support children

- A children and families' board to coordinate ministerial initiatives
- A national agency for children and families which will be responsible for policy on a national basis for children, young people and families
- Local committees for children and families developing collaboration and sound working relationships
- Local authority management boards which will ensure service delivery
- Lines of accountability to run through these organisations which will be inspected and reviewed by government inspectors

Improvements to the exchange of information

- Government should review the free exchange of information
- Staff should be accountable for using information in a clear and unambiguous manner

National children's database

- This would enable a detailed picture of the past history of individual children to be built. This is an important aspect since some parents have deliberately avoided services by moving to different geographical locations

Service funding

- Local authorities should engage with the community and represent their needs
- Local authorities should be funded to provide 24-hour specialist services for children and families
- The use of agency and locum staff is not appropriate

Training and supervision

- This is identified as being essential and should:
  - use the report to promote better practice
  - train staff to protect and care for children and support their families
  - provide child protection training for all staff
  - implement an effective system of supervision in action for all services

Practice guidance and documentation

- Documentation of guidance must be simplified and uniform (Common Assessment Framework)
- Nursing care plans must contain issues of suspected harm
- Health professionals should all contribute to the same set of records for each child

---

The past 2 years have been a very active phase in the development of services for children. Whilst there is still a period of time for the full implementation to take place, it is hoped that at last a network is being provided that will allow children to grow up in a secure environment where there will not be the potential for any one of them to suffer.

SUMMARY

This chapter has explored a number of key concepts which should be considered as the cornerstones of practice for the professional nurse. Although each concept has been dis-cussed as a separate entity, in practice they are interrelated. The nurse has to understand the elements of risk within any situation in order to act as a responsible professional who is accountable to patients, employers and the profession. When providing information to children and parents, the nurse should exclude personal values and opinions and give an unbiased, rational explanation. Practitioners who are able to do this are true advocates for their patients. Advocacy also requires that the practitioner is cognisant of the risks for the patient. Therefore, sound research-based knowledge should underpin the key concepts of this chapter.

The confines of this chapter have only permitted a relatively superficial exploration of the concepts of accountability, informed consent, advocacy, clinical governance, risk management and child protection. It is suggested that readers use the References and Further Reading to explore these issues further.

Finally, many of the issues raised give nurses cause for concern. They are everyday incidents in practice, and nurses should be encouraged to discuss their practice with colleagues. This might happen at the changeover of shifts, during clinical supervision or in the more formal setting of a seminar. Whatever the chosen setting, the importance of dialogue cannot be overestimated. Each nurse should accept responsibility for encouraging colleagues to speak out about their practice, keep themselves updated and share knowledge and skills.

Within this new millennium, nurses now have more opportunity than ever before to develop their knowledge and skills to enhance practice. Nurses should be proud of this practice and be prepared to share what they do well, as the many practices provided in this text prove.

References

Age of Legal Capacity (Scotland) Act 1991 HMSO, Edinburgh

Adoption and Children Act 2002 The Stationery Office Limited, London

Alderson P 2000 The rise and fall of children's consent to surgery. Paediatric Nursing 12(2): 6–8

Altschuler J 1997 Family relationships during serious illness. Nursing Times 93(7): 48–49

Beale H 2002 Respite care for technology dependent children and their families. Paediatric Nursing 14(7): 18–19

Bowden D 1996 Calculate the risk. Nursing Management 3(4): 10–11

British Medical Association 2001 Consent, rights and choices in health care for children and young people. BMJ Books, London

Carter B, Campbell S 1997 Children's nurses as critical thinkers. Journal of Child Health Care 1(1): 5

Casey A 1997 So much to do. Paediatric Nursing 9(9): 3

Chadwick R, Tadd W 1992 Ethics and nursing practice. Macmillan Education, London

Charles-Edwards I 1995 Moral, ethical and legal perspectives. In: Carter B, Dearmun A (eds) Child health care nursing – concepts, theory and practice. Blackwell Science, Oxford

Charles-Edwards I 2001 Children's nursing and advocacy: are we in a muddle? Paediatric Nursing 13(2): 12–15

Charles-Edwards I 2003 Power and control over children and young people. Paediatric Nursing 15(6): 37–43

Children (Scotland) Act 1995 HMSO, Edinburgh

Children's Act (England and Wales) 1989 HMSO, London

Collier J, Robinson S 1997 Holding children still for procedures. Paediatric Nursing 9(9): 12–14

Corby B 2000 Child abuse: towards a knowledge base. Open University Press, Oxford

Cox S J, Robinson S, Murrells T 2003 Planning a career as a children's nurse: the availability of career guidance during the nurse diploma course. Journal of Child Health Care 7(4): 258–275

Coyne I T 1998 Researching children: some methodological and ethical considerations. Journal of Clinical Nursing 7(5): 409–416

Darbyshire P 1994 Living with a sick child in hospital: the experiences of parents and nurses. Chapman and Hall, London

Dearmun A K, Campbell S, Ballow J 1995 Meeting the needs of the child and family with altered gastrointestinal function. In: Carter B, Dearmun A K (eds) Child health care nursing – concepts, theory and practice. Blackwell Science, Oxford

Department of Health 1996 The patient's charter: services for children and young people. HMSO, London

Department of Health 1999 Making a difference: strengthening the nursing, midwifery and health visiting contribution to health and health care. TSO, London

Department of Health 2000a The NHS plan: a plan for investment, a plan for reform. TSO, London

Department of Health 2000b An organisation with a memory: report of an expert group on learning from adverse events in the NHS chaired by the Chief Medical Officer. TSO, London

Department of Health 2001a Consent – what you have a right to expect. A guide for children and young people. TSO, London

Department of Health 2001b Building a safer NHS for patients – implementing an organisation with a memory. TSO, London

Department of Health 2002 Learning from Bristol: The Department of Health's response to the report of the public inquiry into children's heart surgery at the Bristol Royal Infirmary 1984–1995. TSO, London

Department of Health 2003a The Victoria Climbie inquiry: report of an inquiry by Lord Laming. TSO, London

Department of Health 2003b What to do if you're worried a child is being abused. TSO, London

Department of Health 2004a National service framework for children, young people and maternity services. DH, London

Department of Health 2004b Every child matters. DH, London

Department of Health 2004c The Chief Nursing Officer's review of the nursing, midwifery and health visiting contribution to vulnerable children and young people. DH, London

Dimond B 2002 Legal aspects of nursing, 3rd edn. Longman, Harlow

Donaldson S 1997 Atopic eczema: management and control. Paediatric Nursing 9(8): 29–34

Donaldson L 2000 Clinical governance: a concept. In: Van Zwanenberg T, Harrison J (eds) Clinical governance in primary care. Radcliffe Medical Press, Oxon

Gates B 1995 Whose best interests? Nursing Times 91(4): 31–32

Great Britain Parliament 1969 Family Law Reform Act. HMSO, London

Gulam H 2004 Consent: tips for health care professionals. Australian Nursing Journal 12(2): 17–19

Guy J, Persaud J, Davies E, Harvey D 2003 Drug errors: what role do nurses and pharmacists have in minimising risk? Journal of Child Health 7(4): 277–290

Hall D 2003 Protecting children, supporting professionals. Archives of Diseases in Childhood 88: 557–559

Hill P 2000 Reducing risk in primary care. In: Van Zwanenberg T, Harrison J (eds) Clinical governance in primary care. Radcliffe Medical Press, Oxon

Howard R 1997 Grasping the opportunities within evolving nursing boundaries. Journal of Child Health Care 1(2): 81–83

Hughes J M, Callery P 2004 Parents' experiences of caring for their child following day case surgery: a diary study. Journal of Child Health 8(1): 47–58

Kennedy I 2001 Learning from Bristol. The report of the public inquiry into children's heart surgery at the Bristol Royal Infirmary 1984–1995. TSO, Norwich

Kenny G 2003 Skills or skilled? Children's nursing in the context of the current debate around skills. Journal of Child Health Care 7(2): 113–122

Kitson A 2004 Future vision. Royal College of Nursing, RCN Magazine Autumn 2004

Kohrman A, Clayton E W, Frader J E et al 1995 Informed consent, parental permission and assent in pediatric practice. Pediatrics 95(2): 314–317

Lowden J 2002 Children's rights: a decade of dispute. Journal of Advanced Nursing 31(1): 100–107

Lugon M, Secker-Walker J 1999 Clinical governance: making it happen. Royal Society of Medicine Press, London

Mallik M 1997 Patient representatives: a new role in advocacy. British Journal of Nursing 6(2): 108–113

Marshall K 1998 New law on children and medical consent [advice leaflet]. University of Glasgow/Yorkhill NHS Trust, Glasgow

Martin E A 2004 Oxford dictionary of nursing. Oxford University Press, Oxford

Mullaly S 2003 Address to the Joint Professional Committee for Nurses, Midwives and Health Visitors meeting at the Department of Health, London

National Patient Safety Agency 2003 Seven steps to patient safety – your guide to safer patient care. NPSA, London. Online. Available: www.npsa.nhs.uk/sevensteps

National Society for the Prevention of Cruelty to Children 2003 Child protection awareness in health. NSPCC EduCare, Leamington Spa

Nursing and Midwifery Council 2002a Supporting nurses and midwives through lifelong learning. Online: Available: www.nmc-uk.org

Nursing and Midwifery Council 2002b Guide for students of nursing and midwifery. Online: Available: www.nmc-uk.org

Nursing and Midwifery Council 2004 The NMC code of professional conduct. NMC, London

Ondrusek N, Abramovitch R, Pencharz P, Koren G 1998 Empirical examination of the ability of children to consent to clinical research. Journal of Medical Ethics 24(3): 158–165

Orr F E 1999 The role of the paediatric nurse in promoting paediatric right to consent. Journal of Clinical Nursing 8(1): 291–298

Phillips T 1994 Children and power. In: Lindsay B (ed.) The child and family: contemporary nursing issues in child health and care. Baillière Tindall, London

Protecting Children 2003 Protecting children – a shared responsibility. Scottish Executive, Edinburgh

Pursell E 1995 Listening to children: medical treatment and consent. Journal of Advanced Nursing 21(4): 623–624

Pyne R 1998 On being accountable. Health Visitor 61: 173–175

RCN 1999 Restraining, holding still and containing children. Guidance for good practice. RCN, London

RCN 2004 Children and young people's mental health– every nurse's business. RCN, London

Rennick J 1986 Re-establishing the parental role in a pediatric intensive care unit. Journal of Pediatric Nursing 1(1): 40–44

Richardson J, Webber I 1995 Ethical issues in child health care. Mosby, London

Rushton C H, Armstrong L, McEnhill M 1996 Establishing therapeutic boundaries as patients' advocates. Pediatric Nursing 22(3): 185–189

Russell-Johnson H 2004 Parental responsibility: preparing for the change in the law. Paediatric Nursing 16(1): 28–29

Russell S 1995 Risk management. British Journal of Nursing 4(10): 607

Smallman S 2003 Keeping children safe in the healthcare system. Paediatric Nursing 15(8): 20–22

Smith F 2003 Safeguarding the young. Paediatric Nursing 15(10): 24–25

Stower S 2000 Keeping the hospital environment safe for children. Paediatric Nursing 12(6): 37–42

Symons J 1995 Making staff aware of risks. Health Manpower Management 21(4): 15–19

Tingle J 1995 Clinical supervision is an effective risk management tool. British Journal of Nursing 4(14): 794

United Nations 1989 Convention on the rights of the child. UN, Geneva

Ward Platt M P, Brown K 2004 Evaluation of advanced neonatal practitioners: confidential enquiry into the management of sentinel cases. Archives of Diseases in Childhood Fetal and Neonatal edition. Online. Available: www.archdischild.com

Whiting M 1997 Community children's nursing: a bright future? Paediatric Nursing 9(4): 6–8

Wilson J, Tingle J 1999 Introduction to clinical risk management and modification. In: Wilson J, Tingle J (eds) Clinical risk modification: a route to clinical governance. Butterworth-Heinemann, Oxford

Woodrow P 1997 Nurse advocacy: is it in the patient's best interests? British Journal of Nursing 6(4): 225–229

Further Reading

Alderson P 1990 Choosing for children: parents consent to surgery. Oxford University Press, Oxford

Alderson P 2000 Young children's rights: exploring beliefs, principles and practice. Jessica Kingsley, London

Atherton T M 1994 The rights of the child in health care. In: Lindsay B (ed.) The child and family: contemporary issues in child health and care. Baillière Tindall, London

Bijsterveld P 2000 Competent to refuse? Paediatric Nursing 12(6): 33–35

Brykczynska G M 1989 Ethics in paediatric nursing. Chapman and Hall, London

Burns F 1998 Information for health: an information strategy for the modern NHS 1998–2005. DH, Wetherby

Candy D, Davies G, Ross E 2001 Clinical paediatrics and child health. W B Saunders, Edinburgh

Chambers M A 1992 Who speaks for the children? Journal of Clinical Nursing 1(2): 73–76

Curtin L, Flaherty M J 1982 Nursing ethics: theories and pragmatics. Prentice-Hall International, Englewood Cliffs, NJ

Dickenson D 1994 Children's informed consent to treatment: is the law an ass? Journal of Medical Ethics 20: 205–206

Dimond B 1996 The legal aspects of child health care. Blackwell Science, Oxford

Dineen M 1995 Clinical risk management – a pragmatic approach. British Journal of Health Care Management 1(14): 724–727

Donaldson M 1987 Children's minds. Fontana Press, London

Gillick V 1985 Dear Mrs Gillick. Marshall, Basingstoke

Hanks P 1987 The new Collins concise dictionary of the English language. Guild Publishing, London

Heywood Jones I 1990 The nurse's code. Macmillan, London

Loftus-Hills A 2004 How sound is your child protection practice? Royal College of Nursing, London

Nicholson R (ed.) 1986 Medical research with children: ethics, law and practice. Oxford University Press, Oxford

Nitschke R, Humphrey B, Sexauer C, Catron B, Wunder S, Jay S 1982 Therapeutic choices made by patients with end stage cancer. Journal of Pediatrics 101(3): 471–476

Smith F 2003 'Getting the right start': the Children's National Service Framework. Paediatric Nursing 15(4): 20–21

Solon M 1995 How not to go to court – keep the record straight. British Journal of Health Care Management 1(14): 719

Weithorn L A, Campbell S B 1982 The competency in children and adolescents to make informed treatment decisions. Child Development 53: 1589–1598

Control of infection

Susan Macqueen

INTRODUCTION

The prevention and control of healthcare-associated infection (HCAI) is the responsibility of all those involved in the care of patients. Many practical procedures are carried out by clinicians (nurses, doctors and people in professions allied to medicine) and can be a source of infection.

Infection control is an important part of risk management and there is a legal obligation to take appropriate precautions (Public Health (Infectious Disease) Regulations (HMSO 1988, NHS QIS 2001)). A controls assurance standard (DoH 2003a) on infection control, first produced in 1999, provides a checklist of measures for acute hospitals to ensure that the environment is managed so as to minimise the risk of infection to patients, staff and visitors. The Department of Health (DoH) document *Getting Ahead of the Curve* (2002a) outlines the changing patterns in communicable diseases and anti-microbial resistance and emphasises the need for their control. The increasing emergence of serious infections with meticillin-resistant *Staphylococcus aureus* (MRSA) in the paediatric population is cause for concern (Khairulddin et al 2004). The report on *Winning Ways* (DoH 2003b) aims to bring infection control into the mainstream of health care by setting out a strategy (see Box 1). With the advent of new and emerging infectious diseases it is important that there are written management procedures with formal risk assessment and audit trails where there may be hazards from infection towards patients, visitors or staff in the workplace. This includes all healthcare institutions within the hospital and community settings. National evidenced-based guidelines for preventing HCAI have been published for hospitals (Pratt et al 2001) and the community (Pellowe et al 2003, Thames Valley University 2003). A clean, well-maintained environment plays an essential part

---

Box 1   Winning ways – working together to reduce healthcare–associated infection

- Action one: active surveillance and investigation
- Action two: reducing the infection risk from use of catheters, tubes, cannulae, instruments and other devices
- Action three: reducing reservoirs of infection
- Action four: high standards of hygiene in clinical areas
- Action five: prudent use of antibiotics
- Action six: management and organisation
- Action seven: research and development

---

in minimising infection. The *NHS Healthcare Cleaning Manual* (2004) supports the *'Matron's Charter'* (NHS Estates 2004) and empowers senior nurses – modern matrons – to ensure the environment is safe to nurse patients.

The Health Protection Agency (HPA)/ Health Protection Scotland (HPS) provides an integrated approach to protecting the health of the public against infectious diseases and chemical and radiological hazards by working with the NHS and local authorities. Their website provides up-to-date epidemiological data and guidelines on infectious diseases including healthcare-associated infection (www.hpa.org.uk and www.hps.scotland.nhs.uk). Newly emerging or newly identified diseases such as severe acute respiratory syndrome (SARS) is an example of how rapidly the world's communicable disease network (through the World Health Organisation) can communicate essential information.

About 9% of hospital inpatients acquire an infection while in hospital and between 50 and 70% of surgical wound infections occur after discharge. Between 15 and 30% of hospital-acquired infection could be prevented by better application of knowledge and implementation of realistic infection control policies (DoH 2002a). The incidence of nosocomial infection in children is higher and proportional to their age with the highest incidence in neonates and infants under 1 year of age. The cost to the NHS has been estimated as £1 billion per year. For example, for

hospital-acquired bacteraemia this equates to an extra £6209 per case (National Audit Office 2000).

Medical and nursing cultural influences may play a part in non-compliance with evidence-based infection control practice. Ethnographic studies (Macqueen 1995) have indicated that nurses wash their hands more frequently before aseptic procedures than after 'dirty' tasks, and that they perceive babies as being 'less dirty' than older children. Ongoing education, training and support for all staff must therefore be an integral part of an infection control programme.

THE CHAIN OF INFECTION

The chain of infection consists of the microorganism, a source, a susceptible host, a portal of entry and a means of transmission.

The microorganism

Most nosocomial infections are caused by bacteria and viruses but problems with fungi are increasingly being identified, especially in immunosuppressed patients.

The most important characteristics of the organism are:

- pathogenicity – ability to produce disease
- infectivity – ability to spread from person to person
- invasiveness – ability to spread within the host
- virulence – the severity of the illness
- properties of adherence to synthetic materials such as implanted devices, e.g. *Staphylococcus epidermidis* adheres well to some synthetic material.

When the body's natural defences are invaded, either by a pathogenic microorganism for which the body is not immune or through invasive technology (e.g. insertion of medical devices or surgery), the risk of infection increases. When foreign material is inserted into the body, the material interacts with the host's natural defence mechanism and the risk of infection increases. The surface of the foreign body (e.g. a plastic catheter) is covered with host-derived proteins such as albumin, fibrinogen, fibronectin, collagen, laminin, vitronectin and immunoglobulins. Some of these components (e.g. albumin) may serve to retard microbial adherence, whilst others such as fibronectin may serve as receptors for bacteria. This complex of host and bacterial constituents is known as a biofilm (Bisno 1995). It is important that nurses are aware of different catheter materials in order that the most appropriate for the procedure may be selected to reduce the risk of infection. Considerations of availability, cost, site and length of time of insertion, and chemicals with which the material may come in contact, such as drugs or intravenous solutions, must be taken into account.

The antigenic make-up of an organism may also change through the use of antibiotics and disinfectants. Outbreaks of multiply antibiotic-resistant Gram-negative bacteria such as *Klebsiella*, *Escherichia coli* and *Pseudomonas* and Gram-positive bacteria such as methicillin-resistant *Staphylococcus aureus* (MRSA) are becoming more common in both the hospital and the community setting (Kelly & Chivers 1996, O'Brien 1997). Reports on MRSA bacteraemia in the UK indicate the problem is increasing amongst children less than 15 years of age (Khairulddin et al 2004).

The source of infection

Microorganisms are carried on inanimate or animate objects from a reservoir to a source. The reservoir is the place where the organism maintains its presence, metabolises and replicates. The source is the place from which the infectious agent passes to the host either by direct or indirect contact through a vehicle as the means of transmission.

The infection may be endogenous, arising from the child's own flora, or exogenous, arising from the environment. Exogenous sources may be other children, parents, staff or visitors, animals (Cotton et al 2000), equipment or a dirty environment (Dancer 1999). The source may include:

- those with acute disease
- those who are not infectious

- persons who are colonised with an infectious agent but who do not have the disease (asymptomatic carriers)
- those who are chronic carriers of an infectious agent.

Environmental transmission of the organism may be increased through air movement and dust.

The following have all been cited as environmental sources of hospital-acquired infections:

- lack of adherence by healthcare workers to basic infection control guidelines
- overcrowding of patient beds (Harbarth et al 1999)
- a badly maintained environment, e.g. torn chairs or mattresses, soiled curtains, cracked tiles
- inadequate decontamination and maintenance of equipment
- inadequate disposal of clinical and household waste
- lack of pest control, e.g. the sighting of cockroaches, mice or rats
- inadequate food hygiene practice
- improper air flow
- lack of isolation facilities.

Mode of transmission

Transmission may occur by one or more of five different routes.

Contact

- Direct contact as in person-to-person spread when nursing or turning a child or between two children physically playing together (e.g. scabies or antimicrobial-resistant microorganisms)
- Indirect contact such as inadequate decontamination of equipment or the environment (e.g. contaminated needles or noroviruses causing acute diarrhoea and vomiting).

Droplet

Droplets are generated by the source person during sneezing, coughing or talking and during procedures such as suctioning or bronchoscopy. Transmission occurs when small particles (>5 μm) of residue-containing organisms are propelled a short distance through the air and deposited on the host's conjunctivae, nasal mucosa or mouth. Droplets do not remain suspended in the air and therefore this should not be confused with airborne transmission. Examples of droplet infection are pertussis (whooping cough) and influenza.

Airborne
Dissemination via this route is of either airborne droplet nuclei (small particle residue of evaporated droplets ≤5 μm in size that remain suspended in the air for long periods of time) or dust particles containing the infective organism. Organisms can be widely dispersed by air currents and inhaled by susceptible hosts either in the same room or over a further distance, therefore special air-handling and ventilation may be required to prevent airborne transmission. Varicella (chickenpox), measles virus and *Mycobacterium tuberculosis* are examples of organisms transmitted by the airborne route.

Foodborne
This applies to organisms transmitted by contaminated items such as food, water, medications, devices and equipment (e.g. salmonella or cholera).

Vector-borne
Organisms may be carried by vectors such as flies, cockroaches, mice, rats and other vermin.

Bloodborne,
This is where infection is transmitted through blood or blood products (e.g. HIV, hepatitis C).

The host

Host factors that influence the development of infections are the site of deposition of the organism and the host's defence mechanism (see Table 1).

PRECAUTIONS TO BE TAKEN

The application of source isolation or protective precautions (barrier nursing) was revised by the Communicable Disease Center in Atlanta, USA, in 1996 and the terms 'standard' precautions and 'transmission' precautions are now felt to be more appropriate (Garner 1996). However, within the UK universal precautions, source and protective isolation continue to be terms in widespread use. This encompasses the need to control healthcare-associated infections which includes the increasing emergence of multiple antibiotic-resistant organisms, common outbreaks of viral diarrhoeal illnesses, infections with implanted devices and the recognition of blood-borne viruses. Although local practices may vary, the principles of infection control remain the same.

Standard precautions
These precautions are designed to reduce the risk of transmission of microorganisms from both recognised and unrecognised sources of infection (EPIC 2001). They should be practised in both hospital and the community when care may involve coming into contact with:

- blood
- all body fluids, secretions and excretions regardless of whether they contain blood
- non-intact skin
- mucous membrane.

The key principles include:

- hand hygiene before and after patient contact
- regular maintenance and appropriate cleaning, disinfection or sterilisation of equipment
- position of the patient within the ward/clinical area
- wearing protective clothing to avoid contamination of the skin or mucosal surfaces – gloves, aprons, face protection as appropriate
- safe handling and disposal of sharp instruments and needles
- safe disposal of clinical waste
- safe disposal of foul and infected linen
- safe handling and transportation of specimens
- maintaining a clean environment.

Transmission–based precautions
These precautions are designed for:

1. children known or suspected to be infected or colonised with pathogens for which additional precautions are required to interrupt

Table 1 Common risk factors for infection

Risk factors	Reasons

Gestational age: <32 weeks	The stratum corneum is very scant and permeable to bacteria. The skin is an effective barrier by 37 weeks' gestation
	  The skin of babies born full term has a pH of 6.4 which reduces to 4.9 over a few days as the body develops its protective acid mantle, a natural antibacterial protection. This can take up to 3 weeks in preterm infants
	  Humoral defence mechanism–complement activation is only 20–40% of adult values (full-term newborn is 50–80% of adult value)
	  Maternal IgG begins passing transplacentally at approximately 15 weeks' gestation but does not reach the optimum until about 33 weeks. The fetus begins to synthesise IgM at about 30 weeks' gestation

Low birth weight	Risk of infection is increased in babies weighing <1000 g and reduced in babies >2500 g
Method of nutrition	Infection occurs less in breastfed babies because of protection from maternal antibody transference Infection occurs more in bottle-fed babies because of lack of hygiene in equipment, preparation and storage
Umbilical cord stump	Associated with infection, especially after placement of umbilical vein catheters or delayed separation of cord
Congenital abnormalities	Such as abnormal immune function (severe combined immune deficiency, DiGeorge syndrome, Down syndrome), congenital infection (rubella, cytomegalovirus, hepatitis) or congenital cardiac or renal disease
Acquired disease processes	Other infections or chronic disease processes
Invasive devices	External devices such as intravascular, urinary, endotracheal tubes, nasogastric, gastrostomy, drainage systems. Internal devices such as ventricular atrial/peritoneal shunts, heart valves and artificial patches
Surgery	Type and length of surgery
Chemotherapy	Antibiotic therapy has been associated with *Clostridium difficile* and necrotising enterocolitis. Certain drugs such as steroids alter immunity
Length of stay in hospital	Increases the risk of colonisation/invasion with pathogenic organisms
Increased handling by hospital staff	Hands of staff have been associated with cross-infection of pathogenic organisms in hospitalised patients
Equipment	Equipment includes suction apparatus, respiratory equipment, humidifiers, feeding utensils, thermometers, pedal bins, incubators, scalp electrodes, stethoscopes, laryngoscopes, surgical instruments, communal ointments

transmission; this may include one or more of airborne, droplet or contact transmission
2. children who are immunosuppressed and require an environment with a filtered clean air system to prevent the risk of acquiring airborne fungal infections such as *Aspergillus* (MMWR 2000).

Children who have or are suspected of having highly transmissible or epidemiological important pathogens for which additional precautions are required should preferably be isolated in a single cubicle. A risk assessment should be made to include the causative organism, the route of transmission, the need for a special environment such as a negative-pressure room or clean, filtered air and resources available. The child may need to be:

- nursed in an individual cubicle, preferably with hand hygiene and en suite toilet facilities
- cohorted (placed with other children) in a separate area on the ward with others who are infected/colonised with the same pathogen
- nursed in a room with negative pressure with at least ten exchanges of air per hour. There is usually an air-lock and the door must be kept closed (NHS Estates 2005)
- nursed in a room with high-efficiency filtered positive air pressure. There is usually an air-lock and the door must be kept closed. This is usually reserved for severely immunosuppressed children such as those undergoing transplantation
- nursed at home away from susceptible people if the risk factor of infection to others is felt to be high, such as small babies or those with significant immunosuppression.

Hand hygiene

Hand hygiene is the single most cost-effective method of reducing cross-infection (APIC 1995, Boyce & Pittet 2002). The purpose of hand hygiene is to remove dirt, organic material and transient microorganisms (Gould 1991). Healthcare workers (HCWs) can contaminate their hands with pathogenic microorganisms by performing 'clean procedures' or touching intact areas of skin of hospitalised patients (Boyce & Pittet 2002). Transient hand carriage, especially of Gram-negative organisms, has been reported in 20–30% of hospital staff and may persist for several weeks. Sneddon's (1990) study demonstrated that Gram-negative organisms were isolated from 44% of nurses' hands before washing and from 12% after washing; 40% of hands sampled after dirty activity and 25% after clean activity were contaminated. Only 52% of the handwashes were considered good. Pittet et al (1999) reported that hand hygiene decreased with higher workload and higher-risk patients. Increasing hand hygiene frequency among hospital staff has

been associated with a decrease in hospital-acquired infection (Pittet et al 2000).

Cuts and abrasions of any exposed areas of skin must be covered with a dressing that is semi-permeable and an effective bacterial and viral barrier. Healthcare workers with exfoliating skin lesions must report to an occupational health department.

Requirements
- A hand basin with running warm water.
- An appropriate liquid soap, antiseptic detergent and/or alcohol hand-rub. Alcohols effectively reduce bacterial counts on hands provided they are not visibly contaminated with proteinaceous material (body fluids, dirt, grease, etc.). Personalised alcohol hand-rubs can be attached to the individual to encourage hand decontamination during high-risk tasks or busy periods.
- Disposable towels. A clean, laundered non-disposable towel can be used in the home setting.
- Where the above is not possible, an alcohol rub will suffice where hands are not heavily contaminated.

Handwashing method
The correct method of handwashing is shown in Figure 1. Table 2 lists types of hand hygiene practice – the method used will depend on the type of practice to be undertaken.

Risk factors for infection
- Skin lesions, e.g. eczema, paronychia, cuts and abrasions.
- Nail polish, artificial nails or long nails including nail art.
- Not washing hands after removal of gloves.
- Jewellery, e.g. rings, watches, bracelets. These may harbour pathogenic organisms.
- Non-compliance – hand hygiene occurs in approximately half of the instances in which it is indicated.
- Communal hand lotion.
- Cloth hand towels in an institutional setting.
- Large reusable containers and 'topping up' antiseptics and liquid soap.
- Communal bar soap.

1.Wet hands, apply soap and use the following procedure

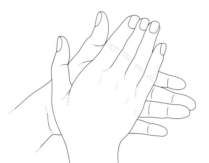 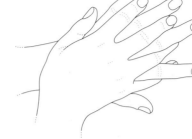

2. Rub palm to palm   3. Rub back of both hands

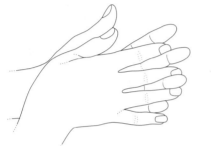

4. Rub palm to palm with fingers interlaced   5. Rub backs of fingers (interlocked)

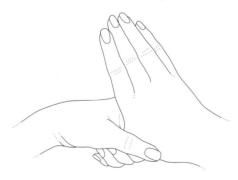 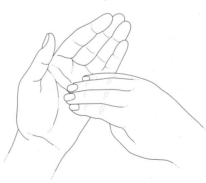

6. Rub all parts of both hands   7. Rub both palms with finger tips

7. Rinse hands under running water and dry thoroughly on a clean towel

Figure 1   Methods of handwashing.

- Alcohol hand-rub is not as effective in the presence of physical dirt.
- Moisturising agents and surfactants may interfere with the residual activity of chlorhexidine.
- Lack of sufficient hand hygiene facilities.

- Waste pedal bins with broken lids which have to be opened with the hand.

Protective clothing

Personal protective equipment must be made available for all HCWs. A risk assessment of

Table 2   Methods of hand hygiene practice

Description	Purpose	Method
Social hand-wash	To remove soil and transient microorganisms	Liquid soap or detergent for at least 10–15 seconds
Hand antisepsis	To remove or destroy transient microorganisms	Antimicrobial soap or detergent or alcohol-based hand rub for at least 10–15 seconds
Surgical hand-scrub	To remove or destroy transient microorganisms and reduce resident flora	Antimicrobial soap or detergent preparation with brush (sterile) to achieve friction for at least 120 seconds or alcohol-based preparation for at least 20 seconds

the task to be performed must be made (Fig. 2) in order that the correct protective clothing may be worn. The assessment may differ between parents and HCWs who are more exposed to a variety of pathogens during their duties. However, risk factors in association with blood-borne viruses such as HIV, hepatitis B or C, for example, may be the same. The increasing recognition of latex allergy in both patients and HCWs must be taken into consideration (Markey 1994, Johnson 1997). Manufacturers are being asked to minimise or abolish the use of latex in medical equipment and consumables.

Any blood or body secretions/excretions may contain microbial pathogens and must be handled as potentially infectious. In young children, especially in the nappy-wearing age, the bowel flora is commonly distributed over the skin and in the upper respiratory tract.

Disposable gloves

- Gloves provide added protection when the risk of microbial contamination is increased such as during nappy changing or when handling contaminated material as in specimen collection.
- Non-sterile gloves must be worn for direct contact with blood or body fluids, non-intact skin and mucous membrane.
- Wear gloves for all care if intact skin is a source of contamination, such as when the child is colonised with multiply antibiotic-resistant organisms. Certain pathogens such as *Klebsiellae* have increased adherence properties to the skin and may be found on the hands after social hand hygiene (Casewell & Phillips 1977).
- Gloves should be disposable and discarded between patients or contaminated body sites.
- Hands have become contaminated even when wearing gloves and therefore a soap

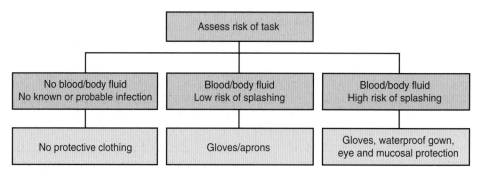

Figure 2   Risk assessment for protective clothing

and water handwash or alcohol hand-rub is recommended after removal of gloves.

- Wear gloves when handling disinfectants or cleaning.

Risks factors for infection

- Quality of gloves – leakage has been reported in 4–63% of vinyl gloves and 3–52% of latex gloves (Korniewicz et al 1989).
- Petroleum-based or oil emollients may affect the integrity of latex.
- Dermatitis due to allergy to latex or glove powder.
- Not removing stoned rings, watches and jewellery before hand hygiene.

Plastic aprons

Cotton gowns offer minimal microbial protection (Donowitz 1986) and therefore should be replaced with single-use disposable plastic aprons. Hands must be washed after removal of the apron.

Aprons should be changed between clean and dirty tasks and should be worn for:

- all patient care
- aseptic techniques
- serving meals and feeding patients
- performing dirty tasks
- bedmaking.

Facial protection

Masks, eye protection and face shields should be worn to protect mucous membranes of the eyes, nose and mouth during procedures and patient care activities which are likely to generate splashes, sprays or aerosols of blood, body fluids and secretions or excretions.

Masks may also be worn to protect the HCW from droplet or airborne infectious diseases. There are different size filters in masks and the appropriate one must be chosen for the correct protection. There are filter face pieces (FFP) class 1 (low efficiency), 2 (medium efficiency) and 3 (high efficiency). For example, a FFP 3 filtered mask should be worn when dealing with patients with diseases such as SARS. The Health and Safety Executive (2003) describes fit testing of respiratory protective equipment face pieces.

Surgical masks are worn in theatre to protect the patient against large particle droplets from the surgical team immediately over the operation site (Belkin 1997). More research is required as to the risk of infection to the patient from members of the circulating theatre team, especially during prolonged surgery where the risk may be higher.

Factors to consider

- Compliance with wearing the protective device correctly.
- Type of filter in mask.
- Procedures which generate aerosols, e.g. bronchoscopy or suctioning.
- Risk of splattering of blood or other body fluids.
- Open pulmonary tuberculosis and multiply antibiotic-resistant tuberculosis (MRTB).
- Risk to and from the child and HCW.

Protective gowns and headwear

These should not only be made of appropriate material to minimise 'strike through' or leakage of blood and body fluids, but also be comfortable to the wearer. Hair should be covered by the hood/hat. They should be available where the risk of contamination with blood and body fluids is increased such as in the operating theatre, intensive care or accident and emergency units.

Foot protection

Contamination of the feet with blood/body fluids will be minimised if boots/theatre shoes are worn in high-risk areas such as the operating theatre, intensive care or accident and emergency units. Theatre footwear should not be worn outside the theatre complex. Overshoes have not been shown to reduce infection and may indeed increase the risk by contaminating hands on application or removal.

Waste disposal

Revised waste regulations have been updated by the Environmental Agency (2004, 2005). This includes further segregation of special waste including prescription-only medicines. All contaminated clinical waste must be placed into yellow clinical sacks. It must be secured and the source area identified, i.e. the responsible local health authority (check local policy for hospitals and the community), before it is removed from the premises for incineration.

Sharps

Needles, blades and other sharp instruments must be placed in a rigid, puncture-proof sharps container immediately after use. Discard needles and syringe as one unit into the sharps box. Do not resheath contaminated needles as this increases the risk of injury (Jagger et al 1990). Never fill the container more than two-thirds full and ensure that it is securely closed and labelled before disposal and incineration (BMA 1990).

Uncontaminated paper and other household waste should be placed in a black bag, secured ready for collection.

Risk factors for infection
- Resheathing needles.
- Breaking the hub of the needle to take blood from neonates.
- Leaving sharps lying around and not disposing of them immediately into a sharps bin.
- Overfilling sharps bins or clinical waste bags.
- Handing sharp instruments to another person instead of laying them down safely so that they can be picked up, especially in the operating theatre where the risk of injury may be increased.
- Leaving contaminated waste unbagged or available to the public which may encourage pests and indiscriminate searching for hypodermic needles.

Disposal of infected linen

Local policies for the handling of laundry must be followed (HSG(95)18). Foul and infected linen should be segregated and placed in a red water-soluble bag contained in an outer bag and labelled 'danger of infection' as per local policy.

Soiled linen may also be contaminated with pathogenic microorganisms and should be placed directly into appropriate laundry containers. Baby clothes, blankets, etc. should be laundered centrally in an institution. If performed at local level, a separate room with adequately maintained washing and drying facilities must be available.

Risk factors for infection
- Washing baby clothes in the kitchen or dirty utility room in an institution.
- Not maintaining adequate washing temperatures for disinfection (70–71°C for at least 3 minutes or 65°C for 10 minutes).
- Inadequate maintenance of washing/drying machines.
- Transporting dirty linen on the same trolley as that used for transporting and serving food.
- Storing clean linen in unhygienic conditions.

Eating utensils such as dishes, cups, glasses, baby bottles

Eating utensils carry a risk of transmitting infection.

Factors to note
- All feeding utensils should be washed in a well-maintained dishwasher. They should be placed in the dishwasher immediately after use and not left lying around.
- Where dishwashers are not available, feeding utensils should be thoroughly washed in hot water and detergent, rinsed in hot water and dried.
- Baby feeding bottles and equipment should be washed in a well-maintained dishwasher or a commercial steam steriliser. It is not necessary to sterilise them in an autoclave in hospital.
- Feeding utensils for severely immunosuppressed children, such as those undergoing transplantation, should be washed in a dishwasher, thoroughly dried and stored separately. Sterilisation by autoclave is not considered necessary.
- Where a heat process is not available, baby bottles and feeding equipment should be thoroughly cleaned before immersion in a chemical sterilant such as hypochlorite or dichloroisocyanurate for the recommended time and stored in a clean container afterwards.

- Equipment for expressing breast milk should be sterile and single use, and breast pumps should be decontaminated and maintained regularly.
- It is not considered necessary to use disposable utensils if the above facilities are available.

Risk factors for infection

Food poisoning microorganisms and Candida can be associated with poor hygiene and the inadequate decontamination of teats and dummies.

The use of disinfectants in the environment and with equipment

Up-to-date information can be found at www.decontamination.nhsestates.gov.uk.

Cleaning must always be undertaken before disinfection or sterilisation. The following definitions (Ayliffe et al 1993, Wilson 2002) are used to standardise different methods of decontamination.

Sterilisation

A process used to render an object free from all living organisms.

Disinfection

A process used to reduce the number of microorganisms but not usually of bacterial spores. The process does not necessarily kill or remove all microorganisms but reduces the number to a level which is not harmful to health.

Cleaning

A process that removes contaminants including dust, soil, large numbers of microorganisms and the organic matter (e.g. faeces, blood) that protects the organisms. Cleaning is always necessary before sterilisation or the use of disinfectants.

The risks to patients from the environment and equipment may be classified as follows:

1. High risk – items in close contact with a break in the skin or mucous membrane or introduced into a normally sterile body area should be *sterile*.
2. Intermediate risk – items in contact with mucous membrane or other items contaminated with particularly virulent or readily transmissible organisms, or items to be used on highly susceptible patients should be *disinfected*.
3. Low risk – items in contact with normal and intact skin should be *cleaned* and dried.

Advice on the use of disinfectants should be followed (Rutala 1996, Ayliffe et al 1993) and local policies adhered to. The use of disinfectants in the paediatric setting should be kept to a minimum to ensure safety. Care must be taken to keep them locked away out of reach of children.

Hot water and detergent with thorough drying is considered adequate for most environmental cleaning. The environment must be kept clean and a high standard of housekeeping maintained. However, studies have shown that viruses (e.g. noroviruses including Rotavirus) causing diarrhoea can remain viable on inanimate surfaces for several days (Satter et al 1994). Touching contaminated surfaces can transfer infectious viruses to the hands and aid spread. Chlorine-based agents are an effective disinfectant against these viruses.

Factors to note

- Equipment must be cleaned with hot water and detergent before sterilisation or disinfection. Always follow manufacturers' instructions regarding decontamination. Chemicals may react adversely on some materials, for example alcohol will produce opaqueness on Perspex material or hypochlorites may rust metals.

- Always use moist heat sterilisation and heat disinfection where possible. Some materials are heat labile and chemical sterilisation or disinfection may need to be used, such as with endoscopic equipment. Outbreaks of infection with contaminated endoscopes are not uncommon and appropriate guidelines must be followed. Equipment may require to be sent to a local decontamination unit or centre.

- A risk assessment to the child and health care worker must be made with any chemical used in accordance with the Control of Substances Hazardous to Health (COSHH) Regulations.

- The use of phenolic disinfectants has been associated with neonatal hyperbilirubinaemia (Wysowski et al 1978).

- Care must be taken with hypochlorite disinfectants on urine spillages as they can create toxic fumes.

- Hypochlorite disinfectant is used for:

  - 1.0% (10 000 ppm available chlorine) – disinfection of heavy spillages of blood

  - 0.1% (1000 ppm available chlorine) – general cleaning when disinfection is required

  - 0.0125% (125 ppm available chlorine) – disinfecting babies' bottles, teats, dummies.

- Walls should be cleaned if visibly dirty.

- After cleaning a room which has housed a child with an infection, it is unnecessary to leave it to air for a set period of time.

Risk factors for infection
- Not cleaning equipment before using chemical disinfection. Many disinfectants are inactivated in the presence of organic matter such as blood, dirt or grease.
- 'Topping up' bottles of disinfectant or antiseptics.
- Not making up fresh solutions or using the correct dilution.
- Hypochlorite solutions are unstable and must be renewed every 24 hours.
- Mixing incompatible chemicals.
- A poorly maintained environment encourages infestation and inhibits adequate cleaning.

Equipment

It is preferable that all equipment is cleaned and maintained in a central unit where documentation and quality control can be monitored. Manufacturing guidelines must be followed according to the type of equipment and level of decontamination required, e.g. sterilisation, disinfection or cleaning (Fuller 1992).

Factors to note
- Equipment must be decontaminated before service or repair; see HSG(93)26 (DoH 1993).
- Single-use items must not be reused unless the health authority have in place an adequate quality assurance programme and accept liability (MDA 2000).
- Equipment such as wooden spatulas have been used as splints for intravenous cannulation sites, a purpose for which they were not designed, and consequentially caused serious fungal infection (Holzel et al 1998).

Risk factors for infection
- Torn mattresses, pillow covers and chairs causing difficulty in cleaning.
- Poorly maintained equipment such as suction apparatus, breast pumps or blood gas machines.
- Inadequately cleaned equipment such as urine- or stool-testing equipment, thermometers, laryngoscopes, incubators and respiratory ventilators/humidifiers.

Occupational health

All health care workers should have access to an occupational health department and should report:

- For a pre-employment health review and to be advised on immunisations and relevant immunity status such as after vaccination against hepatitis B. A small percentage of people do not produce antibodies to some immunisations and therefore remain susceptible to the disease (Salisbury & Begg 1996, www.dh.gov.uk). If they are doing exposure-prone procedures (EPP) then they must provide evidence that they are not carrying the hepatitis B or C virus (DoH 2002b).
- If they have not had varicella (chickenpox), a varicella vaccine is available to HCWs.
- If on immunosuppressive therapy or pregnant, when appropriate advice to reduce the risk of infection can be given (Advisory Committee on Dangerous Pathogens 1997).
- If they have suffered from an infectious disease and have been at work or wish to return to work.
- If they feel that they are likely to be or are infected with a blood-borne virus such as human immunodeficiency virus, hepatitis B or C and are performing exposure-prone procedures during their work (HSG(93)40

(NHSME 1993) and Addendum (DoH 1996); RCN 1997).

- For all accidents, including those involving:
  - sharps injuries or contamination of mucosal surfaces of the eyes, nose or mouth with blood or body fluids
  - blood or body fluids on non-intact skin (guidance on HIV post-exposure prophylaxis (DoH 2004) must be followed).
- When allergic reactions occur such as with latex or chemicals.

Risk factors for infection
- Not adhering to hand hygiene procedures.
- Not wearing recommended protective clothing.
- Working with exfoliating skin lesions or uncovered broken skin.
- Working with children who have certain infectious diseases such as chickenpox and not being immune.
- Not being protected from infectious diseases where immunisation is available.
- Travelling abroad and not taking healthcare advice.
- Not reporting when you have an infectious disease or an infected skin lesion.

Surveillance of infection and auditing practice

Surveillance of infection and ongoing audit of hospital-acquired infection should be seen as a collaborative multidisciplinary activity undertaking between the infection control team, clinical staff and managers (DoH 2003b).

Documentation of increased risk factors, such as insertion and removal of devices including intravascular and urinary catheters, respiratory intubation or any invasive procedure, must be maintained (DoH 2003b). Surveillance methods vary and should be discussed with the local infection control team.

The role of the nurse as a health educator can be of particular importance to the child and family when explaining about infectious diseases. Nurses must feel confident in their knowledge and be able to individualise care safely and explain basic hygiene precautions. Children and their families should have a right to expect that their health will be protected as well as promoted when receiving healthcare services.

The Scottish Surveillance of Healthcare Associated Infection Programme (SSHAIP) also outlines associated epidemiological data (see www.show.scot.nhs.uk/scieh).

The Health Protection Agency has a steering group on healthcare-associated infections (see www.hpa.org.uk).

References

Advisory Committee on Dangerous Pathogens 1997 Infection risks to new and expectant mothers in the workplace. HSE, London

Association for Professionals in Infection Control and Epidemiology (APIC) 1995 APIC guideline for hand-washing and antisepsis in health care settings. American Journal of Infection Control 23: 251–269

Ayliffe G A J, Coates D, Hoffman P N 1993 Chemical disinfection in hospitals, 2nd edn. Public Health Laboratory Service, London

Belkin N L 1997 The evolution of the surgical mask: filtering efficiency versus effectiveness. Infection Control and Hospital Epidemiology 18: 49–57

Bisno A L 1995 Molecular aspects of bacterial colonization. Infection Control and Hospital Epidemiology 16: 648–657

Boyce J M, Pittet D 2002 Guidelines for hand hygiene in health-care settings: recommendations of the Healthcare Infection Control Practitioners Advisory Committee and the HICPAC/SHEA/APIC/ IDSA Hygiene Task-force. MMWR 51(RR16): 1–44

British Medical Association (BMA) 1990 A code of practice for the safe use and disposal of sharps. BMA, London

Casewell M, Phillips I 1977 Hands as a route of transmission for *Klebsiella* species. British Medical Journal 2(6098): 1315–1317

Cotton M F, Wasserman E, Pieper C H et al 2000 Invasive disease due to extended spectrum beta-lactamase-producing *Klebsiella pneumoniae* in a neonatal unit: the possible role of cockroaches. Journal of Hospital Infection 44: 13–17

Dancer S J 1999 Mopping up hospital hygiene. Journal of Hospital Infection 43: 85–100

Department of Health 1993 Decontamination of equipment prior to inspection, service or repair. HSG(93)26. HMSO, London

Department of Health 1996 Addendum to HSG(93)40: protecting health care workers and patients from hepatitis B. DH, Wetherby

Department of Health 2004 HIV post-exposure prophylaxis: guidance from the UK Chief Medical Officer's Expert Advisory Group on AIDS. DH, London

Department of Health 2002a Getting ahead of the curve: a strategy for combating infectious diseases. A report by the Chief Medical Officer. DH, London

Department of Health 2002b Hepatitis C infected health care workers. DH, London

Department of Health 2003a Controls assurance standard. Infection control. Online. Available: www.dh.gov.uk; search for Controls Assurance

Department of Health 2003b Winning ways: working together to reduce healthcare associated infection in England. A report by the Chief Medical Officer. DH, London

Donowitz L G 1986 Failure of the overgown to prevent nosocomial infection in a paediatric intensive care unit. Pediatrics 77: 35–38

Environmental Agency 2004, 2005 Waste regulations Online. Available: www.environment-agency.gov.uk

EPIC 2001 EPIC guidelines: standard principles for preventing hospital-acquired infections. Journal of Hospital Infection 47(Suppl): S21–S37

Fuller A 1992 Sterilising instruments. Journal of Infection Control Nursing, Nursing Times 88(50): 64–65

Garner J S 1996 Guidelines for isolation precautions in hospitals. American Journal of Infection Control 24: 24–52

Gould D 1991 Nurses' hands as vectors of hospital-acquired infection: a review. Journal of Advanced Nursing 16: 1216–1225

Harbarth S, Sudre P, Dharan S, Cadenas M, Pittet D 1999 Outbreak of *Enterobacter cloacae* related to understaffing, overcrowding and poor hygiene practices. Infection Control and Hospital Epidemiology 20(9): 598–603

Health and Safety Executive 2003 OC 282/28. HSE, London

HMSO 1998 Public Health (Infectious Disease) Regulations (SI 1988: 1546). HMSO, London

Holzel H H, Macqueen S, MacDonald A et al 1998 *Rhizopus microsporus*: a major threat or minor inconvenience? Journal of Hospital Infection 38: 113–118

HSG (93) 26 (DoH 1993) Health Service Guidelines. Decontamination of equipment prior to inspection, service repair. DoH, London

HSG(95)18: Hospital laundry arrangements for used and infected linen. DoH, London

Jagger J, Hunt E H, Pearson R D 1990 Sharp object injuries in the hospital: causes and strategies for prevention. American Journal of Infection Control 18: 227–231

Johnson G 1997 Time to take the gloves off. Occupational Health 49: 25–28

Kelly J, Chivers G 1996 Built-in resistance. Journal of Infection Control Nursing, Nursing Times 92(2): 50–54

Khairulddin N, Bishop L, Lamagni T L, Sharland M, Duckworth G 2004 Emergence of methicillin resistant *Staphylococcus aureus* (MRSA) bacteraemia among children in England and Wales, 1990–2001. Archives of Disease in Childhood 89: 378–379

Korniewicz D M, Laughton B E, Butz A, Larson E 1989 Integrity of vinyl and latex procedure gloves. Nursing Research 38(3): 144–146

Macqueen S 1995 Anthropology and germ theory. Journal of Hospital Infection 30(Suppl): 116–126

Markey J 1994 Latex allergy: implications for healthcare personnel and infusion therapy patients. Journal of Intravenous Nursing 17(1): 35–39

Medical Devices Agency (MDA) 2000 Single-use medical devices: implications and consequences of reuse. MDA DB2000 (04). MDA, London

MMWR 2000 Guidelines for Preventing Opportunistic Infections among Hematopoietic Stem Cells. Transplant Recipients: Recommendations of CDC, The Infectious Disease Society of America and The American Society of Bone and Marrow Transplantation 2000/49 (RRIO) 1–128. www.cdc.gov/mmwr

National Audit Office 2000 The management and control of healthcare associated infections in acute NHS Trusts in England. London, The Stationery Office.

National Health Service Management Executive (NHSME) 1993 Protecting health care workers and patients from hepatitis B. HSG(93)40. DH, London

NHS Estates 2004 A matron's charter: an action plan for cleaner hospitals. Online. Available: www.nhsestates.gov.uk

NHS Estates 2004 The NHS Healthcare Cleaning Manual. Online: www.nhsestates.gov.uk

NHS Estates 2005 HBN supplement 1: Isolation facilities in acute settings. Online: www.nhsestates.gov.uk

NHS QIS 2001 Standards for healthcare associated infection (HAI). Infection Control. NHS Quality Improvement Scotland, Edinburgh

O'Brien T F 1997 The global epidemic nature of antimicrobial resistance and the need to monitor and manage it locally. Clinical Infectious Diseases 24(Suppl 1): S2–S8

Operational Circular 2003 OC282/28. HSE, London

Pellowe C M, Pratt R J, Harper P et al 2003 Infection control: prevention of healthcare-associated infection in primary and community care. Journal of Hospital Infection 55(Suppl 2): S1–127. Online. Available www.richardwellsresearch.com

Pittet D, Mourouga P, Pernege T V 1999 Compliance with hand washing in a teaching hospital. The members of the Infection Control Programme. Annals of Internal Medicine 130: 126–130

Pittet D, Hugonnet S, Harbarth S et al 2000 Effectiveness of a hospital-wide programme to improve compliance with hand hygiene. Lancet 356: 1307–1312

Pratt R J, Pellowe C, Loveday H P et al 2001 The epic project: developing national evidence-based guidelines for preventing healthcare associated infections. Phase 1: guidelines for preventing hospital-acquired infections. Journal of Hospital Infection 47(Suppl): S1–S82. Online. Available: www.richardwellsresearch.com

Royal College of Nursing (RCN) 1997 Hepatitis guidelines. RCN, London

Rutala W A 1996 APIC guidelines for selection and use of disinfectants. American Journal of Infection Control 24: 313–342

Salisbury D M, Begg N 1996 Immunisation against infectious diseases. HMSO, London. Online: www.dh.gov.uk

Satter S Y, Jacobson H, Rahman H, Cusack T M, Rubino J R 1994 Interruption of rotavirus spread through chemical disinfection. Infection Control and Hospital Epidemiology 15: 751–756

Sneddon J G 1990 A preventable course of infection: carriage of Gram-negative bacilli on hands. Professional Nurse 6(2): 98–104

Thames Valley University 2003 Infection control: prevention of healthcare-associated infection in primary and community care. Clinical guidelines 2. National Institute for Clinical Excellence, London

Wilson J 2002 Infection control in clinical practice. Baillière Tindall, London

Wysowski D M, Flynt J W Jr, Goldfield M, Altman R, Davis A T 1978 Epidemic neonatal hyperbilirubinaemia and the use of phenolic disinfection. Paediatrics 16(2): 165–170

Further Reading

Advisory Committee on Dangerous Pathogens 2003 Transmissible spongiform encephalopathy agents: safe working and the prevention of infection. Online. Available: www.advisorybodies.doh.gov.uk/acdp/publications.htm

Auditor General 2000 A clean bill of health? A review of domestic services in Scottish hospitals. TSO, Edinburgh

Boucher I 1998 Third report of group of experts. *Cryptosporidium* in water supply. TSO, London

Department of Health 2000 The management and control of hospital infection. The UK Antimicrobial Strategy and Action Plan. HSC 2000/002. DH, London

Department of Health 2002 Hepatitis C: strategy for England. DH, London

Department of Health 2002 Guidelines for renal dialysis transplantation units: prevention and control of blood-borne virus infections. DH, London

Department of Health 2005 Saving Lives: a delivery programme to reduce healthcare associated infection including MRSA. Online: www.dh.gov.uk

Drews M B, Ludwig A C, Leititis J U, Daschner F D 1995 Low birthweight and nosocomial infection of neonates in a neonatal intensive care unit. Journal of Hospital Infection 30: 65–72

Emmerson A M, Enstone J E, Griffin M, Kelsey M C, Smyth E T M 1996 The second national prevalence survey of infection in hospitals – overview of the results. Journal of Hospital Infection 32: 157–190

Glenister H M, Taylor L J, Bartlett C L R, Cooke E M, Sedgwick J A, Mackintosh C A 1993 An evaluation of surveillance methods for detecting infections in hospital inpatients. Journal of Hospital Infection 23: 229–242

Haley R W, Culver D H, White J W 1985 The efficacy of infection surveillance and control programs in preventing nosocomial infections in university hospitals (SENIC study). American Journal of Epidemiology 121: 182–205

Hunter P R 1991 Application of hazard analysis critical control point (HACCP) to the handling of expressed breast milk on a neonatal unit. Journal of Hospital Infection 17: 139–146

Macqueen S 1996 Think globally, act locally: germ invasion and risk analysis. Journal of Neonatal Nursing 2(1): 20–25

Medical Devices Agency 2001 Safe use and disposal of sharps. MDA SN 2001 (19). MDA, London

Millward S, Barnett J, Thomlinson D A 1993 A clinical infection control audit programme: evaluation of an audit tool used by infection control nurses to monitor standards and assess effective staff training. Journal of Hospital Infection 24: 219–232

NHS Executive 2000 The management and control of hospital infection. HSC 2000/002. NHSE, London

NHS Estates 2003 Standards of cleanliness in the NHS: a framework in which to measure performance outcomes. NHS Estates, Leeds

NHS Quality Improvement Scotland (QIS) 2002 Health care associated infection (HAI): cleaning service standards. NHS Quality Improvement Scotland, Edinburgh

Pasquarella C, Pitzurra O, Savino A 2000 The index of microbial air contamination. Journal of Hospital Infection 46: 241–256

Scottish Office Department of Health 1999 Hospital acquired infection. A framework for a national system of surveillance in Scotland. TSO, Edinburgh

Teare E L, Peacock A 1996 The development of an infection control link-nurse programme in a district general hospital. Journal of Hospital Infection 34: 267–278

Introduction to community

Dawn Moss

CONTENTS

INTRODUCTION

Paediatric care today has been transformed with fewer admissions to hospital and a shorter hospital stay. The emphasis is on primary health and the delivery of health care in the community rather than secondary care based in the hospital (Middleton 2000). Medical advances have seen an increase in the numbers of babies born prematurely and surviving with increasing levels of needs. Children are now being discharged home from hospital earlier and with more complex problems (Fradd 1994). Children with serious illnesses such as cancer and cystic fibrosis now have a significantly improved prognosis. While (1991) considers that parents view the provision of home care to be an acceptable and welcome alternative to hospital-based care. Indeed it can be stated that children and their families have a right to expect appropriate nursing provision in the community (DoH 1991, Audit Commission 1993). Professional collaboration and effective communication with acute and community-based professionals ensures a coordinated approach to facilitating early discharge and reducing admission to hospital (Smith 1995).

MULTIAGENCY WORKING IN THE COMMUNITY

For Scotland's Children (Scottish Executive 2001a) states that better integrated children's services will ensure that services are more responsive, and identifies the need to bring services together to meet the needs of individual children, young people and their families. The *National Service Framework for Children, Young People and Maternity Services* (DoH 2004a) states that everyone who works with children, not only in healthcare settings, but also in schools and the wider community, will be expected to have an understanding of children's needs. The Framework states that future services will need to be designed and delivered around the needs of children and their families, rather than around organisations or professionals. *Every Child Matters* (DoH 2004b) will provide opportunities for health organisations to deliver improved outcomes in new ways and in partnership with other organisations.

The children's nurse working in the community has a role to play to enable each child they come into contact with to achieve these outcomes.

COMMUNITY CHILDREN'S NURSING

Community children's nursing (CCN) is described as specialist nursing that aims to provide high-quality care and support for the child and their family at home (Sidey 1995). CCN services have developed since their inception in 1987 and the majority of areas throughout the UK now have a service. The Royal College of Nursing (2000) states that CCN services tend to have been developed in response to local need and circumstances instead of being based on the most effective model of provision. Models of service delivery vary and include:

- hospital/ambulatory care outreach
- hospital at home
- CCN team based in acute services
- CCN team working within general practice
- community-based, nurse-led clinics
- children's palliative care teams
- multidisciplinary/multiagency working (includes taking on the role of key worker for children with complex healthcare needs and management of complex packages of care).

To understand the healthcare needs of children and families and which services are required to meet these needs, the Royal College of Nursing (2000) advises undertaking a profile of the community and a needs assessment. An effective way of identifying the needs of a population is by community profiling. The gathering of information gives a knowledge of contacts and resources about a defined community, giving the community practitioner the 'know how' of which services are required (Cernik & Wearne 1992). Analysis can then be made to form the basis for the planning and delivery of future health care (Blackie 1998). The information provided within a community profile gives community children's nurses (CCNs) the knowledge of the resources available that may be used to offer support to the families in their care.

CCNs provide a wide range of care options related to the child's individual needs. They will have a caseload for which they provide a specialist or generalist service, including the following:

- Children with life-threatening or terminal conditions (e.g. cancer, degenerative conditions, organ failure)
- Children with complex healthcare needs (e.g. technology-dependent)
- Training, education, support and management of non-parent carers
- Children in schools
- Children with acute illnesses/conditions (e.g. bronchiolitis, postoperative care)
- Children with chronic conditions (e.g. constipation, epilepsy, cystic fibrosis).

The difference between the specialist and generic role is one where the specialist nurse has more focused knowledge about caring for a child with a specific condition (Turner & Penn 1996). Whether in a specialist or generic role, CCNs recognise that it is not only the sick child needing care but that a holistic approach sees each child as part of a family. Alongside this is the philosophy of partnership and collaborative working with each family and the agencies involved (Perkins & Billingham 1997, Whyte 1997, Williams 1998).

TRANSITION FROM HOSPITAL TO HOME

Implementing a successful transition of care from hospital to home needs careful planning. The aim of this planning is to ensure that the child's care is continuous and the parents receive the support and education that enables them to provide safe care without undue stress. For children with complex healthcare needs, discharge planning needs to start some weeks before the child leaves hospital. Ideally the CCN will visit the family in hospital to enable them to develop a relationship and to start to discuss the practical issues of going home. The CCN can become familiar with the care that the child is currently receiving and can identify the resources that will be required in the home. This can be described as 'hospital in-reach' where the CCN takes an active role in the discharge planning process (Royal College of Nursing 2000). Whilst the child is still in hospital, education programmes can be initiated for the child and parents, who should be encouraged to discuss any concerns that they may have so that they are able to give informed consent to the care that they are being asked to undertake. Communication between the hospital and the primary health-care team is essential. The CCN is often ideally placed to act as a liaison and is able to involve the general practitioner and the health visitor at an early stage in the planning process.

Charles-Edwards and Casey (1992) pose ethical issues for children's nurses about parental involvement and voluntary consent. They discuss the need for the benefits of home care being weighed against any potential risks that might occur if the family felt under pressure to take on the caring role, were not confident or competent to undertake the care, or were given insufficient information. The hospital (or general practitioner, if accepting medical responsibility) 'retains the duty of care in the laws of negligence for the safety of the child' (Dimond 1996). It is therefore the responsibility of the individual practitioner to ensure that 'the reasonable standard of the responsible nurse working in those circumstances with those particular patients' (Dimond 1996) has been followed. Documentation should record what has been shown to parents. This should also demonstrate that the instruction has been understood and that the parents are capable of undertaking the procedure confidently and competently, being aware of all the problems that might occur and what action to take. Families should always be given the option of handing back control if they feel that they can no longer cope.

PROVIDING ACCESSIBLE SERVICES

CCN services need to ensure that the child and their family have easy access to services and information (Eaton & Thomas 1998). Team members can be contacted by telephone to provide advice and reassurance to both parents and professionals. Support and advice are vital elements of a CCN service, as well as accessibility, which enable the child to return to the service at any time (Smith 1995). The prime responsibility of the CCN is the duty of care for the child's physical and emotional safety (Sidey 1995). To meet this responsibility CCNs work creatively and flexibly, and implement training where necessary to enable children to live their lives to the full, whatever their illness or prognosis (Whyte 1997). CCNs facilitate family-led packages of care and empower the parents in care partnerships (Gould 2000). The level of care and support varies to ensure that each family is confident and competent in the care they are able to provide.

Many parents need all the available information to enable them to understand the difficulties, know all the available options and to be able to make decisions for their child and for the family (Cook 1999). Davis (1993) states that parents tend to base their decisions on what they already know; they therefore have a need for information to enable them to form their own constructions about their child's condition.

WORKING IN PARTNERSHIP WITH THE FAMILY

A family-centred approach encourages the family to become active partners with health professionals in the management, decision-making, and treatment and care of their child (Sidey 1995). This is supported by parents involved in a research study (Townsley et al 2004) who stated:

If co-ordinating services means reducing gaps, duplication and boundaries, then perhaps what we as families see as obvious, simple and common sense will start to happen.

The study explored the impact of multiagency working on disabled children with complex needs and concluded that interagency working enables families to be supported in managing their children's complex healthcare needs at home. In addition, and perhaps more importantly, children and young people with complex needs have presented their own views on what they expect from healthcare professionals (Stalker et al 2003). This includes the following:

● Being treated as individuals
● To be asked about their care and treatment, to be listened to and to have their wishes acted upon
● To have choices
● To be given information
● To know the staff involved in their care.

As mentioned above, the CCN recognises that a holistic approach sees each child as part of a family. The CCN works together with families as partners in planning holistic packages of care that best meet the needs of the child and family. Whyte (1992) recognises the need for the awareness of family dynamics along with the commitment to the whole family's health. A family nursing approach acknowledges that the needs of the child cannot be met in isolation from the family (Whyte 1997). The Royal College of Nursing (2000) states that CCNs use the networks within the community to facilitate family-centred appropriate care by teaching, supporting, advising, counselling and liaising. This allows children to continue to live their lives in a variety of community settings (Sidey 1995).

COORDINATION OF CARE AND CONTINUING CARE

If there is a lack of coordination between different agencies and professionals, no holistic view of the child is obtained. The more services a child receives, the more coordination is required to ensure services complement each other (Ovretveit 1993). Sloper (2002) states that parents report a 'constant battle' to find out what services are available and know what the roles of different professionals are. Parents can feel frustrated at trying to get professionals to understand their needs. Effective care coordination prevents fragmented care and duplication of services. Sidey (1995) emphasises how established and effective networks of communication should exist between the CCN, child and family, and professionals involved with the family from primary, secondary and tertiary services. Townsley et al (2004) explored the impact of multiagency working on disabled children with complex needs and concluded that well-coordinated interagency working enables families to be supported in managing their child's care at home.

Government policies have consistently advocated that children should be cared for in their own homes and that appropriate services are developed to facilitate this (Ministry of Health 1959, Department of Health and Social Security 1976, DoH 1991, NHS Executive 1996, House of Commons Health Committee 1997). *Every Child Matters* (DoH 2004b) advocates support for parents and carers and the new *National Service Framework for Children, Young People and Maternity Services* (DoH 2004a) further enhances the home care concept for children with complex health needs. In 1998 the Department of Health provided funding for CCN teams in Princess Diana's memory (DoH 1998). More recently in 2003 the New Opportunities Fund provided £48 million of lottery money to expand home-based paediatric palliative care teams in selected primary care trusts across the country.

In order for children with complex health needs or life-limiting conditions and their families to have their needs met, it is essential for 'continuing care' to be planned effectively. Continuing care can be defined as an individualised package of seamless care planned by health, social care and education in partnership with children and their families.

Historically, continuing care for children has always fallen under the auspices of CCN teams. In recent years such teams have begun to develop more robust services to ensure that children with complex health needs and disabilities are having their needs met. Continuing care teams have evolved to provide home-based respite care for children with complex health needs.

There are many continuing care models for children across the country. Carers are trained, assessed, supervised and supported by specialist practitioners in community children's nursing.

Coordinated services should ensure a referral network that can provide a seamless service between hospital and community. One of the key roles of the CCN and continuing care nurse is liaising with other professionals involved with each family from a variety of multidisciplinary teams within the hospital and throughout the community, including social care and education. The movement towards the integration of child health services has shown how hospital and community services can join together, ensuring continuity of care according to need, age and locality (Fradd 1994).

Research (Sloper & Turner 1992, Beresford 1995) has shown the importance to families of key workers who help them to access services, share information and support families. The CCN often takes on the role of key worker and is pivotal in offering direct meaningful support and improving coordination for families (Smith 1995). The Royal College of Nursing (2000) also identifies that it is the CCN who fulfils the key worker role that families ask for; that is, someone who visits regularly, is approachable and easy to access, and someone who listens. As a key worker the CCN will offer the family a single point of contact for any concerns, be an advocate and the source of practical, personal and emotional support and advice.

HEALTH PROMOTION AND HEALTH IMPROVEMENT

In Scotland, *Nursing for Health* (Scottish Executive 2001b) considers the contribution of nurses, midwives and health visitors in the context of the needs of children and young people to achieve optimal, healthy development. It states that nurses have a distinctive contribution to make to improving health based on their 'accessibility, acceptability and local knowledge'. The profound effects of early influences on lifelong health have been well documented. Breastfeeding, nutrition, dental health, immunisation and accident prevention are all major focuses for child health improvement and have been shown to have lifelong influences on the health of the individual. As in other areas, the impact of inequalities on child health is significant, with children living in areas of deprivation having significantly poorer health. To be effective in improving the health of children, nurses need to work not only with children and their families, but also with communities and other agencies.

An identified role of the CCN is to provide opportunistic health promotion for the whole family (Smith 1995). Downie et al (1996) define health as something that can be constantly improved. This acknowledges that many of the children cared for by the CCN may never attain the state of complete physical, mental and social health that is defined by the World Health Organisation (1984). Health promotion can be considered as a separate or 'add-on' activity, but for the CCN this can be viewed as an integral part of everyday practice (Benson & Latter 1998). The CCN offers each family support or assistance in order to improve their health and well-being (Fradd 1994).

The skills needed to be effective in health promotion include up-to-date knowledge, good communication skills and awareness about the resources and systems of support to refer families to (Blackie 1998). The CCN uses these skills to empower independence, moving from active nursing care to a supportive role. Parents may experience a great deal of stress related to the responsibility of caring for their child at home (Smith 1995). Ewles and Simnett (1999) state that, if clients are feeling insecure or anxious, this will affect their ability to learn. Support, advice and encouragement are therefore vital elements of the CCN role. The client-centred approach to health promotion practised by the CCN is emphasised by Blackie (1998) as being more successful than a top-down prescriptive approach. Examples of health promotion topics discussed might include diet and nutrition, dental health, drugs and alcohol, and smoking cessation.

ACCOUNTABILITY

Edwards (1998) identifies that critical thinking and analysis require the ability to discriminate relevant from irrelevant information, to consider information from a variety of sources, to analyse the facts and, as a result, make decisions. As Whyte (1997) indicates, the CCN is often in the position of using professional judgement rather than strict protocols. CCNs frequently make independent decisions within their nursing practice; they need to be sure of professional support to back up the decisions they make (Bradley 1997). CCNs may be involved with children and families on their caseload for many months or even years. At times the CCN can feel 'stuck' with a family within the confines of the available resources. Clinical supervision can enable the nurse to reflect on how effective they consider their contribution to a family to be. The skills needed to practise reflection involve description, critical analysis, synthesis and evaluation (Atkins & Murphy 1993). The practice of reflection can enable the CCN to develop self-awareness by a gradual, continuous process of noticing and exploring aspects of themselves (Burnard 1997). Challenging your attitudes and practice is not always an easy or comfortable thing to do but reflection as a process of clinical supervision is a means for the CCN to become more effective in practice and in meeting the needs of the child and family.

EVALUATION OF COMMUNITY CHILDREN'S NURSING SERVICES

The evidence suggests that CCNs are effective in meeting children's health needs and in promoting psychological health, family health, family unity and parental control (Bradley 1997). CCNs promote care by the family, which enables independence and the integrity of the family unit. This is achieved by teaching, health education, support, guidance, advice and nursing intervention (Smith 1995).

Sidey (1995) states that community children's nursing is not a cheap option, although on analysis it is considerably less than occupying an acute hospital bed. Bradley (1997) suggests measuring efficiency by the collection of quantitative data such as rates of admission and re-admission to hospital. Such data have shown that admission to hospital can be reduced by the provision of a CCN service (Sidey 1995, Smith 1995, Bradley 1997). The reduction in hospital admissions and outpatient appointments reduces travel costs, admission costs and disruption to family life (Bradley 1997).

Facey (2000) presents a system of dependency scoring to enable CCNs to calculate the dependency scores of the patients on their caseload to ensure appropriate use of resources. The Royal College of Nursing (2000) advises evaluation of the nurse's workload by monitoring the following:

- Child's care needs
- Quality of care delivered
- Skill mix within the team
- Time allocated to deliver care.

The Royal College of Nursing (2000) also advises that each CCN team develops a system for monitoring the pressure of work on each nurse including the numbers of:

- highly dependent families
- child protection problems
- children with life-threatening or life-limiting conditions
- development work (non-clinical work)
- time worked over contracted hours
- caseload turnover.

THE FUTURE FOR NURSING CHILDREN IN THE COMMUNITY

Previous recommendations have stated that children should have access to 24-hour, 7-day

CCN services (House of Commons Health Committee 1997) but whilst CCN services have developed it is evident that this level of service is yet to be achieved in many areas of the UK. The CCN is just one of the professionals providing services to children in the community. The emphasis should be about focusing the model of teamworking with the child in the centre. Turner and Penn (1996) emphasise how collaborative working allows the burden of caring for a child at home to be shared.

In England, the *Chief Nursing Officer's Review of the Nursing, Midwifery and Health Visiting Contribution to Vulnerable Children and Young People* (DoH 2004c) states that integration is needed across a number of boundaries – most importantly health, social care and education. There is also a need to overcome the current fragmentation between hospital and primary care, and between nurses, midwives and health visitors. A key theme from this review is the need to 'follow the child', which means providing services as close to home as possible, including schools and the wider community. This means that the demand for children's nursing in the community will increase as children's continuing care needs are provided at home.

References

Atkins S, Murphy K 1993 Reflection: a review of the literature. Journal of Advanced Nursing 18: 1188–1192

Audit Commission 1993 Children first. HMSO, London

Benson A, Latter S 1998 Implementing health promoting nursing: the integration of interpersonal skills and health promotion. Journal of Advanced Nursing 27: 100–107

Beresford B 1995 Expert opinions: families with severely disabled children. Policy Press/Joseph Rowntree Foundation, York

Blackie C 1998 Community health care nursing. Churchill Livingstone, Edinburgh

Bradley S 1997 Better late than never? An evaluation of community nursing services for children in the UK. Journal of Clinical Nursing 6: 411–418

Burnard P 1997 Effective communication skills for health professionals, 2nd edn. Stanley Thornes, Cheltenham

Cernik K, Wearne M 1992 Using community health profiles to improve service provision. Health Visitor 65(10): 343–345

Charles-Edwards I, Casey A 1992 Parental involvement and voluntary consent. Paediatric Nursing 4(1): 16–18

Cook P 1999 Supporting sick children and their families. Baillière Tindall, Edinburgh

Davis H 1993 Counselling parents of children with chronic illness or disability. The British Psychological Society, Leicester

Department of Health 1991 Welfare of children and young people in hospital. HMSO, London

Department of Health 1998 A proposal to develop a national children's community nursing service. DH, London

Department of Health 2004a National Service Framework for children, young people and maternity services: primary care version. DH, London

Department of Health 2004b Every child matters. DH, London

Department of Health 2004c The Chief Nursing Officer's review of the nursing, midwifery and health visiting contribution to vulnerable children and young people. DH, London

Department of Health and Social Security 1976 Fit for the future. Report of the committee on child health services (Chairman: Professor S D M Court). HMSO, London

Dimond B 1996 The legal aspects of child health care. Mosby, London

Downie R S, Tannahill C, Tannahill A 1996 Health promotion: models and values, 2nd edn. Oxford University Press, Oxford

Eaton N, Thomas P 1998 Community children's nursing: an evaluative framework. Journal of Child Health 2(4): 170–173

Edwards S 1998 Critical thinking and analysis: a model for written assignments. British Journal of Nursing 7(3): 159–166

Ewles L, Simnett I 1999 Promoting community health: a practical guide, 4th edn. Baillière Tindall, Edinburgh

Facey S 2000 Dependency scoring in community children's nursing. In: Muir J, Sidey A (eds) Textbook of community children's nursing. Baillière Tindall, Edinburgh, Ch 19

Fradd E 1994 Whose responsibility? Nursing Times 90(6): 34–36

Gould C 2000 Economic evaluation in practice. In: Muir J, Sidey A (eds) Textbook of community children's nursing. Baillière Tindall, Edinburgh, Ch 34

House of Commons Health Committee 1997 Health services for children and young people in the community – home and school. Third Report. TSO, London

Middleton C 2000 A short journey down a long road: the emergence of professional bodies. In: Muir J, Sidey A (eds) Textbook of community children's nursing. Baillière Tindall, Edinburgh, Ch 1

Ministry of Health 1959 The welfare of children in hospital. Report of Central Health Services Council (Platt Report). HMSO, London

NHS Service Executive 1996 A patient's charter: services for children and young people. HMSO, London

Ovretveit J 1993 Co-ordinating community care: multi-disciplinary team and care management. Open University Press, Buckingham

Perkins E, Billingham K 1997 Working together to care for children in the community. Nursing Times 93(43): 46–48

Royal College of Nursing 2000 Children's community nursing: promoting effective teamworking for children and their families. Royal College of Nursing, London

Scottish Executive 2001a For Scotland's children. Scottish Executive, Edinburgh

Scottish Executive 2001b Nursing for health: a review of the contribution of nurses, midwives and health visitors to improving the public's health in Scotland. Scottish Executive, Edinburgh

Sidey A 1995 Competence for community health care nursing (children). In: Sines D (ed.) Community health care nursing. Blackwell Science, Oxford, Ch 11

Sloper P, Turner S 1992 Service needs of families of children with severe physical disability. Child: Care, Health and Development 18: 259–282

Sloper T 2002 Meeting the needs of disabled children. Quality Protects Research Briefings 6. Department of Health, Research in Practice. DH, London

Smith F 1995 Children's nursing in practice: the Nottingham model. Blackwell Science, Oxford

Stalker K, Carpenter J, Phillips R, Connors C, MacDonald C, Eyre J 2003 Care and treatment. Joseph Rowntree Foundation, East Sussex

Townsley R, Abbott D, Watson D 2004 Making a difference? Exploring the impact of multi-agency working on disabled children with complex health care needs, their families and the professionals who support them. Policy Press, Bristol

Turner P, Penn K 1996 Palliative care: the community role of the specialist nurse. Geriatric Medicine, May

While A 1991 An evaluation of a paediatric home care scheme. Journal of Advanced Nursing 16: 1413–1421

Whyte D 1992 A family nursing approach to the case of a child with a chronic illness. Journal of Advanced Nursing 17: 317–327

Whyte D (ed.) 1997 Explorations in family nursing. Routledge, London

Williams Y 1998 Working with parents to promote health. Journal of Child Health Care 2(4): 182–186

World Health Organization 1984 Health promotion: a discussion document on the concepts and principles. WHO, Copenhagen

Practice 1

Administration of medicines

Louise Dyer, Catherine Furze, Christina Maddox, Rachel Sales

Introduction and rationale

The Crown Report (DoH 1999, p. 23) provides a comprehensive review of all aspects of drug administration that includes prescribing, supplying and administering medicines, and clearly states that: 'No health professional should undertake any aspect of patient care for which they are not trained and which is beyond their professional competence.' Therefore, for students undertaking programmes to become registered children's nurses, recognition of personal limits, knowledge, understanding and skills are an essential part of the learning process. This is also endorsed within the Nursing and Midwifery Council (NMC) *Guidelines for the Administration of Medicines* (2002a).

The administration of medicines to infants, children and teenagers requires a complex set of skills that must be grounded in a sound understanding of child development, not only in terms of biophysiological changes but also changes that occur from a psychological perspective (Watt 2003a). Knowledge and skills that are essential for children's nurses include understanding the relevant underpinning theory to support care, being numerically competent and an effective communicator (Nicol & Thompson 2000, 2001, NMC 2002a). For this to happen, registered nurses must have a sound knowledge base regarding the administration of medicines that draws upon the currently available literature and use this to inform everyday practice.

Learning outcomes

After reading this section you should understand:

- the importance of administering medicines safely
- the need to communicate effectively with the child and family
- the importance of preparing children when administering medicines
- the routes for the administration of medicines
- the identification of suitable techniques for administration via each route.

Factors to note

There are two main pieces of legislation that influence the administration of medicines within the UK: the Medicines Act (1968) and the Misuse of Drugs Act (1971). Within the European Union there are approximately 75 million children between the ages of 0 and 16 years, which represents approximately a fifth of the total population (European Commission 2002). Choonara (2000) indicates that European studies investigating the use of medicines for children found fundamental flaws in practice which opposed the manufacturers' guidelines; these included the use of unlicensed medicines and the administration of incorrect dosages. Approximately 50–90% of all medicines administered to children have never been evaluated for use with children (Schaad 2001, European Commission 2002). This has had the effect of children becoming 'therapeutic orphans' which has led to the death of some children (Sutcliffe 2003). As a consequence, the European Commission proposed regulation of orphan medicinal products and this was adopted in December 1999 (European Commission 2002).

Within the UK, marketing authorisation is required from the Medicines Control Agency before medicines can be marketed and promoted (Stephenson 2000); however, it is common practice to prescribe unlicensed medicines (UL), also known as off label medicines (OL), to children; it is not illegal for a doctor to prescribe a medicine with different indicators or to children of different ages (Stephenson 2000, 2001). Prescribing medicines that are off label is necessary when there is no suitable alternative (Watt 2003a). For example, in a neonatal intensive care unit, 90% of infants receive UL or OL drugs (Stephenson 2001); in primary care approximately 11–33% of prescriptions for children are UL or OL (McIntyre et al 2000). *Medicines for Children* (RCPCH 1999) is a relatively new formulary that provides practitioners with consensus views on correct dosages for children of all ages and is an important point of reference for all those involved in prescribing medicines to children.

With reference to the administration of medicines there are two key principles of common law, the first of which is the person's right to self-determination. Griffith et al (2003) cite Lord Goff in Airdale NHS Trust v Bland [1993] and maintain that self-determination requires healthcare professionals to respect the wishes of patients and carers. The second principle involves the practitioner's responsibility when administering medicines in any environment. A medicine that does have a product licence would be deemed to be unlicensed if, for example, tablets are crushed or capsules are opened, in which case the practitioner must be able to justify the reasons why this was done and may find themselves personally liable if harm comes to those receiving the medicine (Griffith et al 2003).

What is a medicine?

A medicinal product may be defined as any substance or combination of substances presented for treating or preventing disease in human beings or animals (Article 1.2 EC Directive 65/65 cited by the Crown Report, DoH 1999, p. 79).

Within the Medicines Act (1968, section 130), there are three legal categories in which medicines can be grouped: according to potency, potential adverse effects and the need for the supply of some medicines to be professionally supervised (cited by the Crown Report, DoH 1999).

- POM: prescription only medicines – This group of medicines is sold or supplied with the signed authorisation of an 'appropriate practitioner'; this may be a doctor, dentist or, in some instances, a nurse prescriber. These medicines must be supplied by or under the supervision of a pharmacist.
- P: pharmacy medicines – These medicines must be supplied or sold by or under the supervision of a pharmacist on registered premises.
- GSL: general sales list medicines – These can be supplied and purchased directly by members of the public at 'any lockable business premises'.

Guiding principles for administering medicines to children

The National Service Framework for Children (DoH 2003) clearly states that the administration of medicines to children must be based on the best available evidence to underpin practice. The Guidelines for the Administration of Medicines (NMC 2002a) clearly indicate that it is not a rule book to be adhered to, covering all potential situations that may be encountered in practice; instead it is a set of guiding principles that must be used in conjunction with local trust/hospital policy (DoH 2003), thereby attempting to reduce the potential for errors in the administration of medicines (Watt 2003b).

According to the NMC (2002a):

The administration of medicines is an important aspect of the professional practice of persons whose names are on the Council's register. It is not solely a mechanistic task to be performed in strict compliance with the written prescription of a medical practitioner. It requires thought and the exercise of professional judgement.

The Guidelines for the Administration of Medicines (NMC 2002a) must be used in conjunction with local trust policies on how to administer and who can administer medicines, as policies and protocols will vary to meet local needs. The NMC (2002a) requires that the registered nurse or midwife be able to administer medicines in a way that is technically safe and that they should also be able to contribute to any decisions regarding the prescription in a clinically competent and professional manner. Nurses are accountable for the drugs that they administer; therefore a prerequisite must be knowledge about drug actions, side-effects and dosages of any drugs that are administered to the child (O'Shea 1999). Kaushal et al (2001) suggest that adverse drug events (ADEs) in children may be more common than had been originally thought.

Watt (2003b) identified the five 'Cs' as important principles to ensure the safe administration of medicines to all children:

- Correct child
- Correct medicine
- Correct dose
- Correct time
- Correct route.

To administer medication safely the nurse must ensure that:

- the *correct child* receives the medication. The identity of the child must be checked. Name bands are used. However, if a parent is available, confirmation of identity by them is a useful resource. If in doubt, ask, because you may encounter children with similar names, or children from multiple births and potentially the patient can be confused with another child if engaging in activities on the ward or play room.

- the *correct medicine* must be given to the child. Hand-written prescriptions must be clear and unambiguous; in addition the label on the medicine to be dispensed must have guidelines that are also clear and easy to follow. There are times when seeing a drug written on a prescription may be assumed to be one thing when, in fact, it is something else (e.g. ceftazidime, cefotaxime). The nurse must be clear and understand exactly what is to be dispensed; if there is any element of doubt the doctor must rewrite the prescription in a clear and legible manner. It is also important that the expiry dates on all medicines are checked for each drug, every time they are given.

- the *correct dose* must be given to the child. It is important that nurses ensure that the child receives the correct dose of medication; if in doubt there are numerous formularies to refer to including *Medicines for Children* (RCPCH 1999). The NMC (2002a) position is clear in that nurses must check the dose to be given. This requires numeracy skills that are not dependent upon the use of a calculator; relying on a calculator and a formula is not sufficient. If there is any element of doubt, *stop* – do not give the medicine. Check with the doctor and pharmacist and read the appropriate drug information. Where there is

more than one checker, calculations need to be completed independently and you should not feel intimidated if you arrive at different answers; check again separately and then with a third person if necessary (Watt 2003b). It is possible to administer an overdose if you do not understand the difference between milligrams (mg) and micrograms (µg). It is important to request that prescriptions are written out in full and abbreviations are not used as this helps to avoid such confusion.

- the *correct time*. It is important that the medicine is given at the correct time; in some instances therapeutic doses need to be maintained. The NMC guidelines (2002a) state that when administering medicines the checking of the route of administration as well as the time that the medicine is given are important parts of the process. Therefore all medicines that are administered must be an integral part of caring for the child and family and considered within the context of the child's current condition and other treatments that the child may be receiving. If there is any doubt that a dose has already been given but there is no evidence to indicate that the medicine has been administered, do not repeat the dose, but check with the person concerned and inform the doctor and ward manager. All events and actions taken must be documented in the nursing records (Watt 2003b).

- the *correct route*. Ensuring that the medicine is administered by the correct route is fundamental to the NMC's principles, which clearly indicate that nurses must consider the method of administration and its appropriateness and that the instructions written by the doctor match the information written on the medicine label (Dimond 2003b). If there are discrepancies, the doctor and pharmacist need to be alerted to the situation and this action documented in the child's nursing care records.

Record keeping

Good record keeping should be regarded as an important part of the process of administering medicines (NMC 2002a; see also local trust policies). It is the duty of the nurse administering the medicine to ensure that a record is made of the dose administered, the time given, the drug given and the administration route (Dimond 2003c). In the event of an error in medication administration being noted, it is important to follow trust policies for such an event; this usually includes ensuring the child is safe, informing the ward manager, doctor, parent and child. If appropriate, an incident form *must* be completed and the error documented in the patient's notes (Watt 2003b).

Dimond (2003c) acknowledges that there is a danger that if a mistake is made by a nurse, they will not acknowledge that it has happened for fear of reprisals. In the event that an error in administration of a medicine occurs, the NMC's position is very clear in terms of advice to practitioners: 'If you make an error, you must report it immediately to your line manager or employer' (NMC 2002a).

For individuals to admit when mistakes have been made, employers need to facilitate an open culture and one in which individuals are not fearful of reprisal. The NMC (2002a) is supportive of critical incident panels as a forum in which lessons can be learnt and improvements made to local practice in light of such incidents (Dimond 2003c). As Dimond (2003c, p. 761) highlights:

> The NMC takes great care to distinguish between those cases where the error was the result of reckless or incompetent practice or was concealed, and those that resulted from other causes, such as serious pressure of work, and where there was immediate, honest disclosure in the patient's interest.

Employers should therefore be encouraging a work culture in which it is considered to be normal working practice to challenge and question all members of the healthcare team, irrespective of who or what they do as a member of that team.

Storage of medicines

The manufacturers of medicines will usually indicate the type of storage conditions required, for example avoid sunlight or store at low temperatures, to ensure that drugs do not lose therapeutic effectiveness. There are legal obligations that each trust or care setting must adhere to as in cases where the manufacturer of a medicine is not known then the last person in the supply chain will be deemed to be the manufacturer and can be held liable for any damages against the person (Griffith et al 2003). It is essential that all trusts/hospitals/care settings where medicines are administered keep accurate details of all supplies of medicines and ensure that they are securely stored (Griffith et al 2003).

The storage of all medicines is subject to legal requirements and statutory instruments (Dimond 2003a) and to local trust/hospital policies; therefore all practitioners working within a trust are responsible for familiarising themselves with those policies. These will include the following guiding principles, as adapted from Griffith et al (2003):

- Medicines should be stored and assembled in temperatures that remain below 25°C.
- Medicines for taking orally (by mouth) should be stored in a locked trolley, cupboard or room.
- All controlled drugs must be stored in a locked cabinet.
- A locked refrigerator must be employed for the exclusive use of storing medicines and should have a thermometer to monitor the temperature on a daily basis.

Self–administration of medicines

The NHS Plan (DoH 2000a) has, as a central theme, the importance of empowering patients to take an active role in their own care. The Audit Commission (2001) clearly indicates that patients are given the opportunity to learn about and take responsibility for their own medicines. Self-administration of medicines is not a new concept within the realms of adult care (DoH 2000a), with many parts of the UK fully embracing this as everyday practice. However, self-administration in children's nursing is a less established practice. Wright et al (2002) maintain that the role of the nurse in terms of administering medicines to children is not that of a 'traditional role of administering'; adversely, it is now becoming a role that involves children and families managing their own medicines, with nurses focusing on education and facilitation of the child and family.

Nurse prescribing

To date, doctors, dentists and certain nurses are legally authorised to prescribe medicines. The Crown Report (DoH 1999) recommended the further development of the prescribing role and *The NHS Plan* (DoH 2000a) highlights that the prescribing of medicines and treatments is a key role for nurses. The Crown Report (DoH 1999) has also identified that there needs to be training for the preparation of specific practitioners (Dimond 2003d, Hutchinson & Hall 2003).

Gibson et al (2003) have been able to demonstrate how nurse prescribing can be seen as a means of improving care delivery to children and families, and the expansion of the role of the clinical nurse specialist (CNS) as a 'logical development' in the expanding role of nurses. Whilst it is anticipated that nurses are the most likely group of healthcare professionals to develop prescribing skills, it is also important to note that other health professionals such as physiotherapists may be accommodated within the legislation in the future (Dimond 2003d).

Developmental issues for consideration

As students you will be constantly reminded of the fact that children are not 'mini adults'. This is a complex phenomenon that includes social, cultural, ethnic, biological and physiological differences which all impact on the ways in which children understand and make sense of their world and communicate with others. Therefore, gaining the child's trust and cooperation to effectively and safely administer medicines requires a sound understanding of the forces at play.

There is an abundance of literature that explains the developmental progression of the infant through to adolescence, and this work has provided the basis for researchers to explore how children understand their bodies,

health, illness and the experiences of being in hospital.

There is a growing body of evidence to suggest that healthcare professionals may be offering inadequate explanations of children's and families' experiences of the healthcare system; this may include the administration of medicines because this is an integral part of care (Alderson 1993, Holaday et al 1994, Alderson & Montgomery 1996, Rushforth 1996, 1999).

Preparation of children for any procedure is vital; this includes the giving of medicines and remembering to assess the child's understanding (Rushforth 1999, Sleath et al 2003). It is only by communicating effectively with children and families that you will gain their trust, understanding and cooperation, not only when administering medicines but in all other aspects of care.

Routes of administration

The administration of medicines to children is frequently an aspect of nursing care that causes concern for the child, family and nurse. Medicines may vary in form and are given by a range of routes (see Table 1.1). The child's dignity, individuality and understanding need to be paramount when giving medicines (NMC 2002a), and whenever possible the family needs to be fully involved to reduce any trauma experienced by the child (DoH 1996). Additional consideration needs to be paid by the children's nurse to the individual child's cognitive development, communication and understanding throughout the whole procedure.

Principles of medicine administration

When administering any medicine to a child, certain key principles apply regardless of route. It is also important to note that in some hospitals/trusts the local policy will require two people to check all medicines given.

For all routes the following key aspects of technique/method apply:

● Full explanations need to be given to the child and family, prior to and during the procedure, which outline the ideal

Table 1.1   Medication administration routes

Route	Form
Gastric tube (via naso/oropharyngeal/direct)	Solutions, suspensions, syrups, elixirs, emulsions, oils
Inhaled (into the lung)	Compressed air nebulisers, metered dose inhalers, powder devices, sterile liquids
Injected: Subcutaneous (under the skin)	Dependent on route: aqueous solutions, suspensions, lipid (fat) solutions, dilutions
Intramuscular (into the muscle)	
Intravenous (into the vein)	
Intrathecal (into the cerebrospinal fluid)	
Intraosseous (into the bone)	
Arterially (into the artery)	
Intra-aural (into the ear)	Solutions, suspensions, drops
Intraocular (into the eye)	Solutions, suspensions, drops, ointments
Intravaginal (into the vagina)	Pessaries, liquids, solutions, ointments, creams, lotions
Nasally (into the nose)	Solutions, suspensions, drops, ointments, sprays
Orally (by mouth)	Liquid: solutions, suspensions, syrups, elixirs, emulsions, oils
	Solid: tablets, capsules, granules, lozenges, beads
Rectally (into the rectum)	Enemas, aqueous solutions, suspensions, oils, suppositories, ointments
Sublingual (beneath the tongue)	Capsules, beads, granules, tablets, drops
Topically (onto the skin)	Solutions, suspensions, ointments, sprays, creams, lotions, pastes, powders, shampoos, soaps, liquids

Adapted from Royal College of Paediatrics and Child Health 1999.

positioning, action to be taken and reason for the administration of the medication. It is also important that the nurse is honest about how the medication is to be given, including the possibility of pain, and any after-effects that may be experienced.

- Education of the child and family and the sharing of information are important roles which are the nurse's responsibility (NMC 2002b).
- Prior to any intervention the nurse should undertake a thorough handwash and wear gloves to reduce the possibility of cross-contamination and recurrent exposure to the medication.
- The medication should be prepared according to the manufacturer's instructions and checked in accordance with the NMC *Guidelines for the Administration of Medicines* (2002a) and individual NHS trust guidelines.
- All contaminated equipment should be disposed of immediately following the procedure.
- Following any intervention the nurse should undertake a thorough handwash to reduce the possibility of cross-contamination.
- The administration of medication, and site of injection where applicable, should be recorded in the child's health records (i.e. drug chart) (NMC 2002c).

- The child must be monitored following medication administration to ensure recognition of any reaction to the medication and prompt treatment to deal with this.

ORAL MEDICATION

In children the most common route for administration of medicines is the oral route, i.e. medication administered by mouth. Most medications come in a choice of tablet or suspension form, and there are frequently a number of different strengths and flavours. If suspensions are unavailable, tablets can be crushed and mixed with sterile water, using a tablet crusher; however, advice should be sought from the pharmacist about whether such methods are suitable and which diluents are appropriate.

Some suspensions have a high sugar content, or the medication itself can cause damage to gums and teeth if used over a prolonged period (e.g. phenytoin); rinsing the mouth with water after administration and good oral hygiene are essential.

Some tablets cannot be crushed or dissolved, for example those with enteric coating, or slow-release tablets. Care should be taken if dividing tablets to ensure as accurate a dose as possible.

Medicines can be administered by spoon, syringe or cup; however, when using a syringe care must be taken not to force the syringe into the mouth or between the teeth, as trauma can result and the action may have the potential to trigger an oral aversion in the child. Oral syringes are available with connectors that cannot be fitted to intravenous equipment, thus making the risk of administering oral drugs through the intravenous route less likely.

Equipment

- Medication
- Medicine pots or cups, with measured volumes
- Oral syringes: various sizes
- Medicine spoons, again with measured graduations

- Tablet crusher
- Tablet divider
- Water (sterile water is required for babies)
- Formulary
- Prescription/medicine chart.

Technique

When administering oral medications, solutions should be shaken before use and measured into an appropriate container at eye level and on a solid flat surface, or drawn up into a syringe to ensure accurate medication volume measurement. Advice should be sought from the pharmacist when tablets need to be cut or crushed. Following the administration of the medication the child needs to be observed closely for any signs of aspiration or choking.

Young infants
The young infant is likely to have a strong attachment to a parent and may become anxious with a 'stranger'. The nurse's role is to encourage parental involvement, provide positive reinforcement and promote sensory soothing measures (i.e. cuddling and stroking the infant) throughout the procedure (Watt 2003b).

- Ask the parent to hold the infant firmly on their lap in a semi-reclining position.
- Encourage the infant to open their mouth, and place the syringe onto their tongue.
- Gently introduce the suspension into the infant's mouth.
- Depressing the infant's tongue slightly with the syringe or gently stroking their cheek and under the chin will encourage the sucking and swallowing reflex and aid administration of the medication.
- Record the medication administration in the child's health records (i.e. drug chart) (NMC 2002c).

Toddlers
As a toddler, the child is considered to be developing autonomy and striving for independence (Watt 2003b). Characteristically, the toddler will need clear instructions and a firm direct approach. The toddler is likely to have a strong bond with their parents but may be interested in exploring new tastes and

sensations; therefore, whenever possible, allow the child to participate and take the medication independently. Promote the full involvement of the parents and the use of positive reinforcement, encouragement and praise. Toddlers can be encouraged through play and fun; however, medications should not be disguised in a drink, such as a milk shake, as the full volume may not be taken and the child may feel betrayed if they discover the deception, and refuse to drink at all.

Older children

Older children need to be encouraged to participate fully in the administration of medicines. The sharing of information, communication and encouragement will encourage the child to cooperate fully and self-administer the oral medication. Children learn to swallow tablets at different ages, and this does require some coordination, but learning to swallow tablets is a skill worth encouraging, as tablets can be far easier to swallow and taste less bitter than suspensions. Swallowing tablets can also represent a welcome sign of growing up and learning new skills, especially important for children with chronic illness who may struggle to attain any independence.

NASOGASTRIC, OROGASTRIC OR GASTROSTOMY MEDICATION

Medication administration via the nasogastric, orogastric or gastrostomy route is directly into the stomach via a tube (see Enteral Feeding, p. 180).

For the child who has an indwelling tube placed directly into the stomach, medications may be prescribed via this route instead of orally. However, there are a number of precautions associated with this route.

Guidelines and precautions (Whaley & Wong 1999)

- Always check for correct placement of the tube.
- Always monitor the child for any sign of aspiration, distress or deterioration.
- Use an elixir or suspension preparation of the medication.

- Avoid the use of tablets whenever possible.
- If using tablets, crush to a fine powder and mix with sterile water.
- Never crush enteric-coated or sustained-release tablets.
- Avoid the use of fat/lipid-based medicines, as they tend to cling to the sides of the tube.
- Do not mix any medication with another solution, as interactions may occur (check with a pharmacist for compatibility).
- Administer medications at room temperature.
- Flush the tube with (sterile) water between medications and following use (utilise a flush volume appropriate to the size of the child and length/gauge of the tube) to avoid blockages and medication interactions.
- Record the medication administration in the child's health records (i.e. drug chart) (NMC 2002c).

INTRAVENOUS MEDICATION

Intravenous medication (medication administered directly into the vein) may be given by intermittent bolus injection, continuous or intermittent infusion, or via peripheral or central access devices (see Aseptic Non-Touch Technique, p. 75 and Intravenous Therapy, p. 211). The choice of technique will depend on the pharmacological characteristics of the medication (half-life, preferred plasma levels) and the lifestyle of the child (e.g. intermittent bolus injections may be preferable to continuous infusion in children who are at school).

Intravenous medication has the following benefits:

- It can sustain high plasma drug levels.
- It can be used in an emergency when a child cannot swallow, and will have an immediate effect.
- The drug will reach the 'target' rapidly when transported in the bloodstream.
- The drug can be absorbed if gastrointestinal absorption is impossible.
- It requires fewer needles than other forms of injection as it uses an in-situ cannula, and is therefore less traumatic.

- The intravenous route is the preferred route if the child is critically ill.

However, intravenous medication also carries with it the following potential complications:

- Anaphylaxis
- Once injected, reversal is almost impossible unless an antidote exists
- Contamination: microorganisms, foreign matter (e.g. latex from a rubber bung, drug precipitate)
- Extravasation (or 'tissuing', as the vein walls break down)
- Phlebitis (inflammation of the vein, causing localised pain)
- Air embolism
- Incompatibility if several infusions/bolus drugs are given at the same time
- Needlestick injury to child or nurse
- Fluid overload.

Equipment

The following should be available to the nurse administering intravenous medication:

- Clean surface: trolley, table top, etc.
- Medication
- Reconstitution solution if needed (see below)
- Sterile saline or heparinised saline for flush (see below)
- Needles
- Syringes
- Alcohol swabs
- Giving sets, connectors, bungs and lines: a large variety of types and sizes are available
- Gloves
- Infusion pump or syringe pump
- Medication chart
- 'Drug additive' or 'date and time' labels for line, syringe or burette.

Normally, intravenous medication will be given in an environment where emergency and resuscitation equipment is available. Because of the risk of anaphylaxis, epinephrine should be available to nurses administering intravenous injections. Community nurses will usually carry packs of epinephrine, but must ensure that they are covered by local policy and appropriately trained to administer it in an emergency without a prescription or medical supervision.

Method

Reconstitution, dilution and length of infusion will all vary according to the drug being used. Nurses should refer to drug information sheets supplied with the medication as a first point of reference. These will often be the most up-to-date source of information, but recognised paediatric formularies (e.g. Guy's, Lewisham and St Thomas' NHS Trust 1999, Royal Liverpool Children's Hospital 2000) should be used as further guidance. Some hospital pharmacies supply their own drug information (e.g. with data about displacement volumes).

Displacement values/volume must be taken into account when reconstituting intravenous medications for children as failure to calculate the displacement value/volume will lead to an incorrect dose being given to the child (Ellis 1995). The displacement value/volume is the volume occupied by the powder in a vial; for example the displacement value of a 250 mg vial of amoxicillin is 0.2 ml. If 4.8 ml of diluent is added to this vial the resulting volume would be 5 ml; however, if 5 ml of diluent is added the resulting volume would be 5.2 ml. Awareness of displacement values/volumes in children's nursing is important because children are often prescribed small doses which need to be part-drawn from a vial.

Administration (see also Intravenous infusions, p. 211)

Many drugs require reconstitution. Some pharmacy departments offer a reconstitution service or centralised intravenous additives services (CIVAS) especially for cytotoxic or other potentially toxic drugs. In such a service, drugs are prepared under strict aseptic conditions, using lamina flow chambers. CIVAS reduce waste, and therefore expense, and have the clinical benefits of reducing the incidence of phlebitis, extravasation, contamination and drug errors (Rodkin 1987, Williams 1996). However, there will still be circumstances when drugs are reconstituted on the wards. This must be done in a clean environment, using a sterile technique and equipment.

Method

This is a role that should only be undertaken by a registered nurse and with appropriate trust/hospital training and assessment of skills.

- Medication may be added to a volume of fluid for infusion via bag or burette, or directly into the intravenous tubing or cannula through a bung near the entry site.
- If infusion lines are used, the amount of prime solution required should be considered when calculating the drug volume.

Doctors may sometimes administer medication directly into the vein through a hypodermic or 'butterfly' needle. This latter technique may only be used in an emergency or on induction of anaesthetic and can vary between hospitals and trusts.

Flush solutions (e.g. normal saline) are used in the following circumstances:

- to check before intravenous administration whether the line is patent
- between sequential injections or infusions, to ensure that incompatible drugs do not mix
- at the end of administration to ensure that no drug remains in the line, and to ensure that the vein remains patent.

In larger cannulae, normal saline (0.9%) is as effective as and cheaper than heparinised solutions (Danet & Norris 1992, Kotter 1996, Le Duc 1997).

Intravenous pumps should always be used to deliver infusions. There are many different types and makes of pump on the market. Nurses must ensure that they are familiar with each type of pump used in practice; evidence suggests that many drug errors occur because of staff's unfamiliarity with equipment (MDA 1995, Quinn 2000).

INTRAMUSCULAR MEDICATION

Intramuscular (IM) injections (medication administered directly into the muscle) are rarely used routinely in children's care (Hemsworth 2000). Despite the fact that most medicines can be administered into the muscle, the IM route is now used only when other routes are not viable or do not allow effective absorption of the medication.

Sites for injection

Certain factors need to be considered when selecting an injection site, including:

- The size and age of the child; the site recommended may depend on the age/weight of the child.
- The child's ability to maintain the required position safely.
- The size and condition of the muscle; an accessible, well-developed, vascular muscle that will tolerate the volume of medication being administered should to be used.
- The frequency or number of injections; a more developed muscle will preferentially be chosen for frequent use.
- The type of medication being given and the manufacturer's instructions.

Three sites are used for the administration of IM injections (see Fig. 1.1):

- *Deltoid muscle* (lateral aspect of the upper arm) – This site is commonly used for small-volume IM injections (i.e. vaccinations) but caution must be exercised when using this site in children less than 5 years of age (RCPCH 1999) and is not recommended for repeated use or large volumes (Hemsworth 2000).
- *Quadriceps muscle* (lateral aspect of the thigh) – This is a traditional site commonly used for IM injections, especially for children under 6 months of age.
- *Gluteus maximus muscle* (upper, outer quadrant of the buttock) – This site's popularity has diminished following reported damage to the sciatic nerve (RCPCH 1999). Furthermore, there is some concern about the

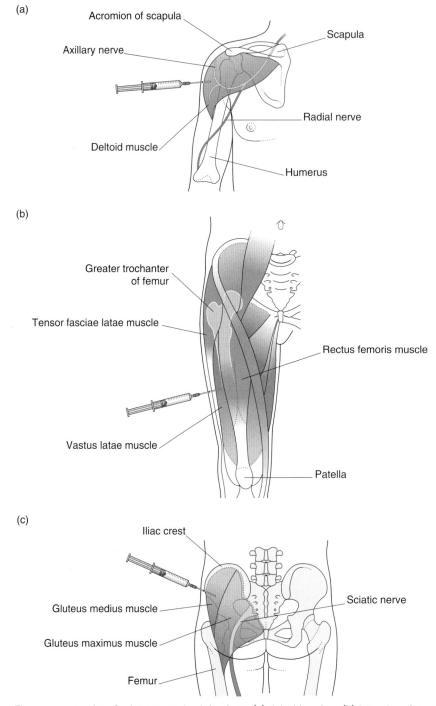

Figure 1.1 Three common sites for intramuscular injections: (a) deltoid region; (b) lateral surface of the thigh; (c) buttock. (Reproduced with permission from the Resuscitation Council (UK) 2002a,b.)

viability of the site in infants and children prior to walking (Whaley & Wong 1999); therefore the site is not recommended for general use in children (RCPCH/RCN 2002).

Volume

The exact volume that can be injected into each muscle is unclear and depends on the muscle development, medication used and viscosity of the solution.

The maximum volume recommended for adults is 5 ml (Beyea & Nicoll 1995), with 1–2 ml for less-well-developed muscles (Beyea & Nicoll 1995). In children, especially those under the age of 2 years, a maximum of 1 ml is advisable (Skale 1992).

Potential complications (RCPCH 1999, Hemsworth 2000, RCPCH/RCN 2002)

Attention needs to be paid to the possible complications of administration of a medication via the IM route. Potential complications include:

- Nerve damage – ranges from foot drop to paralysis.
- Muscle fibrosis and contractures – mainly reported following multiple injection site use.
- Necrosis and gangrene – rare but has occurred in neonates following large-volume injections.
- Intramuscular haemorrhage – especially when IM injection is used for children with a clotting disorder.
- Septic and sterile abscesses – secondary to large-volume injections.
- Infection – relating to poor technique and multiple-use equipment.
- Pain – necessitating the use of topical analgesics.
- Allergic or anaphylactic reaction.
- Needle phobia and mistrust – following poor technique and patient preparation (Whaley & Wong 1999).

Equipment

- Dish or tray
- Medication and reconstituent solution (where appropriate)
- Prescription chart
- Needle – to 'draw up' the solution
- Syringe (size appropriate to the volume of solution)
- Needle – to 'give' the solution (usually a 25G1 or a 23G1) (RCPCH/RCN 2002).

Technique

- Local anaesthetic (e.g. Ametop gel, EMLA cream, ethyl chloride spray or ice-packs) may block superficial pain but deep muscular pain, bruising, stiffness or 'soreness' may still occur.
- The cleansing of the skin, prior to injection, is not necessary when administering IM medications (RCPCH/RCN 2002); however, some conflicting advice exists (Beyea & Nicoll 1995) and referral to individual NHS trust guidelines is recommended.
- The position of the child is essential in the safe, effective delivery of an IM medication and may help the child to relax, thereby decreasing the pain and anxiety experienced.
- Once the medication is fully prepared, a new needle must be used to administer the solution.
- The needle should be inserted into the skin and muscle at a 90° angle. The needle should not be deep enough to touch bone but must penetrate deep into the muscle.
- Following insertion, the syringe should be aspirated to ensure that a blood vessel has not been punctured. If the aspirate is clear, then the medication can be given slowly at a maximum rate of 1 ml/10 seconds (Soanes 2000). However, if blood is withdrawn into the syringe, *stop* and then recommence the procedure. It is important to inform the nurse in charge of what has happened.
- After administration of the medication the needle should be removed slowly whilst maintaining the 90° angle.
- Gentle pressure should be applied to the site using a sterile cotton wool ball or gauze pad.
- The IM site needs to be reviewed regularly for signs of bruising or any other complication.

- Record the medication administration in the child's health records (i.e. drug chart) (NMC 2002c).

SUBCUTANEOUS MEDICATION

Subcutaneous (SC) injection or infusion (medication administered under the skin into the subcutaneous tissues) is frequently used in caring for children, especially for the administration of anticoagulants, analgesia, insulin and some anticancer drugs.

Site

Certain factors need to be considered when selecting an injection site, including:

- The size and age of the child; the site recommended may depend on the age/weight of the child.
- The frequency or number of injections; a more frequently used site may become fibrosed over time.
- The type of medication given and manufacturer's instructions.

Common sites for the administration of SC injections are chosen for their deep fat layer and accessibility; these include the upper thigh, abdomen, upper arm and buttocks. Sites should be rotated, as a frequently used site may become fibrosed, which could reduce the absorption of the medication.

Potential complications

Attention needs to be paid to the possible complications of administration of a medication via the SC route. Possible complications include:

- Tissue fibrosis – following multiple use of one site.
- Infection – relating to poor technique and multiple-use equipment.
- Pain – necessitating the use of topical analgesics.
- Allergic or anaphylactic reaction.
- Needle phobia and mistrust – following poor technique and patient preparation (Whaley & Wong 1999).

- Medication errors – due to confusion between syringes measured in units (i.e. heparin, insulin) and those measured in millilitres (ml) (i.e. analgesia).

Equipment

- Dish or tray
- Medication and reconstituent solution (where appropriate)
- Prescription chart
- Needle – to 'draw up' the solution
- Syringe (size appropriate to the volume of solution)
- Needle – to 'give' the solution.

Technique

- Local anaesthetic (e.g. Ametop gel, EMLA cream, ethyl chloride spray or ice-packs) may block superficial pain but bruising, stiffness or 'soreness' may still occur.
- The cleansing of the skin, prior to injection, is not necessary when administering SC medications (RCPCH/RCN 2002); however, some conflicting advice exists (Beyea & Nicoll 1995) and referral to individual NHS trust guidelines is recommended.
- Once the medication is fully prepared, a new needle must be used to administer the solution.
- The needle should be inserted into the skin and muscle at a 45° angle.
- Following insertion, the syringe should be aspirated to ensure that a blood vessel has not been punctured. If the aspirate is clear then the medication can be given slowly at a maximum rate of 1 ml/10 seconds (Soanes 2000). However, if blood is withdrawn into the syringe, *stop* and then recommence the procedure. It is important to inform the nurse in charge of what has happened.
- After administration of the medication the needle should be removed slowly whilst maintaining the 45° angle.
- Gentle pressure should be applied to the site using a sterile cotton wool ball or gauze pad.
- The SC site needs to be reviewed regularly for signs of bruising or any other complication.

- Record the medication administration in the child's health records (i.e. drug chart) (NMC 2002c).

Subcutaneous infusions can be used to administer analgesia, especially in palliative care situations. Subcutaneous infusions can be administered through butterfly needles or purpose-designed subcutaneous infusion cannulae. Portable infusion sets are used to ensure that the child has as free a lifestyle as possible. The needle or cannula should be resited every 2–7 days (Jody et al 1993). All equipment needs to be disposed of safely in accordance with local and national guidelines concerning the safe disposal of hospital waste and sharps (Health and Safety Commission 1999, May & Brewer 2001).

INTRAOSSEOUS ADMINISTRATION

Intraosseous (IO) administration (medication administered directly into the bone) is usually undertaken by medical staff; however, in some hospitals/trusts, nurses with PALS training may also use IO methods in an emergency situation. This technique is used for quick vascular access primarily in emergency situations, especially when veins are collapsing due to shock. The Advanced Paediatric Life Support (APLS) (2001) guidelines recommend that this route is used if venous access fails, or if it will take more than 1.5 minutes to achieve in life-threatening situations. The IO needle is inserted aseptically into the upper tibia or lower femur, allowing fluids introduced into this vascular marrow space via IO administration to be absorbed.

Equipment

- Skin disinfectant.
- Intraosseous 18G needle with trocar (at least 1.5 cm in length).
- Local anaesthetic.
- 5 ml syringe.
- 20 ml syringe.
- Infusion fluid.

Method

When identifying the site for an IO needle, the anterior aspects of the upper tibial or lower femoral plate sites should be used. Fractured bones must be avoided as should the tibia if the femur is fractured on the same side (APLS 2001). The skin is cleaned and a local anaesthetic used. The needle is inserted at 90° to the skin and advanced until a 'give' is felt as the needle penetrates the cortex of the bone. The correct position of the needle is confirmed by aspirating blood using a 5 ml syringe. When confirmed, the needle is secured in place with sterile gauze and strapping. Intraosseous infusions should only be used in emergency situations and, to prevent infection, should be replaced as soon as a normal vein can be cannulated.

EPIDURAL INFUSIONS

Continuous epidural infusions, along with other forms of spinal nerve block, are becoming more commonly used in children, as they provide effective major pain relief without the side-effects of systemic opiates (see Pain Management, p. 271). The catheter is usually sited preoperatively in theatre under anaesthetic, by the anaesthetist or surgeon. Epidural infusions should be supervised by nursing and medical staff experienced and knowledgeable in their use. They should be used in conjunction with regular pain assessment.

Epidurals may use a local anaesthetic agent (e.g. bupivacaine hydrochloride) and/or opiates for analgesia. If opiates are used, the patient should be observed closely for signs of respiratory depression. Other side-effects of opiate epidural analgesia include nausea and vomiting, or excessive sedation; therefore naloxone should always be available. If analgesia is insufficient, a technical cause such as local leakage or catheter disconnection should be sought before automatically increasing the infusion.

Side-effects common in older patients with epidurals, such as hypotension and lower limb paraesthesia, may be caused by an epidural haematoma. They appear to be less common in children, but nurses must nonetheless remain alert for such signs (Campbell & Glasper 1995). Nurses should also observe for urinary retention as a result of local anaesthetic or opiate.

INTRATHECAL MEDICATION

The intrathecal route of administration allows medications that cannot pass through the blood–brain barrier (a semi-permeable membrane that acts as a natural filter for substances from the blood to the brain) to enter cerebrospinal fluid via an implantable port or lumbar puncture. This method is commonly used within cancer treatments, pain management and severe spasticity/mobility problems.

CHEMOTHERAPY

Chemotherapy is the name given to a group of cytotoxic (cyto = cell; toxic = poison) drugs that are used mainly in the treatment of cancer. There are many different types of chemotherapy which fall naturally into a number of classes, each with characteristic cytotoxic activity, site of action and toxicity. Nevertheless, they all have the same role of destroying cancerous cells by damaging them so that they cannot divide and grow. However, they also affect normal non-cancerous cells, thereby producing side-effects. The handling of cytotoxic drugs has been acknowledged as an occupational hazard (Valanis et al 1993); therefore hospital and trust policy surrounding chemotherapy is essential, as these drugs can be given by many different routes including oral and subcutaneous.

RECTAL MEDICATION

The rectal route (medication inserted into the rectum) is used when drugs cannot be absorbed orally, when the child is nil-by-mouth or when a local effect is required (see Bowel Care, p. 115). Diarrhoea or impacted faeces are contraindications to the use of this route.

In some countries the rectal route is commonplace (e.g. France). However, in the UK there is a reluctance to administer via this route, perhaps owing to child protection concerns and cultural or sexual taboos. Because of these concerns nurses must exercise great sensitivity in using this route, especially with older children and adolescents who may be totally unaware that this technique exists. Consent should be sought from the child and family, especially if the suppository is to be inserted in the recovery room or while the child is sedated, and a chaperone, preferably the parent, should be present (Rogers & Irwin 2003).

Potential complications

Attention needs to be paid to the possible complications of administration of a medication via the rectal route. These include:

- pain and discomfort
- allergic or anaphylactic reaction
- mistrust – following poor technique and patient preparation.

Equipment

- Medication chart.
- Gloves.
- Dish or tray containing:
  - suppository.
  - lubricating gel.
  - swab or tissue.

Site

The child should be on their side, with legs curled up in a fetal position. With babies it is possible to lift the legs and flex the knees, as for changing a nappy.

Technique

- Prior to any intervention the nurse should undertake a thorough handwash to reduce the possibility of cross-contamination and put on a pair of clinical gloves.
- The suppository should be lubricated with a water-soluble gel (i.e. aqueous gel).
- The suppository should be gently inserted into the anus, just beyond the anal sphincter (Addison 2000).
- It may be necessary to hold the buttocks together for several minutes to prevent the immediate expulsion of the suppository.
- Record the medication administration in the child's health records (i.e. drug chart) (NMC 2002c).

- Product literature will either recommend suppositories are inserted apex-first or make no recommendations at all; product details and hospital/trust policy must be checked when deciding which way a suppository should be inserted (Moppett 2000). According to Moppett (2000) there are no significant differences in expulsion rates when suppositories are inserted either blunt end or apex first; however, there is currently very little evidence to support this.

TOPICAL MEDICATION

Topical medication (medication applied directly to the skin) – for example a cream, ointment or topical solution – may be prescribed for a variety of reasons, including:

- the treatment of eczema, dermatitis or Candida
- local anaesthesia
- severe excoriation
- skin trauma (i.e. following a scald or burn).

The absorption of the medication through the skin may vary with age; medications administered topically may be absorbed systemically in neonates and infants (due to reduced skin density and maturity) when a localised response was intended (Prosser et al 2000). In order to prevent skin sensitisation and allergic reactions due to possible local inflammatory responses (Demoly & Bousquet 2001), gloves should be worn when administering any form of topical medication.

Topical medications frequently have a variety of strengths and preparations; the children's nurse needs to be vigilant when checking the strength, dosage and preparation prescribed.

Equipment

- Medication.
- Gloves.
- Dressings/bandages as required.

Technique

- Topical medication should always be single patient use to avoid cross-contamination

and the administration of an incorrect dosage.
- Prepare the child and family.
- It is important that the person administering the medication wears gloves to reduce the potential of absorbing the medication through the skin of the hands.
- Administer the medication to the area stated in the prescription as per product instructions.
- Avoid contamination of the surrounding skin.
- Record the medication administration in the child's health records (i.e. drug chart) (NMC 2002c) (see Skin Care, p. 355).

TRANSCUTANEOUS MEDICATION

The use of patches is increasing within both children's pain management and oncology. Transcutaneous absorption via patches or topical administration is greater in children than in adults (Prosser et al 2000). Although the use of skins patches can be considered, it must be borne in mind that absorption within neonates is altered and topical substances can damage the skin and internal organs (Garcia-Gonzalez & Rivera-Rueda 1998).

Equipment

- Medication.
- Gloves.

Technique

- Prepare the child and family.
- Administer the medication to the area stated in the prescription as per product instructions.
- Record the medication administration in the child's health records (i.e. drug chart) (NMC 2002c).

INTRA-AURAL/OTIC MEDICATION

Intra-aural/otic medication (medication inserted directly into the ear canal) is not a painful procedure; however, it can cause uncomfortable or unpleasant sensations for children. As with the administration of medication via any other route, it is paramount that the child and family are fully prepared and informed prior to the procedure. A potential problem associated with this route is the need to have the full cooperation of the child or to utilise gentle restraint to attain an optimum head position in order to insert the medication.

Equipment

- Medication (frequently single-use ampoules and/or with a dropper attached).
- Syringe or dropper.
- Swab or tissue.

Technique

Medications for the ear often have a short shelf-life once opened, so expiry dates should be checked carefully. To help reduce the unpleasant/uncomfortable sensations associated with this administration route, remove medications stored in the refrigerator a few minutes before use to allow the medication to warm up to room temperature before instillation. If in doubt, check with the pharmacist or the manufacturer's recommendations.

- Lay the child on their back (supine) and turn their head to the appropriate side.
- For children less than 3 years of age, gently pull the pinna downwards and straight back in order to straighten the external auditory canal.
- For children over 3 years of age, gently pull the pinna upward and back in order to straighten the auditory canal.
- Instil the drops, as prescribed, into the ear, without contaminating the dropper.
- After administration, encourage the child to remain still for a few minutes to allow the drops to be absorbed.
- Gentle massage of the area immediately anterior (in front of) the ear may help the droplets to descend and aid in relaxing the child.
- A swab or tissue should be used to absorb any exudate or leakage and to reduce skin contamination or irritation.

- Record the medication administration in the child's health records (i.e. drug chart) (NMC 2002c).

There is some debate whether to use small cotton wool plugs placed into the ear to prevent the leakage of the medication; however, to avoid any complications, it is safer to avoid their use (Campbell & Glasper 1995).

INTRAOCULAR/OPTIC MEDICATION

Intraocular/optic medication (medication administered directly onto the eye) may cause a significant level of discomfort, visual blurring and irritation to the child. As with the administration of medication via any other route, it is paramount that the child and family are fully prepared and informed prior to the procedure. A potential problem associated with this route is the need to have the full cooperation of the child or to utilise gentle restraint to attain an optimum head position in order to insert the medication. Administration of eye drops can be particularly difficult in young children and toddlers, who may struggle and close their eyes protectively. Play, patience and asking the parent to hold the child firmly on their lap, will help.

Equipment

- Medication (frequently single-use ampoules and/or with a dropper attached).
- Syringe or dropper.
- Swab or tissue.

Technique

Medications for the eye often have a short shelf-life once opened, so expiry dates should be checked carefully. To help reduce the unpleasant/uncomfortable sensations associated with this administration route, remove medications stored in the refrigerator a few minutes before use to allow the medication to warm up to room temperature before instillation. If in doubt, check with the pharmacist or the manufacturer's recommendations. Medicines for the eye need to be used exclusively for the left or right eye and not shared between patients.

- Lay the child flat on their back (supine) or sitting with head extended and asked to look upwards, toward the ceiling.
- Use one hand to pull down the lower eyelid; rest the other hand on the child's forehead, so that it moves with the child and is therefore less likely to cause an injury if the child moves suddenly (Campbell & Glasper 1995).
- Drops: instil the prescribed number of drops, not directly onto the eyeball, but to the lower, inner corner of each eye.
- Ointment: squeeze the ointment along the inside of the lower lid.
- Do not touch the eye with the bottle, tube or your fingers, as the eye can easily become contaminated or damaged.
- Encourage the child to close their eyes, not squeeze together, and roll them around to disseminate the medication.
- A swab or tissue should be used to absorb any exudate or leakage and to reduce skin contamination or irritation.
- Record the medication administration in the child's health records (i.e. drug chart) (NMC 2002c).

ANAPHYLAXIS

Anaphylaxis seems to be increasingly common and is almost certainly associated with an increase in the prevalence of allergic disease over the last two or three decades (Resuscitation Council (UK) 2002a).

Anaphylaxis can result from exposure to an agent or substance to which the body has previously been exposed or in which there has been no previous exposure (Jamieson et al 2002).

Causes

Anaphylactic reactions vary in severity and may follow exposure to a variety of agents, the most common of which are:

- medications (and contrast media)
- insect stings
- foods (e.g. peanut and tree nut)
- latex.

Incidence

The speed at which an anaphylactic reaction may occur appears to depend on the hypersensitivity of the child to the agent encountered. Anaphylactic reactions vary in severity and can be rapid, slow or biphasic. A severe reaction will often occur immediately but some cases have been reported up to 24 hours post-exposure (Resuscitation Council (UK) 2002b).

Recognition of anaphylactic reactions

The signs and symptoms of anaphylaxis vary in severity according to the hypersensitivity of the child to the agent encountered. Common signs and symptoms are shown in Box 1.1.

Equipment and treatment

Equipment that should be in place includes oxygen, suction, etc.

Rapid treatment is needed when an anaphylactic reaction occurs (see Fig. 1.2).

Box 1.1   Common signs and symptoms of anaphylactic reactions

- Angio-oedema
- Urticaria
- Dyspnoea
- Hypotension
- Skin colour change – pale or flushed
- Cardiovascular collapse

- Rhinitis
- Conjunctivitis
- Abdominal pain
- Vomiting
- Diarrhoea
- Sense of impending doom

Adapted from Resuscitation Council (UK) 2000c.

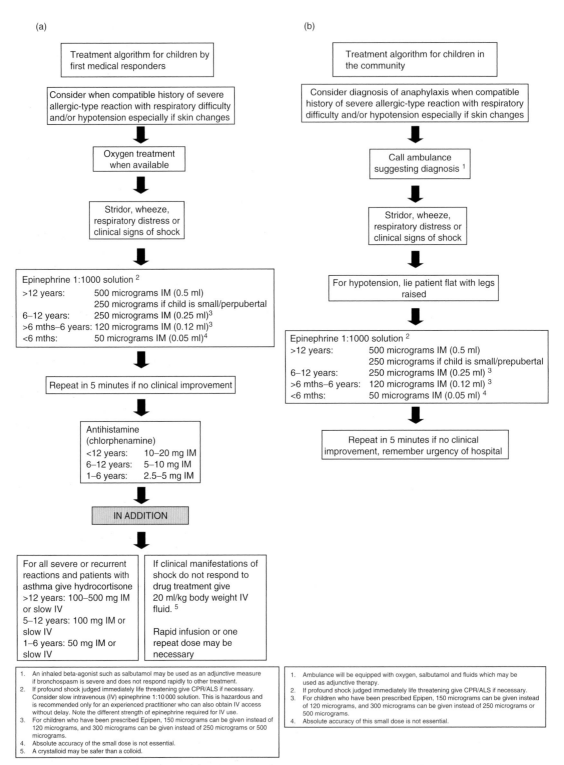

(a)

Treatment algorithm for children by first medical responders

Consider when compatible history of severe allergic-type reaction with respiratory difficulty and/or hypotension especially if skin changes

Oxygen treatment when available

Stridor, wheeze, respiratory distress or clinical signs of shock

Epinephrine 1:1000 solution [2]
>12 years: 500 micrograms IM (0.5 ml)
                   250 micrograms if child is small/perpubertal
6–12 years: 250 micrograms IM (0.25 ml)[3]
>6 mths–6 years: 120 micrograms IM (0.12 ml)[3]
<6 mths: 50 micrograms IM (0.05 ml)[4]

Repeat in 5 minutes if no clinical improvement

Antihistamine
(chlorphenamine)
<12 years: 10–20 mg IM
6–12 years: 5–10 mg IM
1–6 years: 2.5–5 mg IM

IN ADDITION

For all severe or recurrent reactions and patients with asthma give hydrocortisone
>12 years: 100–500 mg IM or slow IV
5–12 years: 100 mg IM or slow IV
1–6 years: 50 mg IM or slow IV

If clinical manifestations of shock do not respond to drug treatment give 20 ml/kg body weight IV fluid. [5]

Rapid infusion or one repeat dose may be necessary

1. An inhaled beta-agonist such as salbutamol may be used as an adjunctive measure if bronchospasm is severe and does not respond rapidly to other treatment.
2. If profound shock judged immediately life threatening give CPR/ALS if necessary. Consider slow intravenous (IV) epinephrine 1:10 000 solution. This is hazardous and is recommended only for an experienced practitioner who can also obtain IV access without delay. Note the different strength of epinephrine required for IV use.
3. For children who have been prescribed Epipen, 150 micrograms can be given instead of 120 micrograms, and 300 micrograms can be given instead of 250 micrograms or 500 micrograms.
4. Absolute accuracy of the small dose is not essential.
5. A crystalloid may be safer than a colloid.

(b)

Treatment algorithm for children in the community

Consider diagnosis of anaphylaxis when compatible history of severe allergic-type reaction with respiratory difficulty and/or hypotension especially if skin changes

Call ambulance suggesting diagnosis [1]

Stridor, wheeze, respiratory distress or clinical signs of shock

For hypotension, lie patient flat with legs raised

Epinephrine 1:1000 solution [2]
>12 years: 500 micrograms IM (0.5 ml)
                   250 micrograms if child is small/prepubertal
6–12 years: 250 micrograms IM (0.25 ml) [3]
>6 mths–6 years: 120 micrograms IM (0.12 ml) [3]
<6 mths: 50 micrograms IM (0.05 ml) [4]

Repeat in 5 minutes if no clinical improvement, remember urgency of hospital

1. Ambulance will be equipped with oxygen, salbutamol and fluids which may be used as adjunctive therapy.
2. If profound shock judged immediately life threatening give CPR/ALS if necessary.
3. For children who have been prescribed Epipen, 150 micrograms can be given instead of 120 micrograms, and 300 micrograms can be given instead of 250 micrograms or 500 micrograms.
4. Absolute accuracy of this small dose is not essential.

Figure 1.2   Anaphylactic reactions: (a) treatment algorithm for children by first medical responders; (b) treatment algorithm for children in the community. (From Resuscitation Council (UK) 2002a,b.)

- A full history and examination of the child should be undertaken.
- The child's health records should be examined for any past sensitivity or reactions.
- Any medications that the patient has received should be disclosed to the healthcare team.
- Assess and monitor the child's condition and any physical symptoms, especially:
  - airway
  - breathing
  - pulse rate
  - blood pressure
  - skin colour
  - temperature
  - check for MedicAlert bracelet or necklace.
- If a severe reaction occurs – 'Call for help' and ring for immediate medical assistance (either from the resuscitation team – in the hospital environment, or from the emergency services (999) – in the community environment).

Epinephrine

Epinephrine is regarded to be the most important medication for the treatment of severe anaphylactic reactions in either children or adults (Resuscitation Council (UK) 2000c). Although there appears to be some conflicting advice regarding the administration of IV epinephrine, the use of IM epinephrine is consistently recommended as the treatment of choice for all patients with clinical signs of shock, airway swelling or definite breathing difficulty (Resuscitation Council (UK) 2000c, Moor & Jennison 2004). IM epinephrine is most effective when given early after the onset of symptoms, is likely to be rapidly absorbed and is very rarely associated with adverse reactions or side-effects (see Box 1.2 for recommended dosages).

As the likelihood of a child experiencing an anaphylactic reaction continues to be a relatively rare occurrence, the majority of healthcare practitioners may not be familiar with the management and treatment of anaphylaxis. Therefore, pre-filled, dose-specific injection devices, such as the junior Epipen, are recommended for use in those children over 6 months of age (Moor & Jennison 2004). Although anaphylaxis is extremely rare in infants under the age of 6 months, IM epinephrine continues to be the recommended treatment but would need to be administered in specialist areas by practitioners trained in this field. Unlike most other medications, the use of epinephrine for the treatment of anaphylaxis does not routinely require a medication prescription; however, the event should be documented in the child's records and local trust policy and guidance should detail the qualified (registered) children's nurses' responsibilities regarding the administration of medications in an emergency and outline any specific training requirements.

INHALED THERAPY DEVICES

Inhalation therapy is the most effective way to administer preventative and symptom-relieving drugs as used in the treatment of lung conditions such as asthma and cystic fibrosis (NICE 2000a,b, O'Connor 2001, Madge 2002). Through inhalation the drug will reach the lungs directly, requiring a lower dose and minimising any systemic side-effects (Watt 2003a).

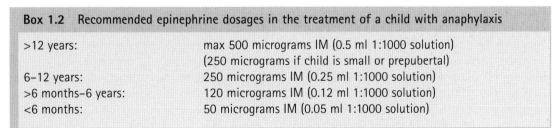

Box 1.2   Recommended epinephrine dosages in the treatment of a child with anaphylaxis

>12 years:	max 500 micrograms IM (0.5 ml 1:1000 solution)
	(250 micrograms if child is small or prepubertal)
6–12 years:	250 micrograms IM (0.25 ml 1:1000 solution)
>6 months–6 years:	120 micrograms IM (0.12 ml 1:1000 solution)
<6 months:	50 micrograms IM (0.05 ml 1:1000 solution)

From Resuscitation Council (UK) 2000c, p. 6.

There are a variety of inhaled drugs, the pharmacology of which will not be discussed here. The nurse should refer to one of the formularies for drug and inhaler device clarification, prior to prescribing or using them.

Guidelines

Prescribing an inhaler suited to the child's cognitive and psychomotor ability is important. It is suggested that all children use an inhaler with a spacer device, because using the pressurised metered dose inhaler (pMDI) alone is complicated, requires high-level coordination and is least efficient (NICE 2000a,b, Lissauer & Clayden 2002, SIGN 2004). Effective inhalation therapy and good symptom control are dependent upon adequate preparation of the child and parent. The spacer device will improve efficacy, increase the amount of drug reaching the lungs and reduce the amount of medication remaining in the throat (Jordan & White 2001, Child et al 2002). The NICE (2000a,b) guidelines state that a pMDI with spacer device should be prescribed in the first instance. Only when the child has a high non-compliance rate when using the inhaler plus spacer device should other types of inhaler, such as dry powder (DPI) or breath-actuated inhalers, be considered. Although less cumbersome, both the DPI and breath-actuated inhaler require a significant inspiratory breath, which precludes their effectiveness during an exacerbation of symptoms (Child et al 2002, Roberts 2002). O'Callaghan and Barry (2000) maintain that there is no evidence to suggest that changing from a pMDI with spacer to DPI or breath-actuated inhaler will improve compliance and that they are not suitable for children under age 6 years; they also argue that as the inhaler plus spacer is mainly used on waking and going to bed, the size of the spacer should not be problematic as the device can remain at home.

Nurses need to be aware of and teach children and families that plastic spacer devices such as the Volumatic and Babyhaler (see Fig. 1.3) produce a positive charge that will attract the drug particles to the spacer walls, thus reducing the amount of drug inhaled. The

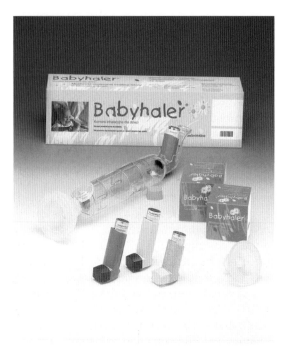

Figure 1.3   Babyhaler and Volumatic plastic spacer devices. (Reproduced courtesy of Glaxo Wellcome, UK).

best way to minimise this effect is to wash the spacer once a week in detergent and allow to air dry. This will leave a detergent coating on the spacer and reduce the electrostatic charge (Le Souif 1999, NICE 2000a).

There are a number of different inhalers with different operating methods. It is important that nurses learn the correct technique for each type of inhaler, when used alone or with a spacer device. Teaching the child and family good inhaler technique and reviewing this regularly improves treatment adherence and symptom control and reduces the incidence of acute episodes (Francis, 2001, O'Connor 2001, Roberts 2002).

In the case of asthma, a treatment plan should detail what medication is to be inhaled, the dosage, frequency, type of inhaler, how to monitor symptoms and what to do in the event of symptom exacerbation. Self-management plans have been developed for school-age children with the emphasis on improved symptom control and using peak flow measurement (Harrop 2002, Roberts 2002, Milnes & Callery

2003). The peak flow meter is a diagnostic and assessment tool that measures the peak expiratory flow rate.

Assessment should include observation of respiratory rate and effort (see Assessment, p. 86–87). Skin colour and general well-being should be noted. Signs of increasing effort may include intercostal recession or using accessory muscles to aid breathing. The child may seek a position with the chest upright and head forward to increase lung expansion. Peak flow measurement (see below) is a useful test of lung function. Oxygen saturation measurement may give an early indication of any hypoxia. X-rays and other more detailed lung function tests can be performed. The history of the illness should be noted, especially as classic signs of chronic respiratory distress – chronic night-time coughing and shortness of breath after exercise (Caldwell 1998) – are still often ignored by parents and GPs.

Peak flow measurement

The peak expiratory flow rate (PEFR) is the fastest rate at which air can be expelled from the lungs and is measured in litres per minute. Regular PEFR measurement assists with good symptom control, gives early indication of disease exacerbation and can assist in identifying allergens (Singel & Lira 2001).

In order to monitor PEFR a 'normal' peak flow value is calculated using the child's height. This is plotted on a nomogram, which details height on one axis and predicted peak flow on the other axis of the graph (Godfrey et al 1970, cited by Lissauer & Clayden 2002, p. 398). The child will also have a personal baseline rate, which is best measured when the child is in optimum health. The PEFR should be measured before inhalation and again 15 minutes after inhalation (Lissauer & Clayden 2002).

Several types of peak flow meter are available for different age groups and the nurse must ensure the one used is suitable for the child as children will vary in their ability to understand according to their age and stage of development (Rushforth 1999, Sleath et al 2003). To ensure understanding the nurse

should clarify this by asking the child and/or parent(s) to repeat what is expected of them.

Measuring peak flow
The child should be taught the following steps:

1. Move the measurement bar on the meter to zero.
2. Ask the child to stand up.
3. Hold the meter horizontally.
4. Open mouth, and slowly inhale as large a breath as possible.
5. Put mouthpiece in the mouth, ensuring tongue is clear and seal with the lips.
6. Blow out: a short, hard and fast breath.
7. Relax and note reading.
8. Repeat steps 1–7 three times.
9. Record the best reading.

The reading should be compared to the child's own baseline measurement and the normal values for a child of their height, as detailed. Changes in PEFR will indicate an increase or decrease in the child's state of health.

Older children who are being taught self-management of their asthma may benefit from peak flow guidelines (Milnes & Callery 2003); these set levels above and below which certain medication should be taken or increased. While it is quite normal for morning readings to dip, variation above 15% may be significant.

Inhalers

Equipment
Tables 1.2 and 1.3 summarise the different features of common devices. As can be seen from these tables, children should be assessed individually to determine which device would be most suitable (see also Fig. 1.3).

Aerosol inhalers used to contain chlorofluorocarbons (CFCs), gases which contribute to the depletion of the ozone layer. As from 2003, all inhalers must be CFC-free (Lissauer & Clayden 2002). Hydrofluroalkanes replaced CFCs but there may be some adjustment in switching from the older inhalers to the new CFC-free inhalers; they may look, feel, smell and taste different, but patients can be assured that they are equally effective (Shapiro et al 2000).

Table 1.2 Summary of features of dry powder inhalers (positive attributes in bold)

Device features	Capsule inhalers	Diskhalers	Multidose dry powder inhalers
Preloading required	Yes	Yes	No
Multiple doses available	No	Yes 8/4 doses	Yes 50, 100, 200 doses
Indicator of doses taken/remaining	N/A	Yes	Yes (last 20 only)
Inspiratory flow rate (1/min)	60	60	30 (60 = optimum)
Lactose carrier	Yes	Yes	Varies with manufacturer

None of these devices is suitable for children under 5 years old.
All the devices have the following attributes:

- discreet and portable
- do not contain CFCs
- do not need shaking before use
- do not require hand–lung coordination
- no time lapse between actuations required.

Adapted from Warner & Gregson (1995)

Table 1.3 Summary of features of aerosol inhalers (positive attributes in bold)

Device features	Metered–dose inhaler (MDI)	Large spacer and MDI	Breath–actuated MDI	Spinhaler
Discreet and portable	**Yes**	No	**Yes**	**Yes**
Require hand–lung synchronisation	Yes	**No**	**No**	Yes
Time lapse between actuations	Yes (30 s)	Yes (30 s)	Yes (60 s)	Yes (60 s)
Oropharyngeal impaction leading to inhibition of inhalation	Yes	**No**	Yes	Yes
Minimum age for use	7 years	**Infant**	7 years	No studies
Inspiratory flow rate (1/min)	30	22 (tidal volume breathing)	28–30	30
Medications available	**All**	Product specific	6	3

In addition, these devices have the following characteristics:

- no preloading required
- multiple doses available
- number of doses remaining/taken indicated
- require shaking before use.

Adapted from Warner & Gregson (1995).

Method

The following common principles apply to all devices:

- Drugs should be checked and administered according to local policy and NMC guidelines (2002a).
- Always check expiry date of drug canister and inhaler.
- Always remove the protective mouthpiece before use.
- Ensure spacer device, if used, is clean, dry and assembled.
- Record the medication administration in the child's health records (i.e. drug chart) (NMC 2002c).

Spacers for babies and young children

A large-volume spacer (such as Volumatic) should not be used with babies as the amount of drug absorption will be reduced. Instead the smaller-volume, purpose-made Babyhaler has been shown to increase drug deposition in the lungs and uses special valves that require minimum inspiratory volume to release drug particles, thus allowing the spacer to be used at any angle (Glaxo Wellcome; see Fig. 1.3). Contrary to popular belief, keeping the baby quiet, preferably sleeping, during inhalation gives the highest possible drug deposition (Iles et al 1999, O'Callaghan & Barry 2000).

Method
1. The medication should be checked against the prescription as per policy for administration of medications.
2. Remove the mouthpiece cover from the metered dose inhaler.
3. Shake the inhaler.
4. Insert the inhaler into the inhaler holder of the Babyhaler.
5. Place the facemask gently and securely over the baby's nose and mouth; try to keep the baby calm.
6. Hold the Babyhaler at an angle that is comfortable for the baby and the person administering.
7. Press down on the canister once to release a puff of medication into the Babyhaler.
8. Keep the Babyhaler facemask over the nose and mouth until the baby has taken at least 5–10 breaths.
9. Repeat steps 2 to 7 if necessary and check with the pharmacist if there is any doubt.
10. Remember to wipe the face of the baby after administration of inhaler.
11. Record the medication administration in the child's health records (i.e. drug chart) (NMC 2002c).

Nebulisers

Nebulisers can be used at home, in hospital during acute episodes, or to treat respiratory infections with inhaled antibiotics (e.g. cystic fibrosis). Depending on the child's ability, using a mouthpiece rather than a mask gives higher lung deposition, as much of the drug is lost through the mask vents (O'Callaghan & Barry 2000). Nebulisers do have the advantage that oxygen can be administered simultaneously, which is important if the child is hypoxic. The use of an inhaler plus spacer device is as effective at treating acute asthma exacerbation as the nebuliser (O'Callaghan & Barry 2000, Cates et al 2003) and nurses should check the local trust protocol for treatment of acute asthma exacerbation in children.

Equipment
- Nebuliser unit or oxygen point.
- Nebuliser pot and mask or mouthpiece.

Different sizes are available to suit all ages. O'Callaghan and Barry (2000) found that a mouthpiece gives higher lung deposition of nebulised drug. Some nebuliser types are better for specific drugs than others. If the child is ventilated, special connectors are available to connect the nebuliser to the ventilator tubing. The gas can be administered via a compressor, or via a bottled or piped gas supply. Oxygen should be used in acute asthma, as the child is likely to be hypoxic.

Method
- The medication should be checked against the prescription as per policy for administration of medications.
- To ensure adequate droplet formation, the nebuliser solution should be diluted to volume as recommended by the nebuliser manufacturer, for example 2.5 ml for Medic Aid nebulisers (Medic Aid 1995). Even though some medications come in prepacked nebules, they may need further dilution if the volume is too small, for example when a small baby receives only a small proportion of the nebule, as a small volume of the fluid always remains in the pot (O'Callaghan & Barry 2000). Rees and Price (1995) recommend 4 ml minimum volume. The oxygen or airflow should reach 8–10 litres/minute to create a vapour (Rees & Price 1995).

- The child should be sitting comfortably, either in bed, on a chair, or on a parent's or nurse's lap.
- Tap the nebuliser during nebulisation to ensure that large droplets are shaken down.
- Observe the child's condition during and after using the nebuliser.
- After the nebuliser has finished, dry tubing using driven gas (use oxygen or air to run through the tubing to help dry), and wash and air dry nebuliser pot and mask. Store for that patient only.
- Record the medication administration in the child's health records (i.e. drug chart) (NMC 2002c).

Summary of possible complications

The number of medications that may be given by inhaler precludes a comprehensive list of side-effects being given here. A thorough knowledge of pharmacology is, however, necessary to understand and identify these side-effects. Jordan and White (2001) and Roberts (2002) offer a good description of drugs used in asthma and their potential side-effects. It must be remembered that complications may occur, due both to the side-effects of the therapy and the natural history of the respiratory condition. Rinsing the mouth after the use of an inhaler may help to lessen any potential systemic side-effects (Jackson & Lipworth 1995).

Factors to note

- Children with asthma should carry their relievers at all times.
- Regular and repeated teaching and follow-up checks of inhaler technique should improve compliance.
- Familiarise yourself with features of different devices in order to advise on the most suitable.
- Encourage mouthwashing/gargling in patients who use inhalers, especially if inhaled steroids are prescribed (Caldwell 1998, Roberts 2002).
- Ensure effective interprofessional liaison with all healthcare professionals involved in the child's care (Campbell 2002).

COMMUNITY PERSPECTIVE

The role of the community children's nurse (CCN) may range from supporting parents giving oral medication to administering complex drug regimens.

If it is necessary for the CCN to carry drugs, these should be transported in a sturdy container or cool box. If drugs have to be left in the car between visits, care must be taken to leave them unobtrusively in a securely locked car. Nurses must work within local guidelines in regard to the transport or carrying of controlled and cytotoxic drugs (RCN 2001).

Drugs must be stored at the recommended temperatures. It may be necessary to supply the family with a drug refrigerator or freezer.

A recommended resource is *Administering Intravenous Therapy to Children in the Community* (RCN 2001). As nurses are increasingly asked to undertake pioneering clinical work in the home, each practitioner must consider their own accountability.

All drugs must be administered according to local policy. Control of Substances Hazardous to Health (COSHH) Regulations (HSE 2002) apply in the home and the CCN is responsible for ensuring safe practice. This may include providing protective clothing for the administering nurse or parent and provision of spillage kits as appropriate.

The safety of the home environment for the preparation and administration of intravenous drugs will need to be assessed. Some homes may prove to be unsafe, either through inadequate standards of hygiene or lack of space, but this is the exception. The nurse will need to be able to create an aseptic field (see Aseptic Non-Touch Technique, p. 78).

COMMUNITY PERSPECTIVE

Where parents are undertaking administration of drugs by injection, it is the responsibility of the CCN to ensure that appropriate training, supervision and written guidelines are in place. These must include information about side-effects and possible complications of therapy, including anaphylactic rescue.

Anaphylaxis kits containing adrenaline, chlorphenamine and hydrocortisone should be available to the nurse. These drugs should be prescribed and documented in the child's records by the hospital or GP.

Wherever possible, two people should check intravenous drugs. The parent or an older child may be involved. However, preloaded syringes, prepared in a hospital pharmacy, are preferable.

When electrically powered syringe drivers or intravenous pumps are used, it is essential to ensure that they are capable of running on their own batteries, in case of power failure. Parents should know what they should do if the pump/driver fails to work, as it may be unrealistic to have spare pumps available. All equipment should be serviced regularly.

When opioids are administered subcutaneously by syringe driver or intravenously via a pump, it may be necessary to have naloxone in the home as an antidote to respiratory depression. This is unlikely to occur as the majority of children on opioids are terminally ill and will have had their dosages increased gradually.

Any clinical waste should be disposed of according to local policy.

Parents must know who to contact at any time should they have problems and the CCN must be aware of any potential problems that may occur with any of the devices in use, or the medication being administered.

Do and do not

- Do be careful.
- Do allow sufficient time.
- Do ask for help if unsure of what you are being asked to do.
- Do not become rushed or distracted.
- Do not take 'short cuts' with checking procedures.
- Do your own calculations; if you disagree, say so.
- Do check with the doctor or pharmacist if unsure.
- Do check that the correct child receives the correct medication, in the correct dose, at the correct time, via the correct route.
- Do ensure that all medicines administered are recorded in the child's health records (i.e. drug chart) (NMC 2002c).
- Do be familiar with equipment used in drug administration, e.g. pumps and nebulisers.
- Do emphasise that children with asthma should carry their relievers with them at all times.
- Do offer regular teaching sessions to check the use of inhalation devices.
- Do communicate with the school nurse regarding children's medications.
- Do encourage mouth washes in patients who have steroids via inhalers.

References

Addison R 2000 How to administer enemas and suppositories. Nursing Times 10(96): Supplement 3–4

Advanced Paediatric Life Support Group (APLS) 2001 Advanced paediatric life support: the practical approach, 3rd edn. BMJ Publishing Group, London

Alderson P 1993 Children's consent to surgery. Open University Press, Buckingham, UK

Alderson P, Montgomery J 1996 What about me? Health Service Journal 11th April, 22–24

Audit Commission 2001 A spoonful of sugar: medicines management in the NHS hospitals. Audit Commission, London

Beyea S C, Nicoll L H 1995 Administration of medicines via the intramuscular route: an integrative review of the literature and research-based protocol for the procedure. Applied Nursing Research 8(1): 23–33

Caldwell C 1998 Management of acute asthma in children. Nursing Standard 12(29): 49–54

Campbell A 2002 Inter-professional collaboration and children with asthma. Paediatric Nursing 14(10): 32–34

Campbell S, Glasper E A (eds) 1995 Whaley and Wong's children's nursing. Mosby, London

Cates C, Bara A, Crilly J, Rowe B 2003 Holding chambers versus nebulisers for beta-agonist treatment of acute asthma [systematic review]. Cochrane Airways Group, Cochrane Database 3

Child F, Davies S, Clayton S, Fryer A, Lennay W 2002 Inhaler devices for asthma: do we follow the guidelines? Archives of Disease in Childhood 86(3): 176–179

Choonara I 2000 Clinical trials of medicines in children: US experience shows how to ensure that treatment of children is evidence based. British Medical Journal 321(7269): 1093–1094

Danet G D, Norris E M 1992 Paediatric IV catheters. Efficacy of saline flush. Pediatric Nursing 18(2): 111–113

Demoly P, Bousquet J 2001 Epidemiology of drug allergy. Current Opinion in Allergy and Clinical Immunology 1(4): 305–310

Department of Health 1996 Immunization against infectious disease. HMSO, London

Department of Health 1999 Review of prescribing, supply and administration of medicines. Final Report. TSO, London

Department of Health 2000a The NHS Plan. TSO, London

Department of Health 2000b Pharmacy in the future – implementing the NHS plan. TSO, London

Department of Health 2003 Getting the right start: National Service Framework for children. Standard for hospital services. DoH, London

Dimond B 2003a The statutory framework for the control of medicines. British Journal of Nursing 12(7): 443–446

Dimond B 2003b Principles for the correct administration of medicines: 1. British Journal of Nursing 12(11): 682–685

Dimond B 2003c Principles for the correct administration of medicines: 2. British Journal of Nursing 12(12): 760–762

Dimond B 2003d The introduction of nurse prescribing 2: final Crown Report. British Journal of Nursing 12(16): 980–983

Ellis J 1995 Administering drugs. Paediatric Nursing 7(4): 29–39

European Commission Enterprise Directorate-General 2002 Better medicines for children. Proposed regulatory actions on paediatric medicinal products. European Commission, Brussels

Francis C 2001 Setting up a school-based clinic to improve adolescent asthma. Community Nurse July/August, 19–22

Garcia-Gonzalez E, Rivera-Rueda M 1998 Neonatal dermatology: skin care guidelines. Dermatology Nursing 10(4): 274–275, 279–281

Gibson F, Khair K, Pike S 2003 Nurse prescribing: children's nurses' views. Paediatric Nursing 15(1): 20–25

Godfrey S, Kamburoff P, Nairn J 1970 Spirometry, lung volumes and airway resistance in normal children aged 5 to 18 years. British Journal of Diseases of the Chest 64: 15–24

Griffith R, Griffiths H, Jordan S 2003 Administration of medicines part 1: the law and nursing. Nursing Standard 18(2): 47–54, 56

Guy's, Lewisham and St Thomas' NHS Trust 1999 Paediatric formulary, 5th edn. Guy's, Lewisham and St Thomas' NHS Trust, London

Harrop M 2002 Self-management plans in childhood asthma. Nursing Standard 17(10): 38–42

Health and Safety Commission 1999 Control of substances hazardous to health regulations. Approved code of practice. TSO, London

Health and Safety Executive (HSE) 2002 Control of substances hazardous to health regulations. TSO, London

Hemsworth S 2000 Intramuscular injection technique. Paediatric Nursing 12(9): 17–20

Holaday B, La Monagne L, Marciel J 1994 Vygotsky's zone of proximal development: implications for nurse assistance of children's learning. Issues in Comprehensive Pediatric Nursing 17: 15–27

Hutchinson F, Hall C 2003 Nurse prescribing: issues for neonatal nurses. Journal of Neonatal Nursing 9(6): 203–206

Iles R, Lister P, Edmunds A 1999 Crying significantly reduces absorption of aerolised drugs in infants. Archives of Disease in Childhood 81(2): 163–165

Jackson C, Lipworth B 1995 Optimising inhaled drug delivery in patients with asthma. British Journal of General Practice 45: 683–687

Jamieson E M, McCall J M, Blythe R 2002 Clinical nursing practices, 4th edn. Churchill Livingstone, Edinburgh

Jody A, Charnow N A, Fandek P H, Johnson G A, Sloane G (eds) 1993 Medication administration and I.V. therapy. Springhouse Corp., Springhouse, PA

Jordan S, White J 2001 Bronchodilators: implications for nursing practice. Nursing Standard 15(27): 45–55

Kaushal R, Bates D W, Clapp M et al 2001 Medication errors and adverse events in pediatric inpatients. JAMA 285: 2114–2120

Kotter R W 1996 Heparin vs saline flush for intermittent intravenous device maintenance in neonates. Journal of Neonatal Nursing 15(6): 55–59

Le Duc K 1997 Efficacy of normal saline solution vs heparin solution for maintaining patency of peripheral intravenous catheters in children. Journal of Emergency Nursing 23(4): 306–309

Le Souif P 1999 Asthma in children. Medicine 27(9): 54–58

Lissauer T, Clayden G 2002 Illustrated textbook of paediatrics, 2nd edn. Mosby, London

Madge S 2002 Cystic fibrosis. Professional Nurse 17(6): 343–344

May D, Brewer S 2001 Sharps injury: prevention and management. Nursing Standard 15(32): 45–54

McIntyre J, Conroy S, Avery A et al 2000 Unlicensed and off label drug use in general practice. Archives of Disease in Childhood 83: 498–501

Medic Aid 1995 Information pack on nebulisers. Medic Aid, Pagham, Sussex, UK

Medical Devices Agency (MDA) 1995 Infusion systems. Device Bulletin DB9503. MDA, London

Milnes L, Callery P 2003 The adaptation of written self-management plans for children with asthma. Journal of Advanced Nursing 41(5): 444–453

Moor J, Jennison N 2004 A trust-wide strategy for the management of anaphylaxis. Nursing Times 100(15): 32–34

Moppett S 2000 Which way is up for a suppository? Nursing Times, NTPLUS 96(19): 12–13

NICE 2000a Guidance on the use of inhaler systems (devices) in children under the age of 5 years with chronic asthma. Technology Appraisal Guidance No. 10. National Institute for Clinical Excellence, London

NICE 2000b Inhaler devices for routine treatment of chronic asthma in older children (aged 5–15 years). Technology Appraisal Guidance No. 38. National Institute for Clinical Excellence, London

Nicol M, Thompson B 2000 Causes of medication errors. Nursing Progress 8: 9–11

Nicol M, Thompson B 2001 Causes of medication errors. Part II. Nursing Progress 10: 17–19

Nursing and Midwifery Council (NMC) 2002a Guidelines for the administration of medicines. NMC, London

Nursing and Midwifery Council (NMC) 2002b Code of professional conduct. NMC, London

Nursing and Midwifery Council (NMC) 2002c Guidelines for records and record keeping. NMC, London

O'Callaghan C, Barry P 2000 How to choose delivery devices for asthma. Archives of Disease in Childhood 82(3): 185–187

O'Connor B 2001 Inhaler devices: compliance with steroid therapy. Nursing Standard 15(48): 40–42

O'Shea E 1999 Factors contributing to medication errors: a literature review. Journal of Clinical Nursing 8(5): 496–504

Prosser S, Worster B, MacGregor J, Dewar K, Runyard P, Fegan J 2000 Applied pharmacology. An introduction to pathophysiology and drug management for nurses and health care professionals. Mosby, London

Quinn C 2000 Infusion devices: risks, functions and management. Nursing Standard 14(26): 35–41

Rees J, Price J 1995 Asthma in children: treatment. British Medical Journal 310: 1522–1527

Resuscitation Council (UK) 2002a Anaphylactic reactions: treatment algorithm for children in the community. Resuscitation Council (UK), London. Online. Available: www.resus.org.uk

Resuscitation Council (UK) 2002b Anaphylactic reactions: treatment algorithm for children by first medical responders. Resuscitation Council (UK), London. Online. Available: www.resus.org.uk

Resuscitation Council (UK) 2002c The emergency medical treatment of anaphylactic reactions for first medical responders and for community nurses. Resuscitation Council (UK), London. Online. Available: www.resus.org.uk

Roberts J 2002 The management of poorly controlled asthma. Nursing Standard 16(21): 45–53

Rodkin S 1987 Monitoring of phlebitis during and after CIVA trial at Wellesley Hospital. Official Journal of the Canadian Intravenous Nurses Association 3(2): 11

Rogers J, Irwin K 2003 Digital rectal examination. Guidance for nurses working with children and young people. Royal College of Nursing, London

Royal College of Nursing (RCN) 2001 Administering intravenous therapy to children in the community. RCN, London

Royal College of Paediatrics and Child Health (RCPCH) 1999 Medicines for children. RCPCH, London

Royal College of Paediatrics and Child Health (RCPCH) and Royal College of Nursing (RCN) 2002 Position statement on injection technique. RCPCH and RCN, London

Royal Liverpool Children's Hospital 2000 Paediatric injectable therapy guidelines. Royal Liverpool Children's Hospital, Liverpool, UK

Rushforth H 1996 Nurses' knowledge of how children view health and illness. Pediatric Nursing 8: 23–27

Rushforth H 1999 Practitioner review: communicating with hospitalised children. Review and application of research pertaining to children's understanding of health and illness. Journal of Child Psychology and Psychiatry 40(5): 683–691

Schaad U B 2001 Drug therapy in children: still more art than science. Current Opinion in Infectious Diseases 14(3): 301–302

Scottish Intercollegiate Guidelines Network (SIGN) 2004 The British Thoracic Society. British guideline on the management of asthma. Quick reference guide. Royal College of Physicians, Edinburgh

Shapiro G, Bronsky E, Murray A, Barnhart F, Vanderleer A, Reisner C 2000 Clinical comparability of Ventolin formulated with hydrofluoroalkanes or conventional chlorofluorocarbon propellants in children with asthma. Archives of Pediatrics and Adolescent Medicine 154(12): 1219–1225

Singel L, Lira R 2001 'Yes, you can!': nurses create a template for teaching school-aged children to live with asthma. American Journal of Nursing 101(8): 24a–24c

Skale N 1992 Manual of paediatric nursing procedures. J B Lippincott, Philadelphia, PA

Sleath B, Bush P J, Pradel F G 2003 Communicating with children about medicines: a pharmacist's perspective. American Journal of Health-System Pharmacy 60(6): 604–607

Soanes N 2000 Injection site safety. Nursing Standard 14(25): 55

Stephenson T 2000 Implications of the Crown Report and nurse prescribing. Archives of Disease in Childhood 83(3): 199–202

Stephenson T 2001 Medicines for children – the last century and the next. Archives of Disease in Childhood 85(3): 177–179

Sutcliffe A G 2003 Testing new pharmaceutical products in children: a positive step, but ethical concerns remain. British Medical Journal 326(7380): 64–65

Valanis B G, Vollmer W M, Labuhn K T et al 1993 Acute symptoms associated with antineoplastic drug handling among nurses. Cancer Nursing 16(4): 288–295

Warner J O, Gregson R K 1995 Asthma inhalers: developments or distractions? Maternal and Child Health (Dec): 383

Watt S 2003a Safe administration of medicines to children: part 2. Paediatric Nursing 15(5): 40–44

Watt S 2003b Safe administration of medicines to children: part 1. Paediatric Nursing 15(4): 40–43

Whaley L F, Wong D 1999 Whaley & Wong's nursing care of infants and children, 6th ed. Mosby Year Book, St Louis, MO

Williams A 1996 How do you avoid mistakes in medication administration? Nursing Times 92(14): 40–41

Wright A, Falconer J, Newman C 2002 Self-administration and reuse of medicines. Paediatric Nursing 14(6): 14–17

Further Reading

Dougherty L, Lamb J (eds) 1999 Intravenous therapy in nursing practice. Churchill Livingstone, London

Taylor C M 1999 An examination of the development of language in the normal child. Journal of Child Health Care 3(1): 35–38

Practice **2**

Aseptic non-touch technique

Stephen Rowley, Heather Laird

Every year it is estimated that as many as 5000 patients die unnecessarily in the UK from hospital-acquired infection (National Audit Office 2000). Many of these infections are due to poor aseptic technique. Aseptic non-touch technique (ANTT) is an evidence-based aseptic technique developed in the paediatric setting to provide healthcare workers with a practical guide to safe aseptic practice (Rowley 1996). The principles of ANTT are applicable to all clinical procedures, such as wound dressing, catheterisation and intravenous (IV) therapy. Intravenous therapy is particularly important as it is the most commonly performed aseptic procedure in hospitals today and often provides the most direct infection risk to the patient.

What is ANTT?

ANTT is a clinical practice founded upon a comprehensive theoretical framework (Fig. 2.1). There are two main components to ANTT: the evidence underpinning the technique and the work involved in ensuring staff actually comply with it. This chapter is primarily concerned with the former. The latter is, however, very important to those concerned with implementing ANTT into clinical teams, and involves standardised assessment, audit, education and training. By following this approach aseptic practice can be more easily standardised. Standardised practice is key as it facilitates audit of compliance, smoother skills acquisition and an increased feeling of patient safety. In addition, and significantly, the method becomes instantly recognisable to other staff and patients which helps maintain compliance as well as providing greater reassurance to patients and families. ANTT dispenses with much of the mythology of aseptic technique and provides straightforward clear guidance that has been tested in the clinical setting.

Why does ANTT work?

The easy-to-follow clinical guideline approach helps provide a simple and effective tool which signposts best practice, helping to establish safe, standardised aseptic technique.

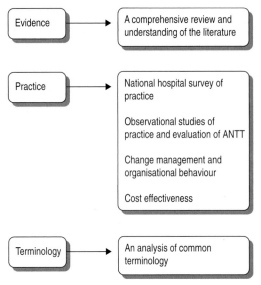

Figure 2.1 Theoretical framework (Rowley 2005)

First, staff are taught to identify and protect the key parts of any procedure, perform effective handwashing, institute a non-touch technique, wear only the appropriate infective precautions and practise in a logical order. Second, by introducing ANTT as an audit cycle using quality resources, staff are trained and re-trained on an ongoing basis. In typical ward-based teams, these two approaches combined with patient involvement have the added value of creating a degree of peer pressure which further helps promote standardised practice.

Learning outcomes

By the end of this section you should:

- understand the principles of achieving asepsis
- apply the principles of the non-touch technique to any particular aseptic procedure
- understand why it is important to use the correct and thus achievable terminology when referring to aseptic techniques.

Terms used

Infective precautions
Equipment used to help maintain asepsis, e.g. gloves, aseptic towels, aprons, etc.

Key parts/key sites
Those parts or sites that if contaminated by infectious material increase the risk of infection. In IV therapy, key parts are usually parts of equipment which come into direct or indirect contact with the liquid infusion.

Aseptic non-touch technique (ANTT)
An aseptic technique which prevents direct and indirect contamination of key parts and key sites, by a non-touch method and by other appropriate infective precautions (Rowley 2001).

Factors to note

Correct use of terminology
Other terms, such as 'sterile' and 'clean technique', are often used inaccurately and can confuse practitioners (see Box 2.1).

Equity in intravenous care
In intravenous therapy, ANTT should be used for both central and peripheral line care (see Intravenous infusion, p. 212).

Healthy, sick and handicapped children
The definition or principles of the aseptic non-touch technique are not dependent on the diagnosis of the child. However, although the principles should always remain constant, infective precautions may change depending on the type of procedure or condition of the child. This is not to say that nurses should categorise perceived high-risk groups such as immunosuppressed children and always insist on using a high level of infective precautions for all procedures. In many cases this would be an unnecessary waste of resources. According to Jones (1987), an ideal aseptic technique for intravenous catheter care is one that is safe and effective yet requires a minimal amount of time and equipment. Choosing appropriate infective precautions for any particular procedure is achieved by an effective assessment of 'risk'. If the nurse considers that asepsis of key parts/sites cannot be maintained by a non-touch method, further steps must be taken to minimise the risk of contamination. This

---

Box 2.1   Terminology should accurately reflect practice

Sterile techniques – are not achievable

The word sterile means 'free from microorganisms' (Weller 1993). Therefore, due to the natural multitude of microorganisms in the atmosphere it is not possible to achieve a true sterile technique for procedures in typical ward/home environments.

Aseptic techniques – are achievable

For infections to occur in the bloodstream (in IV therapy) or local sites (in wound care etc.), key parts or sites must be contaminated by a sufficient number of virulent, pathogenic organisms (Hendrick 1988). Therefore, a

technique that prevents this level of contamination is safe. Such a technique is most accurately termed an 'aseptic technique', as the word asepsis means 'freedom from infection or infectious (pathogenic) material' (Weller 1993).

Non-touch techniques – are paramount!

Pathogenic organisms cannot always be removed by effective handwashing (Church 1986). Additionally, handwashing is not always effective (Mallett & Dougherty 2000). Therefore, a non-touch technique is perhaps the single most important component in achieving asepsis.

---

might entail the use of extra precautions such as forceps or sterile gloves.

A review of the literature indicated that aseptic techniques have evolved more from anecdotal evidence and ritualistic practice than from empirical research. In addition, the principles of aseptic technique require reappraising in nursing practice (Lund & Caruso 1993). These two factors underpin the theoretical framework and need for ANTT.

Evidence: important components of ANTT

Handwashing

Handwashing is a central component of ANTT. On each square centimetre of the skin there may be as many as three million bacteria (Gould 1991a). Some are normal or resident skin flora and some are transient organisms that can be carried on the skin for weeks or months (Gould 1991a). Studies have demonstrated the ability of pathogenic organisms to survive and breed on the hands of healthcare workers (Adams & Marrie 1982, Bauer et al 1990). Effective handwashing can significantly decrease bacterial counts (Leonard 1986, Rossoff et al 1995, Pittet et al 1999, 2000, Girou et al 2002, Lucet et al 2002). Effective hand hygiene is important both before and after

glove use when bacterial counts will have rapidly risen (increased) in the warm humid environment created under gloves (Larson 1989, Gould 1991a, Pittet et al 1999). Stringer et al (1991) found that failure to wash hands after the removal of gloves was one of the most common breakdowns in universal precautions.

Hand cleansing has been identified as the single most significant procedure in preventing cross-infection (Maki et al 1973, Thomlinson 1990, Gould 1991a, Girou et al 2002, Cochrane 2003). Paradoxically, it is also poorly complied with by healthcare workers (Thomlinson 1990, Gallagher 1999, Pittit et al 1999). The reasons for this are multifactorial and include:

● environmental factors such as heavy workload (Gould 1991a, Gallagher 1999, Pittet et al 2000)
● inadequate handwashing facilities (Gould 1991a, 1994, Gallagher 1999, Pittet et al 2000, Girou et al 2002, Cochrane 2003)
● lack of knowledge regarding infection control.

Practice issues such as failing to wash hands before and after wearing gloves (Stringer et al 1991, Pittit et al 2000) or use of a poor handwashing technique have also been identified (Mallett & Dougherty 2000).

In terms of improving compliance, the use of bedside alcohol hand-rubs has been shown to be effective (Rossoff et al 1995, Gallagher 1999, Pittet et al 2000, Lucet et al 2002) and is more successful in decreasing bacterial counts than conventional soap and water (Pittet et al 1999, Girou et al 2002).

ANTT recommends a combination of effective handwashing with soap and water (Ayliffe et al 1978) be used interchangeably with alcohol hand-rub during aseptic non-touch technique procedures. Hand cleansing before and after glove use is another important recommendation. It is perfectly possible for hands to be washed effectively this way in just 20–40 seconds (ICNA 2002) (see Control of Infection, p. 26).

Gloves – should they be worn and what type?

Choosing between sterile, non-sterile or no gloves at all is often debated in aseptic technique. In the absence of empirical research, sterile gloves seem to have been advocated simply on a 'safer rather than sorry' basis. Aseptic non-touch technique recommends the use of non-sterile gloves for nearly all aseptic procedures. The rationale for this is based on the following:

- There is no substantial evidence demonstrating that any particular type of glove reduces the incidence of IV-related infection.

- Even sterile gloves cannot always be considered 100% sterile, due to a small but significant micropermeability (DeGroot-Kosolcharoen & Jones 1989).

- Key parts/sites should *never* be touched either by gloved or non-gloved hands, thus reducing the necessity for sterile gloves.

- Gloves should be worn in order to protect the healthcare worker from hazardous substances (drugs and body fluids) and to comply with COSHH regulations (1988). The wearing of gloves for all procedures involving potential exposure to body fluids such as blood and urine was recommended by the Expert Advisory Group on AIDS (HMSO 1990) and by the Centers for Disease Control (1988).

- Ojajarvi (1990) established that colonisation of skin by transient bacteria is the likely outcome when skin is repeatedly moist or damaged. Shredded skin caused by such damage can transmit bacteria via the contact route (Gould 1991b). Practitioners often have moist and damaged hands due to frequent washing and drying. Gloves may serve as a barrier to prevent de-scaling of bacteria onto key parts and sites.

- It has been reported that excessive precautions contribute to a false sense of security and thus a reduction in sensible precautions (Lund & Caruso 1993). This is supported by observations of staff who thought it was acceptable to touch key parts when wearing sterile gloves (Rowley 1996).

- A study conducted by Anderton and Aidoo (1991) revealed no contamination in any enteral feed samples gathered from systems assembled while wearing non-sterile gloves, indicating that non-sterile gloves are aseptic.

Environmental/air contamination

Due to airborne microorganisms, a flawless sterile technique is not possible in healthcare and home settings. Airborne infections in hospital account for only 10% of all endemic infections (Eickhoff 1994). Therefore, the potential for harmful contamination of key parts and sites by air is insignificant compared to contamination by direct contact. It is possible to reduce the potential for environmental infection by taking 'sensible measures', i.e. not practising aseptic procedures at the bedside immediately after activities like bed making and wound dressing – when the level of airborne bacteria is at its highest.

Aseptic fields

The nurse must decide what kind of aseptic field is required to maintain the asepsis of equipment and key parts. The need for sterile towels, dressing packs, etc. for all procedures is overly extravagant. For the majority of aseptic procedures, asepsis of only one or two small key parts/sites needs to be maintained. This can be achieved simply and effectively by a non-touch method and ad hoc aseptic fields (e.g. using the inside of equipment packaging).

In IV therapy a large plastic or disposable tray is ideal. Such trays should be aseptic, large enough to provide an organised working space, be flat and have high sides in order to en-house sharps safely and to protect the nurse and child from spillages.

Reuse of this equipment between patients is acceptable with appropriate cleaning as guided by local policy.

Risk assessment and equipment

It is impossible to provide a definitive list of equipment for all aseptic procedures. It is, however, possible to break down any aseptic procedure into five broad stages (see Fig. 2.2) which require either a specific action, or a choice of infective precautions. It can be seen that components 1, 4 and 5 are compulsory for all procedures. However, for some procedures the nurse

must make choices regarding the use of gloves and an aseptic field. These will differ depending on how difficult each procedure is, i.e. the degree of risk involved. Risk assessment is simple. The practitioner should simply ask whether it is possible to perform the procedure without contaminating key parts. Most aseptic procedures can be completed without touching any equipment that will be in direct contact with the patient. In ANTT such equipment is called key parts. An example of a key part in IV therapy is parts of equipment that will come into contact with the liquid infusate such as the syringe end, the needle used for drawing up the liquid, the inside of the syringe and so on. If it is not possible to complete the procedure without touching key parts due to the complexity, the length or the type of procedure, then more infective precautions will become necessary including the use of sterile gloves (see Box 2.2). It should be noted, however, that such procedures in IV therapy are rare and sterile gloves should never be worn as a shortcut to asepsis.

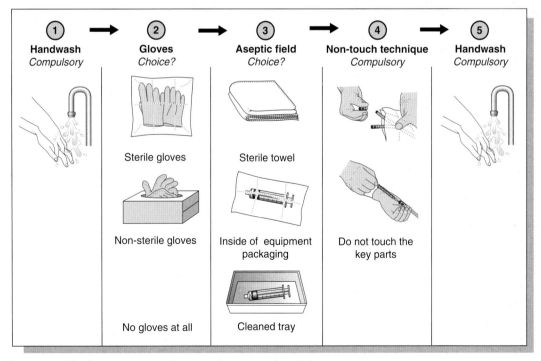

Figure 2.2   The five core stages of an aseptic non-touch technique

Box 2.2   The five core stages of ANTT – a practice example

Aim: to prepare and administer an intravenous drug into a peripheral cannula.
Setting: a typical hospital preparation room or the child's bedside.

Method	Notes
Enter the prep room or at the bedside with clean hands, i.e. just washed	
Clean your aseptic field according to local policy – making it 'aseptic', e.g. a good-sized plastic tray with sides (alternatively, a clean cardboard tray may be used)	A good-sized aseptic field will help you protect the key parts; a tray is also nicely portable
Whilst the tray dries, gather all the equipment you need and lay around the aseptic field	You need to get all these 'dirty' activities done before you clean your hands again
Clean your hands with alcogel or soap and water	
Put on non-sterile gloves	Gloves are used here in accordance with COSHH regulations, i.e. to protect the nurse from repeated drug exposure
Prepare drugs and equipment using a non-touch technique	Maintains asepsis
Do not touch any key parts but *do* touch non-key parts with confidence	Touching non-key parts with confidence will help the user develop good, safe handling skills
Remove gloves and wash hands	
When ready, go straight to the patient without delay	Helps ensure the right patient gets the right drug
Check patient's identification bracelet	
Prepare the patient, and gain free access to the IV site:	
● Explain procedure to the child and involve the child's carer in this reassurance/consenting process	
● Prepare the site (remove bandage etc.)	
● Ensure the IV site shows no signs of infection or trauma. In the event of complications seek help and document in the nursing notes	
Put on a pair of non-sterile gloves	
Clean all key parts (in this case, the cannula port) and wait for it to dry (20 seconds)	A key part is not aseptic until dry
Administer drugs according to policy	
Dispose of all sharps and used products safely	
Remove gloves and wash hands	
Document as appropriate	

Observations and complications

If key parts/sites are inadvertently contaminated, remedy the situation by cleaning with appropriate agents or by changing equipment.

COMMUNITY PERSPECTIVE

The principles remain the same within the home environment.

CCNs need to be aware that handwashing facilities may be inadequate in some homes and they will therefore need to carry appropriate hand-cleansing equipment and disposable towels.

A simple way to form an aseptic field is to clean a plastic tray with an alcohol solution immediately prior to the procedure.

In situations where families perform aseptic procedures, the CCN will need to ensure that they understand the rationale for, and methods of achieving, aseptic non-touch techniques as part of maintaining a safe environment.

In some instances it may be appropriate for the CCN to arrange for disposal of clinical waste, according to local policies.

Do and do not

- Do not confuse your practice. For example, don't try to keep one hand 'clean' and the other 'dirty' as this will only make things more difficult.
- Do touch non-key parts with confidence – this will make the procedure easier.
- Do concentrate on the key parts and key sites. As long as they are not touched/contaminated by you or anything else, you are practising safely.
- Do take time to develop your own handling technique. As long as it meets the principles of the aseptic non-touch technique, you are practising safely and efficiently.
- Do clean away from the wound in wound care. Only uncontaminated gauze, forceps, gloves, etc. should make direct contact with the wound.
- Do remember the importance of hand cleansing.
- Do not use unnecessary infective precautions as this only wastes time and resources.

References

Adams B G, Marrie T J 1982 Hand carriage of aerobic gram-negative rods by health care personnel. Journal of Hygiene 89(1): 23–31

Anderton A, Aidoo K E 1991 The effect of handling procedures on microbial contamination of enteral feeds – a comparison of the use of sterile vs nonsterile gloves. Journal of Hospital Infection 17: 297–301

Ayliffe G A J, Babb J R, Quoraishi A H 1978 A test for hygienic hand disinfection. Journal of Clinical Pathology 31: 923

Bauer T M, Ofner E, Just H M, Just H, Daschner F D 1990 An epidemiological study assessing the relative importance of airborne and direct contact transmission of microorganisms in a medical intensive care unit. Journal of Hospital Infection 15(4): 301–309

Centers for Disease Control 1988 Nosocomial infection surveillance. MMWR CDC Surveillance Summaries 1986, 35(1): 17SS–29SS

Church J 1986 Spread of infection: direct contact. Nursing 3(4): 136–137

Cochrane J 2003 Infection control audit of hand hygiene facilities. Nursing Standard 15(17): 33–38

COSHH 1988 Control of substances hazardous to health. HMSO, London

Degroot-Kosolcharoen J, Jones J M 1989 Permeability of latex and vinyl gloves to water and blood. American Journal of Infection Control 17(4): 196–201

Eickhoff T C 1994 Airborne nosocomial infection: a contemporary perspective. Infection Control and Hospital Epidemiology 15(10): 663–672

Gallagher R 1999 This is the way we wash our hands. Nursing Times 95(10): 62–65

Girou E, Loyeau S, Legrand P, Oppein F, Brun-Buisson C 2002 Efficacy of handrubbing with alcohol based solution verses standard hand washing with antiseptic soap: randomised clinical trial. British Medical Journal 325: 362–364

Gould D 1991a Nurses' hands as vectors of hospital-acquired infection: a review. Journal of Advanced Nursing 16: 1216–1225

Gould D 1991b Skin bacteria: what is normal? Nursing Standard 18(5): 25–28

Gould D 1994 Infection control. Making sense of hand hygiene. Nursing Times 90(30): 63–64

Hendrick E 1988 Infectious waste management: will science prevail? Infection Control and Hospital Epidemiology 9: 488–490

HMSO 1990 Guidance for clinical health care workers. Protection against infection with HIV and hepatitis viruses. Recommendations of the Expert Advisory Group on AIDS. HMSO, London

ICNA 2002 Hand decontamination guidelines. Infection Control Nurses Association in partnership with Regent.

Jones P M 1987 Indwelling central venous catheter related infections and two different procedures of catheter care. Cancer Nursing 10(3): 123–130

Larson E 1989 Hand washing: it's essential – even when you use gloves. American Journal of Nursing Jul: 934–941

Leonard M 1986 Handling infection. Journal of Infection Control Nursing 82: 81–84

Lucet J C, Rigaud M P, Mentre F et al 2002 Hand contamination before and after different hand hygiene techniques: a randomised clinical trial. Journal of Hospital Infection 50: 276–280

Lund C, Caruso R 1993 Nursing perspectives: aseptic techniques in wound care. Dermatology Nursing 5(3): 215–216

Maki D G, Goldman D A, Rhama F S 1973 Infection control in IV therapy. Annals of Internal Therapy 79: 869–880

Mallett J, Dougherty L 2000 The Royal Marsden Hospital manual of clinical nursing procedures, 5th ed. Blackwell Science, Oxford, Ch 3

National Audit Office 2000 The challenge of hospital acquired infection. NAO, London

Ojajarvi J 1990 Effectiveness of hand washing and disinfection methods in removing transient bacteria after patient nursing. Journal of Hygiene 85: 193–203

Pittet D, Dharan S, Touveneau S, Sauvan V, Perneger T V 1999 Bacterial contamination of the hands of hospital staff during routine patient care. Archives of Internal Medicine 195: 821–826

Pittet D, Hugonnet S, Harbarth S, Mourouga P, Sauvan V, Touveneau S 2000 Effectiveness of a hospital-wide programme to improve compliance with hand hygiene. Lancet 356: 1307–1312

Rossoff L J, Borenstein M, Isenberg H D 1995 Is hand washing really needed in an intensive care unit? Critical Care Medicine 23(7): 1211–1216

Rowley S 1996 A safe and efficient handling technique for IV therapy: aseptic non-touch-technique. (Unpublished)

Rowley S 2001 Aseptic non-touch technique. Nursing Times 97(7). Infection Control Supplement

Stringer B, Smith J A, Scharf S, Valentine A, Walker M M 1991 A study of the use of gloves in a large teaching hospital. American Journal of Infection Control 18(5): 233–236

Thomlinson D 1990 Time to dispense with the rituals: changing infection control practice. Professional Nurse May: 421–425

Weller B (ed.) 1993 Encyclopedic dictionary of nursing and health care. Baillière Tindall, London

Practice **3**

Assessment

Kerry Cook, Hermione Montgomery

Paediatrics is speciality bound by age and not by system.

Gill & O'Brien (1998, p. 41)

Introduction

Assessment forms a key part of the acute, episodic healthcare journey for the infant, child, young person and their family. It can provide practitioners with important clinical, physical, social, psychological and emotional information; it can help to promote the child's understanding of their body *and* it can educate and provide health promotion (Vessey 1995) as well as assisting in detecting potential health risks and problems. These could be:

- developmental
- psychological
- nutritional
- intellectual (Byrnes 1996).

With the growing recognition of advanced nursing roles, detailed health assessments are increasingly being undertaken by advanced nurse practitioners and nurse consultants who

have expert clinical examination skills (Hamric et al 1996, Barnes 2003). However, despite this role development, the physical assessment skills of inspection, palpation, percussion and auscultation are not commonly utilised by nurses in general (Rushforth et al 1998). Assessment skills are necessary not only for the paediatric nurse working in the acute setting, but also for all practitioners that come into contact with children, for example, in GP practices, walk-in clinics, NHS Direct, NHS 24, health visitors, school nurses and others. This chapter aims to assist these practitioners in developing an appropriate approach to the physical assessment of the child. In this chapter the term 'child' refers to infants, children and young people. All nurses should follow the principles of good practice, particularly when the examination is of an intimate nature as outlined by the RCN guidance regarding the protection of nurses working with children and young people (RCN 2001).

Assessment of the child's physical wellbeing will be demonstrated using the SOAP model (Weed 1964, 1968, 1969, Epstein et al

1997, Bond & Uzelac 2004, Uzelac et al 2004) as a systematic assessment tool.

Learning outcomes

By the end of this section you should be able to:

- assess the child's physical well-being by using a systematic assessment tool
- interpret, document and communicate the findings and take appropriate action
- recognise when vital signs do not fall within the expected limits for the child's age, condition and developmental level
- evaluate the child's physical well-being during an episode of care.

Rationale for assessment

To obtain information via observation, history taking and physical examination, which will form a baseline for immediate action and ongoing assessment, and assist in developing your plan of action. Assessments are undertaken at various times such as on admission, on an acute or ongoing needs basis, from shift to shift.

Model of assessment

Assessment of the child can reveal a plethora of information, which will be used towards formulating a provisional diagnosis and a plan of action. However, without a structured approach crucial information may be missed. Using a model will ensure that the assessment and subsequent documentation is structured and incorporates all key elements, including observation, history taking and the physical examination. Most nursing models provide assessment tools to guide the practitioner in making the assessment, for example Orem (Cavanagh 1991) and Roper, Logan and Tierney (2000). However, nursing models of assessment tend to be holistic, covering physical and psychological parameters, spiritual, social and cultural differences. For this reason they are too broad to use as a framework for this chapter, which aims specifically to explore the development of physical examination skills.

Nurses throughout the UK are expanding their skills and responsibilities in line with the Chief Nursing Officer's 10 key roles for nurses (DoH 1999), which is in keeping with role expansion across all four countries of the UK. Proficient physical examination skills are synonymous with the increase in autonomy and advanced practice that this brings. The development of skills required for this integral aspect of holistic assessment is therefore important for practitioners wishing to expand their practice. The changes that these 10 key roles will bring to nursing as a whole could mean that, in the future, development of these skills will become a fundamental part of pre-registration education. In the meantime, this chapter will provide a guideline for students wishing to enhance their assessment skills by developing a systematic approach to clinical examination.

The SOAP model – the Subjective Objective Assessment Plan – was originally described by Lawrence L. Weed in the 1960s as an integral part of the patient-oriented medical record (POMR) (Weed 1964, 1968, 1969, Epstein et al 1997), and has been universally adopted in the medical field since its inception. It was chosen as a structure for this chapter as it provides a rigorous and systematic framework that can easily be adapted by nurses. Application of the model is taught as a fundamental part of paediatric physical examination courses and is successfully used by other professional groups (nurses, physiotherapists and paramedics) in clinical practice.

Approaching the examination

No matter why you are undertaking an examination, the first action you take before formal evaluation is to visually appraise the well-being of the child. This will provide immediate information regarding the severity of the condition, the demeanour of the child, interactions with parents and general characteristics such as developmental milestones; for example, you would expect a 2–5 month old to smile and coo and to grasp a rattle; a 6–9 month old to transfer objects from one hand to another; at 10–12 months to pull up to stand; and at 13–18 months to walk alone with heels flat on the floor

(Bee 2000). Your plan of action may be determined by the information gained during this brief episode, which should be communicated to the appropriate professionals and agencies and must be documented in the child's records (DoH 2003a). If at this point urgent action needs to be taken, the airway, breathing, circulation (ABC) approach should be used (APLS 2001); if urgent attention is not required, the assessment should continue as below.

Before commencing the formal examination, ensure that the environment is private and comfortable for the child and their parents. Providing a variety of toys and games will help the child to feel more at ease and to cooperate during the physical examination. Maintaining a non-judgemental approach is essential, recognising and respecting the individuality of the family including culture and the religious beliefs of various ethnic groups (Byrnes 1996, Barnes 2003). Confidentiality and consent need to be taken into consideration at all ages but particularly for the young person, as they may wish to give information and undergo physical examination without their parents being present. You should refer to your local consent policy (DoH 2001).

Subjective information (history)

Subjective information refers to that obtained from the child and their parents. The child and their parents have the most intimate knowledge of the problem and are therefore the best source of data.

It may be clearer to substitute 'history' for 'subjective' (Donnelly 1997) as here you are attempting to build a profile of the child and their problems using information regarding the presenting complaint, previous hospital admissions, their prenatal, birth and neonatal history, allergies, current medications (including any over-the-counter preparations), immunisations, personal habits, nutrition, hygiene, elimination, developmental history (Bee 2000), family and cultural history (Wong 2003), significant life events, psychosocial history, education, physical activity and home circumstances (Byrnes 1996, Epstein et al 1997, Barnes 2003). Remember that the history provides about 80% of the data required when making an assessment, so this is a vital part of the process. Questioning needs to be sensitive so as not to cause undue alarm or embarrassment for the child or parents. It also needs to be delivered at the child's and parents' level of understanding, avoiding the use of medical jargon (Byrnes 1996).

Objective information (physical examination/observation)

Objective information refers to that obtained by the practitioner. It may be more accurate to substitute 'observation' for 'objective' (Donnelly 1997) as here you are gaining information through the physical examination and any investigative tests. The younger the child, the more important it is to observe their well-being and any physical signs from a distance; sleeping children should be observed before waking them up to examine them (Epstein et al 1997). You can learn a lot before touching without abruptly handling or invading with an instrument. Examination should be approached using your eyes and hands before your ears, using the standard format of inspection, palpation, percussion and auscultation (Archer & Burch 1998). Some aspects of respiratory function and the musculoskeletal and neurological systems can be assessed whilst the child plays, or mobilises, around the room. For example, children with respiratory distress may exhibit the tripod position to make breathing easier; this is exhibited as an extension of the arms forward and downwards whilst the back is arched (Thomas 1996). The child's breathing can be observed – is it rapid, laboured, noisy or shallow? If the child is coughing, wheezing or stridulous, this may indicate respiratory distress (Thomas 1996). For the musculoskeletal system, one could observe the shape and contour of the body and assess the gait. One can also observe for knock-knee and bowleg (Wong 1997). Asking the child to reach for an object such as a toy would uncover neurological information about coordination (Wong 2003).

Age-specific approaches

Infants are usually easier to examine and care must be taken to prevent hypothermia when exposed (Vessey 1995). The examination is best approached in a top to toe fashion, starting with the head and encompassing the entire body down to the feet in a systematic fashion whilst linking the systems together, auscultating the heart, lungs and abdomen whilst the infant is quiet. Palpation and percussion of areas should be conducted together. Reflexes can also be elicited whilst the body is being examined, but generalised primitive reflexes should be determined last. Traumatic procedures should be performed at the end of the examination, for example checking the mouth for intact palate. Many sick infants will exhibit distress and deterioration in their condition when handled to measure vital signs. In these infants taking recordings using equipment such as blood pressure monitors can cause more harm than good; visually observing for changes will be a much more accurate indication of well-being. For example, the nurse should visually observe for changes in the respiratory rate such as increasing effort, efficacy and efficiency of breathing; grunting, wheeziness and stridor; changes in skin and mucosal colour; and changes in movement and responsiveness before measuring rate (see Table 3.1).

The older infant/toddler will prefer to be sitting on the parent's lap during examination. The advantage of this position is that the parent can also gently hold the child still if necessary (RCN 2003) since this age group strongly object to being held in one position even when non-invasive examination is taking place, for example placing a temperature probe under the arm. It may be worthwhile gaining the assistance of a play specialist or another person to provide distraction with toys whilst the child is being examined. Infants from 6 months upwards may demonstrate stranger and separation anxieties (Bee 2000) which could impede your ability to assess them. These anxieties peak at 9 and 13 months respectively and by the age of 2 years have usually significantly reduced. This may be overcome by having someone with the child that is familiar to them, such as one or both of their parents or another familiar caregiver. These children prefer minimal physical contact initially and so equipment should be introduced slowly. Areas of the body could be inspected through play, such as tickling toes, or asking toddlers to point to different parts of their body; this will also assist in gaining cooperation. Parts of the physical examination where cooperation is required can then be conducted, such as auscultating the apex beat, although it may be best to perform these when the child is quiet. Again, traumatic procedures should be left until the end of the examination (Vessey 1995). Unless the examination is being undertaken rapidly because of the severity of the child's condition, time should be taken to ensure that the child and parents feel sufficiently relaxed in order to gather a thorough history before proceeding onto the examination.

Preschoolers are more obliging and like to follow simple instructions. By this age they will know most external body parts and possibly three to five internal body parts. They will prefer to be standing or sitting close to their parents, but are likely to want to undress themselves. The examination can be approached in a top to toe direction if they are cooperative, or as above if not. These children like stories about the task and to examine the equipment before it is used. You should offer the child choices to assist in gaining their cooperation.

The school-age child is more knowledgeable about internal body parts and understands simple scientific explanations. They are likely to be cooperative in most positions, although prefer sitting. The older child may prefer their parents

Table 3.1 Normal respiratory rates	
Age of child	Respiratory rate in breaths per minute
Newborn	30–60
6 months	30–45
1–2 years	25–35
3–6 years	20–30
> 7 years	20–25

Reproduced by kind permission from Hull & Johnston 1993.

not to be present. The examination should follow the top to toe pattern, leaving examination of genitalia (if necessary) until last. The school-age child will like to be given an explanation of the rationale for examination and the equipment used (Vessey 1995, Wong 1997).

The adolescent will generally prefer privacy; however, you should offer the option of having their parents present. They will have a basic knowledge of anatomy and physiology and hence will like to be told findings of the examination throughout. Although the top to toe pattern can be used, it is best to expose only the area being examined, thus allowing privacy to be maintained (Vessey 1995, Wong 1997).

Examining the systems (obtaining the objective information)

The examination may be undertaken using a system-based approach as suggested below. This is by no means an exhaustive explanation of factors to consider but offers some suggestions as to the approach that could be taken.

Respiratory examination

Respiratory disorders in infancy can be acute, life threatening or chronic. In the acute, life-threatening situation, e.g. epiglottitis, early assessment of airway and breathing is vital if the child is to be treated effectively (APLS 2001).

The most common reason for infants and toddlers to attend the GP surgery is an acute respiratory tract infection, normally upper, i.e. ear, nose, mouth and throat (Gill & O'Brien 1998). It is much better to stand back and observe rather than to immediately get your hands and stethoscope onto the child. The good observer will often be able to distinguish between an upper and lower respiratory tract infection by carefully looking and listening. Observation is also the most useful since auscultation is frequently drowned by environmental noise.

Inspection

You should observe the pattern, work and rate of breathing. The respiratory rate should be counted over a full minute to ensure accuracy. In infants and children under the age of 6–7

years the abdominal movements should be counted, as they are primarily abdominal and diaphragmatic breathers (Wong 1997) (see Tables 3.1–3.5 for normal age-related vital signs). The nurse should observe for respiratory distress, for example nasal flaring, grunting, wheezing, dyspnoea, recession, use of accessory and intercostal muscles, chest shape and movement. What is the child's colour? Is there finger clubbing? Are there traumatic petechiae around the eyelids, face and neck following a severe bout of coughing? Remember that infants are nose breathers; therefore any form of nasal obstruction will also cause problems with feeding.

Palpation and percussion

A more experienced practitioner, who has undertaken a nurse practitioner programme, a paediatric physical examination course or an advanced programme of education (e.g. Advanced Nursing Practice) may perform this aspect of the examination. Alternatively, these advanced assessments could be covered by in-house competency-based training.

Auscultation

A stethoscope with a paediatric diaphragm and bell should be used. The bell is much more useful for infants, toddlers and children because it is smaller, warmer and less surface noise penetrates, making it easier for the operator to hear the breath sounds (Gill & O'Brien 1998).

Pulse oximetry and oxygen saturation (see also Oxygen Therapy, p. 257)

The child or infant who presents with any kind of respiratory distress should have a baseline recording of arterial saturation of oxygen (SaO_2) taken with a pulse oximeter. In the healthy child the percentage saturation of oxygen should be 95–98% (Sims 1996). In the child with cardiac or chronic respiratory problems their normal oxygen saturation levels may be lower. The nurse should discuss the acceptable range of oxygen saturation levels with the paediatrician, paediatric cardiologist or senior nurse/advanced nurse practitioner. Parents may also provide valuable information about their child's normal levels. Pulse oximetry is a non-invasive, painless and reliable technique for measurement of the SaO_2 (Hanna 1995). When used properly, it will detect hypoxaemia before clinical signs become evident (Hanna 1995).

A sensor (or probe) is placed around a fleshy part of the body, e.g. a fingertip in the older child, around the nailbed of the toe in the infant or around the ball of the foot in a neonate under 3 kg in weight. Exactly which sensor to use depends on where on the body it is sited and the child's weight. The sensor packaging will clarify the weight range of child for which it is to be used.

The sensor emits red and infrared light and has a photodetector, which detects the amount of light that is absorbed by the tissues. The different colours of oxygenated and deoxygenated blood absorb different amounts of infrared light. This information is then converted into an average value, which is displayed as a percentage saturation. Pulse oximeter measurements have been shown to correlate closely to arterial blood gas values (Coull 1992).

Limitations. There are limitations to the use of an oximeter. For example, if the child's peripheral perfusion is poor (the blood supply to the extremities may be reduced under some circumstances, e.g. when the child is shocked), the readings may be inaccurate. The sensor cannot read accurately if there is excessive motion. The sensor cannot detect the difference between haemoglobin molecules saturated with oxygen and those saturated with other gases such as carbon monoxide (Carroll 1993). It is therefore not safe for use in cases of carbon monoxide poisoning. Accuracy of pulse oximetry can also be affected by the presence of direct, bright light on the sensor.

If the machine records an abnormal saturation, first look at the child. Do the physical signs fit with what the machine is telling you? Remember though, that the main reason why the pulse oximeter is used is because it can detect changes before clinical signs become evident. However, if the child's condition indicates that no ̃changes have occurred, next check that the machine is recording properly

and that the sensor is placed and secured appropriately.

If a pulse oximeter is used for prolonged periods, there is a risk of pressure sores (Coull 1992, Carroll 1993), and Sims (1996) suggests that there is a risk of burning the skin if a faulty sensor is applied. Sensors must be used in accordance with the manufacturers' instructions and the site of the sensor should be changed at least 8-hourly when continuous monitoring is in progress and more frequently in neonates or the very sick child.

Cardiovascular examination

Inspection
Inspection would include observing for dysmorphic features, growth, skin colour (e.g. cyanosis, mottling, anaemia or polycythaemia), oedema, clubbing of the upper and lower extremities, respiratory difficulty, and chest and spine abnormalities (Engel 1997, Archer & Burch 1998, Gill & O'Brien 1998). The nurse should then move onto palpating the pulse, assessing the capillary refill time and taking the blood pressure.

Palpation – pulse
Palpate the arterial pulse over the radial, brachial and femoral arteries, preferably using your fingers rather than thumbs, as the practitioner's own pulse may interfere with the reading. The pulse should be counted for at least 1 minute, particularly in infants and young children as there may be irregularities in rhythm (Wong 1997). In the neonatal period it is important to palpate and compare the brachial or axillary pulse, the femoral arterial pulse and the dorsalis pedis in the foot in the context of possible coarctation of the aorta (Archer & Burch 1998). The standard grading for pulses is:

0 = absent pulse
1 = weak, thready pulse
2 = normal pulse
4 = bounding pulse.

The brachial pulse is best felt in children under 2 years of age as an infant's neck is generally short and fat and therefore the carotid artery may be difficult to palpate (APLS 2001). When palpating the pulse, information should be obtained regarding rate, rhythm, volume and character. Pulses can be graded according to the criteria in Table 3.2.

Auscultation

Auscultation of the heart sounds is more commonly used to assess the heart rate of the infant and younger child, using a stethoscope, over the 4th intercostal space inside the nipple under 5 years of age. The apex can be auscultated over the 5th intercostal space at or inside the nipple in the over 5 year olds (Archer & Burch 1998). It may also be necessary to prioritise the order of examination, performing auscultation of the heart sounds before the baby cries. The nurse should primarily listen for the first and second heart sounds (lub dub). If any additional sounds are heard the nurse should discuss the findings with relevant colleagues. Table 3.3 provides data on normal heart rates.

Blood pressure taking and recording blood pressure. It can be very difficult to gain an accurate blood pressure (BP) reading in an infant using a conventional sphygmomanometer. It is extremely hard to reliably auscultate the child's pulse beat in the cubital fossa (de Swiet et al 1989). The child is also unlikely to cooperate and hold completely still. For this reason, an electronic machine that measures blood pressure (e.g. Dinamap by Critikon, Nellcor by Hewlett Packard) by oscillometry is recommended for use in infants and younger chil-

Table 3.2 Grading of pulses

Grade	Description
0	Not palpable
+1	Difficult to palpate, thready, weak, easily obliterated with pressure
+2	Difficult to palpate, may be obliterated with pressure
+3	Easy to palpate, not easily obliterated with pressure
+4	Strong, bounding, not obliterated with pressure

After Wong 1997.

dren. However, it is important to remember the limitations of such equipment. Movement in the patient adversely affects the accuracy of an electronic blood pressure machine. It is therefore imperative that the manufacturer's instructions are followed. Unless very sick or well sedated, few children (particularly the younger ones) will hold still for the duration of the procedure. In addition, accurate recordings will only be obtained if the correct size of cuff is used.

Selection of cuff. The cuff should not be chosen dependent upon the manufacturer's age range printed on the cuff, e.g. infant cuff/adult cuff (Wong 1997); it is the cuff size that is important. There are discrepancies in the research about cuff size (Iyriboz et al 1994, Clausen et al 1999, Bur et al 2000, 2003, Clark et al 2002); however, the main school of thought is that the width of the cuff should be two-thirds

Table 3.3 Normal heart rates

Age of child	Heart rate in pulse beats per minute	
	When child awake	When child asleep
Newborn	100–180	80–160
< 3 months	100–220	80–180
3 months–2 years	80–150	70–120
3–10 years	70–110	60–100
10 years–adult	55–90	50–90

Reproduced by kind permission from D L Wong 1995, *Paediatric quick reference*, 2nd edn. Mosby, St Louis.

of the distance from the elbow to the shoulder, the inflatable part (bladder) of the cuff should reach almost all of the way around the arm, whilst the length of the cuff should be sufficient to cover the whole circumference of the arm (Archer & Burch 1998, Wong 1997) (see Fig. 3.1). The nurse should document the size of cuff used to ensure that the same cuff is used on future occasions. If the cuff is too small a false high pressure would be given and vice versa. False readings will also be gained if the infant or child is crying or very restless.

Once you have recorded the BP, consider whether it is higher or lower than expected. Remember a low BP is a late sign of shock. A raised BP could be because the child is in pain or experiencing rising intracranial pressure. The latter would be a particular concern if the child simultaneously demonstrated a falling pulse rate. As with temperature, a single abnormal recording must be re-checked. See Table 3.4 for normal blood pressure values.

Neurological examination (see also Neurological Observations and Coma Scales, p. 243)

Full neurological examination will be undertaken by the medical clinician, including assessment of the cranial nerves, reflexes, behaviour, movement, gait and coordination (Engel 1997, Epstein et al 1997). However, the nurse needs to undertake some aspects of the examination as part of the general assessment of the infant, child or young person. Once again this can be performed initially just by observing (inspection). Are they alert, how are they behaving, are they responding to their mother/father in an appropriate way? Is their cry normal and are they moving their limbs normally? On examination, if asleep do they wake up; if not, do they react to more robust stimulus/pain? If the child's level of consciousness is causing concern, or if there is a history of a head injury, or a fall, a full neurological assessment using the Glasgow

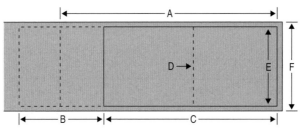

Figure 3.1 Blood pressure cuff dimensions. Dimensions of bladder and cuff in relation to arm circumference. (A) Ideal arm circumference; (B) range of acceptable arm circumferences; (C) bladder length; (D) midline of bladder; (E) bladder width; (F) cuff width. (Reproduced from Perloff et al 1993 with permission from www.americanheart.org. © 2005, American Heart Association.)

Table 3.4 Normal blood pressure values

Age of child	Systolic blood pressure in mmHg	Diastolic blood pressure in mmHg
Neonate	60–85	20–60
Infant (6 months)	75–105	40–70
Toddler (2 years)	75–110	45–80
School age (7 years)	75–115	45–80
Adolescent (15 years)	100–145	60–95

After Hull & Johnston 1993.

Note: Blood pressure values are expressed as a range, because there are variations according to sex and the child's position on the centile chart for growth.

Coma Scale must be carried out immediately (APLS 2001).

Palpation

When examining an infant's head (lying flat on the back or sitting upright), is the anterior fontanelle depressed? This is a sign that a feed may be due or of hypovolaemia if the infant is vomiting or has diarrhoea. If this fontanelle is bulging and the infant is not coughing or crying and appears irritable, this could indicate raised intracranial pressure due to infection, injury or a number of other reasons, which need to be recorded and reported. When handling the infant, do they exhibit abnormal signs of distress, are they floppy or stiff and are they difficult to placate? This could indicate that they are acutely unwell (Gill & O'Brien 1998).

Examination of the skin (see also Hygiene, p. 187)

Inspection

Observation of the skin will yield pertinent information and is a valuable part of the assessment procedure. Inspect the colour and pigmentation of the skin, preferably in natural daylight and especially when observing for jaundice. Blue discolouration may be a result of cold or anxiety; however, it could be an indication of central cyanosis, in which case the child's nails, lips, mouth and trunk will be involved and oxygen needs to be administered. Pallor of the nails, mouth, face and conjunctivae may indicate fever, anaemia and, with clamminess, may be associated with shock. Dry mucous membranes and lack of skin turgor, accompanied with a capillary refill of more than 2 seconds (following cutaneous pressure of a digit or preferably the sternum for 5 seconds), may be a sign of dehydration (Mackay-Jones et al 2001). Observe for bruises; those of the soft tissue (e.g. on the forearm and buttocks) may be a sign of child abuse.

Palpation

Examine the skin's texture and palpate for lesions and rashes, document shape, size, colour and consistency (refer to Engel 1997, pp. 99–107). Oedematous areas should be gently pressed with the thumb to determine their nature; oedema of the lower extremities and sacrum may result from cardiac or renal disease. Petechiae that are flat, round purple/red pin-like marks, blotches or bruises, which do not blanch when gently touched, may indicate meningococcal disease and the child will require immediate treatment.

Using the back of the hand, feel the temperature of the skin for hypo- and hyperthermia. The nurse also needs to consider the racial variations in skin colour and the effect that this will have on the interpretation of signs such as cyanosis and bruises.

Taking and recording a temperature (see also Temperature Control, p. 391)

In spite of various studies to determine the optimal site and temperature device to be used, there is no one correct way and it will differ according to the age of the child and other factors. Glass and mercury thermometers are not used routinely because of the risk of injury due to glass being broken and contamination with mercury. Rectal temperature recordings are not recommended for general use (McQueen 2001) because the thermometer needs to be inserted to a depth of at least 5 cm to obtain core temperature, which could cause injury to the fragile mucosa of the anus as well as rectal perforation (Wong 1997). They are also not recommended for ethical reasons as this can relate to rectal intrusion when continuous monitoring is in progress. When rectal temperatures are required a dedicated rectal electronic probe should be used (McQueen 2001).

Tympanic recording of temperature is fast, easy to use and acceptable to children (Pickersgill et al 2003, Rush & Wetherall 2003); however, it should not be used in newborn infants and young children as the earpiece is too large for the ear canal which could result in inaccurate readings. Usage is not recommended when precision is required such as in situations of hypothermia (McQueen 2001). Rush and Wetherall's (2003) review of the literature suggests that two recordings be performed using the same ear once the child has been in an even temperature for 20 minutes. Tempadot is now generally accepted as a reliable way of recording temperature, especially for those children over 2 years of age and can be used under the axilla although Rush and Wetherall (2003) suggest using it sublingually where possible. The strip should be held sublingually for 1 minute and axillary for 3 minutes; after removing the strip wait 10–15 seconds before reading the colour changes (Wong 1997). These strips must be stored in a cool environment. The nurse should refer to the manufacturer's guidelines for more details. Where possible, the child or young person should be given a choice of whether tympanic or Tempadot recording is used (DoH 2003a, Pickersgill et al 2003). See Table 3.5 for normal temperature values.

Abdominal examination

Inspection

Much of the nurse's general examination of the abdomen can be undertaken by observation. Most toddlers and young children will have an abdomen that protrudes when standing and is often associated with exaggerated lordosis (exaggeration of the lumbar curvature). Since respiration in the younger child involves the use of the abdominal muscles, movement of the abdomen with inspiration and expiration is normal. The rectus muscle may be noted as being slightly separated (divarication) but this is normal. Small umbilical hernias are frequently noted; one might see distended veins and sometimes loops of bowel in malnourished infants. Abdominal distension is often gaseous, but can be distinguished with simple percussion.

Palpation

Examination of the genitalia is unnecessary in older children unless the presenting condition indicates the need. In infants and younger children examination of the genitalia may be conducted through observation, for example when changing the nappy. One is looking for normality or deviation from this, such as hypospadias, undescended testes, intersex organs, size of clitoris/labia majora and male and female circumcision. If the child urinates whilst this is being done then the nurse could observe for direction of flow as this may indicate whether the urethral orifice is at the normal position. A rectal examination should be performed only by doctors if the condition warrants it; this procedure should not be performed routinely.

As it is beyond the scope of this chapter to discuss child sexual abuse in detail, we therefore recommend that the nurse communicates any concerns regarding sexual abuse to the medical staff (Gill & O'Brien 1998).

Growth and nutrition information

Growth is a key indicator of normal health and development. The World Health Organization identifies growth assessment as the best single measure for defining the nutritional status and health of children, as well as being an indicator for populations as a whole for quality of life (Holden & MacDonald 2000, p 161). It is therefore essential that the nurse should take a detailed history of the eating practices of the child, determining whether the child has a special diet, any known food allergies, typical dietary intake of the child and family, recent weight loss or gain, cultural, ethnic or religious influences (Engel 1997), exercise taken and any concerns that the parents may have such as food refusal, obesity and feeding problems (Holden & MacDonald 2000). Nurses are in an ideal position to educate children and their families about nutrition, particularly since obesity is currently on the increase generally, due to lifestyle and food availability.

All children being admitted to hospital or attending any healthcare setting should have their height and weight measured and plotted on a centile chart, as currently recommended (Hall 2000). The measurements should be recorded on the appropriate centile chart produced by the Child Growth Foundation as

Table 3.5 Normal temperature	
Age of child	Core temperature in degrees centigrade (°C)
< 6 months	37.5
7 months–1 year	37.5–37.7
2–5 years	37.2–37.0
> 6 years	36.6–36.8

After Wong 1995.

endorsed by the Royal College of Paediatrics and Child Health (2002); these charts correspond with those used in the child's parent-held record. Head circumference should also be measured and recorded in infants.

When weighing children under 2 years of age, the child should be naked. Electronic scales should be calibrated following the manufacturer's instructions; the weight should then be measured to the nearest 10 g. When weighing children over 2 years, the child should be in vest and pants and weighed on sitting or standing electronic scales. When measuring height, children who are unable to stand unaided should be measured supine (under 2 years); those that can stand upright unaided (over 2 years) can have a standing height measured. Measurements should be taken to the nearest millimetre to ensure accuracy (Patel et al 2003). Further information can be gained from the Child Growth Foundation. The weight and height should be recorded along with the date and the practitioner's signature on the centile chart, medical/nursing notes and in the child's parent-held record.

There are a number of additional methods of measuring that provide a non-invasive means of assessing nutrition (e.g. the degree of obesity). Body mass index (BMI) is an alternative method of assessing nutritional status, particularly since weight and height are affected by a number of factors. This is calculated by dividing the weight (in kg) by the square of the height (in meters) (w/h^2). The BMI varies during childhood and therefore there can be some problems associated with using it (Holden & MacDonald 2000). Skin fold thickness gives an indication of subcutaneous fat and therefore an idea of nutritional status. The skin is pinched between two fingers and then the thickness of the skin fold is measured using specialised callipers (Holden & MacDonald 2000).

Pulling it all together

Pulling together a smooth assessment can be quite demanding as there is no single right way to perform a physical examination. The ultimate aim is to create a method that works for you. The examination should cover all aspects so that you have a realistic chance of identifying any problem that may in fact be present. Try to link together areas that are connected spatially, even if they are detached physiologically. This allows you to be economical and efficient and also reduces the number of times the patient has to get up and down. Being effortlessly replicable ensures that you perform the examination in the same way all of the time (Goldberg 2002).

Assessment (provisional diagnosis)

The assessment stage refers to the overall impression gained by the practitioner from the subjective and objective information obtained, i.e. the provisional diagnosis. The overall impression will indicate whether immediate action should be taken or whether the needs of the child are ongoing. The practitioner should accurately document and communicate the findings of the examination to the relevant members of the multidisciplinary team (Vessey 1995, Wong 1997, DoH 2003b).

Plan (treatment options)

In the case of a child requiring immediate treatment, your plan of action may have been determined by the information gained during the brief episode of visually appraising the child pre-assessment. Alternatively, the plan of action may be decided upon once the examination has been undertaken, a provisional diagnosis or impression has been formed and this information has been communicated to the relevant multidisciplinary team members, incorporating, for example, investigations, treatments and monitoring. Again the plan should be documented clearly and updated as necessary (Vessey 1995, Wong 1997).

Complications

There are few risks associated with assessment or taking observations. The biggest problem arises when the individual performing the task does not recognise the importance of the results obtained, misinterprets the results and takes an inappropriate action in consequence, or does not act on them at all (DoH 2003b).

The nurse must:

1. have an idea of whether or not the information obtained is normal or abnormal
2. be able to assess if the result obtained was due to malfunction or misuse of equipment (if used)
3. know how to act on the results – what must be done and who must be informed.

Failure in any of these three areas could adversely affect the child.

COMMUNITY PERSPECTIVE

Whilst assessment of the child is integral in the role of the CCN, consideration must be given to the necessity of formal monitoring of vital signs, remembering that the aim of care is to make the home as unclinical an environment as possible whilst maintaining the safety of the child.

When the child's condition requires this monitoring, the parents should be given a full explanation.

Do and do not

- Do ensure that you have been properly trained in the use of electrical equipment such as pulse oximeters and blood pressure machines.
- Do note and inform medical staff of any bruising or anything unusual.
- Do remember to *record* and *report* your information.
- Do ensure that assessments are undertaken in a safe environment.
- Do ensure that consent has been obtained.

Conclusion

This chapter has aimed to demonstrate assessment of the child's holistic well-being using the SOAP model (Weed 1964, 1968, 1969, Epstein et al 1997) as a systematic assessment tool. Following assessment, the nurse should ensure that the findings are interpreted, documented and communicated to the appropriate party and that appropriate action is taken. Normal limits have been included to enable nurses to recognise when vital signs do not fall within the expected limits for the child's age, condition and developmental level. Finally, the nurse should evaluate the effect of any action and hence the child's holistic well-being during the healthcare episode.

References

Advanced Paediatric Life Support Group (APLS) 2001 Advanced paediatric life support: the practical approach, 3rd edn. BMJ Publishing Group, London

Archer N, Burch M 1998 Paediatric cardiology. An introduction. Chapman and Hall Medical, London

Barnes K (ed) 2003 Paediatrics: a clinical guide for nurse practitioners. Butterworth-Heinemann, London

Bee H 2000 The developing child, 9th edn. Allyn and Bacon, London

Bond M, Uzelac P S 2004 SOAP for emergency medicine. Blackwell Publishing, Oxford

Bur A, Hirschl M M, Herkner H et al 2000 Accuracy of oscillometric blood pressure measurement according to the relation between cuff size and upper arm circumference in critically ill patients. Critical Care Medicine 28(2): 371–376

Bur A, Herkner H, Vlcek M et al 2003 Factors influencing the accuracy of oscillometric blood pressure measurement in critically ill patients. Critical Care Medicine 31(3): 793–799

Byrnes K 1996 Conducting the pediatric health history: a guide. Pediatric Nursing 22(2): 135–137

Carroll P 1993 Clinical application of pulse oximetry. Pediatric Nursing 19(2): 150–151

Cavanagh S 1991 Orem's model in action. Palgrave Macmillan, London

Clark J A, Lieh-Lai M W, Sarnaik A, Mattoo T K 2002 Discrepancies between direct and indirect blood pressure measurements using various recommendations for arm cuff selection. Pediatrics 110(5): 920–923

Clausen L R, Olsen C A, Olsen J A, Mortensen P E, Nielsen P E 1999 Influence of cuff size on blood pressure among schoolchildren. Blood Pressure 8(3): 172–176

Coull A 1992 Making sense of pulse oximetry. Nursing Times 88(32): 42–43 de Swiet M, Dillon M J, Littler W, O'Brien E, Padfield P L, Petrie J C 1989 Measurement of blood pressure in children – recommendations of a working party of the British Hypertension Society. British Medical Journal 299: 497

Department of Health 1999 The NHS plan. DoH, London

Department of Health 2001 Seeking consent: working with children. DoH, London

Department of Health 2003a Getting the right start: National Service Framework standard for hospital services. DoH, London

Department of Health 2003b The Victoria Climbie inquiry. Report by Lord Laming. TSO, London

Donnelly W J 1997 The language of medical case histories. Annals of Internal Medicine 127(11): 1045–1048

Engel J 1997 Pocket guide to pediatric assessment, 3rd edn. Mosby, St Louis, MO

Epstein O, Perkin G D, de Bono D P, Cookson J 1997 Pocket guide to clinical examination, 2nd edn. Mosby, London

Gill D, O'Brien N 1998 Paediatric clinical examination, 3rd edn. Churchill Livingstone, Edinburgh

Goldberg C 2002 A practical guide to clinical medicine: pulling it all together. University of California, San Diego, CA

Hall D M B 2000 Growth monitoring. Archives of Disease in Childhood 82: 10–15

Hamric A B, Spross J A, Hanson C 1996 Advanced nursing practice. An integrative approach. W B Saunders, Philadelphia, PA

Hanna D 1995 Guidelines for pulse oximetry use in pediatrics. Journal of Pediatric Nursing 10(2): 124–126

Holden C, MacDonald A 2000 Nutrition and child health. Baillière Tindall and RCN, London

Hull D, Johnston D I 1993 Essential paediatrics, 3rd edn. Churchill Livingstone, Edinburgh, ch 8, p 117

Iyriboz Y, Hearon C M, Edwards K 1994 Agreement between large and small cuffs in sphygmomanometry: a quantitative assessment. Journal of Clinical Monitoring 10(2): 127–133

Mackay-Jones M J, Molyneux E, Phillips B, Wieteska S 2001 Advanced paediatric life support. A practical approach, 3rd edn. BMJ Books, Bristol, UK

McQueen S 2001 Clinical benefit of 3M Tempadot thermometer in paediatric settings. British Journal of Nursing 10(1): 55–58

Patel L, Dixon M, David T J 2003 Growth and growth charts in cystic fibrosis. Journal of the Royal Society of Medicine 96(Suppl 43): 35–41

Perloff D, Grim C, Flack J et al 1993 Human blood pressure determination by sphygmomanometry. Circulation 88: 2460–2470

Pickersgill J, Fowler H, Bootham J, Thompson K, Wilcock S, Tanner J 2003 Temperature taking: children's preferences. Paediatric Nursing 15(2): 22–25

Roper N, Logan W, Tierney A J 2000 The Roper–Logan–Tierney model of nursing: the activities of living model. Churchill Livingstone, London

Royal College of Nursing 2001 Protection of nurses working with children and young people: guidance for nursing staff. RCN, London

Royal College of Nursing 2003 Restraining, holding still and containing children. RCN, London

Royal College of Paediatrics and Child Health (RCPCH) 2002 Growth reference charts for use in the UK. RCPCH, London

Rush M, Wetherall A 2003 Temperature measurement: practice guidelines. Paediatric Nursing 15(9): 25–28

Rushforth H, Warner J, Burge D, Glasper E A 1998 Nursing physical assessment skills: implications for UK practice. British Journal of Nursing 7(16): 965–970

Sims J 1996 Making sense of pulse oximetry and oxygen dissociation curve. Nursing Times 92(1): 34–35

Thomas D O 1996 Assessing children – it's different. RN 59(4): 38–45

Uzelac P S, Moon R W, Badillo A G 2004 SOAP for internal medicine. Blackwell Publishing, Oxford

Vessey J A 1995 Developmental approaches to examining young children. Pediatric Nursing 21(1): 53–56

Weed L L 1964 Medical records, patient care and medical education. Irish Journal of Medical Science June: 271–282

Weed L L 1968 Medical records that guide and teach. New England Journal of Medicine 278: 593–600, 652–657

Weed L L 1969 Medical records, medical education and patient care: the problem-oriented medical record as a basic tool. Case Western University, Cleveland, OH

Wong D L 1997 Whaley & Wong's essentials of pediatric nursing, 5th edn. Mosby, St Louis, MO

Wong D L 2003 Essentials of paediatric nursing. Mosby, St Louis, MO

Further Reading

Bee H 1997 The developing child, 8th edn. Addison-Wesley, New York

Frisch N A, Coscarelli W 1986 Systematic instructional strategies in clinical teaching: outcomes in student charting. Nurse Educator 11(6) 29–32

Hanning C D, Alexander-Williams J M 1995 Pulse oximetry: a practical review. British Medical Journal 311: 367–370

Hazinski M 1992 Nursing care of the critically ill child, 2nd edn. Mosby Year Book, St Louis, inside cover

http://medicine.ucsd.edu/clinicalmed/together.htm

http://www.chiro.org/documentation/ABSTRACTS/Maximizing_the_Effectiveness.html

Langlois J P, Thach S 2000 Managing the difficult learning situation. Family Medicine 32(5): 307–309

McPhee A 1987 Teaching students how to chart . . .
SOAP notes, Nurse Educator 12(4): 33–36

Stoneham M D, Saville G M, Wilson I H 1994 Knowledge about pulse oximetry among medical and
nursing staff. Lancet 344: 1339–1342

Welk D 2001 Teaching students a pattern of reversals
eases the care plan process. Nurse Educator 26(1):
43–45

Practice **4**

Bereavement care

Bernadette McGarry

Introduction

Nurses are at the forefront of delivering needs-led health care in a changing society. Advances in maternal and child health have influenced patterns of illness, promoting growth in community and palliative care services for children with chronic and life-limiting illnesses (ACT & RCPCH 2003). Child health involves not only physical care but also religious and spiritual care (Scottish Executive Health Department 2002). The diversity offered by a multicultural society, incorporating an increasing number of asylum seekers and migrant workers, presents many challenges to nurses at all stages of life/death continuum.

Bereavement care of a child and family is perhaps one of the most complex and demanding aspects of children's nursing. Nurses require knowledge of current legislation, an awareness of cultural preferences relating to preparation of the child's body and insight into the psychosocial effects of a child's death on the family. The role of the family in caring for sick children cannot be overemphasised and involving family is essential not only in life but also in death (Hindmarch 2000).

Learning outcomes

By the end of this section you should:

- be aware that a child and family may choose where the child dies and is cared for after death
- be able to describe the principles of caring for the child's body after death with reference to cultural and religious customs and legal requirements
- be able to help distressed relatives and staff to follow the procedures that are necessary when a child has died
- be able to identify resources which may help family and staff begin to accept the death of a child and understand and manage their own grief process
- be able to explain under which circumstances there may be a need for a post-mortem.

Rationale for bereavement care

In the UK, childhood death occurs infrequently (Whittle & Cutts 2002) but the impact on the family is profound (Davies & Connaughty 2002). The nurse's professional experience of childhood death may be limited; however, when it does occur, compassionate, professional and effective management of the situation may positively influence the family's ability to grieve (Hindmarch 2000) and assist staff in obtaining a balance between professional and personal loss (Read 2002).

Retention of organs and post-mortem (PM)

Bereavement care includes determining the need for post-mortem in discussion with the medical team and obtaining informed consent from the child's next of kin for the procedure. Obviously, this is a time of great stress and sadness for everyone and detailed discussions should be handled with sensitivity. Following the Royal Liverpool Children's Inquiry (2001) into the retention of organs, changes in the whole concept of gaining consent have taken place and have shaped the current process.

- The possibility of a coroner's PM must only be mentioned if the death is reportable to the coroner.
- If the coroner declines a PM, but the clinician wishes a hospital PM to be undertaken, the next of kin must be made aware that no compulsion exists for this to be carried out.
- The full procedure must be explained to the next of kin including opening the body, removal and weighing of organs and if any

organs or tissue will be retained (Human Tissue Act 1961).

Box 4.1 details some of the major categories relating to the death of a child which indicate that the case must be referred to the coroner, by law (Regulation 51 of the Registration of Births, Deaths, and Marriages Regulations 1968). In these circumstances, the coroner will usually order a post-mortem.

Sometimes local practice requires a post-mortem to be performed in additional circumstances to those required by law, for example, if the death was within 24 hours of admission to hospital or if the deceased was detained under the Mental Health Act (Ellis & Edwards 1995). It is important to establish what local policy and practice require. Ethically, medical staff should always obtain consent for post-mortem from parents, but it is not legally required for a coroner's post-mortem (Ellis & Edwards 1995).

Post-mortem is a very emotive subject for families and Ellis & Edwards (1995) stress the importance of a sensitive, positive, multidisciplinary approach to the family when seeking consent for post-mortem. Careful explanation of the need for the examination and the actual procedure should be given. It must be stressed that the body will be treated with the utmost respect and the same care as for a living patient. Parents may be concerned that the body will be disfigured by the procedure and should be reassured that suture lines on the torso and above the hair line will be the only evidence of the post-mortem and will not be unduly disfiguring. Parents should be given

---

Box 4.1   Deaths to be referred to the coroner

- There is an element of suspicious circumstances or history of violence
- The death may be linked to an accident (whenever it occurred)
- The death is linked with an abortion
- The death may be related to a medical procedure or treatment

- The death occurred during an operation or before full recovery from the effects of anaesthesia or was in any way linked to the effects of anaesthesia
- The actions of the deceased may have contributed to his or her own death, e.g. self-neglect, drug or solvent misuse

Adapted from Ellis & Edwards 1995.

the opportunity to view the body afterwards. It is generally accepted that having this opportunity helps families to grieve (Haas 2003). However, evidence exists which suggests that this may not be the case in the neonatal death experience (Skene 1998). Therefore, caution should be shown and each case treated as individual (Davies & Connaughty 2002).

The inability to stop a coroner's post-mortem may cause extreme distress to some families, particularly those whose religion expressly forbids such a procedure (see Box 4.2). These parents will need a lot of support, and advice should be sought from their religious or spiritual advisors concerning special procedures for handling the body during post-mortem and returning organs to the body. Jewish and Islamic faiths require that any organs removed from the body during a legally required post-mortem examination be returned to it for burial (Green & Green 1992). When post-mortem is required, any cannulae, drains or tubing should not be removed from the body without discussion with medical staff (Green & Green 1992).

Organ donation

In some cases, the question of organ donation may arise. Suitability for organ donation will depend on the child having no evidence of major untreated systemic infection, malignancy (excepting primary brain tumour),

chronic severe hypertension or positivity to Australia antigen (hepatitis B) or human immunodeficiency virus antibodies (Browne & Waddington 1993). A child who is maintained on mechanical ventilation must have met the brain stem death criteria before organ donation can occur.

Browne and Waddington (1993) suggest approaching parents when the first set of tests has been completed and the criteria met. It may be possible to broach the subject earlier than this if someone who is experienced in discussing the subject with parents, e.g. a transplant coordinator, handles it sensitively. Ensure that when parents are approached regarding organ donation someone with whom they have been able to build a relationship, for example a member of the medical or nursing staff, is present. Organ donation must always be broached sensitively and by someone who has a positive attitude towards transplantation but is not seen as biased.

If parents agree to organ donation, the transplant coordinator will help support them and explain forthcoming procedures. Parents should be aware that they can see their child after donation. They should be warned that their child will be white, cold and, depending on which organs have been retrieved, may have large scars.

Religious objection to organ transplantation is not the inevitable consequence of the laws and beliefs of the different faiths (Ethnicity Online 2004). However, the following examples illustrate how some find it a very difficult issue:

- Jehovah's Witnesses because other transfused blood will circulate through the organ
- Christian Scientists because they prefer the body to be inviolate and to rely on the healing power of prayer
- Orthodox Jews because of their beliefs in the sanctity of the body and physical resurrection.

Once parents have consented and the coroner has agreed, organ donation can take place. Table 4.1 lists the organs which can be used.

Box 4.2 Religious/spiritual perspectives on post-mortem

- Religions which absolutely forbid post-mortem: Jews, Muslims, Zoroastrians (Parsees)
- Religions which strongly object to post-mortem: Christian Scientists
- Religions which would prefer post-mortem not to occur if at all possible: Rastafarians
- Religions which do not have specific views on the post-mortem examination: Christians, Jehovah's Witnesses, Mormons, Buddhists, Hindus, Sikhs

From Green & Green 1992.

Table 4.1 Organs which can be donated from children (Browne & Waddington 1993)

Organ	Minimum age of donor	Special requirements of donor's condition	Treatment necessary to maintain organ in good condition prior to removal
Kidney	2 years	No renal disease, good renal function	Inotrope infusion and intravenous fluids to maintain perfusion of kidneys
Liver	3 months	No liver diseases, drug abuse or alcoholism. Good liver function	–
Heart	6 months	No cardiac defect or disease. Donor's condition should be stable without excessive inotropic support	–
Heart and lung	6 months	No cardiac defect or disease or pulmonary dysfunction. No heavy smoking. Good arterial blood gases and lung compliance. Ventilation should not have been prolonged	–
Pancreas	14 years	No history of diabetes. If the liver is also being retrieved, patient must have spleen still intact	–
Cornea	Any age	No corneal scarring. No infectious eye disease	Eye care extremely important. Eyes must be closed and protected after death
Heart valves	6 months	–	Can be retrieved up to 72 hours after death

Reproduced with the permission of Stanley Thornes Publishers Ltd from *Manual of Paediatric Intensive Care Nursing*, B Carter, 1993.

Special religious needs of the dying child and the care of the child's body after death

Information contained within this section pertaining to religious customs and death is taken from Green and Green (1992), Bull (2004) and Ethnicity Online (2004). There are several common themes between some religions relating to rituals after death. These are summarised in Box 4.3. Other special considerations are as detailed below.

Christian families

Many Christians will want their child to be baptised if death is imminent. If this is not possible before death, a priest may conduct a naming and blessing ceremony after death. In an emergency, any Christian may conduct a baptism. Baptism is important to Roman Catholics to the extent that they will allow even a non-believer to conduct an emergency baptism if a priest is not available. Roman Catholic families may also want a priest to perform the Sacrament of the Sick and Sacrament of the Dying (extreme unction). Holy Communion will be important if the child has taken their first Holy Communion.

Jewish families

Traditionally, the body is not to be touched for 20 minutes after breathing has stopped. After 10 minutes, a feather is then placed over the mouth and nose to ensure that breathing has stopped. The body should be touched as little as possible and gloves should be worn to do so. Close the child's eyes and straighten out the body, lying flat with feet together and arms by the sides. The body should be covered in a plain white sheet and should never be left alone or in the dark. A light should be left on as a mark of respect.

Muslim families of the Islamic faith

The dead child's extended family are likely to visit to pay respects and support the immediate family. The parents may wish the body to be

Box 4.3 Rituals surrounding care of the body after death common to the Jewish, Muslim, Hindu and Sikh religions

- The child will not be left unattended whilst dying, nor must the body be left unattended after death
- Cleansing of the child's body after death is only to be performed by special individuals:
  - specially trained members of the community of the same sex as the dead child perform Jewish last offices
  - a non-Muslim must not touch the body of a Muslim child, but if it is unavoidable, a non-Muslim should wear disposable gloves
  - a non-Hindu should preferably not touch the body of a Hindu child
  - family members of the same sex as the child care for the body of a Sikh child.
- Therefore, the body of a child of any of these religions should simply be straightened,

limbs straightened and the eyes closed, then covered with a clean sheet until further instructions can be obtained from the family. If a family member is not able to be present, it may be appropriate to ask if they wish a member of staff to remain with the body
- It is important that the funeral should take place within 24 hours of death. It can be possible to arrange, even if there has to be a post-mortem
- Any religious emblems (bracelets or necklets made from Holy thread) and jewellery on the body of a Hindu or Sikh child must be left in place on the body

placed with the face facing towards Mecca (south-east). Muslims believe that flexing the elbows, shoulders, knees and hips before straightening will help delay the onset of stiffening. Often Muslim families do not wish their child to go to the hospital mortuary but arrange for the body to go straight to the mosque for cleansing or to a Muslim undertaker.

Hindu families

A Hindu family is likely to prefer that their child die at home and may wish a priest to be present at the child's bedside to perform holy rites. In addition to Holy thread (Yagyopavit) around the child's limbs or body, the skin may be marked with paste or a sacred leaf (Tulsi) or ghee (butter) placed in the mouth. Gloves should be worn if the child's body is touched. A light should be left on near the child's head as a mark of respect and to comfort the soul. Children under 5 years are buried and not cremated.

Sikh families

It may be inappropriate to remove underclothing as this may have religious significance. If the child wears a turban, this must also be left in place after death. The face may be cleansed

if it is dirty. Touch the body as little as possible. Wear gloves if the body is touched. Wrap the child's body in a plain white sheet.

Guidelines

Family care when a dying child has to undergo resuscitation

In an emergency situation such as resuscitation, parental presence may be seen as inappropriate. In one research study, Back and Rooke (1994) found that doctors raised concerns that families would be more likely to complain if they witnessed resuscitation, e.g. complain that not enough or too much was done, nurses and doctors seemed uncaring or that inappropriate comments were made. Staff may also fear that relatives might display uncontrollable grief which could hinder the resuscitation. However, research in America (Renzi-Brown 1989, Hanson & Strawser 1992) would dispute this. Hanson and Strawser found that relatives wished to be present during resuscitation. Throughout this 9-year trial, staff concerns that relatives' grief could hamper the resuscitation attempts were not well founded. On the contrary, they discovered that relatives who had been present during resuscitation felt that it brought a sense of reality to their loss and helped them in their grieving process. A more recent study whereby relatives were supported by a family facilitator reports similar findings (Meyers et al 2000).

Including families in resuscitation may reassure them that everything was done that could have been done (Meyers et al 2000, Vanderbeek 2000) and, to quote Back and Rooke (1994), when the need for resuscitation arises: 'It seems absurd that the person who has been so involved in care is immediately ushered away to another room and not given the choice of whether or not to stay with his or her kin.' Notably, nurses' attitudes towards relatives being present during resuscitation change significantly if they or their relative were the patient (Ellison 2003).

Most research into the presence of relatives during resuscitation relates to general emergency settings, not specifically paediatrics. However, Back and Rooke (1994) found that staff were more in favour of parents being present during paediatric resuscitation than of relatives being present during adult resuscitation. They suggest that this is reflective of parental involvement in care within paediatrics. Kelly (1992) suggests that parents have more right to be in the resuscitation room than staff.

Connor (1996) concludes that although parents should not be excluded during resuscitation, it is of vital importance that they must:

- be given the choice of whether or not to stay
- not be left on their own to witness the events
- be supported by someone who can explain what is happening to their child.

Specially trained pastoral care staff as well as nurses and doctors have been used as suitable supporters for relatives witnessing resuscitation (Hanson & Strawser 1992). In paediatrics, there may often be other relatives with the child and the parents who will also need help, support and information. Hanson and Strawser (1992) describe the inclusion of family members other than the next of kin during resuscitation, something that may need consideration.

Family care when death is expected and planning can take place

The family may wish to consider alternatives about where their child spends the last days of their life. There should be several options from which they may choose the one most suitable to their individual needs (Soutter 1994). There are three main choices: hospital, home or hospice. A hospital ward may be too noisy, busy and lacking in privacy, but some parents find comfort in being in the hospital environment. This may be due to their fears about how their child will die: Will he be in pain? Will he bleed or choke to death? Careful discussion about their reasons for wanting to be in hospital may uncover these fears. Explanation and reassurance will help to allay them. Parents may then decide that hospital is not their first choice. Some areas are fortunate to have children's hospices where it may be possible for the child and family to spend the last hours. This can be arranged days or weeks in advance where circumstances allow, but many hospices can be of assistance at very short notice. Some hospices will care for children who have already died (e.g. on a hospital ward). They take the child's body into the hospice so that the family may spend some time with the child in a setting which is not part of a mortuary or Chapel of Rest but more like home.

In a non-emergency situation, parents may choose who else should be present when their child is dying. Some families like to have the dying child surrounded by the whole family – parents, siblings and grandparents, uncles and aunts. Other parents may wish to be on their own with their child. The nurse may offer to tactfully refuse visitors for parents if they wish to have privacy. It can be difficult for parents to be assertive about numbers and timing of visits and visitors when their child is dying.

Other family members

Siblings and grandparents will also need a lot of support at the time of a child's death. This can be a particular issue for nurses if the parents are concentrating entirely on the dying child and dealing with their own grief. Other agencies may help provide support for these groups, e.g.

play therapists for siblings, religious figures to help grandparents.

When parents are not present when their child dies

If parents have not been present at the death of their child, they must be informed as soon as possible after death. Someone who has access to accurate information about the circumstances of the child's death and the experience and confidence to inform the relatives should perform this task. It is important to be gentle but direct. Using simple language such as 'she has died', rather than euphemisms such as 'she has passed away', will avoid misunderstandings and help parents to acknowledge their child's death – the first step towards acceptance (Nelson 1995). Do not be afraid of silence once the news of the death has been given. In a study of bereaved parents, Soutter (1994) was told by them that 'words were not necessary because the pain was too great and could not easily be assuaged'. However, the same study also highlighted the comfort that was afforded to parents by the physical contact of an embrace. In some cultures, relatives are expected to show their grief by wailing and keening. This can be very noisy and possibly cause distress to staff and any other patients or relatives who may be nearby (in a hospital setting). Explanation that this is their way of expressing their grief should be given.

Bereavement care after a child has died

Parents

Invite parents and family to help with washing and dressing their child after death. This need not be rushed. Some parents will not want to be involved; others may welcome the opportunity (Browne & Waddington 1993). When parents wish to be involved, be sensitive as to whether or not your presence is required. Gentle explanation should be given to parents who choose to be involved. They should know that as their child is moved, air may escape from the lungs and result in a noise which may sound like a groan. They should also be aware there may be leakage of body fluids and that blood will pool according to gravity and may make their child's skin appear a strange colour.

Support beyond the time immediately following death

Brown (1993) stresses the vital importance of advice, counselling and support for bereaved parents. Care and ongoing support for bereaved parents is becoming more widely available with ever-increasing numbers of bereavement groups established. Examples of national groups are those such as the Compassionate Friends, SANDS (the Stillbirth and Neonatal Death Society), the Child Bereavement Trust and the Child Death Helpline. There are also many groups related to specific illness such as the Children's Liver Disease Foundation and SPOCC (Society of Parents of Children with Cancer). Often, there are local groups established in response to an identified need, such as the Forget-Me-Not Club described by Walters and Nelson (1997). It is useful to have a resource which lists all the available agencies, for example the Contact-a-family Directory. Parents should not be pushed into counselling. In the early stages of grief, they may not yet feel able to address counselling. They should also be told that access to counselling can be at any time, even years after the death of their child.

Siblings and friends of the child

Although the need to support parents is now well recognised, help for siblings or the dead child's friends may not be so readily available. Simmons (1992) describes how, as a school nurse, she encountered bereaved children who were not receiving adequate support to help them deal with their grief. It is important that these children are not forgotten. The school nurse, health visitor and relatives such as the grandparents and aunts and uncles may be enlisted to help support these children if there are no established bereavement groups for their benefit.

Staff

Anonymous (1993) and Brown (1993) highlight the issue of 'who cares for the carers' and suggest that all nurses involved in the death of a child should be offered some sort of counselling, if only to evaluate the impact of the event. However, surely this sentiment should be extended further. The whole multidisciplinary team cares for a child and the whole multidisciplinary team may therefore be affected by the death of that child. The possibility of a multidisciplinary forum, facilitated by a trained counsellor, to discuss feelings surrounding the child's death should be considered. Suitable facilitators may be found from the clinical psychology department, the clergy or occupational health service. It is also important to be aware if there are any members of the team who might require individual support.

Equipment needed for caring for a child after death

- Warm water for washing the child
- Soap
- Towels
- Clean nappy (if child still in nappies)
- Clean clothing which can be day or night-clothes according to the parents' preference
- Dressings if necessary (if there are cannulae, percutaneous lines or drains to be removed), e.g. small adhesive, waterproof plasters and gauze swabs or padding in case of leakage of body fluids from any wounds
- Spigots or plugs to cap the end of cannulae, drainage tubes, etc. if they are to be left in situ for a post-mortem
- Gauze swabs in case the child's eyes need to be covered to help them remain closed
- Clean bed linen
- Linen skip for dirty linen
- Brush or comb
- Identity band with child's name and hospital registration number or labels which concur with local policy, e.g. Notice of Death Certificate and tape or safety pin to secure it to the sheet covering the body
- Clean sheet, big enough to wrap around the child's body
- Toy to place with the body if parents request it
- Flowers, if available, may be placed in the child's hand or nearby if suitable to the child's age and sex.

The following may also be needed:

- Documentation to list and record the child's belongings
- Scissors and a suitable container for obtaining and keeping a lock of the child's hair
- Equipment for taking hand and feet prints or casts
- Camera for photograph.

Photographs taken after death can be very important. Hawley (1997) describes that 'photographs taken at that time are among our most precious reminders [of the dead child]'. If it is a neonate who has died, it may be the only picture of their child that the parents will ever have.

Note: Some hospitals provide bereavement packs. They may include prompts to provide mementoes such as footprints, photographs, and information about how to register the death, people who could offer help and support groups.

Some hospitals have special Moses baskets, cots or prams in which to place an infant's body.

A body bag made of heavy, waterproof plastic with zip, of a size suitable to contain the body, will be necessary if the child was suffering from hepatitis B, AIDS or was HIV positive.

Method

1. Washing and laying out of the body should be considered within 2–3 hours of death. This is because rigor mortis can begin as soon as 2 hours after death, especially if the child's temperature was high at the time of death (Green & Green 1992). This may not always be the case, however, but it may be aesthetically more pleasing if the child has been washed. It is much more difficult to handle a body when rigor has commenced. Once washed, the child can be given back to parents to cuddle if they wish.

2. Remove the bedclothes and straighten the body as far as possible without using force. This may not be possible if the child has a physical deformity such as severe scoliosis, or severely retracted limbs. Support the

head with one small pillow. If the cot is too small for a pillow, consider using a folded, soft towel. Cover the body with a sheet to preserve the child's privacy and dignity.

3. Remove the child's clothing; observe the body for any bruising or signs of injury. Any findings should be noted in the nursing documentation. Cover the body with the sheet.

4. Clean the child's eyes if necessary and close them. If they will not close of their own accord, it may be necessary to place dampened gauze swabs over each eye to help keep them shut. Sometimes a small piece of tape can be used, but it must be of a type which will not cause trauma to the skin when it is removed. Micropore tape is ideal for this.

5. Clean the child's mouth carefully. Often the jaw may be slack and leave the mouth gaping. This can be distressing for parents and presents a risk of leakage of body fluids. If it is gaping, it may be necessary to support the jaw (temporarily) with a small pad (e.g. a rolled face towel) under the chin. It may be acceptable to use a piece of cotton bandage tied gently around the head, but again be careful not to cause any trauma to the skin. Usually, once rigor starts to establish, the mouth will remain closed, unsupported.

6. Leakage of body fluids represents a potential hazard to those who have to handle the body after death (Green & Green 1992). Therefore, empty the bladder by applying gentle pressure to the lower abdomen. If there is a lot of leakage from the bowel or vagina, ensure that a nappy or incontinence pad is used. In any child who wore nappies when alive, the parents will find nothing odd in seeing them in a nappy after death and this will cope with most leakages. An incontinence pad may be more appropriate for an older child.

7. If there is to be a post-mortem, in accordance with instructions from medical staff, lines, drains, catheters and cannulae should be left in situ (Green & Green 1992). Any drainage bags, infusion tubing, etc. must be removed and the lines, drains, catheters and cannulae spigoted to prevent leakage of body fluids.

8. If there is no post-mortem, then everything except tunnelled intravenous catheters should be removed and carefully disposed of according to local policy. Removing tunnelled catheters would cause significant trauma, which is why they should be left in situ. Any wounds left by removing cannulae, drains, etc. should be covered with waterproof tape. Any stoma or wound which could continue to leak should be covered with padding and then waterproof tape to prevent leakage. Any removable sutures or clips should be left in place.

9. If required, cut a lock of hair from the back of the child's head (where it will not be obvious that it has been removed). Take plaster casts or foot and handprints from the child's hands and feet.

10. The child's body should then be washed all over and carefully dried. Applying a little petroleum jelly to the lips will help prevent the skin drying out and prevent any corrosion from gastric juices (Green & Green 1992).

11. If there is jewellery on the body, it is usual to remove it unless it has religious significance. If a nurse removes jewellery, it must only be done in the presence of a witness and its removal must be recorded in the documentation.

12. Make up the bed or cot with fresh linen and dress the child. Comb the hair. Place the child in the bed or cot and add a toy and/or flowers as appropriate. Cover the child with a sheet. Some areas will require that a child who has to be put into a body bag must be placed in it as soon as possible after death. If this has to be done, it is possible to leave the zip part way down so that parents may view the body, but it

should be argued that there is no need for the body to be placed in the bag until it has to go to the mortuary or funeral parlour. The child is no more infectious after death than before and so parents should have the right to hold and cuddle their child in death as they did in life.

13. If parents are unsure whether or not to have photographs of their child, it may be a good idea to take them now. Explain to parents that even if they feel they do not want photographs now, they may subsequently change their minds. Explain that it is possible to take them and place them in the child's medical records so that they may be retrieved for the family at a later date if they do change their minds. **You may not take photographs without the parents' consent.**

14. Ensure that the child has a clearly legible identity name band in situ on the wrist or ankle. Some areas require there to be a name band on both wrist and ankle.

15. Tidy up. Dispose of linen, sharps and clinical waste carefully and safely to prevent injury or cross-infection and in accordance with local policy.

16. Document the child's property, noting if any jewellery was removed and reserve the property for the family to take home if they wish.

17. If parents have not been involved in the laying out of their child, it is at this point that it would be appropriate to ask them to return to spend time with their child. Encourage them to hold and cuddle their child. Do not be afraid to cry in front of the relatives, but ensure that they do not feel that they have to support you. Be aware that in some cultures it is a mark of respect to grieve loudly and obviously after a death.

    Parents should be allowed to spend as much time with their child as possible. If circumstances (e.g. on a busy ward) make this difficult, explain to them beforehand that at this stage they will have limited time. Offer them a private place where they may see their child. This may need to be the hospital chapel or holy room. Some hospitals have special viewing rooms which are decorated like a bedroom and the child's body is placed in a bed, crib or cot according to age. Once the child has gone to the funeral director, the parents should be able to see their child there without any problem. The only exception to this is if the child is in a body bag because of a potential risk of infection. Be aware that, in many cases, once a potentially infectious body has left the hospital, it can only be seen from a distance if at all, and it may be impossible for the parents to hold and cuddle their child again. In this case, it is kindest to hold the body as long as possible where the parents can still have access.

18. When it is time to take the child to the mortuary or the child is to be collected by the funeral director, the body should be wrapped securely in a clean, white sheet, unless the parents specifically request otherwise. If the body has to be placed in a body bag, it must be done before the body goes to the mortuary or funeral parlour. The sheet or bag should be labelled according to local policy.

19. The Notification of Death certificate must accompany the body to the mortuary and is commonly pinned to the sheet. Obviously, pins must not be used on a body bag, as this would damage the integrity of the bag. Sticky tape would suffice. Some areas require a name band label to be attached to the outside of the sheet. The Notification of Death certificate must state if the child has a pacemaker in situ (it must be removed if the body is to be cremated as it is liable to explode during cremation), or if the body is potentially infectious.

20. Ensure that the parents have clear, preferably written instructions about what they must do to register the death, organise the funeral and so on. Verbal instructions may not be assimilated when parents are

distressed. If there is a bereavement pack for parents, give this to them. If there is a bereavement counsellor, they will be able to support the parents through this process and will be able to help parents access support from other agencies such as bereavement groups.

21. Finally, check who has to be informed about the child's death and who is responsible for doing so. Again, bereavement counsellors may do this as part of their role. A checklist such as that illustrated in Table 4.2 may be utilised.

Observations

As previously described, the nurse should observe the child's body for unusual marks and bruising and these should be recorded. The presence of jewellery on the body or the removal of jewellery from the body should also be observed and recorded.

Complications

Complications should not arise in caring for the body as long as careful thought and preparation are exercised. Without thorough preparation, complications that could arise include:

- inappropriate handling of the body in relation to legal requirements (post-mortem), religious custom or the parents' own wishes
- nurses inexperienced in managing the death of a child are left without support or resources to tell them what to do
- additional distress caused to parents who were not made aware of the risk of vocal-type noises emitting from the body or leakage of body fluids
- additional distress caused to parents who are not made fully aware of the procedures surrounding the death of their child, e.g. having to wait for a death certificate leading to a delay in the funeral.

Table 4.2 Checklist of those who may need to be informed of the death of a child

Person/agency to be informed	To be informed by
Named nurse	Nursing staff
Medical records	Nursing staff
General practitioner	Medical staff
Health visitor	Nursing staff
Paramedical staff (physiotherapist, play therapist)	Nursing or medical staff
Religious/spiritual advisor	Nursing staff
Social worker	Nursing staff
Liaison nurse	Nursing staff
Community nurses	Nursing staff
Bereavement counsellor	Nursing staff
School: head, form teacher and school nurse	Hospital school/nursing staff
Siblings' school	Nursing staff
Hospice	Nursing staff

COMMUNITY PERSPECTIVE

CCNs are likely to have been involved with the families of children with life-limiting illnesses during their treatment phase and will have had the opportunity to develop a trusting relationship. They may have met members of the extended family and close friends and will therefore be aware of the family dynamics. They may also have had the opportunity to discuss the family's spiritual beliefs.

When a child enters the palliative stage of illness, the parents should be reassured that this does not mean that no active treatment will take place. Treatment options will change, but symptom control in palliative care is often active treatment. A multidisciplinary approach, involving the CCN, general practitioner and the health visitor will be of the greatest benefit to the family. The primary healthcare team will be dealing with the family for many years after the death of the child. It is also important for the CCN to liaise with school nurses and teachers involved with either the dying child or the child's siblings. School friends may also need help to deal with the situation.

Discussion should take place within the family as to how and where the child will be cared for. So much control has been taken away from the family because of the child's illness that it is imperative that their wishes during the last period of life are valued. It is important to remember that no two families will cope with grief in the same way (ACT & RCPCH 1997).

The decision that the family reaches must be adhered to as closely as resources permit. It is not possible to guarantee that one particular team member will be present at the time of death and the family need to be aware of this. However, they can be reassured that they will, wherever possible, be supported 24 hours a day should they decide to care for their child at home. The government has consistently advocated that children should be cared for in their own homes and that appropriate services are developed to facilitate this (Health Committee 1997, DoH 2003, 2004). In 1998 the Department of Health provided funding for community children's nursing teams in memory of Diana, Princess of Wales (DOH 1998a,b) and in 2003 the New Opportunities Fund provided £48 million of lottery money to expand home-based paediatric palliative care teams in selected primary care trusts across the country. Although these initiatives have greatly improved palliative care options, some small CCN teams may not be able to provide 24-hour cover all the time, depending on their caseload commitment and whether there is more than one child needing palliative care. The family need to have a list of contact numbers and be aware of who is on call. They also need to know the available respite care options should they feel unable to cope at any time. The CCN must be able to recognise that some families need time on their own, away from professional input. The CCN needs to be sensitive to this and to appreciate that, by visiting more than the family wish, the CCN may be answering personal needs, rather than the family's.

The CCN is ideally placed to empower the family to care for their child and maximize the quality of the child's life. This can be an important time for the family to collect mementoes, photographs, video recordings, items made by the dying child, etc. It is a period of adjustment, during which the family may be able to address the reality of impending loss and decide how and what to tell younger children, including the dying child. The CCN plays a crucial role in providing emotional support to the family and in turn will need opportunities to off-load, be this in the form of peer support or more formal clinical supervision (ACT& RCPH 1997, NHS Executive 1998).

During the final period of terminal care, ideally the CCN team will be available to the family at all times. Respite care in the home may be offered. Symptom management, including pain control, is vital and a team member or alternative appropriate cover needs to be accessible at all times, in case treatment regimes need changing or the family require help with nursing care. Regular visits from familiar faces will help to reassure the family.

Community Perspective continues

The CCN will be able to offer guidance on issues surrounding the actual death of the child and the days immediately following. She will be able to discuss:

- the likely manner of death
- the importance of involving siblings and preparing for the death (Dyregrov 1996)
- the long-term benefits of those closely involved seeing and holding the body after death (Dyregrov 1996)
- that parents can wash and dress their child in favourite clothes following death, if they wish
- where the child's body should rest before the funeral: the child's body may remain at home providing certain procedures have been undertaken by the funeral director; alternatively the body can be taken to a Chapel of Rest or a hospice
- how to register the death
- funeral arrangements and what form this important ritual will take. The parents can be encouraged to allow the siblings some choice. Older children who have come to terms with their impending death may have had strong views on funeral arrangements.

In the months following death, many families need to maintain contact with the professionals involved in their child's care (Goldman 1998). Bereavement visiting should continue for as long as both parties feel to be appropriate. Work with siblings can be undertaken, for example collecting together items which remind them of the child and putting them in a memory box. It may be years before the family are ready to place the lid on that box and it is important for them to realise that this is perfectly acceptable. This is something over which they do have control.

CCNs may be involved where children die unexpectedly, for example as a result of major surgery. The CCN may have been involved with the family prior to the hospitalisation which resulted in death. In this situation, bereavement visiting and maintaining contact may be appropriate.

Do and do not

- Do consult the parents about their wishes for their child after they have died.
- Do remember to maintain the privacy and dignity of the child at all times after death.
- Do establish whether there is to be a post-mortem.
- Do establish if there are any special religious needs associated with care of the child after death.
- Do remember that the parents may not be the only family members who require support.

- Do remember to warn parents helping to wash and dress their child after death of how the child may appear, possible noises the body may make and leakage of body fluids.
- Do be aware if there are other staff who may be adversely affected and require support because of the death of a child.
- Do not remove lines, cannulae, etc. if there is to be a post-mortem.
- Do not be afraid to show grief and cry with parents after a child has died, but do not allow your own grief to overshadow any situation or make parents feel that they must comfort and support you.

References

Anonymous 1993 A cry for help. Nursing Times 89(4): 29–30

Association for Children with Life Threatening or Terminal Conditions and their Families (ACT) and Royal College of Paediatrics and Child Health 1997 A guide to the development of children's palliative care services. ACT, Bristol, UK

Association for Children with Life Threatening or Terminal Conditions and their Families (ACT) and Royal College of Paediatrics and Child Health 2003 A guide to the development of children's palliative care services. ACT, Bristol, UK

Back D, Rooke V 1994 The presence of relatives in the resuscitation room. Nursing Times 90(30): 34–35

Brown P 1993 Saying goodbye. Nursing Times 89(4): 26–29

Browne J, Waddington P 1993 Care of the dying child. In: Carter B (ed.) Manual of paediatric intensive care nursing. Chapman and Hall, London, ch 10, p 299

Bull A 2004 Culture and belief system information manual. Yorkhill Division, Greater Glasgow NHS, Glasgow

Carter B 1993 (ed.) Manual of paediatric intensive care nursing. Chapman and Hall, London

Connor P 1996 Should relatives be allowed in the resuscitation room? Nursing Standard 10(44): 42–44

Davies B, Connaughty S 2002 Pediatric end-of-life care: lessons learned from parents. Journal of Nursing Administration 32(1): 5–6

Department of Health 1998a Diana, Princess of Wales Memorial Committee. Preliminary advice. TSO, London

Department of Health 1998b A proposal to develop a national children's community nursing service. DoH, London

Department of Health 2003 Every child matters. DoH, London

Department of Health 2004 National Service Framework for children, young people and maternity services. DoH, London

Dyregrov A 1996 Children's participation in rituals. Bereavement Care 15(1): 2–4

Ellis J, Edwards J 1995 Part of a learning process: the paediatric post-mortem. Child Health 2(6): 244–246

Ellison S 2003 Nurses' attitudes toward family presence during resuscitative efforts and invasive procedures. Journal of Emergency Nursing 29(6): 515–521

Ethnicity Online 2004 Cultural awareness in healthcare. www.ethnicityonline.net

Goldman A 1998 Palliative care for children. In: Fauld C, Carter Y, Woof R (eds) Handbook of palliative care. Blackwell Science, London

Green J, Green M 1992 Dealing with death. Practices and procedures. Chapman and Hall, London, chs 13, 16–31, p 115–123, 149–230

Haas F 2003 Bereavement care: seeing the body. Nursing Standard 17(28): 33–37

Hanson C, Strawser D 1992 Family presence during cardiopulmonary resuscitation: Foote hospital emergency department's nine-year perspective. Journal of Emergency Nursing 18(2): 104–106

Hawley R 1997 Seasons of grief. Nursing Times 93(8): 24–26

Health Committee 1997 House of Commons Select Committee. Health services for children and young people in the community: home and school. Third Report. TSO, London

Hindmarch C 2000 On the death of a child. Radcliffe Medical Press, Oxon, UK

Human Tissue Act 1961 HMSO, London

Kelly E 1992 Encouraging shared care. Nursing Standard 6: 42

Meyers T, Eichhorn D J, Guzzetta C E et al 2000 Family presence during invasive procedures and resuscitation: the experience of family members, nurses and physicians. American Journal of Nursing 100(2): 32–43

Nelson L 1995 When a child dies. American Journal of Nursing 95(3): 61–64

NHS Executive 1998 Evaluation of the pilot project programme for children with life threatening illnesses. TSO, London

Read S 2002 Loss and bereavement: a nursing response. Nursing Standard 16(37): 47–55

Registration of Births, Deaths, and Marriages Regulations 1968 HMSO, London

Renzi-Brown J 1989 Risk management specialist. Nursing 19(2): 43–46

Royal Liverpool Children's Inquiry 2001 TSO, London

Scottish Executive Health Department 2002 Guidelines on Chaplaincy and Spiritual Care in the NHS in Scotland. Scottish Executive Health Department, Edinburgh

Simmons M 1992 Helping children grieve. Nursing Times 88(50): 30–32

Skene C 1998 Individualised bereavement care. Paediatric Nursing 10(10): 13–16

Soutter J 1994 A strategy for caring for families in bereavement. Nursing Times 90(30): 37–39

Vanderbeek J 2000 Till death do us part. American Journal of Nursing 100(2): 44

Walters C, Nelson P 1997 Never too late. Nursing Times 93(8): 27

Whittle M, Cutts S 2002 Time to go home: assisting families to take their child home following a planned hospital or hospice death. Paediatric Nursing 14(10): 24–28

Practice 5

Blood glucose estimation

Mark Denial

Introduction

Blood glucose estimation may be needed for a number of medical reasons within both the acute setting and the community.

Within the hospital the nurse may need to check a child's blood glucose level if the child is undergoing treatment which may *potentially* cause a rise in the blood glucose level, e.g. during the use of steroids. If the child is susceptible to hypoglycaemia or is unconscious, the blood glucose level will also be taken. Neonates in particular may be prone to hypoglycaemia and consequently may require regular blood glucose monitoring when cared for within the neonatal unit (Baumeister et al 2001).

The most common reason for the monitoring of blood glucose may be associated with the management of diabetes mellitus, which also involves the education of the child and their parent/guardian.

At both ward-based level and within the child's home blood glucose monitoring is undertaken using blood glucose meters. There are many types of blood glucose meter in use within the National Health Service and selec-

tion of the meter should be based on the age of the child and the skills level of the parents (Page et al 2001). In practice, however, each hospital will have its own selection of blood glucose meters for use.

These guidelines are related to one specific method of blood glucose estimation using the Accu-Chek Advantage blood glucose meter, but the principles are the same for the majority of meters.

Learning outcomes

By the end of this section you should:
- be able to identify when an estimate of blood glucose level is needed
- appreciate the need to use a finger-pricking device to obtain a sample of blood
- appreciate the need to use the sides of the fingers for obtaining a capillary blood sample
- be able to use the Accu-Chek Advantage blood glucose meter
- be able to interpret the result, record it and liaise with other healthcare professionals when appropriate.

Rationale for blood glucose monitoring

Monitoring of blood glucose can give vital information on the current physiological status of the acutely ill child and also inform us of the effectiveness of the treatment that the child is receiving (Fain 2004). Capillary blood glucose measurement should only be performed by staff who have undertaken a training programme and been regularly updated, as the results obtained may affect the treatment of the child (Page et al 1996, Harrop et al 1999).

Factors to note

Educating the child and carer

Whenever possible, the diabetes specialist nurse, the diabetes ward link nurse or a nurse who has undergone appropriate education/training will teach the child and parent how to monitor the blood glucose levels. In some instances other ward/department nurses will need to carry out this procedure as long as they have undertaken the appropriate training (SIGN 2001). This may be necessary when a child is diagnosed with insulin-dependent diabetes mellitus, or for children who are receiving treatment, or have a condition which affects their blood glucose level and who therefore require ongoing measurement within the home.

When children or carers are being taught a practical skill, they need to know the importance of the procedure and how to interpret the results.

It is vital to the well-being of the child and family that adequate education is provided, as studies have shown that failing to meet the needs of the family increases the stress they feel and therefore the parents are less able to support their child (SIGN 2001).

To provide an appropriate teaching programme, the nurse has to assess the child and the child's family separately before undertaking an education plan for blood glucose measurement. Even young children have the ability to learn, and be competent in doing, blood glucose monitoring. Play is often a fun way of educating a young child (Hatcher 1990).

Guidelines

It is vital that the principles of performing a capillary blood glucose measurement are followed both within the acute setting and during patient and carer education. When using a blood glucose meter the manufacturer's instructions should be adhered to.

Equipment

- Accu-Chek Advantage blood glucose meter (see Fig. 5.1)
- Advantage 2 test strips
- Finger-pricking device for multiple patient use or single patient use
- Appropriate lancet for finger pricker
- Cotton wool/gauze
- Latex-free disposable gloves
- Sharps bin.

Method and rationale

1. Explain the procedure to the child (if appropriate) and the family. This will help to alleviate any anxiety they may have.
2. Prepare all the equipment as listed. This will encourage a smooth procedure.
3. Ensure the meter has been quality controlled. If not, carry out this procedure first following the manufacturer's instructions.
4. Check the expiry date of the test strips. Out-of-date strips will give inaccurate results because of contamination, but as long as the

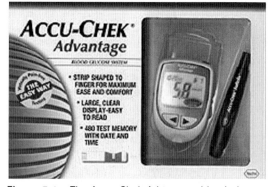

Figure 5.1   The Accu-Chek Advantage blood glucose meter. (Reproduced with permission from Roche Diagnostics Ltd.)

strips have been stored correctly they will remain stable until the expiry date.

5. The person taking the blood sample should wash and dry their hands with soap and water to reduce the risk of cross-contamination.

6. Wash the child's hands with soap and warm water, remembering to rinse and dry thoroughly.

7. The nurse should wear gloves according to hospital policy.

8. Put the test strip into the meter and check the code on the screen with the code on the side of the box. If different, change the test strips and coding chip for new as per the manufacturer's instructions as any results will be inaccurate.

9. Check that the length of the needle is appropriate for the child and prick the side of the finger, or heel, with either the child's own device or the one recommended by the hospital.

10. Milk the finger in a downward stroke until there is a reasonable hanging drop of blood. A drop of blood is needed to ensure full coverage (see Fig. 5.2).
    Note: The manufacturer's instructions recommend using the *first* drop of blood acquired.

11. Move the blood glucose strip towards the drop of blood (strip will soak up blood).
    Note: Insufficient covering of the test strip will give an inaccurate result as will smearing or blotting the blood onto the pad.

12. When the strip takes up sufficient blood, the meter will beep. Countdown will then commence.

13. A second beep will be heard when the result is ready. If the meter reads 'Hi', the result is over 33.3 mmol/l; if the meter reads 'Lo', the result is under 0.6 mmol/l.

14. Record the result in a record book or on a ward/department recording sheet and report any abnormality to the medical staff if appropriate (refer to local guidelines for normal parameters).

15. Dispose of sharps immediately, according to local policy, to prevent needlestick injuries.

Factors to note during the procedure

- Alcohol-based wipes should not be used as they will react with reagents in the strip and give a false reading.
- Washing hands and wearing gloves reduces the risk of cross-infection and removes any glucose from the skin.
- Warm water will also help promote blood flow to the fingers.
- A finger pricker should always be used because, owing to the measured depth of the device, it reduces the pain to the finger or heel.
- Heel pricks are needed in babies and young children to obtain a capillary sample.
- The sides of fingers should be used. Avoid using the pads of fingers as this reduces sensation. Young children use the pincer action for picking up objects and repeatedly pricking finger pads will cause more discomfort (Page et al 1999).
- If there is not enough blood, the meter will read 'ERROR'. You will need to re-check all of the above and re-test.

Observations and complications

The normal range for blood glucose level should be 4–7 mmol/l (Page et al 1999).

It is important to clarify with the medical staff at what point they should be informed if the blood test result falls outside of this range; depending on hospital policy, it may be necessary to send a blood sample for estimating true blood glucose level. This will also depend on the child's condition and treatment.

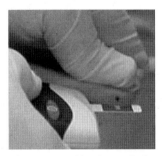

Figure 5.2   *Obtaining a blood sample for checking*

Do and do not

- Do explain the procedure to the child and the family and the reason for the test.
- Do give the family adequate instruction and written instructions on the practice if they are to continue checking the glucose levels at home.
- Do explain the range that the blood glucose level should fall between, giving contact numbers for advice if the result is abnormal, if the family are to continue to monitor the blood glucose levels at home.
- Do ensure that the strips are stored at room temperature and the bottle is kept sealed at all times. Contamination is caused by moisture in the air and incorrect storage affects the readings.
- Do perform control tests on meters following manufacturers' instructions. This should be performed once a week if the child is cared for at home using a meter and as per local policy for meters in hospital.
- Do not change strips from one tube to another; all bottles have their own code number on the side of the bottle. This is especially important when using a blood glucose sensor for the reading of the strip. There is also an expiry date on each bottle.
- Do not use Mediswabs as they harden the skin and cause discomfort when the finger is pricked.
- Do not cut the strips as this allows the chemicals to leak out and contaminate the rest of the strips.

References

Baumeister F A M, Rolinski B, Busch R, Emmrich P 2001 Glucose monitoring with long term subcutaneous microdialysis in neonates. Pediatrics 108(5): 1187–1192

Fain J A 2004 Helping your patient carefully weigh the available options so he can choose wisely. Nursing 34(11): 48–51

Harrop M, Thornton H, Woodhall C, Ratcliff J 1999 Improving paediatric diabetes care. Nursing Standard 13(51): 38–43

Hatcher T 1990 Learning is fun. Paediatric Nursing (March): 10–12

Page N, Mackowiak L, Bratt K 1999 Identifying and caring for the child with new onset Type 1 diabetes. JSPN 4(3): 128–130

Page N E, Mackowiak L, Bratt K 2001 Identifying and caring for the child with new onset type 1 diabetes. 'Ask the expert' JSPN 4(2): July–September

Page S R, Scholey K, Clarke P et al 1996 The effect of a quality assurance scheme and compulsory training programme on the performance of ward-based blood glucose measurements. Practical Diabetes International 13(5): 144–147

SIGN 2001 Scottish Intercollegiate Guidelines Network management of diabetes. National Clinical Guideline No. 55. SIGN, Edinburgh

Further Reading

Bannister M 1996 Promotion of diabetes self-care through play. Professional Nurse 12(2): 109–112

Selekman J, Scofield S, Swenson-Brousell C 1999 Diabetes update in the pediatric population. Pediatric Nursing 25(6): 97–105

Seley J 2000 Blood glucose testing. American Journal of Nursing 100(8): 24A–24G

Practice 6

Bowel care

Louise Dyer

Introduction

The concept of what a 'normal' bowel movement is varies considerably between individuals. Parents are no different and some will become concerned if their child has not had a bowel movement every day (Thompson 2001c). There is now a growing body of literature indicating that nurses have an important role in the prevention and management of constipation in children and young people (Rogers 1997, 2000, Allen 1998, Day 2001, Thompson 2001c); however, there is a general lack of empirical research-based evidence demonstrating the importance of the role of the nurse in care delivery (Farell et al 2003).

The RCN (2003a) guidelines on digital rectal examination (DRE) highlight the fact that many nurses are concerned about DRE and the manual evacuation of faeces. These are invasive procedures that do not form part of the normal assessment and delivery of care for infants, chil-

dren and young people with bowel problems. However, for some children and young people, especially those with spinal injuries, these procedures can become an important part of their bowel management (RCN 2003a). The RCN (2003b) also recommend that all trusts/hospitals develop a strategy to ensure that when DREs are required, care is delivered by those on the children's nurses registers (Part 8 or Part 15) of the Nursing and Midwifery Council's register. Carrying out a DRE and other related procedures requires the skill and expertise of an expert practitioner; this is not a procedure that should be considered as a part of routine practice (RCN 2003a). The DRE guidelines (RCN 2003a) also clearly outline the need to listen to children and young people and the importance of informed consent from them and their family members before carrying out all such invasive procedures; this includes all aspects of bowel care.

Learning outcomes

By the end of this section you should be able to:

- list the potential causes of constipation/diarrhoea
- identify the role of the children's nurse in preventing constipation
- discuss health promotion strategies used to promote normal bowel habits
- identify the potential consequences of abnormal bowel habits for the child and family.

Definitions of terms

- The word 'constipation' has Latin origins and means 'constipare' or to crowd together (Rogers 2003); constipation is now generally defined as difficulty or a delay in the passage of stools that may not necessarily be hard in consistency (Buchanan 1992, Rogers 2000).
- Encopresis is referred to as the movement of stools in a place that is not considered to be socially acceptable and that the underlying reason is not one of constipation (Rogers 2000).
- Diarrhoea is referred to as a change in bowel habit that results in frequent and/or loose(er) stools (Armon et al 2001).
- Soiling is the passage or leaking of fluid or semi-solid stool into the underclothing; this is usually as a result of overflow from a rectum that is loaded with faeces (Enuresis Resource and Information Centre 2001, Burnett & Wilkins 2002).

Factors to note

Growth and development issues

According to Felt et al (1999) and Rasquin-Weber et al (1999) the daily frequency of defaecation of infants and children varies with age. The issue of what is normal in terms of defaecation is further compounded by the fact that very little is known about the normal bowel habits of children, particularly those of school age (Yong & Beattie 1998). This is further compounded when the infant or child has disabilities (Bosch et al 2002).

The Department of Health (1997) and Murphy (2001) note that, for community children's nurses, infants and children with constipation can represent 36% of their caseload. Therefore nurses and other healthcare professionals have an important role to play in terms of promotion of healthy bowel habits (Farrell et al 2003). For this to occur it is essential that the children's nurse understands the need for a healthy diet balanced with adequate fluid intake, together with an understanding of the normal physiology of the bowel and the mechanisms of defaecation.

There is a clear relationship between dietary fibre intake and constipation which implies there is some parental control or lack in terms of the dietary fibre that children and young people consume, thus suggesting a lack of parenting skills. This may result in feelings of guilt and the expectation that healthcare professionals will blame the parents for the child's condition (Cavet 1998, Day 2001, Farrell et al 2003).

Psychosocial issues

Constipation in children can result in significant levels of stress for the family and needs effective treatment and management (Elshimy et al 2000). Farrell et al (2003) report that healthcare professionals can underestimate the impact of childhood constipation on all members of the family; if left untreated, this can be significant and can impact upon the relationships between parents and within families (Muir & Burnett 1999). Other potential problems include social isolation, which may result in a negative impact upon the child's self-confidence and a subsequent lack of self-esteem (Goh et al 2001). This can result in failure to achieve at school and has the potential for being a precursor to mental ill health (Bond & Bond 1992, Murphy 2001).

Vernon et al (2003) highlight the importance of the need of children to use the toilet regularly whilst at school in order to encourage normal processes of elimination. The findings of this pilot study demonstrated that a significant number of children deliberately avoid the use of the school toilets and resist the need to have a 'poo'. The children cited a lack of privacy, poor hygiene of the actual toilets, a lack of handwashing facilities and the threat of being bullied as the reasons for avoidance of use of school toilets. Improvements in standards of toilets in schools would be cost effective, not only in terms of preventing infectious diseases but also in the prevention of urinary tract infections and bowel problems (Barnes & Maddocks 2002, Vernon et al 2003). These issues are a cause for concern, not only for those that set the standards for school toilets but also for those healthcare professionals working with children in schools; Barnes and Maddocks (2002) advocate that the standards set for toilets in the workplace should also be applied to schools. The Bog Standard Campaign calls for minimum standards in both drinking water and toilet facilities as a prerequisite to child health (Enuresis Resource and Information Centre 2003).

NORMAL BOWEL MOVEMENTS

Infants (see also Feeding, p. 159)

- Within the first weeks of life the infant produces approximately four stools a day. This reduces to two per day when the infant reaches 4 months of age (Felt et al 1999).
- There are also differences between stools of breast-fed and formula-fed babies; for example, breast-fed babies may have twice as many stools as formula-fed babies. Alternatively, there may be a gap between bowel movements of breast-fed babies. In some instances this can be a week or longer; however, the stools are still soft (Hymans et al 1995).
- Hard stools may be more prevalent in infants that are formula fed due to differences in fat digestion and absorption between breast milk and formula feeds (Forsyth et al 1999).
- The transfer from breast to formula feeding may also be associated with 'functional constipation', i.e. a combination of associated factors that may be closely related (Clayden 1992, Rasquin-Weber et al 1999).

Children

- Most children achieve bowel control before or simultaneously with bladder control (Brazelton 1962, cited by Loening-Baucke 1998).
- The average age for toilet training to be completed is approximately 28 months of age (Brazelton 1962, cited by Loening-Baucke 1998).
- A small survey conducted by Yong and Beattie (1998) indicates that in their sample of primary school children at least 60% opened their bowels once a day.
- Anything less than three bowel motions per week indicates the child should be considered 'at risk' from developing constipation (Leung et al 1996).
- Approximately 34% of 4–11 year olds experience constipation, with 5% experiencing chronic constipation, i.e. lasting more than 6 months (Yong & Beattie 1998).

Children with developmental delay

- Del Giudice et al (1999) noted that 74% of children with cerebral palsy have chronic constipation.
- For these children, bowel and bladder control may not occur simultaneously (Bosch et al 2002).
- Tse et al (2000) identified that 50% of children with developmental delay had chronic constipation.
- Children with Down syndrome are also prone to constipation (Buie & Flores Sandoval 1995, cited by Bosch et al 2002).

POTENTIAL CHANGES IN BOWEL MOVEMENTS

CONSTIPATION

Possible causes of constipation include:
- *Diet* – a lack of fibre can result in a lack of agents to bulk the faeces, causing a decrease in peristaltic movement; this is often found to be a direct consequence of being a 'faddy eater' and/or having a poor appetite (Rogers 2003).

- *Fluid intake* – drinking too much milk and inadequate solid food consumption (Iacano et al 1998). Poor fluid intake or excessive loss through diarrhoea/vomiting or a high temperature, therefore causing stools to harden (Clayden 1992, Leung et al 1996).
- *Lifestyle changes* – many children have lifestyles that are sedentary in nature because of the increased popularity of computer and video games (Burnett & Wilkins 2002).
- *Physiological problems* – for example Hirschsprung's disease (congenital megacolon). This occurs in 1:5000 infants and is diagnosed by rectal biopsy which will indicate a lack of parasympathetic ganglion cells in the wall of the large bowel (Thompson 2001b). Treatment involves a surgical resection of the affected gut, usually in the first year of life (Thompson 2001b). Approximately 3–10% of children with Down syndrome also have Hirschsprung's disease (Buie et al 1995, cited by Bosch et al 2002).
- *Drug-induced constipation* – some medication can cause constipation, for example antihistamines, some anticonvulsants and pain medication (opiates) (Di Lorenzo 2000, Nurko et al 2001).
- *Metabolic disorders* – for example hypothyroidism, hypercalcaemia and hypokalaemia (Nurko et al 2001).
- *Perineal or rectal pain when defaecating* (Borowitz et al 2003 cited by Rogers 2003) – for example an anal fissure or possible child sexual abuse (Rogers 2003).
- *Delays in defaecation* (Taylor 2000) – can be due to associated pain on defaecation; for example ignoring the need to have a 'poo' because of the poor provision of facilities at school (Vernon et al 2003).
- *Familial tendencies* – constipation in parents may result in constipation in one child or siblings (Keuzenkamp-Jansen et al 1996, Burnett et al 2004).

Implications for nursing practice

Ideally any treatment and/or bowel management for children and their families should take place in the community with healthcare professionals that are appropriately qualified; it is also important to have the needs of the child and family central to delivering care (Farell et al 2003, Rogers 2003). Treatment in the community has been proven to be more effective and less expensive when compared to treatment in the acute care sector (DoH 1997). Burnett et al (2004) acknowledge that clinical nurse specialists have an important role in the management of constipation, not only within the acute care setting but within primary care as well.

Families need to be reassured that their needs and concerns are taken seriously and interventions are planned to meet their actual, not perceived, needs. Most children that suffer from faecal soiling benefit from well-managed supportive interventions; when parents understand the problem they are then able to realise that soiling is not deliberate and this in turn can help to reduce some of the stress and strain families find themselves under (Lucy 1999). Likewise, helping children to understand the problem can help them to be motivated to help themselves (Rennie et al 1997); an initial assessment that is detailed and traces the child's history of bowel habits is therefore essential (Rogers 2003).

Principles in managing functional constipation

- *Soften and clear any impacted faecal matter* – this may involve the use of a hypertonic phosphate enema and is best given in a clinic by an appropriately qualified healthcare professional. There have been some reported cases of severe electrolyte imbalances and fatalities in children under 4 years of age; therefore it is vital that close medical supervision is available (Loening-Baucke 1998). If the child has retained a large faecal mass then the only option possible is to carry out an evacuation under general anaesthetic (Rogers 2000).

- *Dietary and fluid advice* – children should be encourage to take regular water-based drinks throughout the day, with extra fluid taken when the weather is hot; if the child is reluctant to take extra fluids an alternative could be ice lollies or jellies. Whilst there is no recommended daily intake of fibre for children there is a general consensus that this is calculated using the given formula (Rogers 2003, p. 552).

Child's age + 5 = daily amount of fibre intake in grams (up to age 13 years).

Dietary fibre increases water retention and any increase in intake must be accompanied by an increase in fluid intake (Loening-Baucke 1998, Rogers 2003). The increased consumption of high-fibre, insoluble foods is more effective than advocating the increase of fluid intake on its own, for example, fruits, vegetables and cereals (Yong & Beattie 1998, Burnett & Wilkins 2002).

● *Establish regular pain-free patterns of defaecation* – encourage the child to sit on the toilet with legs well supported (Loening-Baucke 1997, Rogers 2003) for 5 minutes up to three or four times a day. Attempts to defaecate should follow meals to maximise the use of the gastric–colonic reflex (Loening-Baucke 1998, Rogers 2003).

● *Maintenance of regular bowel movements* – this may require the use of laxatives that should be based on individual assessment of need and may include softening agents such as lactulose or a stimulant such as senna (Rogers 2000). There is general consensus that laxative use may have to continue for at least a year (Loening-Baucke 1998, Rogers 2003). After regular bowel habits have been established then the dosage of laxatives can be gradually reduced (Loening-Baucke 1998).

● *Ongoing support* – this is vital and some studies have indicated that children can have ongoing problems with constipation and encopresis for up to 12 months following initial treatment and care management (Clayden 1992, Loening-Baucke 1998). Procter and Loader (2003) have reported in their study that some children had persistent problems with constipation 6 years later, suggesting that constipation is not something that children can 'grow out of'.

● *Exercise* – whilst there is little scientific evidence to support the benefit of exercise as a means of reducing the incidence of constipation, exercise is useful in reducing obesity and other diseases, e.g. type 2 diabetes (Burnett & Wilkins 2002); the increase in non-sedentary play activities should therefore be encouraged.

Factors to note

Medication used to treat constipation
Within the UK the treatment of constipation is well established; however, there is no definitive set of guidelines to inform treatment protocols and the laxatives that should be used to treat constipation in children. This is further compounded by the fact that many of the drugs that are prescribed are not licensed for use for children or are used in doses that exceed manufacturers' recommendations (Price & Elliott 2004). For further discussion of drug licensing, see Administration of Medicines, p. 47.

Rectal examination is an invasive procedure and should only be used for infants and children when a part of a prescribed regime of treatment (Winnett 1999, RCN 2003a). Enemas should therefore only be used with a high degree of caution and administered by an appropriately qualified nurse specialist (Rasquin-Weber et al 1999, RCN 2003a). The preferred choice of medication is the use of oral preparations (Thompson 2001c).

Softening agents
● *Docusate sodium* (Dioctyl) – this is available as a suspension for children and helps to reduce the surface tension of the hard stools, therefore allowing water to .be absorbed to soften the stool (Burnett & Wilkins 2002).
● *Lactulose* – this osmotic laxative can be given up to three times a day and over long periods of time.
● *Liquid paraffin* – the use of this is debatable because of side-effects such as the absorption into the circulatory system and it is not recommended for children under 12 months of age (Sharif et al 2001). The main problem associated with the use of liquid paraffin is the potential of oil leaking through the anal sphincter (Burnett & Wilkins 2002).

Agents used for the evacuation of the bowels

- *Senna* – this stimulates the contraction of smooth muscle in the colon and the transport of fluids and electrolytes and leads to defaecation (Burnett & Wilkins 2002, Rogers 2003). Senna is often used as an alternative when the child refuses other medication such as lactulose or sorbitol. The laxative dose should be adjusted to result in one or two bowel movements per day that are loose enough not to cause the child pain upon defaecation (Loening-Baucke 1998).
- *Movicol* – a glycol preparation with added electrolytes known as polyethylene glycol 3350 (PEG) (Rogers 2003). According to Vincent and Candy (2001) Movicol has been found to be a safe and effective treatment and is generally well tolerated by children; unlike some medication, Movicol has been licensed for use for children aged 2 years and older since September 2003 (Rogers 2003). Polyethylene glycol without electrolytes is also licensed for use for children aged 8 years and older and can be used to manage care for children with constipation in the long term; it can be dissolved in any clear liquid drink of the child's choice (Pashankar & Bishop 2001, Loening-Baucke 2002).
- *Bisacodyl* (Dulco-lax) – is often preferred for older children if they are able to swallow tablets (Burnett & Wilkins 2002).

Administration of enemas and suppositories

The administration of medications via the rectum is a procedure frequently performed by nurses and does carry with it potential risks, which can be fatal (Rasquin-Weber et al 1999, Addison et al 2000). Consequently, any nurse undertaking these procedures must have the relevant knowledge and skills to carry out these procedures safely and effectively (Addison et al 2000). Any nurse required to carry out DRE or to administer medications via the rectum must refer to the trust/hospital's policies and procedures and should also consider personal professional development and additional training needs (Dowse 2000, cited by Willis 2000).

Suppositories

Which way up to administer suppositories is debated. Moppett (2000) maintains that current recommendations from manufacturers either suggest apex (pointed end) first insertion or make no recommendations at all. Mallett and Bailey (1996) suggest that medication that is to be absorbed from the rectum should be inserted blunt end first; however, according to Campbell (1993) suppositories used for bowel evacuation should be inserted pointed end first. Moppett (2000) concludes by suggesting that the lack of evidence to currently inform these practices highlights deficits in the research-based literature and more studies are needed to advocate either blunt end or pointed end insertion. For further details of how to administer suppositories, see Further Reading.

Enemas

When administering enemas they should be at room temperature or warmed to minimise shock and to prevent bowel spasm (Mallett & Bailey 1996). Steroid enemas should be given after defaecation, ideally at bedtime with the bed elevated to aid retention (Mallett & Bailey 1996). It is important that the contents of the enema are not forced in the rectum but to allow gravity to aid the process, otherwise this could result in bowel spasm (Mallett & Bailey 1996).

DIARRHOEA

Possible causes of diarrhoea include:

- Infections: enteral infections, e.g. viral (commonest cause), bacterial, parasitic; non-enteral infections, e.g. otitis media, pneumonia, urinary tract
- Appendicitis, intussusception, short bowel syndrome
- Malabsorption syndromes: coeliac disease, cystic fibrosis
- Constipation with overflow
- Drug induced, e.g. antibiotics
- Food allergy/intolerance (of lactulose or cow's milk protein)
- Child abuse: Münchausen by proxy, sexual (Source: Armon et al 2001)

- Eating contaminated foods or water (undercooked or raw foods) (Jones 2002)
- Faecal/oral route – as a consequence of poor handwashing technique and contaminated toys (Jones 2002)
- Chronic non-specific diarrhoea (CNSD) or toddler diarrhoea (Thompson 2001a).

Toddler diarrhoea

Patterns of bowel movements in healthy toddlers vary in terms of consistency and the number of stools. The stools in toddler diarrhoea are different and are often reported as being offensive in terms of smell and paler colour when compared to normal stools and may be so loose that the stool contains mucus and undigested food substances (Thompson 2001a). Toddler diarrhoea may be intermittent, and often occurs following a bout of gastroenteritis. Toddler diarrhoea is the most frequent cause of chronic diarrhoea in developed Western countries (Hoekstra 1998).

Toddler diarrhoea is attributed to the changes in diet now offered to children; this includes a constant fluid intake, which can often result in excessive amounts of fruit juices being consumed, in addition to a low-fat and low-fibre diet (Thompson 2001a). Hoekstra (1998) argues that toddler diarrhoea is more of a nutritional disorder than a disease and advocates the four 'Fs' (fat, fluid, fruit, fibre) as being central to management; this involves normalising feeding patterns.

- *Fat intake* – parents need to be aware of the fact that fat restriction in the diet of infants and toddlers is inappropriate, because a diet with a normal fat intake will help to reduce gastric emptying (Thompson 2001a). It is therefore recommended that fat intake is increased to 35–40% of total energy levels (Thompson 2001a).
- *Fluid intake* – children with CNSD often drink excessive amounts of fluid (Thompson 2001a).
- *Fruit juices* – the drinking of water has been replaced with the consumption of fruit juices or squashes (Hoekstra 1998). Hymans and Leichtner (1985) found that clear apple

juice is associated with the symptoms of toddler diarrhoea; however, cloudy apple juice appears to be well tolerated (Hoekstra et al 1995).
- *Fibre intake* – convenience foods contain inadequate amounts of fibre to meet minimum dietary recommendations (Hoekstra 1998); encouraging a balanced diet containing grains, fruit and vegetables will help to rectify the situation (Thompson 2001a).

Factors to note

- Diarrhoea is defined as a change in bowel habit that results in the child having more frequent and/or looser stools; acute diarrhoea is often caused by infectious intestinal disease (IID) (Armon et al 2001).
- Diarrhoea with or without vomiting occurs, on average, twice per year for children under the age of 5 years (Jones 2002). Of all the children who attend an Accident and Emergency Department, 16% present with symptoms of diarrhoea (with or without vomiting) (Armon et al 2001). Djuretic et al (1999) estimated that approximately 526 000 children aged under 5 years have an IID resulting in the parents (carers) seeking advice from a healthcare professional.
- Gastroenteritis admission rates are reported to be higher when the child(ren) comes from a deprived area (Olowokure et al 1999).
- Normalising feeding patterns, avoiding excessive use of fruit juices and increasing fat and fibre intake should be the most effective way of managing toddler diarrhoea (Hoekstra 1998, Thompson 2001a).

Assessment of dehydration

For the purposes of assessment, dehydration can be classified as mild, moderate or severe and children rarely fall into one category or another (Jones 2002). Table 6.1 describes the symptoms associated with dehydration.

For the management of dehydration and gastroenteritis in infants and children, see Armon et al (2001) and Jones (2002).

Table 6.1 Symptoms associated with dehydration

Symptom	Minimal or no dehydration (<3% loss of body weight)	Mild to moderate dehydration (3–9% loss of body weight)	Severe dehydration (>9% loss of body weight)
Mental status	Well, alert	Normal, fatigued or restless, irritable	Apathetic, lethargic, unconscious
Thirst	Drinks normally	Thirsty, eager to drink	Drinks poorly, unable to drink
Heart rate	Normal	Normal to increased	Tachycardia, with bradycardia in most severe cases
Quality of pulses	Normal	Normal to decreased	Weak, thready or impalpable
Breathing	Normal	Normal, fast	Deep
Eyes	Normal	Slightly sunken	Deeply sunken
Tears	Present	Decreased	Absent
Mouth and tongue	Moist	Dry	Parched
Skin fold	Instant recoil	Recoil in <2 seconds	Recoil in >2 seconds
Capillary refill	Normal	Prolonged	Prolonged, minimal
Extremities	Warm	Cool	Cold, mottled, cyanotic
Urine output	Normal to decreased	Decreased	Minimal

Sources: Adapted from Morbidity and Mortality Weekly Report 2003, p 5; Duggan et al 1992; WHO 1995.

COMMUNITY PERSPECTIVE

The CCN has a vital role in the management of children with constipation. The CCN is ideally placed to support the child and family in the community with home visits and telephone calls to provide holistic advice and support for the child and family (Rogers 2005). The child's home is an ideal venue to assess their feelings surrounding toileting.

Although disempaction can occur fairly quickly, a child 'may need maintenance therapy for up to 24 months and may suffer a number of relapses before their constipation is resolved' (Cross et al 2005). It is extremely important that the child and family have open access to advice during this period to enable early recognition of potential problems or relapse, facili-

tating a prompt response. CCNs are in an ideal position to offer this support.

The CCN will liaise with the child's school or school nurse with the child's approval to ensure that the toilet facilities are satisfactory and to promote the importance of the child being allowed access to fluids and a private toilet when required. Play specialists can enhance the community support for the child and family.

The role of the CCN is expanding in some areas. Nurse-led clinics are being developed in hospital and in the community, with the CCN receiving direct referrals from GPs, health visitors and school nurses. There are some nurses undertaking nurse prescribing courses, enabling nurse-led clinics to function efficiently.

Do and do not

- Do take the concerns of the family regarding changes in bowel movement of their child seriously.
- Do consider the child's school environment, the locality and the standards of school toilets as this may inhibit defaecation.

- Do complete a full assessment of the child including dietary habits and patterns of defaecation.
- Do check trust/hospital policies and procedures for digital rectal examination and the administration of medications per rectum.
- Do not undertake a digital rectal examination as a student; this must be undertaken by a qualified competent practitioner.

References

Addison R, Ness W, Abulafi M, Swift I 2000 How to administer enemas and suppositories. NTPLUS 96(6): 3–4

Allen C 1998 Management of constipation in children. Community Nurse 4: 39

Armon K, Stephenson T, MacFaul R, Eccleston P, Werneke U 2001 An evidence and consensus based guideline for acute diarrhoea management. Archives of Disease in Childhood 85(2): 132–141

Barnes P M, Maddocks A 2002 Standards in school toilets – a questionnaire survey. Journal of Public Health Medicine 24(2): 85–87

Bond J, Bond S 1992 Sociology and health care. Churchill Livingstone, London

Bosch J, Mraz R, Masbruch J, Tabor A, Van Dyke D, McBrien D 2002 Constipation in young children with developmental disabilities. Infants and Young Children 15(2): 66–77

Buchanan A 1992 Children who soil. Assessment and treatment. Wiley, London

Burnett C, Wilkins G 2002 Managing children with constipation: a community perspective. Journal of Family Health Care 12(5): 127–132

Burnett C A, Juszczak E, Sullivan P B 2004 Nurse management of intractable functional constipation: a randomised controlled trial. Archives of Disease in Childhood 89(98): 717–722

Campbell J 1993 Skills update: suppositories. Community Outlook 3(7): 22–23

Cavet J 1998 People don't understand: children, young people and their families living with a hidden disability. National Children's Bureau Enterprises, London

Clayden G 1992 Management of chronic constipation. Archives of Disease in Childhood 67: 340–344

Cross J, Elbadri A M, Emery R et al 2005 Impact paediatric bowel care pathway. Norgine Ltd, Harefield, Middlesex, UK

Day A 2001 The nurse's role in managing constipation. Nursing Standard 16: 41–44

Del Giudice E, Staiano A, Capano G et al 1999 Gastrointestinal manifestations in children with cerebral palsy. Brain and Development 21(5): 307–311

Department of Health 1997 Health services for children and young people in the community: home and school. Health Committee, Third Report. TSO, London

Di Lorenzo C 2000 Childhood constipation. Journal of Pediatrics 136: 4–7

Djuretic T, Ramsay M, Gay N, Wall P, Ryan M, Fleming D 1999 An estimate of proportions of diarrhoeal disease episodes seen by general practitioners attributable to rotavirus in children under five years of age in England and Wales. Act Paediatrica Suppl. 426: S38–S41

Duggan C, Santosham M, Glass R I 1992 The management of acute diarrhea in children: oral rehydration, maintenance, and nutritional therapy. MMWR 41(RR-16): 1–20

Elshimy N, Gallagher B, West D, Stringer M D, Puntis J W L 2000 Outcome in children under 5 years of age with constipation: a prospective follow-up study. International Journal of Clinical Practice 54: 25–27

Enuresis Resource and Information Centre (ERIC) 2001 Childhood soiling. Minimum standards of practice for treatment and service delivery. ERIC, Bristol

Farell M, Holmes G, Coldicutt P, Peak M 2003 Management of childhood constipation: parents' experiences. Journal of Advanced Nursing 44(5): 479–489

Felt B, Wise C, Olson A, Kochlar P, Marcus S, Conran A 1999 Guideline for the management of pediatric idiopathic constipation and soiling. Archives of Pediatric and Adolescent Medicine 153(4): 380–385

Forsyth J S, Varma S, Colvin M 1999 A randomized controlled study of the effect of long chain polyunsaturated fatty acid supplementation on stool hardness during formula feeding. Archives of Disease in Childhood 81: 253–256

Goh J, Bryne P, McDonald G, Stephens R, Keeling P 2001 Severe juvenile chronic constipation. Irish Medical Journal 94: 81–82

Hoekstra A 1998 Toddler diarrhoea: more a nutritional disorder than a disease. Archives of Disease in Childhood 79(1): 2–5

Hoekstra A, van den Aker J H L, Ghoos Y F, Hartemink R, Kneepkens C M F 1995 Fluid intake and industrial processing in apple juice induced chronic non-specific diarrhoea. Archives of Disease in Childhood 73(2): 126–130

Hymans J S, Leichtner A M 1985 Apple juice. An unappreciated cause of chronic diarrhoea. American Journal of Diseases of Children 5: 503–505

Hymans J S, Treem W R, Etienne N L et al 1995 Effect of infant formula on stool characteristics of young infants. Pediatrics 95: 50–54

Iacano G, Cavataio F, Montalto G et al 1998 Intolerance of cow's milk and chronic constipation in children. New England Journal of Medicine 339(16): 1100–1104

Jones S 2002 A clinical pathway for pediatric gastroenteritis. Gastroenterology Nursing 26(1): 7–20

Keuzenkamp-Jensen C W, Fijnvandraat C J, Kneepkens C N F, Douwes A C 1996 Diagnostic dilemmas and results of treatment for chronic constipation. Archives of Disease in Childhood 75(1): 36–41

Leung A K C, Chan P Y H, Cho H Y H 1996 Constipation in children. American Family Physician 54(2): 611–618

Loening-Baucke V 1997 Fecal incontinence in children. American Family Physician 54(9): 611–618

Loening-Baucke V 1998 Toilet tales: stool toileting refusal, encopresis, and fecal incontinence. Journal of Wound, Ostomy, and Continence Nursing 25: 304–313

Loening-Baucke V 2002 Polyethylene glycol without electrolytes for children with constipation and encopresis. Journal of Pediatric Gastroenterology and Nutrition 34(4): 372–377

Lucy J 1999 The role of health promotion in childhood soiling. Journal of Community Nursing 13: 4

Mallett J, Bailey C 1996 Bowel care. In: The Royal Marsden NHS Trust manual of clinical nursing procedures. Blackwell Science, London

Moppett S 2000 Which way is up for a suppository? NTPLUS 96(19): 12–13

Morbidity and Mortality Weekly Report 2003 Managing acute gastroenteritis among children. Oral rehydration, maintenance, and nutritional therapy. MMWR 52(RR-16): 1–16

Muir J, Burnett C 1999 Setting up a nurse-led clinic for intractable childhood constipation. British Journal of Community Nursing 4(8): 395–399

Murphy W 2001 Constipation and soiling: a community approach. Paediatric Nursing 13(8): 31–35

Nurko S, Baker S, Colletti R, Di Lorenzo J, Ecotor W, Liptak G 2001 Managing constipation: evidence put to practice. Contemporary Pediatrics 18(12): 56–65

Olowokure B, Hawker J, Weinberg J, Gill N, Sufi F 1999 Deprivation and hospital admission for infectious intestinal diseases. Lancet 353: 807–808

Pashankar D, Bishop W 2001 Efficacy of optimal dose of daily polyethylene glycol 3350 for treatment of constipation and encopresis in children. Journal of Pediatrics 139(3): 428–432

Price K J, Elliott T M 2004 Stimulant laxatives for constipation and soiling in children (Cochrane Review). In: The Cochrane Library, Issue 3. Wiley, Chichester, UK

Procter E, Loader P 2003 A 6-year follow-up study of chronic constipation and soiling in a specialist paediatric service. Child: Care, Health and Development 29(2): 103–109

Rasquin-Weber A, Hyman P E, Cucchiara S et al 1999 Childhood functional gastrointestinal disorders. Gut 45(Suppl 11): 1160–1168

Rennie A, Sim J, Denholme N, Tappin D 1997 Home based management of constipation and soiling. Ambulatory Child Health 3: 219–224

Rogers J 1997 Childhood constipation and the incidence of hospitalisation. Nursing Standard 12: 40–42

Rogers J 2000 The causes and management of constipation in children. Community Nurse 6: 39–40

Rogers J 2003 Management of functional constipation in childhood. British Journal of Community Nursing 8(12): 550–553

Rogers J 2005 Reducing the misery of constipation in children. Practice Nursing 16(1): 12–16

Royal College of Nursing (RCN) 2003a Digital rectal examination. Guidance for nurses working with children and young people. RCN, London

Royal College of Nursing (RCN) 2003b Preparing nurses in the care of children and young people. RCN, London

Sharif F, Crushell E, O'Driscoll K, Bourke B 2001 Liquid paraffin: a reappraisal of its role in the treatment of constipation. Archives of Disease in Childhood 85: 121–124

Taylor P 2000 Managing constipation in children. Drug Therapy Bulletin 38: 57–60

Thompson J 2001a Toddler diarrhoea. Community Practitioner 74(5): 195–196

Thompson J 2001b Intussusception, pyloric stenosis and Hirschsprung's disease. Community Practitioner 74(8): 312–313

Thompson J 2001c The management of chronic constipation in children. Community Practitioner 74(1): 29–30

Tse P, Leung S, Chan T, Sien A, Ahk C 2000 Dietary fibre intake and constipation in children with severe developmental disabilities. Journal of Paediatric Child Health 36: 236–239

Vernon S, Lundblad B, Hellstrom A L 2003 Children's experiences of school toilets present a risk to their physical and psychological health. Child: Care, Health and Development 29(1): 47–53

Vincent R, Candy R M 2001 Movicol for the treatment of faecal impaction in children. Gastroenterology Today 11(2): 50–52

Willis J 2000 Bowel management and consent. NTPLUS 96(6): 7–8

Winnett M 1999 Rectal examination in paediatric trauma care. Accident and Emergency Nursing 7(1): 3–7

Yong D, Beattie R M 1998 Normal bowel habit and prevalence of constipation in primary-school children. Ambulatory Child Health 4: 277–282

Further Reading

Addison R, Ness W, Abulafi M, Swift I 2000 How to administer enemas and suppositories. NTPLUS 96(6): 3–4

Enuresis Resource and Information Centre 2001 Childhood soiling: minimum standards of practice for treatment and service delivery: benchmarking guidelines. ERIC, Bristol, UK

Jones S 2002 A clinical pathway for pediatric gastroenteritis. Gastroenterology Nursing 26(1): 7–20

Moppett S 2000 Which way is up for a suppository? NTPLUS 96(19): 12–13

Royal College of Nursing 2003 Digital rectal examination. Guidance for nurses working with children and young people. Royal College of Nursing, London

Thompson J 2001 Intussusception, pyloric stenosis and Hirschsprung's disease. Community Practitioner 74(8): 312–313

World Health Organization 1995 The treatment of diarrhoea: a manual for physicians and other senior health workers. WHO, Geneva, Switzerland

Young R, Beerman L, Vanderhoof J 1998 Increasing oral fluids in chronic constipation in children. Gastroenterology Nursing 21(4): 156–161

Websites

www.eric.org.uk

Practice **7**

Cardiopulmonary resuscitation

Fiona Clements

Introduction

While few resuscitation situations involving children arise without warning, it remains imperative that children's nurses are skilled in the area of basic life support (Simpson 1994, Carter & Dearmun 1995). Paediatric basic life support (BLS) is described as the provision of cardiopulmonary resuscitation (CPR) with no devices or with bag–valve–mask ventilation or barrier devices, until advanced life support (ALS) can be provided (International Guidelines 2000). However, 'if basic life support is not effectively delivered to the child attempts at advanced life support are likely to prove futile' (Simpson 1994, p. 39).

As accidents remain the commonest cause of death in children and as the life expectancy of children with a variety of chronic illnesses is increasing, the need for parents, and also other members of the general public, to learn basic paediatric life support is becoming increas-

ingly important (Carter & Dearmun 1995, Whitton 1995).

It is important to recognise that practising CPR using a baby or child manikin is the most effective way of ensuring that children's nurses have appropriate skills to help an infant or child in need. In addition, these skills, in order to be fresh, require to be updated regularly.

All nurses must be aware of the emergency call telephone number and procedure for their individual clinical areas.

Learning outcomes

By the end of this section and following further reading and simulated practice the nurse should be able to:

● assess responsiveness in infants and children
● use appropriate airway opening techniques
● assess respiration by looking, listening and feeling for expired breath

- provide rescue breathing using both mouth-to-mouth techniques and use of a bag–valve–mask system
- pulse check using appropriate sites
- provide chest compressions
- identify priorities in advanced life support.

Rationale

Commentators on both sides of the Atlantic acknowledge the importance of resuscitation as a nursing skill (American Heart Association 2000, Resuscitation Council (UK) 2000).

Cardiac arrest in children is often the terminal event of progressive shock or respiratory failure; early signs of shock or respiratory failure must be recognised and treated to prevent cardiac arrest (International Guidelines 2000, Resuscitation Council (UK) 2000).

Many children die or suffer permanent neurological impairment each year because of sudden infant death syndrome, infections or trauma. Appropriate prompt action can help avoid many of them.

Advanced life support will be futile if basic life support is not delivered effectively.

Factors to note

Babies and children differ from adults in a number of ways:

- The causes of their cardiopulmonary arrest are different, with adults tending to suffer from *primary* cardiac arrest, whereas children, who predominantly have healthy hearts, tend to have *secondary* cardiac arrest following a period of hypoxia, often associated with an airway or breathing emergency. This fact suggests that cardiac arrest in children may be preventable if appropriate measures are taken to deal with the airway or breathing problem. The presence of hypoxia also explains why children fare so poorly following cardiopulmonary arrest. If the heart is deprived of oxygen to the point where it can no longer function, then similar effects must be seen in the brain and other vital organs (Hampson-Evans & Bingham 1998).

- Respiratory infection and sepsis are the primary causes of cardiopulmonary arrest in children under 5 years of age, with trauma being the major cause in the 5- to 14-year age group (Williams 1994).

- Babies and children differ from each other in resuscitation terms. The term 'infant' refers to the under 1 year old including the neonatal period, the term 'child' is defined as being from the age of 1–8 years and the term 'adult' applies to those over 8 years of age through adult years (International Guidelines 2000).

- The surface area of the face is smaller in babies.

- The paediatric larynx is funnel shaped, not cylindrical. This renders the larynx more susceptible to impaction of foreign objects.

- The larynx of the child is soft and the trachea is short. The tongue of the infant or child is large in comparison and, as such, increases airway obstruction and obscures the view of the glottis (Williams 1994, Bishop-Kurylo & Masiello 1995).

- Infants have poorly developed accessory muscles and an immature bronchial tree, the diaphragm being the major muscle of respiration (Hazinski 1992).

- The pressure required for chest compression is less in babies.

- Chest compressions should be initiated in children under the age of 8 years if the pulse is absent or the heart rate is less than 60 beats per minute with signs of poor perfusion (International Guidelines 2000, Resuscitation Council (UK) 2000).

- Basic life support should be initiated before the administration of any drugs, or other intervention, is considered.

- Cardiac arrest is defined as the absence of palpable central pulses. Four cardiac arrest rhythms may be identified on electrocardiograph (ECG) monitoring in children: asystole, pulseless electrical activity (PEA), ventricular fibrillation (VF) and pulseless ventricular tachycardia (VT).

- The presenting rhythm in most paediatric cardiac arrests is asystole or extreme brady-cardia (Sirbaugh et al 1999, Young & Seidel 1999).

- VF/VT has been reported in 10–20% of pae-diatric cardiac arrests (Mogeyzel et al 1995, Young & Seidel 1999). It is most likely to occur in children who are hypothermic, have structural cardiac disease or have taken an overdose of tricyclic antidepres-sants.

- Defibrillation takes precedence in the treat-ment of ventricular fibrillation. Shocks should be given in sets of three. Paediatric paddles should be used in children below 10 kg (International Guidelines 2000).

BASIC PAEDIATRIC LIFE SUPPORT

Method

The following has been agreed as the basis for one-rescuer basic life support in infancy and childhood (International Guidelines 2000, Resuscitation Council (UK) 2000).

1. Assess the environment surrounding the infant or child; move the child if the envi-ronment is dangerous. It is also important that the nurse does not become the next vic-tim of whatever fate befell the child. If neck injury is suspected, all attempts should be made to move the child with the spinal col-umn intact.

2. Assess the level of responsiveness by gently shaking or pinching the child's fingers or toes. Tactile and verbal stimulation should be used. Care should be taken to avoid vig-orous shaking as this may cause brain injury.

3. If the child is unresponsive, call for help but do not leave the child alone. It is possible that this unconsciousness may cause air-way obstruction. Opening of the airway may be the only resuscitative action that is required.

Opening the airway

- The airway can be opened in either of two ways:

  - *Head tilt/chin lift* – one hand is placed on the child's forehead, and a finger of the other hand is placed on the bony tip of the chin. The head is then tilted back and the chin lifted upwards and forward (see Fig. 7.1). It is important to avoid overextension of the neck and compression of the soft tissues under the chin as either of these can cause obstruction of the air passages.

  - *Jaw thrust* – this technique is the preferred choice where neck injury is suspected because it allows the airway to be opened without moving the neck. In this instance the index fingers of both hands are placed behind the angles of the jaw and the mandible is lifted upwards carrying the tongue forward. This manoeuvre may close the mouth, however, so the thumbs should be placed on the tip of the chin (Hampson-Evans & Bingham 1998).

- If impaction of the airway by a foreign body is suspected or witnessed, this must be removed.

- Once the airway is open, assess breathing.

- Assess breathing by looking for the rise and fall of the chest, listening for breath sounds at the child's mouth and nose, and feeling for evidence of expired breath with your cheek, taking no more than 10 seconds. Care should be taken to differentiate effective

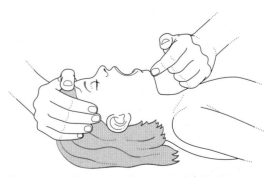

Figure 7.1 Airway opening: head tilt/chin lift

breathing from ineffective gasping respiratory effort (Noc et al 1994, Poets et al 1999).

● If there is no breathing, artificial ventilation should be commenced without delay.

● For infants, deliver breaths to lungs via the mouth and nose. It has been suggested that in some infants it is not possible for an adult to effectively cover both mouth and nose for ventilation (Tonkin et al 1995), but the American Heart Association (2000), International Guidelines (2000) and the Resuscitation Council UK (2000) continue to recommend mouth-to-mouth-and-nose rescue breathing for the infant under 1 year old; this is further supported by Nadkarni et al (1997).

● For the child, breathing should be by the mouth-to-mouth route.

● Maintain the airway in an open position throughout ventilation.

● Deliver breaths slowly, 1–1$\frac{1}{2}$ seconds each, to minimise the possibility of gastric distension and optimise filling of lungs (McCrory & Downs 1990, Resuscitation Council (UK) 1997).

● Observe the chest during rescue breathing to ensure that it rises and falls. This movement confirms the patency of the airway.

● Deliver two effective breaths, taking up to five attempts to achieve this (International Guidelines 2000, Resuscitation Council (UK) 2000). If chest movement is not witnessed, reposition the airway. If this is unsuccessful, the possibility of a foreign body should be considered.

Checking the pulse

● Assess circulation by palpation of the pulse and observing for any other signs of life, e.g. swallowing, moving, breathing (Resuscitation Council (UK) 2000).

● In the child, the carotid artery should be palpated.

● In the infant, palpation of the brachial artery on the inside of the middle section of the upper arm (see Fig. 7.2) is indicated as the carotid artery is difficult to locate owing to the short nature of the neck.

● If no pulse is palpated or the pulse rate is less than 60 beats per minute with signs of poor perfusion, chest compressions should be commenced.

● In both infants and children, the lower half of the sternum should be compressed in the midline.

● In infants, identify this mark as follows:

– place the tips of two fingers, one finger's breadth below an imaginary line joining the infant's nipples (Resuscitation Council (UK) 2000) taking care to avoid compression of the xiphoid process or abdomen (Clements & McGowan 2000).

● In infants, compress by one-third to one-half of the depth of the chest (International Guidelines 2000, Resuscitation Council (UK) 2000).

● In the child, identify this mark as follows:

– locate the lower half of the sternum and place the heel of one hand over it, ensuring

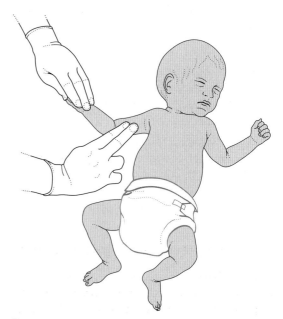

Figure 7.2 Palpation of the brachial pulse

that there is no compression over the xiphoid process; the fingers should be lifted to avoid pressing on the child's ribs (International Guidelines 2000, Resuscitation Council (UK) 2000).

- In the child, compress for one-third to one-half of the depth of the chest (International Guidelines 2000, Resuscitation Council (UK) 2000).

- In the older child, compression with one hand may not provide sufficient force. Two-handed compression may be necessary. This is more commonly associated with adults. The sternum should be compressed one-third to one-half of the depth of the chest.

- In both the infant and the child, five compressions of the chest should be followed by one breath (ratio for older children 15:2). Compression at a rate of 100 per minute should be attempted.

Do and do not

- Do practise locating brachial and carotid pulses.

- Do attend to the needs of the child before telephoning. The cause of the emergency is probably airway or respiratory in nature and quick attention to this may prevent the heart from stopping.

- Do not assume that you are competent in life support because you have read about it. It is imperative that you take time to practise using appropriately sized manikins.

- Do not blindly sweep fingers around an infant's, or child's, mouth. Remember that the paediatric larynx is not cylindrical but funnel shaped and it is possible that blind finger sweeps may impact an object in the larynx, causing harm.

ADVANCED PAEDIATRIC LIFE SUPPORT

Effective basic paediatric life support is a prerequisite for advanced life support, which aims at providing continued perfusion of the coronary and cerebral arteries with oxygenated blood through the use of additional equipment and medication, thus enabling the heart to regain its effectiveness as a pump (European Resuscitation Council 1994, Hampson-Evans & Bingham 1998).

Advanced paediatric life support inevitably will be performed and continued within the clinical setting where it is important that all staff involved are updated frequently on the techniques that are used in both types of life support, thus being familiar with paediatric practice (Williams 1994, Bishop-Kurylo & Masiello 1995).

What must be remembered is that basic life support techniques will continue despite the introduction of advanced life support.

The emergency trolley

Emergency equipment for use during advanced life support should always be readily available within all clinical areas. Although the type and style of emergency trolley will differ between clinical and community areas, the basic contents of the trolley should be similar. In comparison to emergency trolleys used within the adult setting, the trolley within the paediatric setting will carry a wide range of equipment in order to meet the needs of the wide age range and corresponding differences in body proportions of children. Box 7.1 identifies the basic requirements of the paediatric emergency trolley.

The contents of the emergency trolley should be checked on a regular basis, as per local policy, to ensure that all equipment is functional. Expiry dates should be checked on all drugs, intravenous fluids and disposable equipment; batteries and spare bulbs for the laryngoscope should also be checked.

MAINTENANCE OF AIRWAY

A secure and effective airway is essential if ventilation is to be maintained.

Equipment

- Face masks
- Self-inflating bag–valve–mask device with reservoir attached

---

Box 7.1   Basic contents of the paediatric emergency trolley

Airway maintenance

- Selection of oropharyngeal airways: variety of sizes ranging from infant to adult
- Endotracheal tubes: variety of sizes from infant to adult
- Laryngoscope with selection of blades straight and curved, spare handle, spare batteries and bulbs; McGill forceps
- Ventilation face masks: variety of sizes and types
- Self-inflating bag–valve–mask system with reservoir
- Re-breathing set
- T-piece/anaesthetic circuit
- Oxygen tubing, face masks, nasal prongs and portable oxygen supply
- Suction tubing, catheters and portable suction unit
- Oxygen saturation monitoring equipment

Cardiac monitoring

- Cardiac monitor electrodes
- Cardiac monitor
- Blood pressure cuffs

Drugs and intravenous fluids

- Emergency drug box containing epinephrine, sodium bicarbonate, atropine, anticonvulsant drugs, lidocaine and other drugs as per local pharmacy policy
- Saline/dextrose 500 ml bags of fluid: variety of concentrations
- Protein plasma solution
- Fluids used for intravascular volume expansion, e.g. Ringer's lactate solution

Other equipment

- Intravenous infusion equipment
- Selection of intravenous cannulae
- Intravenous cut-down set
- Intraosseous needles, spinal needles
- Syringes, hypodermic needles
- Splints
- Selection of urinary catheters and nasogastric tubes
- Stethoscope
- Silver swaddler
- Scissors
- Mediswabs
- Lubricant gel (water-based)
- Surgical tape
- Blood specimen bottles, labels

- T-piece anaesthetic circuit
- Oxygen supply
- Oxygen tubing
- Selection of oropharyngeal airways
- Selection of endotracheal tubes
- Laryngoscope
- Blades for laryngoscope
- Zinc oxide tape for securing endotracheal tube
- Water-based lubricant jelly
- Scissors
- Suction source and catheters
- Stethoscope.

Method

1. Effective ventilation should be provided using a self-inflating bag–valve–mask with reservoir and face mask. This is connected to the oxygen supply, thus providing a higher concentration of oxygen, which is preferential in advanced life support (European Resuscitation Council 1994).

2. The face mask should provide a good seal around the nose or nose and mouth to enable optimal ventilation. A mask of an appropriate size should be chosen. The

mask should fit snugly around the child's nose and mouth. A mask that is too large will allow carbon dioxide to accumulate and be delivered back to the child (McCrory & Downs 1990, Williams 1994).

3. Where the child's airway cannot be maintained adequately, an oropharyngeal airway should be inserted.

4. The size of the oropharyngeal airway is determined by positioning the airway next to the child's face. A correctly sized airway should extend from the centre of the mouth to the angle of the jaw (European Resuscitation Council 1994, MacNab 1996).

5. In infants, insert the airway with the convex side upwards. The tongue should be guided out of the way using a tongue depressor or the blade from a laryngoscope (MacNab 1996).

6. In the child, insert the airway with the concave side upwards; when the tip reaches the soft palate rotate the airway through 180° and slide over the tongue.

7. Oropharyngeal airways should be used with caution. Airways that are too small will cause additional obstruction, while those that are too large may damage the posterior pharyngeal wall (Williams 1994).

8. Once the airway has been inserted, bag–valve–mask ventilation should be continued.

Endotracheal intubation

Performed by experienced medical staff, endotracheal intubation remains the most effective method of securing and maintaining the airway. This should be performed as soon as possible when effective ventilation cannot be otherwise obtained (Williams 1994, International Guidelines 2000). However, it must be remembered that oxygenation is the priority.

- The size of the endotracheal tube is very important. This can be estimated by a number of methods:

  – in infants, the size of endotracheal tube usually required is 3.0–3.5 mm for the newborn, while infants from 6–9 months require size 4.0 mm (MacNab 1996)

  – in the child, the size of the endotracheal tube can be estimated by use of the following equation:

  Size of endotracheal tube in mm $= \dfrac{\textit{Age in years} + 4}{4}$

  – Broselow tape is a specifically designed tape measure, which can be used to identify the correct size of endotracheal tube (Begg 1995)

  – Another useful guideline is to use a tube of about the diameter of the child's little finger or of a size that will just fit into the nostril (European Resuscitation Council 1994)

  – These measurements provide an estimate of the internal diameter of the tube.

- Endotracheal tubes used in children less than 8 years old are normally uncuffed, as the cuff may cause damage to the soft airway tissue; also the narrow cricoid cartilage forms a sufficient seal (Williams 1994).

- Before intubation, the child is oxygenated with 100% oxygen.

- In infants and young children a straight-blade laryngoscope is normally used during insertion.

- In older children a curved-blade laryngoscope is normally used.

- The endotracheal tube is frequently inserted via the nasal route within the intensive care setting; the laryngoscope and McGill forceps are used to help visualise and direct the insertion of the tube. Once inserted, the tube is fixed in place using zinc oxide tape. This route of insertion is technically more difficult in the emergency situation.

- Once the tube has been inserted, oxygenation can be performed by attaching the re-breathing equipment directly to it, or by the use of a mechanical ventilator.

● Symmetrical chest movement and equal lung air entries should be observed and heard.

VASCULAR ACCESS

Speed is vital when administering fluid or drugs in the advanced life support situation. The method and equipment used for administration will vary with the type of access that is used.

Equipment

● 70% isopropyl alcohol-impregnated swabs (Mediwipes) and/or antiseptic solution appropriate to local area
● Intravenous cannulae (varying sizes)
● Syringes (varying sizes)
● Central venous cannulae
● Intraosseous cannula
● Intravenous administration sets
● Sterile latex-free gloves
● Sterile dressing pack.

Method

Venous access
● Where possible, peripheral venous access should be attempted; however, this is often difficult to achieve in the critically ill child.
● If central venous access is already established, this should be used, but if it is not, only peripheral access should be attempted, as attempting central access is hazardous in the emergency situation (European Resuscitation Guidelines 1994).
● As establishing vascular access in paediatric cardiac arrest is difficult, immediate insertion of an intraosseous cannula may be preferable (International Guidelines 2000).

Intraosseous access
● This is a safe, simple, rapid means of access in all children.
● An intraosseous cannula is a fine screw-like needle which is inserted into the anterior tibial bone marrow; alternative sites include the distal femur, medial malleolus or anterior superior iliac spine (International Guidelines 2000).
● Fluids and drugs can be rapidly infused using this type of access; however, it is not for long-term use.

If access is impossible to obtain, some drugs, e.g. adrenaline (epinephrine) and atropine, can be given via the endotracheal tube. The drug should be injected via a narrow-bore suction catheter beyond the tracheal end of the tube and then flushed in with 1–2 ml normal saline (Resuscitation Council (UK) 2000). The endotracheal dose of adrenaline (epinephrine) is 10 times that of the intravenous dose; the endotracheal dose of atropine is 0.02 mg/kg (International Guidelines 2000). This route is not suitable for fluid administration.

DRUGS AND FLUID THERAPY

Artificial ventilation with oxygen and fluid replacement therapy may re-establish cardiac output without the need for drug therapy. Paediatric emergency resuscitation trolleys should include a variety of crystalloid and colloid intravenous fluids. These would include saline solution in varying concentrations, Ringer's lactate solution, access to human albumin and plasma. The type of solution used is dependent on the cause of the arrest.

These drugs and intravenous fluids should be available within the emergency resuscitation trolley.

Drug therapy
The action of drugs used in resuscitation, and their metabolism, is poorly understood in children. The following examples are those recommended in the guidelines produced by the Resuscitation Council (UK) 2000.

Adrenaline (epinephrine)
This is the first-line drug of choice in paediatric resuscitations (International Guidelines 2000). Adrenaline (epinephrine) will cause an increase in peripheral vascular resistance without constricting coronary or cerebral vessels. This raises systolic and diastolic pressures during cardiac compressions (Simpson 1994).

Recommended doses are as follows (Resuscitation Council (UK) 2000):

● First dose: 10 µg/kg of body weight (0.1 ml of 1:10 000 solution) repeated every 3–5 minutes.

● Second and subsequent doses: There is no evidence that increasing the dose of adrenaline (epinephrine) has any beneficial effects in cardiac arrest in children. Current recommendations are 10 μg/kg, increasing to 100 μg/kg where the cardiac arrest is thought to be secondary to circulatory collapse (Resuscitation Council (UK) 2000).

Sodium bicarbonate

Sodium bicarbonate has been routinely used in paediatric resuscitations for many years. The rationale for its use is the reduction of the metabolic acidosis, which occurs during cardiac arrest. However, a concern with the use of bicarbonate is that it produces more carbon dioxide, because of its buffering action, and thus acidosis is increased. Therefore, if used, it could be considered following ventilation, basic life support and adrenaline (epinephrine) in the patient in prolonged cardiac arrest, or a cardiac arrest that has been associated with a severe metabolic acidosis (Resuscitation Council (UK) 2000).

The dose of sodium bicarbonate is recommended as 1 mEql/kg (1 ml/kg of 8.4% solution) (International Guidelines 2000, Resuscitation Council (UK) 2000).

Atropine

Although there is no clear evidence that atropine is a useful drug in cardiac arrest and paediatric resuscitation, it may be considered as part of the ongoing management of haemodynamically significant bradycardia and after adequate oxygenation (International Guidelines 2000).

The recommended dose is 0.02 mg/kg with a minimum recommended dose of 0.1 mg and a maximum single dose of 0.5 mg in a child and 1 mg in an adolescent. The dose may be repeated in 5 minutes up to a maximum total dose of 1.0 mg in a child and 2 mg in an adolescent (International Guidelines 2000).

Amiodarone

Amiodarone is now recommended in shock-resistant VF/pulseless VT. The recommended dose is 5 mg/kg via rapid intravenous bolus (Resuscitation Council (UK) 2000).

Glucose

Sick children and especially infants may develop hypoglycaemia. Blood glucose should be assessed as soon as possible and treated promptly with glucose solution (Williams 1994).

DEFIBRILLATION

Defibrillation is not commonly required in paediatric resuscitation. It is the term used for the stimulation of the heart muscle using electric currents and is normally performed by experienced medical staff and appropriately trained registered nurses. Used primarily for ventricular fibrillation and pulseless ventricular tachycardia, the energy applied is initially 2 J/kg for the first two shocks and 4 J/kg for subsequent shocks (European Resuscitation Council 1994, Williams 1994). Ventilation and chest compressions should be continued except when shocks are being delivered. Shocks should be delivered in sets of three, where necessary.

Paediatric paddles (4.5 cm) are used in children less than 10 kg in weight, with adult paddles being used for larger children.

Equipment should be readily available to all clinical areas. Often, however, the defibrillation equipment is shared between areas.

Equipment should be checked on a regular basis to ensure that it is charging and discharging properly. This should be performed by appropriately trained registered nurses. Bioengineering departments should check defibrillator equipment regularly as per local policy.

Do and do not

● Do familiarise yourself with the location of the emergency trolley and equipment within your clinical area.
● Do ensure that you know the emergency call number for cardiac arrest.
● Do ensure that you attend a regular resuscitation update. A minimum of yearly is essential.
● Do familiarise yourself with the layout and contents of the emergency resuscitation trolley.
● Do ensure that parents are supported.
● Do not panic, as chaos within an emergency situation can cost valuable time. An

organised person will help focus and calm the rest of the team.

- Do not exclude parents and relatives from the resuscitation room unless it is at their request.

SUMMARY

Resuscitation must begin immediately and not wait until equipment arrives. All personnel working with children require to learn about both basic and advanced life support. It is imperative that the children's nurse is aware of the different techniques for both basic and advanced support and is competent in both.

It remains vital that basic life support skills and techniques are well taught and updated, as ineffective delivery of basic life support will render advanced life support futile. With further scientific evidence, resuscitation guidelines will continue to change, and it is important that nursing staff continually update and revise their practice in resuscitation techniques.

References

American Heart Association 2000 Supplement to Circulation 102(8)

Begg J E 1995 A pediatric care and resuscitation cart: one community hospital's ED experience. Journal of Emergency Nursing 21(6): 555–559

Bishop-Kurylo D, Masiello M 1995 Pediatric resuscitation: development of a mock code program and evaluation tool. Pediatric Nursing 21(4): 333–336

Carter B, Dearmun A K 1995 Child health care nursing – concepts, theory and practice. Blackwell Science, Oxford

Clements F, McGowan J 2000 Finger position for chest compressions in cardiac arrest in infants. Resuscitation 44: 43–46

European Resuscitation Council 1994 Guidelines for paediatric life support. British Medical Journal 308: 1349–1355

Hampson-Evans D C, Bingham R M 1998 Paediatric resuscitation. The European Resuscitation Council Guidelines 1998. Care of the Critically Ill 14(6): 188–193

Hazinski M F 1992 Nursing care of the critically ill child, 2nd edn. Mosby, St Louis, MO

International Guidelines 2000 International guidelines for CPR and ECC – a consensus on science. Resuscitation 46(1–3): 301–333

MacNab R 1996 Paediatric life support. Paediatric Nursing 8(4): 28–33

McCrory J H, Downs C E 1990 Cardiopulmonary resuscitation in infants and children. In: Blumer J L (ed.) A practical guide to pediatric intensive care, 3rd edn. Mosby, St Louis, MO, ch 6

Mogeyzel C, Quan L, Graves J R, Tiedeman D, Fahrenbruch C, Herndon P 1995 Out-of-hospital ventricular fibrillation in children and adolescents: causes and outcomes. Annals of Emergency Medicine 25: 484–491

Nadkarni V, Hazinski M F, Zideman D et al 1997 Paediatric life support. An advisory statement by the Paediatric Life Support Working Group of the International Liaison Committee on Resuscitation. Resuscitation 37: 115–127

Noc M, Weil M H, Sun S, Tang W, Bisera J 1994 Spontaneous gasping during cardiopulmonary resuscitation without mechanical ventilation. American Journal of Respiratory and Critical Care Medicine 150: 861–864

Poets C F, Meny R G, Chobanian M R, Bonofiglo R E 1999 Gasping and other cardiorespiratory patterns during sudden infant deaths. Pediatric Research 45: 350–354

Resuscitation Council (UK) 1997 The 1997 resuscitation guidelines for use in the United Kingdom. Resuscitation Council (UK), London

Resuscitation Council (UK) 2000 Resuscitation guidelines 2000. Resuscitation Council (UK), London

Simpson S M 1994 Paediatric advanced life support – an update. Nursing Times 90(27): 37–39

Sirbaugh P E, Pepe P E, Shook J E et al 1999 A prospective population-based study of the demographics, epidemiology, management, and outcome of out-of-hospital pediatric cardiopulmonary arrest. Annals of Emergency Medicine 33: 174–184

Tonkin S L, Davis S L, Gun T R 1995 Nasal route for infant resuscitation by mothers. Lancet 45: 1353–1356

Whitton H 1995 Infant resuscitation in parenthood education. Health Visitor 68(11): 454–455

Williams C 1994 Paediatric cardiopulmonary resuscitation. British Journal of Nursing 3(15): 760–764

Young K D, Seidel J S 1999 Pediatric cardiopulmonary resuscitation: a collective review. Annals of Emergency Medicine 33: 195–205

Further Reading

Quinn T 1998 Cardiopulmonary resuscitation. Nursing Standard 12(46): 49–56

Seidel J, Tittle S, Hodge D III et al 1998 Guidelines for paediatric equipment and supplies for emergency departments. Journal of Emergency Nursing 24(1): 45–48

Practice **8**

Central lines

Barbara Doyle

Introduction

A central line is inserted when a child requires frequent and/or long-term venous access. Reasons for insertion may include the administration of total parenteral nutrition, cytotoxic drugs or frequent intravenous antibiotics. These lines are usually inserted under general anaesthetic in theatre by experienced paediatric surgeons or by experienced anaesthetists. The use of ultrasound imaging is recommended to locate and assist in central venous access device insertion (NICE 2002).

Learning outcomes

By the end of this section you should:

- be aware of the different types of central venous lines currently in use
- understand the reasons for their use and all aspects of their care
- understand the importance of asepsis in central venous line care
- be able to explain all aspects of the care to the child and family
- be able to recognise potential problems and deal with them appropriately.

Rationale

Central venous lines play a crucial role in the administration of treatment to many children with acute and chronic potentially life-threatening illnesses (see Table 8.1 for examples). They reduce the need for frequent venepuncture which is extremely distressing for all children, particularly the very young.

Nurses have a key role in the care of these lines. In addition to performing the practical procedures, they are responsible for the education of the child, family and those in the community who are unfamiliar with central lines. A sound policy for line care, adhered to by all involved, will help to ensure that a line can safely remain in use for as long as required.

Central venous lines and ports will be encountered by community staff as most children will go home with these devices in situ (Hollis 1992). The amount of direct involvement by community staff in the care of these lines is variable, as in many instances the parents will carry out all the care at home.

Factors to note

There are three types of central line in use in paediatrics.

Tunnelled central venous line
Also known as a Broviac, or Hickman line, or often by the child as a 'wiggly'. These are skin-tunnelled Silastic catheters which are inserted, under general anaesthetic, into the subclavian or internal jugular vein (see Fig. 8.1). These lines can be single, double or triple lumen with each lumen having an external clamp. The type inserted depends upon the clinical requirements of the patient.

The Groshong catheter is a similar type of line, but it has an internal valve to prevent the backflow of blood, so does not require an external clamp.

Note: 10 ml or larger syringes are recommended, particularly when confirming patency.

Implanted port
Also known as a Port-a-Cath, Vascuport or TIVAD (totally implantable venous access device). This is a Silastic catheter, inserted into the subclavian or internal jugular vein, which is attached to a metal chamber sealed at the top with a septum of self-sealing silicone. The port (metal chamber) is positioned under the skin on the chest wall. Access to this system is via straight or angled Huber non-coring needles through the septum of the port (Fig. 8.2).

Note: Always use 10 ml or larger syringes with the ports as recommended by the manufacturers.

Non-tunnelled long line
This is a short-term venous access device more commonly used in the intensive care or high-dependency setting. These lines are not skin-tunnelled and can be inserted under local anaesthetic. They are usually held in place with skin sutures. These lines can have a single, double or triple lumen. Peripherally

Table 8.1 Types of line used for various conditions

Central venous line		Port	Long line
Single	**Double or triple**	**Port**	**Long line**
Solid tumours	Bone marrow transplants	Cystic fibrosis	Critically ill, requiring
Chronic malabsorption	Acute myeloid leukaemia	Haemophilia	inotropes etc.
for total parenteral	Acute lymphoblastic	Beta-thalassaemia	
nutrition	leukaemia (ALL)	major and other	
	Non-Hodgkin's lymphoma	transfusion-dependent	
	Neuroblastoma	haemoglobinopathies	
		ALL (low risk)	
		Solid tumours (low-intensity chemotherapy)	

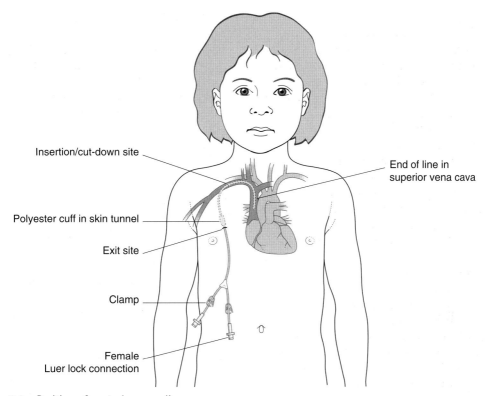

Figure 8.1   Position of central venous line

inserted central catheters (PICC lines) are included in this category of central venous lines.

Note: 10 ml or larger syringes are recommended with PICC lines (www.cc.nih.gov).

The type of line used for a particular child will depend upon various factors:

- the age of the child
- the length of time it will be required
- what treatments it will be used for
- how often it will be used.

This is usually decided by the medical consultants in charge of the individual child's care and is often also dependent upon the treatment protocol. Full details of the line inserted, i.e. make, model and size, should be documented in the child's medical notes. This assists staff to obtain the correct repair kit in the event of a line break. Table 8.1 gives examples of conditions and the type of line used for each condition.

Preparation of the child and family for the insertion of any central line is essential. This includes information from medical and nursing staff, plus preparatory work by the hospital play specialist if available. After discussion with the child and family, it may be useful to introduce them to another child with the same type of line.

Central venous lines can be in situ for months or even years, often in children who are immunocompromised (Vidler 1994, Bravery & Hannan 1997, Tobiansky et al 1997, Tweddle et al 1997, Cesaro et al 2004, Valentino et al 2004). As they provide direct access to the child's central venous system, the major risk is of infection either to the exit site or the line itself with the potential for septicaemia. For this reason alone, strict aseptic procedures need to be maintained when accessing all types of central line (Puntis et al 1990, Hollis 1992, Rumsey & Richardson 1995, Carnock 1996, Harrison 1997, NICE 2003).

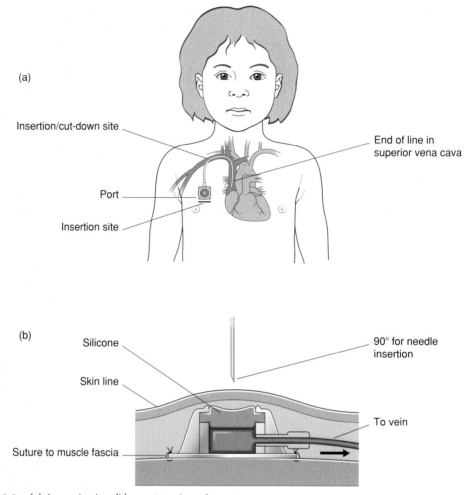

Figure 8.2 (a) A port in situ; (b) cross-section of a port

Many children will go home with these lines in situ so they and their families need to follow the same procedures and be knowledgeable about potential problems and how to deal with them. Community nursing staff may also be involved in their care.

General guidelines

● All staff undertaking these procedures must be knowledgeable about, and adhere to, the relevant hospital policy.

● Thorough handwashing is the single most effective means of improving central line care (Lawrance 1994, NICE 2003). In many centres sterile gloves are worn when performing any procedures involving accessing the central venous system via these lines.

● Before accessing any line, it is important to check for any sign of damage to the line or attachments. It is also necessary to observe for signs of leakage of blood or fluids from the exit site or any attachments or connections when accessing a line.

● When drugs are administered via the system, it must first be flushed with an appropriate solution, i.e. 0.9% sodium chloride. The line must be flushed before and after each drug, and before heparinising the system to maintain patency (see below). The volume of the flush solution should be equal to at least twice the volume of the line and any add-on devices, usually 5–10 ml (INS 2000, NICE 2003). A small number of drugs are incompatible with 0.9% sodium chloride, e.g. amphotericin (AmBisome) and some cytotoxic drugs. In these situations the line must be flushed with an alternative, e.g. 5% dextrose, or as indicated by the pharmacist.

- Lines which are not in use must be heparinised, i.e. flushed with a heparin solution, to maintain their patency. The solution most commonly used is heparin 10 units/ml of normal saline (RCN 2003).

Central venous lines require heparinising weekly when not in use, and after every episode of access. Heparinisation has been shown to significantly reduce bacterial colonisation of central venous lines (Department of Health and Hospital Infection Society 2001). It has also been shown to have a strong non-significant trend towards a reduction in line-related bacteraemia. Some lines with very small lumens will require heparinisation more frequently. There is considerable variation in the frequency of heparinising lines, so local hospital policy must be adhered to.

Ports require a heparin flush every 4 weeks when not in use, as recommended by the manufacturers.

Long lines are rarely not in use, being removed if no longer required. Follow individual hospital policy for heparinising these lines.

According to the manufacturer's instructions, Groshong catheters do not need heparinising. A 0.9% sodium chloride weekly flush is sufficient.

- The distal hub of a central venous line is capped with a Luer lock cap. Various systems are available and the type used will vary depending upon individual hospital preference. Needleless systems are becoming more commonly used to reduce the risk of needlestick injuries to the child, carers or staff. The exact method of accessing the lines will therefore vary depending upon the system used. However, the basic principles will still apply.

The Luer lock cap is changed using an aseptic procedure with the line clamped at all times. The frequency of cap changes will depend on the number of occasions the line is accessed, and the type of cap used, according to the manufacturer's guidelines.

- Cleaning solutions for caps and exit sites also differ between hospitals, usually being determined by the consultant microbiologist based on interpretation of current research. All are alcohol-based, e.g. povidone–iodine solution, industrial methylated spirits, Azowipes and 0.5% chlorhexidine in 70% alcohol (Department of Health and Hospital Infection Society 2001).

- Guidance must be sought from experienced nursing or medical staff if there are any problems with a line, e.g. resistance when flushing a line, or inability to aspirate blood.

- Date of insertion of the Port-a-Cath needle, size of Gripper needle used and date when infusion lines require to be changed should all be documented in the nursing notes.

ADMINISTRATION OF BOLUS DRUGS INTO A HEPARINISED CENTRAL LINE VIA THE CAP

This applies to any type of central line.

Equipment

- Dressing pack and dressing trolley (already cleaned)
- Prescription chart
- Drugs and diluents (if not prepared by pharmacy)
- 0.9% sodium chloride
- Heparin/saline solution (10 units heparin/ml saline)
- Syringes (10 ml syringes required for ports)
- 21G needles
- Filter needle (for any glass ampoules)
- Cap-cleaning equipment, e.g. sterile gauze swabs and povidone–iodine solution
- Sterile latex-free gloves.

Method

1. Wash and dry your hands thoroughly to prevent spread of infection.

2. Open dressing pack, open all syringes and needles, drop onto sterile field. Check and draw up all the prescribed drugs (see Administration of Medicines, p. 47), flushing solution and heparin/saline solution using appropriate syringes and needles. Discard needles, ensuring that the contents of each syringe are identifiable to prevent errors in administration.

3. Pour cleaning solution onto gauze swabs.

4. Take the prepared equipment to the child and explain the procedure to the child and family. Expose the end of the line for easy access.

5. Open the pack of sterile gloves; wash and dry your hands thoroughly; put on gloves. (The sterile inner paper from packaging can be used as a drape if required.)

6. Ask the child or parent to hand you the end of the line.

7. Thoroughly clean the end of the cap with the cleaning solution; allow to dry.

8. Withdraw fluid from the line to observe backflow of blood, so ensuring patency.

9. Administer the drugs over the manufacturer's recommended time, flushing before and after each drug with 5 ml of the correct flushing solution.

10. Heparinise the line. Flush the line with 4–5 ml of heparinised saline, closing the clamp whilst administering the last 0.5–1 ml. Remove the syringe. Continuous positive pressure ensures that the whole line is filled with heparinised saline and has not allowed aspiration of blood into the proximal end of the line. This minimises the risk of a blood clot and subsequent line blockage.

11. Ensure that the child is comfortable and the line is secured (some children wear a wiggly bag, which is a drawstring bag made of washable fabric and worn around the child's neck).

12. Clear away and dispose of all used equipment, as per hospital policy, to maintain a safe environment.

CONNECTING OR CHANGING AN INFUSION SET

Additional equipment

- Intravenous fluid and prescription chart
- Intravenous administration set and filter if required (some centres use 96-hour filters).

Method

1. Wash and dry your hands thoroughly.
2. Prime the administration set with the prescribed intravenous fluid.

3. Follow steps 2–6 of the previous procedure.

4. If the line is heparinised, clean the end of the cap and line thoroughly with cleaning solution and allow to dry. Withdraw 3–5 ml of solution from the line, observing for blood; flush with 5 ml 0.9% sodium chloride and attach the intravenous administration set.

5. If the line is already attached to an infusion, clamp the line, clean the cap, remove the old infusion set and attach the new set. Flush with 0.9% sodium chloride only if the fluid to be administered is different from the previous one.

6. Ensure that the whole system from the child to the intravenous fluid bag is complete and secure, and that the child is comfortable. Open the clamp, set the infusion pump to the prescribed rate and commence infusion.

7. Clear away and dispose of all used equipment.

ACCESSING A PORT FOR USE

This applies to ports only.

A variety of right-angled Huber needles (e.g. Gripper) are available with an integral extension for connection to infusion sets (see Table 8.2). A foam pad or winged plastic section is attached to these needles at the right-angled bend. This section should lie flat against the child's chest when the needle is in place. A dressing is placed over this to keep the needle securely in place. The size of needle chosen will depend upon the viscosity of the fluids to be administered, whilst the length is determined by the size of the child and the amount of subcutaneous tissue over the port.

Equipment

- Dressing trolley
- Dressing pack
- Prescription chart
- Cleaning solution
- Sterile latex-free gloves
- Gripper needle of appropriate size and length
- 10 ml syringes
- 21G needles and filter needle (for any glass ampoules)
- Heparinised saline (the strength used may differ from that used with central venous lines)
- Occlusive dressing.

Local anaesthetic cream, e.g. EMLA or tetracaine (Ametop), should be applied to the skin over the port 1 hour before the procedure to minimise discomfort.

Table 8.2 Gripper needles with extension

Size	Length
20 gauge (0.9 mm)	0.75 inch (19 mm)
20 gauge (0.9 mm)	1.00 inch (25 mm)
20 gauge (0.9 mm)	1.25 inch (32 mm)
22 gauge (0.7 mm)	0.75 inch (19 mm)
22 gauge (0.7 mm)	1.00 inch (25 mm)
22 gauge (0.7 mm)	1.25 inch (32 mm)

When accessing a port, it may be necessary to hold the child securely, especially a young child. The parents and an additional nurse may be required. Preparation for this procedure by the play specialist is invaluable if available.

Method

1. Clean the dressing trolley with alcohol-based solution, e.g. Azowipes, and assemble the required equipment.

2. Explain the procedure to the child and parents; allow them time to ask questions.

3. Wash and dry your hands thoroughly.

4. Prepare a sterile field by opening the dressing pack and emptying other sterile items onto it. Pour cleaning solution into a gallipot within the sterile field.

5. Wash and dry your hands thoroughly and put on gloves.

6. Connect the Luer lock cap to the extension of the Gripper needle. Draw up heparinised saline solution using a syringe and filter needle; prime the extension and Gripper needle; clamp the line; remove the syringe, retaining all items within the sterile field.

7. Ask an assistant or the child or parent to remove the anaesthetic cream.

8. Place a dressing towel over the child's abdomen below the port.

9. Clean the raised port access site and surrounding skin thoroughly with cleaning solution, working in a spiral from the raised centre outwards for at least 10 cm (4 inches). Repeat at least twice; allow to dry.

10. Palpate and locate the port, holding the outer edges through the skin with the fingers. Ensure that the port is secure and non-mobile. Visualise the centre of the port and insert the Gripper needle at an angle of 90° to the skin, through the silicone, until it meets the metal back-plate of the port (see Fig. 8.2).

11. Via the cap, insert the syringe. Unclamp the line, withdraw the plunger until blood is aspirated, then flush with heparinised saline clamping the line whilst administering the last 0.5–1 ml, i.e. under positive pressure.

12. Cover the Gripper needle with an occlusive dressing. It may also be necessary to pad the underside of the needle with sterile gauze if too long a needle has been inadvertently used.

13. Ensure that the child is comfortable and the line is well secured.

14. Clear away and dispose of all equipment.

Note: When a port is in long-term use, the needle must be changed every 2 weeks as recommended by the manufacturers; weekly if the child is neutropenic.

ROUTINE HEPARINISING OF A PORT

Equipment

As for accessing a port for use (above).

Method

1. Follow steps 1–10 of the method for accessing a port for use (above).

2. Via the cap, insert the syringe; unclamp the line; withdraw the syringe plunger until blood is aspirated. Flush with heparinised saline, removing the Gripper needle whilst still injecting the last 0.5 ml. Support the port with thumb and forefinger when removing the needle. (Another pair of hands is required, e.g. parent or another nurse.) This positive pressure manoeuvre prevents backflow of blood into the system, so preventing clot formation and potential occlusion.

3. Immediately wipe the puncture site with gauze soaked in cleaning solution; apply a plaster if requested by the child. Ensure that the child is comfortable.

4. Clear away and dispose of used equipment.

Central line dressings

There are many local variations in the method and frequency of dressings. A small study by Lucas and Attard-Montalto (1996) showed no difference in exit site infection rates between two groups – one with a dressing, the other without. Comparisons between Opsite IV3000 and either conventional film dressings (Keenlyside 1993) or sterile dry gauze (Brandt et al 1996) have also been carried out. Keenlyside found Opsite IV3000 to be highly desirable with reduced moisture accumulation and improved condition of the patient's skin. Brandt and colleagues found no significant difference in infection rates but the Opsite IV3000 was more cost-effective as it was changed weekly as opposed to a daily dressing change with sterile gauze. NICE (2003) guidelines recommend sterile, transparent semipermeable dressings which should be changed aseptically every 7 days unless there is an indication to change them sooner.

Cleaning solutions have also been compared for effectiveness in preventing infections. Maki et al (1991) found that 2% chlorhexidine was the most effective for cleaning exit sites, and for handwashing. A meta-analysis by Chaiyakunapruk et al (2002) of many studies of different cleaning solutions showed that a chlorhexidine gluconate solution was more effective than povidone–iodine solutions for line site care. The current NICE (2003) guidelines recommend the use of an alcoholic chlorhexidine gluconate solution for skin cleaning around central venous line sites.

The main reasons for using a dressing on exit sites, especially in paediatrics, are:

- to prevent contamination with extraneous matter
- to promote patient comfort
- to aid the secure fixation of the central line
- to prevent small children from interfering with the line.

CARE OF CENTRAL VENOUS LINE EXIT SITE

These lines are skin-tunnelled from the entry to a major vein to the exit site on the chest wall.

A few centimetres up the line from the exit site, there is a Dacron cuff around the central line (see Fig. 8.1). This helps to secure the line once the overlying skin has grown into it over the first couple of weeks from insertion, and may act as a partial barrier to ascending infective organisms from the exit site. This exit site is a potential site of infection as it is a long-term break in the skin's integrity. As a potential source of infection, the exit site requires careful monitoring and scrupulous hygiene.

Factors to note

Most children with central venous lines will go home with them in situ (Hollis 1992). The child and parents need to be taught the importance of maintaining a clean exit site. Many parents want to learn how to do the dressing, so nursing staff need to teach them and assess their competency prior to the child's discharge. There will be some parents who do not wish to take on this responsibility, so alternative solutions need to be found. In these situations, dressings may be done on weekly clinic visits or in the home by community staff.

Equipment

- Dressing trolley
- Dressing pack containing sterile towels and swabs
- Chlorhexidine gluconate solution
- Opsite IV3000 (10 × 12 cm)
- Bag for disposal of used equipment
- Additional tape, e.g. Mepore, for securing the line
- Sterile latex-free gloves (as per local policy)
- Swabs if infection at exit site is suspected.

Method

1. Assemble the equipment, take it to the child's bed and pull the curtains for privacy.

2. Explain the procedure to the child and family; allow time for questions and encourage the cooperation of all involved.

3. Wash and dry hands thoroughly, open the dressing pack and prepare all the equipment.

4. Remove the old dressing and discard it in the disposal bag.

5. Examine the exit site for any signs of infection, e.g. redness or exudate. Take swabs for culture if any signs of infection are present.

6. Wash and dry hands thoroughly. Put on sterile gloves if used.

7. Using chlorhexidine-soaked swabs, wipe round the exit site in a circular movement, starting at the centre and working outwards for at least 5 cm. Repeat at least twice with a new swab each time; allow to dry.

8. Clean the line with another swab, from the exit site away from the child for at least 10 cm. Allow the cleaning solution to dry.

9. Coil the line and apply Opsite IV3000 over the exit site, ensuring good adhesion by applying gentle pressure over the whole dressing. If a child is sensitive to Opsite IV3000, another sterile dressing may be required.

10. Loop the hub end of the line up to the chest and secure it with another piece of tape or insert the hub into a wiggly bag if worn by the child. (If a wiggly bag is worn, we suggest that a clean bag is used each day.) Ensure that the child is comfortable.

11. Clear away and dispose of all used equipment.

12. Label swabs and appropriate microbiology forms if required.

13. Record appropriate information in the child's nursing notes.

DRESSING A PORT IN USE

A dressing is only required if a port is in use for treatment. When not in use, the skin's integrity is not broken, as no needle requires to be in situ, so normal personal hygiene is sufficient once the initial insertion wounds have healed.

The dressing on an accessed port need only be changed if it becomes soiled or there is a clinical indication, i.e. potential infection. The recommended weekly or 2-weekly needle change will obviously entail a dressing change as part of that procedure.

Method

The method is the same as for care of the central venous line exit site but extra care should be taken to prevent dislodging the needle.

DRESSING CHANGE ON A LONG LINE

A long line is generally sutured at the exit site at the time of insertion. The long line entry site is protected under Opsite IV3000 for ease of observation. This dressing can remain in place for up to 7 days, but can be changed sooner if required (Brandt et al 1996, NICE 2003). Care must be taken not to dislodge the long line. The hub(s) should be padded to ensure the child's comfort.

The procedure for cleaning the site is the same as for central venous lines.

OBSERVATIONS AND COMPLICATIONS

Infection and potential septicaemia
Of the central line during placement
Sterile conditions in theatre should prevent this, but if the child has a systemic infection at the time of insertion, the lumen of the line can become affected.

Via the infusion system during use
Aseptic handling of the line and any infusions or additives should prevent infection occurring via this route. Filters can also be used, especially for total parenteral nutrition solutions, with different filters being used for the vitamin and lipid solutions.

Of the exit site or skin tunnel
Scrupulous hygiene of the exit site is essential to block this route of infection. Indications of infection are redness and/or exudate at the exit site, and in some instances pain or swelling.

If an infection is suspected, i.e. the child has a fever, blood cultures and exit site swabs should be taken, and then intravenous antibiotics commenced. These can usually eradicate any infection. Only in extreme circumstances

are lines removed because of infection, and then only after lengthy consideration by medical staff in consultation with the child and family. These lines are very precious, especially in the high-risk patients who have them, so prevention of infection is imperative.

Occlusion
Fibrin clot within the line
This is prevented by regular heparinisation, but it is sometimes necessary to dissolve a clot by using an antifibrinolytic agent such as urokinase (5000 units) (Medicines for Children 2003).

A line that does not flush back or bleed back, and has had no obvious kinks in it, is most likely to have an occlusion caused by a fibrin clot.

Drug precipitate
This can occur if certain solutions are not infused correctly, for example etoposide, calcium, diazepam, phenytoin and total parenteral nutrition. Precipitates can be removed by using 90% alcohol or hydrochloric acid, depending upon the likely cause of the occlusion; this must be carried out *only* by experienced senior personnel (Rumsey & Richardson 1995, RCN 2003).

Kinking of the line
This may be either externally or internally within the child's venous system. Visually check all external parts of the line for kinks first, then try altering the child's position. If the line still appears to be blocked, a chest X-ray may be required to check for internal kinks.

Catheter misplacement
Perioperatively
If this occurs there is a potential for pneumothorax, haemothorax, perforation of a vein or dislodgement during surgery. Any of these complications could be apparent in theatre and would be rectified there. The use of ultrasound imaging in theatre during the placement of these lines should reduce the incidence of these complications.

Postoperatively, confirm the correct placement of the line with the medical staff before using the line. Observe the child for any signs of chest pain, dyspnoea, cyanosis or bleeding/haematoma. Notify medical staff if any adverse signs are present.

Line accidentally pulled by the child

Check the exit site for signs of trauma or external appearance of the cuff. If the cuff is not visible or partially visible, check that the line is capable of being aspirated and flushes with no pain or swelling along the tunnel site. Inform medical staff of the situation. A slight misplacement may just require a further restraining suture around the cuff, allowing continued use of the line. A major displacement may result in the line having to be removed.

Superior vena cava syndrome

This can occur at any time because of a thrombus causing obstruction of the venous return to the superior vena cava. Signs include engorgement of head and neck veins, oedema of the head and neck and potential respiratory distress. Medical intervention is required.

Air embolism

This can occur if the line is damaged or left unclamped during a cap change. Careful handling, strict procedures, good staff and family education should prevent this. All caregivers should be taught to clamp the line close to the exit site if it should become inadvertently split or cut. Report the incident immediately to senior medical or nursing staff.

Central line breakage

This can occur if, for example, the line is cut or bitten by the child. The line must be clamped above the break as explained above. Repair kits are available for all central venous lines. The repair is performed under aseptic conditions by experienced senior nurses or medical staff. Details of the child's central venous line should be documented in the medical notes so that the appropriate repair kit is used.

Potential complications are summarised in Table 8.3.

Table 8.3   Summary of potential complications

Observation	Possible cause
Fever	Line infection/septicaemia Exit site infection
Line not flushing or bleeding back	Kink in line Fibrin clot Drug precipitate Displacement of line
Chest pain, dyspnoea, cyanosis	Pneumothorax Haemothorax Superior vena cava syndrome
Fluid leaking out of line	Damage to line, e.g. split or tear Connections not correctly attached

COMMUNITY PERSPECTIVE

The CCN is likely to be involved in the care of tunnelled central venous lines and implanted ports. Hospital visits can be minimised and inpatient time reduced if the CCN undertakes the administration of drugs and blood sampling at home or in school.

Routine flushing of lines can also be undertaken by the CCN if the family do not wish to take on this responsibility.

Although cross-infection is less likely to occur in the home environment, there are other safety aspects that need to be addressed. The CCN may have difficulty in maintaining an aseptic field when there are other siblings or pets in the household. The CCN will also need access to an anaphylaxis kit (see Administration of Medicines, p. 63).

The CCN is also in a position to educate the family about the central lines, enabling them to undertake more of the care themselves if they wish.

Do and do not

- Do ensure that the line is clamped during cap changes.
- Do always wash and dry hands thoroughly.
- Do always maintain strict aseptic techniques.
- Do seek expert advice or help with any problems.
- Do educate the child and family in correct line care and how to clamp the line when it is cut or damaged.

- Do not carry out any procedure for which you have not been trained.
- Do not be afraid to seek help from experienced personnel. These lines are very precious, and with good care can last a long time, greatly aiding in the child's treatment.
- Do not use syringes smaller than 5 ml as they will produce a greater pressure than that of the central line and may result in a fracture if the line is blocked.

References

Brandt B, DePalma J, Irwin M, Shogun J, Lucke J 1996 Comparison of central catheter dressings in bone marrow transplant recipients. Oncology Nursing Forum 23(5): 829–836

Bravery K, Hannan J 1997 Central venous devices in children. Paediatric Nursing 9(10): 29–35

Carnock M 1996 Making sense of central venous catheters. Nursing Times 92(49): 30–31

Cesaro S, Corro R, Pelosin A et al 2004 A prospective survey on incidence and outcome of Broviac/Hickman catheter-related complications in pediatric patients affected by hematological and oncological diseases. Annals of Hematology 83(3): 183–188

Chaiyakunapruk N, Veenstra D L, Lipsky B A, Saint S 2002 Chlorhexidine compared with povidone–iodine solution for vascular catheter-site care: a meta-analysis. Annals of Internal Medicine 136(11): 792–801

Department of Health and Hospital Infection Society 2001 Guidelines for preventing infections associated with the insertion and maintenance of central venous catheters. Journal of Hospital Infection 47(Suppl): 547–567

Harrison M 1997 Central venous catheters: a review of the literature. Nursing Standard 11(27): 43–45

Hollis R 1992 Central venous access in children. Paediatric Nursing 4(6): 18–21

Intravenous Nurses Society (INS) 2000 Infusion nursing standards of practice. Journal of Intravenous Nursing 23(65): Supplement III

Keenlyside D 1993 Avoiding an unnecessary outcome. A comparative trial between IV3000 and a conventional film dressing to assess rates of catheter-related sepsis. Professional Nurse (Feb): 288–291

Lawrance T 1994 Central venous line audit. Paediatric Nursing 6(4): 20–23

Lucas H, Attard-Montalto S 1996 Central venous line dressings: study of infection rates. Paediatric Nursing 8(6): 21–23

Maki D, Ringer M, Alvarado C 1991 Prospective randomised trial of povidone iodine, alcohol and chlorhexidine for prevention of infection associated with central venous and arterial catheters. Lancet 338: 339–343

Medicines for Children 2003 Royal College of Paediatrics and Child Health, Neonatal and Paediatric Pharmacists Group, London

National Institute for Clinical Excellence (NICE) 2002 Ultrasound imaging for central venous catheter placement. NICE, London

National Institute for Clinical Excellence (NICE) 2003 Infection control: prevention of healthcare associated infection in primary and community care (No: 4). Care of patients with central venous catheters. Clinical Guidelines 2. NICE, London

Puntis J, Holden C, Smallman S, Finkel Y, George R, Booth I 1990 Staff training: a key factor in reducing intravascular catheter sepsis. Archives of Disease in Childhood 6: 335–337

Royal College of Nursing (RCN) 2003 Standards for infusion therapy. RCN, London

Rumsey K, Richardson D 1995 Management of infection and occlusion associated with vascular access devices. Seminars in Oncology Nursing 11(3): 174–183

Tobiansky R, Lui K, Dalton D M, Shaw P, Martin H, Isaacs D 1997 Complications of central venous access devices in children with and without cancer. Journal of Paediatrics and Child Health 33(6): 509–514

Tweddle D A, Windebank K P, Barrett A M, Leese D C, Gowing R, on behalf of the United Kingdom Children's Cancer Study Group and the Paediatric Oncology Nursing Forum 1997 Central venous catheter use in UKCCSG oncology centres. Archives of Disease in Childhood 77(1): 58–59

Valentino L A, Ewenstein B, Navickis R J, Wilkes M M
2004 Central venous access devices in haemophilia.
Haemophilia 10(2): 134–146

Vidler V 1994 Use of Port-a-Caths in the management
of paediatric haemophilia. Professional Nurse
10(1): 48–50

Further Reading

Royal College of Nursing (RCN) 2001 Administering
intravenous therapy to children in the community
setting – guidance for nursing staff. RCN, London

Practice 9

Chest drainage

Michaela Dixon

Introduction

Chest drainage may be observed in several practice placement areas, including intensive care, the neonatal unit and accident and emergency departments, as well as the general paediatric ward. It is a common practice that requires a thorough knowledge of research-based principles and pathophysiology to nurse effectively and avoid complications. A systematic review of the nursing management of chest drains in 2001 found that there was lack of rigorous research in all areas of chest drain management, particularly in the under 18s (Charnock 2001). This review also noted that practices varied according to individual institutions and that there were often no written protocols to guide practice. As a consequence of this lack of evidence, most of the information in this chapter is based upon adult studies.

Learning outcomes

By the end of this section you should be able to explain:

- why chest drainage is used
- how it is set up
- how the patient is assessed and drainage monitored
- why some traditional practices are controversial
- complications that may occur.

Pathophysiology

Before learning about chest drainage, it is important to remember some key points relating to the anatomy and physiology of the chest:

- The lungs maintain expansion through diaphragmatic and intercostal contraction during inspiration, causing air to be drawn into the lungs by negative pressure, followed by expiration and elastic recoil of the lungs to their original state (Tortora & Grabowski 2003).

- The heart is positioned in the mediastinum. If blood builds up around the heart, or the lung is pushed over to the wrong side of the chest, the heart will become restricted and its function compromised. This is known as cardiac tamponade (Allibone 2003).
- The pleural cavity is a potential space, lying between the visceral and parietal pleura, the diaphragm and mediastinum. Pressure in the space is normally negative (−4 to −10 mmHg). A small amount of fluid is secreted into the space and acts as a lubricant (O'Hanlon-Nichols 1996).
- Any injury, disease or surgical intervention that may cause accumulation of air or fluid in the pleural cavity may impair ventilation, through firstly reducing elastic recoil of the lung and secondly by compression of the lung (Allibone 2003).

The following conditions require chest drainage.

Pneumothorax
Air is present in the pleural space. A pneumothorax may be termed spontaneous (frequent in neonates who aspirate stomach contents, causing alveolar rupture); tension (the alveoli rupture and leak air into the pleural space – this may occur in critically ill children requiring positive pressure ventilation); or open (through trauma) (Wyatt 1995).

Haemothorax
Blood is present in the pleural space and mediastinum. This can occur after chest surgery such as thoracotomy or sternotomy for repair of congenital heart lesions or trauma.

Pleural effusion
Secretions such as fluid, pus (empyema) or chyle from the thoracic duct (chylothorax) fill the pleural space, often as a complication of surgery, or a pre-existing illness (e.g. cystic fibrosis).

Factors to note

Insertion of a chest drain may be performed as an emergency by the doctor. If this is the case, there is little time to alert and prepare parents or the child for the procedure, but simple, brief explanations should be given. If the parents are not present, it is not usually possible to wait to gain their consent, as a delay could be life threatening, but every effort should be made to contact them and inform them of the situation. If chest drains are expected as a result of surgery, children can be prepared through play, with verbal and visual explanation suitable for their conceptual understanding. There will be more time to give parents and the child fuller information.

The procedure is painful and distressing. Cooperation is likely only in the older child; therefore, if time allows, sedation and analgesia should be given, usually by intravenous injection. Local anaesthesia is normally used around the puncture site. If the child is ventilated, breathing against the ventilator may worsen the condition, therefore the use of muscle relaxants may be indicated. It is important to ensure that the ventilator settings are adjusted, e.g. rate increased, to take into account a child who has received a dose of muscle relaxant.

Full monitoring of the child's respiratory rate and effort, heart rate and oxygen saturations should be in place prior to and for the duration of the procedure.

Resuscitation equipment including Ambu bag or T-piece bagging circuit, appropriately sized face mask, airway adjuncts (e.g. Guedel airway), suction equipment and oxygen must be available.

The child should have an intravenous line, though in an emergency the insertion of the chest tube may have higher priority (APLS 2001).

Equipment

Chest drain
The doctor will specify the size and type of drain dependent on whether air or serous matter needs draining.

For a child with suspected pneumothorax in a resuscitation situation, needle thoracocentesis may be performed using a large intravenous cannula and a 20 ml syringe – this is an emergency procedure and the child will require formal chest drain placement after the initial resolution of the pneumothorax (APLS 2001).

There are a number of proprietary chest drains available, ranging from 8 to 32 French gauge (Fg). These chest drains consist of a PVC catheter, with drainage eyes and radiopaque markings (for visualisation on X-ray), and may include a trocar. Some are specifically designed for neonatal or emergency use. The use of a trocar when inserting chest drains in children is not recommended and indeed in adult practice it is also seen as no longer necessary, due to the potential for secondary trauma within the chest cavity (Tang et al 2002).

Chest drainage system

There are now many systems in use on paediatric units, including the traditional self-assembly sets and the ready-assembled proprietary closed versions (Fig. 9.1). All follow the underwater seal principle, and consist of tubing, a water chamber, collection chamber and suction chamber or connections (Fig. 9.2).

Other equipment

- Large dressing trolley
- Medication as above: local anaesthetic, intravenous analgesia, sedation and muscle relaxants (ventilated children only)
- Sterile or distilled water
- Sterile gloves (latex free)
- Syringes and needles
- Dressing of choice
- Skin disinfecting solution
- A surgical dressing or cut-down pack may be helpful, and should contain the following:
  - sterile drapes
  - gauze swabs
  - suture and needle, suturing forceps
  - sterile scissors
  - small scalpel
  - two chest drain clamps (see below).

Method: insertion of the drain

Position

The child will be positioned either on the back or side, depending on the chosen site for the tube and the reason for chest drainage. Because fluid follows gravity, tubes to drain secretions

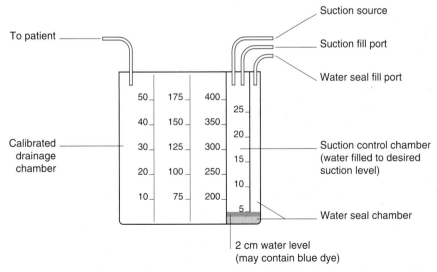

Figure 9.1 Principles of an all-in-one chest drainage unit. Note that it is the level of water in the suction chamber, not the level of suction at source that controls the level of suction in the patient. (Reproduced with permission from Smith et al 1995.)

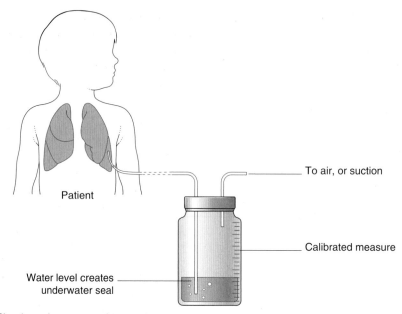

Figure 9.2 Simple underwater seal system

or blood will normally be placed posteriorly, at the lung base. As air normally rises, a tube to drain a pneumothorax will be positioned anteriorly, at the apex of the affected lung (Tang et al 2002, Allibone 2003). Evidence suggests that in most circumstances the actual insertion of the drain within the pleural cavity is more important rather than the precise orientation of the drain (Tang et al 2002).

The nurse is responsible for preparation of the child and equipment, assisting the doctor with the procedure and maintaining asepsis, connecting the system, and comforting and observing the child.

The chest drain should be connected as soon as possible to the underwater seal drainage system. With the all-in-one systems, suction is regulated by the volume of water in the suction chamber (see Fig. 9.1) (Smith et al 1995).

The drainage system should at all times be at least 30 cm below the child's chest (Tang et al 2002, Allibone 2003).

The drain will be sutured to the skin by the doctor. Traditionally a purse-string suture was also used to ease removal; this type of suturing technique is used less often nowadays.

The tubing should be securely attached to the child's skin with adhesive tape to prevent pull on the insertion site. A dry keyhole dressing may be applied to the skin, and secured with tape, or a spray or occlusive dressing used, which allows for visual inspection of the wound.

The child should be positioned comfortably after the procedure, reassured and comforted.

All used equipment should be disposed of according to local polices.

The child should have a chest X-ray to check drain placement.

The procedure and the result of the X-ray should be documented in both the nursing and medical notes.

Complications of chest drain insertion (Tang et al 2002, Allibone 2003)

- Traumatic perforation of the lung
- Traumatic perforation of the mediastinal structures including the heart and major blood vessels
- Traumatic perforation or damage to the diaphragm and intra-abdominal organs
- Trauma to the intercostal neurovascular bundle, which may lead to intercostal neuralgia or haemothorax
- Infection – either at insertion site or within the pleural space

● Subcutaneous emphysema (air collecting in the subcutaneous tissue).

Observations

The child's condition should be observed throughout the procedure and thereafter, especially in the first minutes and hours following insertion, when physiological changes may occur. The frequency of observation will depend on the child's condition, but in the first hour it may be quarter- to half-hourly.

Observation should be systematic starting with the child, then the equipment. All observations should be recorded.

The child

Respiratory system
● Respiratory rate, colour, work of breathing, oxygen saturations.

● Listen to the child's breath sounds, using a stethoscope. Listen to all areas of the chest using a side by side comparison, i.e. listen to the right upper area and then the left upper area, before moving down to the middle area and then the bases. Remember to also listen into the axillary area as air from a pneumothorax may collect in this region. Observe the chest wall for equal movement to each side.

Cardiovascular system
● Heart rate and blood pressure – a fall in blood pressure or rising heart rate may indicate cardiac tamponade, or recurring pneumothorax, and should be reported immediately.
● Skin colour and peripheral perfusion – these should improve after the chest drain is inserted and respiratory function improves.

General
● The child's general condition and responsiveness should be assessed.
● Chest drains are uncomfortable (Gray 2000) and therefore frequent assessment of pain in the child is important with the administration of appropriate analgesia.
● Temperature should be monitored regularly to identify infection.

Care of the equipment
● Identify and label the drains. The child may have more than one, especially after surgery, and it is important to understand their position and intended purpose.

● Observe the insertion site and dressing. There may be signs of fluid or air leakage, or the skin around the site may feel crackly. If so, surgical emphysema may be present and should be reported to the medical staff (O'Hanlon-Nichols 1996). The dressing should be left in place if clean and dry.

● Observe the chest tubes. The connections should be secure. Some units use adhesive tape to ensure that they do not become accidentally separated, though be aware that adhesive tape may actually conceal a loose connection (Godden & Hiley 1998).

● The tubing should be free and unkinked. Excess tubing should not hang in dependent loops from the bed, as this can increase resistance and lessen effective drainage; indeed a column of water accumulating in a loop of tubing may effectively seal the drain and prevent the effective drainage of air (Tang et al 2002); instead it should be positioned in flat loops on the bed (Avery 2000).

● Observe the colour of the drainage and presence of blood (some bloody drainage can be expected immediately after surgery or insertion of a chest drain). Check the volume of fluid drained. It is common practice to mark the level of fluid on the collecting chamber, along with the time and the nurse's initials. The level should be recorded on the fluid balance chart, in accordance with local policy, remembering that drainage represents serous fluid loss, and the doctor may wish to prescribe replacement intravenously, using clear fluid or blood or other blood products. Keep medical staff informed.

● If the drain is a pleural drain, look for the fluid level swinging within the tubing, as the pressures change when the child breathes. Positive pressure ventilation will cause a reverse swing to the negative pressure of spontaneous ventilation. If the fluid is no longer swinging, the air may have completely drained, or the chest drain may have become blocked. This should be reported and discussed with the medical staff (Carroll 1995).

- If the water is bubbling, this may indicate air draining. If the bubbling is continuous, and the child is not receiving positive pressure ventilation, this may indicate an air leak in the drainage system. The system will need to be checked by briefly clamping the chest tube near the patient; if the bubbling continues, there is an air leak. If suction has been applied, the water will bubble gently, but excessive bubbling may indicate too high suction. This will not affect the lungs, but may cause increased water evaporation and disturbing noise for other children and parents (Carroll 1995).

- Check the bottle. It should be well secured, approximately 30 cm below the child's chest.

- Check the fluid level in the drainage chambers; the system will need changing if the chambers are two-thirds full, as too much fluid will increase the resistance to drainage (Allibone 2003). There is little evidence available to be more specific about the frequency of bottle change.

- Check the suction level – suction may not be applied to some intercostal drains; however, if there is a persistent air leak or a large fluid collection, the application of low-pressure suction can expedite the drainage of excessive air or fluid (Tang et al 2002). Drains placed after surgery are normally placed on 'low flow' suction for this reason. There is no definitive evidence about the pressure that should be used; however, the literature suggests that a pressure of 5 kPa or 20 mmHg is usually sufficient (Tang et al 2002). There are some potential problems associated with the application of suction to an intercostal drain – if there is too little suction, it may prevent lung expansion and contribute to infection and atelectasis (Tang et al 1999). If an excessive pressure is used,

there is a risk of damage to the lung tissue (McMahon-Parkes 1997).

Removing the drain

The medical staff will decide to remove the drain on the basis of clinical signs and/or chest X-ray, which will indicate whether the original problem has resolved. Removing the drain can be distressing and uncomfortable. Only the older child will be able to cooperate, so sedation and analgesia may be required.

The tube is removed using an aseptic technique. Any tape holding the tube in position is removed. The tubing is clamped, and any suction discontinued. If the timing can be coordinated, the drain is removed on expiration. If a purse-string suture has been used, the suture is pulled tight to occlude the wound, while the drain is gently and firmly withdrawn. This prevents air being sucked into the pleural space on inspiration. An impermeable dressing is applied to the skin until the wound has healed, so that air cannot enter the pleura through the open drain wound.

The child is made comfortable and observed for recurrence of the problem.

Nursing considerations

Chest drain 'milking'

Chest drain 'milking, when the tubes are stripped with a roller or clamp, has been widely practised in many units and is identified in literature published before the mid 1990s. It was believed to encourage drainage and prevent clots. Its practice is now discouraged, as the negative pressure created can be exceedingly high, up to -400 cmH$_2$O, and cause trauma to the mediastinum or pleural space. It has also been shown that milking has no effect on clot formation, as the pleura have a defibrinating effect on blood (Carroll 1995).

Clamping chest drains

Clamping chest drains when transferring or moving the child is another traditional nursing practice that has been shown to be potentially dangerous. If air is draining, clamping the chest drain can cause a build-up of pressure in the pleural space, leading to tension pneumothorax and sudden lung and circulatory collapse (Avery 2000, Tang et al 2002, Allibone 2003).

The only indications now accepted for possibly clamping underwater seal drains are:

- when changing chest drainage bottles (Allibone 2003)
- in children with pneumothorax, when reinflation of the lung is confirmed by chest X-ray but there is suspicion of an ongoing air leak, allowing for observation of a recurring pneumothorax before the drain is removed. There is a risk of tension pneumothorax developing in this situation and the child must be closely observed during this procedure (Tang et al 2002)
- on accidental disconnection of the chest drain, though it has been argued that a more appropriate response if this has occurred is to submerge the disconnected chest drain under water, while quickly reconnecting the drainage tubes, or reassembling a new drainage system if the previous one has been contaminated (Carroll 1995).

If the bottle is accidentally tipped over or raised above the child's head, it should be immediately returned to its proper position. It should not normally need replacing, as long as the contents of one chamber have not spilled into another.

Do and do not

- Do not milk chest drains.
- Do not clamp drains when moving children – except in specific circumstances.
- Do ask if you are not sure about what you are doing.

Conclusion

The insertion of a chest drain can be a distressing experience for the child and family, therefore the nurse needs to ensure that all aspects of care are explained clearly for all members of the family. If you have any degree of uncertainty, then it is important to seek support and advice from an appropriate member of the care team.

References

Advanced Paediatric Life Support Group (APLS) 2001 Advanced paediatric life support: the practical approach, 3rd edn. BMJ Publishing Group, London

Allibone L 2003 Nursing management of chest drains. Nursing Standard 17(22): 45–54

Avery S 2000 Insertion and management of chest drains. NTPLUS 96(37): 3–6

Carroll P 1995 Chest tubes made easy. Registered Nurse 58(12): 46–56

Charnock Y 2001 The nursing management of chest drains: a systematic review. The Joanna Briggs Institute for Evidence Based Nursing and Midwifery, Adelaide, Australia

Godden J, Hiley C 1998 Managing the patient with a chest drain: a review. Nursing Standard 12(32): 35–39

Gray E 2000 Pain management for patients with chest drains. Nursing Standard 14(23): 40–44

McMahon-Parkes K 1997 Management of pleural drains. Nursing Times 93(53): 48–52

O'Hanlon-Nichols T 1996 Commonly asked questions about chest tubes. American Journal of Nursing 96(5): 60–64

Smith R N, Fallentine J, Kessel S 1995 Underwater chest drainage: bringing the facts to the surface. Nursing 25(2): 60–63

Tang A, Hooper T, Hasan R 1999 A regional survey of chest drains: evidence-based practice? Postgraduate Medical Journal 75(886): 471–474

Tang A, Velissaris T J, Weeden D F 2002 An evidence-based approach to the drainage of the pleural cavity: an evaluation of best practice. Journal of Evaluation in Clinical Practice 8(3): 333–340

Tortora G J, Grabowski S R 2003 Principles of anatomy and physiology. Wiley, New York

Wyatt T 1995 Pneumothorax in the neonate. Journal of Obstetrics, Gynaecology and Neonatal Nursing 24(3): 211–216

Practice **10**

Feeding

Part 1: Breast, bottle and weaning

Teresa Figari, Julia Fearon

Introduction

An adequate diet is vital to promote a child's growth and development. Children are dependent upon adults to feed them safely and appropriately when young and, later, to teach them how and what to provide for themselves when able.

Learning outcomes

By the end of this section you should be able to:

- explain how feeding impacts on a child's development

- describe how to feed a baby/toddler
- list the benefits of breastfeeding
- describe how to calculate a baby's feed requirements.

Rationale

Feeding supplies the baby with food and fluids to aid growth and to promote recovery when ill. It also plays a vital role in development. A children's nurse must be fully aware of how, what and when to feed a child and be able to teach families how to feed their child.

Factors to note

The children's nurse should be familiar with how to assess the child's nutritional status. Being able to plot height and weight on a percentile chart and then interpret the results is an important skill (see 'Assessment', p. 92).

Hands should always be washed thoroughly prior to handling a child's food/feed and before feeding a child. Feeding always presents the risk of cross-infection by introducing bacteria into the body via the intestine. Babies are particularly at risk because of their immature immune system.

Sick infants

Fasting times for procedures

Fasting time is an important consideration, especially for small babies who can dehydrate rapidly and experience hypoglycaemia (Bates 1994). In his article, Bates describes how, further to a research study, fasting times for children have been reduced to 4 hours for solids or milk and 2 hours for clear fluids.

Guidelines

Parental involvement in feeding is not just desirable, but essential. Feeding is one of the basic, vital life functions which parents undertake for their child and is an important part of the bonding process. Parents should always be included.

BREASTFEEDING

The first choice of feed for a healthy baby is breast milk. Breastfeeding secures for the baby optimum health, growth and development, and immunity against illness (Heinig & Dewey 1996, 1997). There is now significant evidence to support the existence of a variety of advantages of breastfeeding both to the infant and mother (British Paediatric Association Standing Committee on Nutrition 1994), which are summarised in Box 10.1.

However, in the UK, breastfeeding rates – although improving – are still relatively low. By the baby's sixth week of life, only 42% of mothers are still breastfeeding, down from 69% who breastfed initially (Hamlyn et al 2002). There is growing evidence of the lifetime benefits of exclusive breastfeeding and consequently the World Health Organization (WHO 2003) recommend that all babies be exclusively breastfed until 6 months of age. This is supported by the UK government (Department of Health 2004a).

A mother whose baby is sick should be given all the information to make a fully informed decision about breastfeeding, especially if she would have chosen to formula feed. The benefits of breastfeeding offer particular advantages to sick babies and, contrary to some thinking, these babies can breastfeed successfully. If the infant is too sick to feed at the breast, the mother can express her milk and it

---

Box 10.1   Advantages of breastfeeding

Advantages to the baby

Reduced risk of developing:
- gastrointestinal illness and gastroenteritis in particular
- middle ear infection
- respiratory system infection
- urinary tract infection
- insulin-dependent diabetes mellitus
- allergies, e.g. eczema

for the preterm baby:
- optimum neurological development

- reduced risk of necrotising enterocolitis

Advantages to the mother

Reduced risk of:
- premenopausal breast cancer
- some forms of ovarian cancer

Social gains:
- ready availability for feeding baby
- unique contact between mother and baby
- may help mother to lose weight naturally

After Heinig & Dewey 1996, 1997.

can be given to the baby via a nasogastric tube, cup and spoon or by bottle.

The reasons why a mother stops breastfeeding vary, but a recurrent issue is the lack of help and support to continue when difficulties are encountered (Hamlyn et al 2002). Social and cultural factors, e.g. early return to work, can also influence a mother's decision to cease breastfeeding. Lack of knowledgeable support can be a particular issue if the baby is admitted to a children's ward, especially straight from a maternity unit, as education about breastfeeding for children's nurses has been sketchy or non-existent in the past. The UNICEF Baby Friendly Initiative (1997) has supported specific guidance for good practice on paediatric units and these should be readily available for paediatric nurses on each unit where babies are admitted.

BREAST MILK

Breast milk changes to reflect the needs of the growing infant. During the first 3 days colostrum is produced which is richer in protein and minerals and lower in carbohydrates, fat and some vitamins than the mature milk that follows. Mature milk changes during the feed: the first milk is called foremilk and is five times lower in fat than the hindmilk which provides the bulk of the calories and is more satisfying to the baby. The foremilk contains high levels of maternal antibodies and immunoglobulins that protect the infant. At 14 days of age the infant ingests approximately 128 kcal/kg while at the age of 3 months the milk yields 70–75 kcal/kg (Riordan 2005).

FREQUENCY AND LENGTH OF BREASTFEEDS

Breastfeeding works on a supply and demand process, so the more the baby feeds the more milk is produced, so baby-led feeding is important for a plentiful milk supply (Chadderton et al 1997). Up to 10–15 times in 24 hours is not an unusual frequency; in the first few days after birth, babies may want to feed for long periods, sometimes up to an hour. As breastfeeding becomes established, the fre-

quency of feeds settles to an average of eight feeds over 24 hours (Hornell et al 1999). If the baby continues to feed frequently and is unsettled after a feed, positioning and attachment could be at fault and the mother should be referred to a breastfeeding specialist. Remember that the baby must be allowed to suckle for long enough in order to receive both high-lactose foremilk and high-fat hindmilk, i.e. not just for a brief 3–5 minutes. Correct positioning and attachment to promote the effectiveness of the baby's sucking are important for effective emptying of the breasts. Baby should be allowed to feed, to come off the first breast automatically (not be taken off) and then offered the second breast. This is then the breast to be offered first at the next feed.

Night feeding is important in a breastfed baby. Maternal prolactin secretion is greater at night and prolactin is the hormone which promotes lactation.

Equipment to breastfeed

- The only 'equipment' necessary for breastfeeding will be a drink for the mother, close to hand.
- Breast pads or tissues may be required to mop any leakage from the breast from which the baby is not feeding.
- The mother must feel comfortable if she is to breastfeed well, so she may require a special chair or pillow in order to find her optimum position.
- Nipple shields should be avoided as they can reduce the mother's milk supply, and also may exacerbate nipple problems, e.g. fissures (Chadderton et al 1997).

Method

This method is based on Chadderton et al (1997).

1. Ensure that the mother is comfortable with a drink close at hand. The mother can either be sitting (see Fig. 10.1) or lying down (see Fig. 10.2).

2. If the baby is calm and relaxed, feeding is likely to progress better.

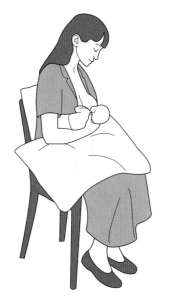

Figure 10.1   Breastfeeding in the sitting position.

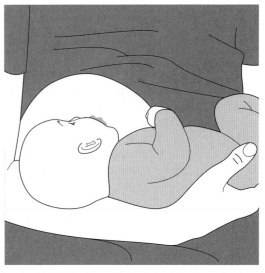

Figure 10.3   Position of the infant during a feed.

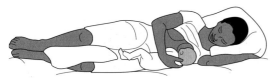

Figure 10.2   Breastfeeding in the lying position.

3. Position the baby to lie comfortably close to the mother with the baby's head and body in line and not twisted. The baby's head should be well supported, but free to move; do not hold the baby's head but support from the shoulders (see Figs 10.3 and 10.4). The baby's nose and mouth should be in line with the nipple.

4. Depending on its size and shape, the mother's breast may need support from her hand (see Fig. 10.5). Place the mother's hand with fingers flat against her rib cage so that the breast is supported by the angle of thumb and forefinger. The breast can also be supported with the hand underneath and thumb lightly on top well back from the areola so that the mother can form her breast into a good shape for the baby to latch on.

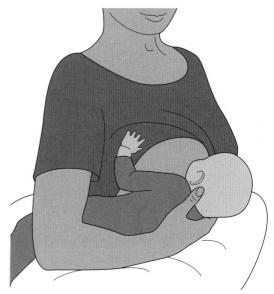

Figure 10.4   Supporting the baby during a feed.

5. Allow the baby to root for the breast, letting tongue and lips touch the nipple (see Fig. 10.6). Allowing the baby's head to tilt back slightly will encourage the baby to open the mouth wide. Then bring the baby back to the breast quickly, but smoothly, aiming the

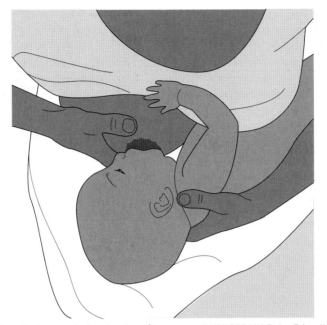

Figure 10.5 Supporting the breast during feeding. (Courtesy of UNICEF UK Baby Friendly Initiative. www.babyfriendly.org.uk)

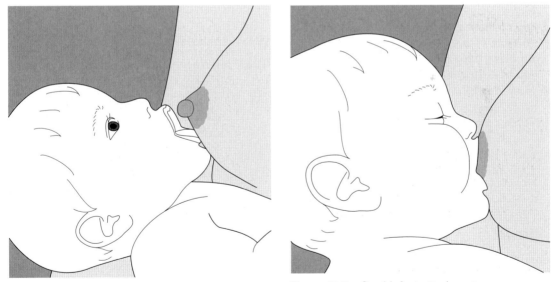

Figure 10.6 Infant rooting to the breast.

Figure 10.7 Good infant attachment.

lower jaw at the base of the areola (see Fig. 10.7). This brings the tongue over the lower lip to scoop up the areola, nipple and as much breast tissue as possible, ensuring that the tongue can reach the lactiferous ducts within the tissue behind the areola. The lactiferous ducts are small reservoirs of milk from which the milk is released.

6. Allow the baby to feed as long as desired from the first breast before moving on to the second, to ensure that both fore- and hind-milks are released. A baby should not have the feed stopped prematurely. While in hospital, any medical or nursing interventions should be timed around feeds and not be allowed to interrupt feeds.

Observations and complications for breastfeeding

Observations (Chadderton et al 1997)

● Observe that the mother and baby are comfortable and relaxed, with baby close to mother with the head and body straight, chin touching her breast (and in the young infant < 6 months, with the bottom supported).
● Observe the baby's responses. Does the baby reach (root in the newborn) for the breast, use the tongue to explore the breast, stay attached? Are there signs of milk ejection (afterpains, milk leakage)?
● Is there evidence of emotional bonding (mother has a secure, confident hold, watches and touches her baby); does the baby watch her?
● Anatomy – are the breasts soft and full, the nipples protractile, skin healthy and breasts round during feeding?
● How does the baby suckle? Is the mouth wide, lower lip turned outward, tongue cupped around the breast? Are the cheeks round? Does the baby produce slow, deep sucks in bursts followed by short pauses? Can you see or hear the baby swallow?
● Note how long the baby feeds and record if required.
● Observe for signs of possible difficulty – see below.

Complications/difficulties

There are no complications of breastfeeding as such, but there may be some difficulties in establishing effective breastfeeding.

● Mother is tense and not relaxed – give the mother time to talk through worries and fears, and provide emotional and practical support. If the baby is uninterested at the start, try cuddling well into the breast, skin to skin between feeds. This will help the

baby become used to the smell, feel and appearance of the breast (Chadderton et al 1997). Do not give dummies, bottles or pacifiers which can confuse a baby trying to learn how to breastfeed (Shore 1998).

● If mother's nipples become sore and/or cracked this is usually due to poor positioning and attachment. Refer to a breastfeeding specialist.

● Be aware that many drugs can be excreted in breast milk and therefore ingested by the baby (Hale 2004).

EXPRESSING BREAST MILK

A mother may need to express milk:

● to relieve her breasts if they are full or uncomfortable
● if her baby is unable to feed because of illness (e.g. too small or sick, or is being starved in preparation for an operation)
● if she is going to be away from her baby for more than an hour or two, or going back to work
● to help the baby attach to a full breast.

There are three ways to express breast milk: by hand (see Fig. 10.8), hand pump (see Fig. 10.9) or electric pump (see Fig. 10.10).

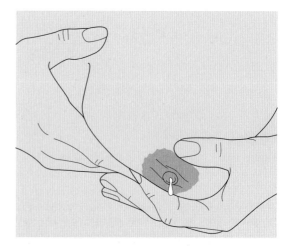

Figure 10.8   Expressing by hand. (Courtesy of UNICEF UK Baby Friendly Initiative. www.babyfriendly.org.uk)

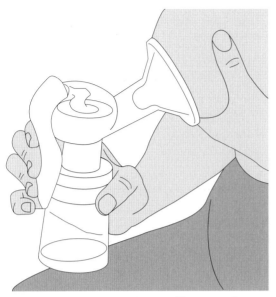

Figure 10.9 Using a hand pump. (Courtesy of UNICEF UK Baby Friendly Initiative. www.babyfriendly.org.uk)

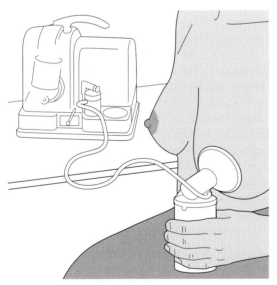

Figure 10.10 Using an electric pump. (Courtesy of UNICEF UK Baby Friendly Initiative. www.babyfriendly.org.uk)

Any equipment used for expressing milk must be sterilised before use and the mother's hands must be washed and carefully dried. In hospital, kits for electric breast pumps can be re-used after autoclaving if recommended for multiple use by the manufacturer, e.g. Egnell breast pump kits. Nurses should familiarise themselves with the type of pump their department offers to mothers to use.

If a mother is expressing milk to maintain a supply whilst her baby is unable to suckle, she should aim to express at least six to eight times in each 24 hours, including once at night.

Breast milk can be stored for up to 24 hours in a refrigerator (which must maintain a temperature of 2–4°C) or up to 3 months in a freezer. However, from an infection control viewpoint, breast milk is a body fluid and therefore should be stored in a refrigerator or freezer containing nothing but breast milk. It must not be stored with any other type of artificial baby milk or any food. The expressed breast milk must be dated to avoid any old milk being given in error. The bottles should also contain the name and unit number of the mother and baby. Always refer to local policies and guidelines.

Breast milk that has previously been frozen then thawed must be stored in the refrigerator and used within 24 hours. If not used, thawed milk must be thrown away.

Do and do not

- Do promote breastfeeding; provide encouragement, help and support to mothers who wish to breastfeed.
- Do ensure that a breastfeeding mother has access to a well-balanced diet and sufficient fluids.
- Do be aware of where to obtain expert help for the breastfeeding mother, if unable to provide it from available staff. Most maternity units and primary care trusts have breastfeeding advisors who are experts in their field.
- Do ensure that a breastfeeding mother has access to facilities to enable her to express milk when necessary.
- Do not give a breastfed baby a dummy or pacifier.
- Do not give a breastfed baby artificial milk, water or juice unless it is medically indicated, with fully informed parental choice and consent.

- Do not give a breastfed baby a bottle. If a breastfed baby has to be given anything by mouth, it should be fed using a cup or cup and spoon.

Eliminating

Breastfed babies should have a good urine output with frequent wet nappies. Their stool can vary but should be soft and yellow without being watery; frequency varies from every nappy to once a day, sometimes even less than this.

ARTIFICIAL FEEDING

Not all mothers will choose or be able to breastfeed their babies. Hull and Johnston (1993) list some contraindications to breastfeeding:

- The very premature infant's inability to suck, but breast milk can be given via nasogastric tube or cup and spoon.
- Some severe abnormalities of an infant's mouth, e.g. severe cleft palate; again breast milk can be given via nasogastric tube.
- Severe maternal ill health may contraindicate breastfeeding, e.g. active tuberculosis and HIV infection can both be transmitted to the infant via breast milk. Fully informed consent from the mother is the factor here; refer to local policies.
- The mother who is severely undernourished or has poor renal function may find breastfeeding an unacceptable drain on her own nutritional reserves.
- The child has a medical condition, e.g. phenylketonuria, which necessitates a special diet that precludes feeding with breast milk (Hull & Johnston 1993).

A children's nurse must be able to undertake and advise on artificial methods of feeding as well as calculate if a baby is taking appropriate amounts of feed to sustain expected growth and development. This is calculated by multiplying the child's body weight by a figure which is determined by age (see Table 10.1).

On the basis of the figures in Table 10.1, a 3-month-old baby weighing 5.2 kg should receive: $5.2 \times 150 = 780$ ml in 24 hours.

Table 10.1 Average fluid requirements of a healthy baby

Age of baby	Average total fluid requirement in 24 hours in ml/kg
Newborn	30
2 days	60
3 days	90
4 days	120
5 days	150
1 week to 8 months	150
9–12 months	120

Exceptions to this calculation are determined by a children's dietitian (if available) or a paediatrician. Exceptional circumstances might include a baby failing to thrive, who requires 200 ml/kg/day, or a child in renal failure or with cerebral oedema, who requires restricted fluids, e.g. 75 ml/kg/day.

It is a matter of parental choice as to which artificial feed their healthy baby is given. They may require guidance from healthcare staff as to the most suitable breast milk substitute, infant formula or follow-on milk, but it should be made clear to all parents that cow's milk is not suitable for children under 12 months of age (Shore 1995). Formula milks are mostly some form of modified cow's milk, containing protein in the form of casein (the protein in cow's milk). Hull & Johnston (1993) summarise the four basic types of formula milk as:

- a whey-based formula with a whey:casein ratio of 60:40 like human milk, e.g. SMA Gold Cap
- a casein-based formula with a whey:casein ratio of 20:80 like cow's milk, e.g. SMA White Cap
- a soya protein-based formula with no milk constituents, e.g. Wysoy
- a follow-on formula for infants who have been weaned; these are iron enriched, with a higher protein content, e.g. Progress.

Vitamin and iron supplements for infants

The Department of Health (1994) advises that vitamin supplements are not necessary for breastfed babies under 6 months, provided that the mother's vitamin intake is adequate, or for formula-fed infants taking more than 500 ml/day. An infant taking less than 500 ml/day or an infant over 6 months whose main source of nutrition is breast milk should receive vitamin A and D supplements.

PREPARING ARTIFICIAL FEEDS

Larger children's units and children's hospitals will usually have a special feed unit or milk kitchen where baby feeds are made under sterile conditions. If feeds are to be made on the wards, very careful attention must be paid to the risk of cross-infection. A separate area should be set aside for feed preparation, away from any other food.

Equipment

- Documentation listing type and quantity of feed to be made
- Washed and sterilised bottles with fluid measure on side
- Washed and sterilised manufacturer-supplied milk powder scoop
- Boiled, cooled water (that has been boiled only once and has not been artificially softened)
- Milk powder of the same brand as the scoop; check that the milk powder is within its expiry date
- Washed and sterilised plastic knife with straight-edged back
- 70% isopropyl alcohol spray or impregnated swab
- Patient identification labels.

Method

1. Wash and dry hands thoroughly; put on disposable plastic apron.
2. Ensure that the work surface is clean and dry; spray or wipe the surface with 70% isopropyl alcohol.
3. Pour the required amount of boiled, cooled water into each of the bottles. The amount required is the total amount of feed per bottle. For example, if the baby requires 125 ml at each feed, put 125 ml of water in each bottle.
4. Using the correct brand of scoop for the type of milk powder being used, scoop up the milk powder. Do not pack the milk tightly into the scoop. Using the flat edge of the knife, level off the top of the powder with the top of the scoop. Add the powder to the water. One scoop of powder is added to each fluid ounce (28.4 ml) of water. Any less powder than this and the baby will be underfed; any more powder than this and the too concentrated feed can lead to diarrhoea and even hypernatraemia.
5. Once all the powder has been added to the feed, put the lid on each bottle and shake well to mix the milk powder and water thoroughly.
6. Label the bottle with the baby's identification label, the type and quantity of feed and the expiry date (24 hours later). All the feeds should then be autoclaved/pasteurised and stored in a refrigerator specifically for milk feeds only.

BOTTLE FEEDING A BABY

Equipment

- Plastic apron
- Sterile bottle of milk of correct formula type and quantity
- Sterile teat
- Jug of hot water with sealable lid or bottle warmer to heat bottle
- Bib
- Comfortable chair with support for arm
- Sterilising unit containing 125 parts per million of hypochlorite in solution
- Documentation to record feed given.

Method

1. Prior to feeding, ensure that the baby's nose is clean and also ensure that the baby has a

clean, dry nappy. The baby is less likely to feed well with a nose blocked with mucus or when uncomfortable from a wet or soiled nappy.

2. Wash hands thoroughly and put on an apron (to prevent cross-infection).

3. If using a proprietary pre-prepared formula milk, first check the cap according to the manufacturer's instructions to ensure that the seal has not been broken.

4. Check that the expiry date of the feed has not passed and check again that the feed is of the correct make and the quantity to be given.

5. If the feed is to be heated (some babies prefer milk at room temperature), a bottle warmer should be used or, if one is not available, then a jug of water taken from the kettle. If the feed has been refrigerated prior to use, this will need to be nearly boiling water. The bottle should be heated in the feed preparation area/ward kitchen and the warmed feed then taken to the infant to avoid any potential hazard from carrying a jug of very hot water through a ward area.

6. After approximately 2 minutes, check the feed to see if it feels warm enough. Test the temperature of the milk by squirting a small amount onto the skin on the underside of the forearm. Ideally the milk should be at approximately blood temperature (37°C), as breast milk would be, therefore it should feel just warm and not hot on contact with the skin. Too hot milk can easily burn the baby's mouth. If it feels hot, it must not be given to the baby until it has cooled down; the temperature must be tested again after cooling, before giving it to the baby.

7. Put the bib around the baby to protect clothing.

8. The baby should be held well supported for feeding, with the head above the stomach. This reduces the risk of accidental aspiration of stomach contents. A baby should never be bottle-fed whilst lying flat because of the increased risk of vomiting and aspiration of feed and vomit into the lungs.

9. Offer the bottle by placing it gently to the lips. Never force a bottle into a baby's mouth. If the baby is reluctant to accept the bottle, it may help to gently stroke the skin just to the side of the baby's mouth. This can stimulate the sucking reflex, as can stroking the baby gently under the chin.

10. Hold the bottle at a sufficiently steep angle to keep the teat filled with milk, to help prevent the baby sucking in too much air which can cause discomfort and vomiting (Hull & Johnston 1993). Most babies can take approximately half of the total amount of feed before requiring to be winded. Winding the baby helps to bring up any air swallowed during feeding (Hull & Johnston 1993), thereby promoting comfort and helping to reduce the incidence of vomiting after feeding.

11. Gently remove the bottle and sit the baby up, supporting the head if the baby is unable to do so. Gently rubbing the baby's back can help to bring up the wind. Some babies like to be put up onto the shoulder to be winded, but take care to protect the shoulder and back in case the baby regurgitates some milk with the wind. Regurgitating a small amount of milk with wind is normal and is known as posseting (Hull & Johnston 1993).

12. Remember that feeding is a time to promote physical contact, eye contact and verbal stimulation for the baby.

13. After the feed is completed, wind again and then make the baby comfortable. Ideally (and particularly if prone to vomiting), the baby should be allowed to sit up for 20–30 minutes after a feed to prevent aspiration and vomiting.

14. Record what feed was offered, how much feed was taken and note if there was any vomiting. If vomiting has occurred, describe the consistency and quantity.

15. Clear away. If the bottle and/or teat (if not a single-use teat) are to be used again, the bottle should be washed thoroughly in warm, soapy water then rinsed carefully.

The teat should be washed thoroughly and salt may be rubbed inside it to remove all traces of milk. It should then be rinsed thoroughly to remove all salt. The clean bottle and teat are then submerged completely in the sterilising solution, ensuring that there are no air bubbles, and left in the sterilising unit for at least 30 minutes. The presence of any organic matter (e.g. milk, saliva) in a hypochlorite solution will destabilise it and render it incapable of sterilising. Hypochlorite solutions should be discarded every 24 hours or if there is evidence of contamination of the solution. It is not necessary to rinse the hypochlorite solution off the teat prior to offering it to the baby.

Observations and complications

Observations

Feeding is a good time to assess whether the baby is developing as expected for age. Be aware of how the baby is on handling. Is head control appropriate for age? Is there any abnormal stiffness or floppiness or does the baby handle as would be expected of a child of that age? Observe the baby's face, expressions, eye movements, eye contact. Check that the baby is achieving developmental milestones, e.g. fixing and following by 4 weeks. Observe how the baby feeds, noting if there is a good, strong suck or if the baby is slow to feed and sleepy or unusually drowsy. If there is vomiting, observe the physical nature of the vomiting and the vomit itself, e.g. is it effortless or projectile, is the vomit milky or bile-stained? Report any unusual findings.

Complications of bottle feeding

As with any calculation, there is the risk of human error, resulting in too much or too little being given. Parents unaware of how much feed they should give their baby could overfeed, leading to excessive weight gain over a prolonged period, or underfeed, resulting in weight loss and dehydration. In addition, a child with medical problems such as congenital heart disease or renal disease may not cope with a feed calculated at the normal quantities. The incorrect feed could be given which may be a problem if special additives are omitted or given accidentally. A feed that has been reconstituted incorrectly may cause hypernatraemia (salt overload) if it is too concentrated, or provide insufficient calories if too dilute.

Do and do not

- Do calculate the feed correctly.
- Do ensure that, if making up feeds, the correct brand of milk scoop is used for the correct type of milk powder.
- Do ensure that exactly one level scoop of milk powder is added to each fluid ounce (28.4 ml) of cooled, boiled water.
- Do ensure that the correct type of formula and amount of feed is given to the right baby.
- Do remember to test the temperature of a feed before it is given to a baby.
- Do not bottle feed a baby which is lying flat.
- Do not reconstitute baby milk powder with water that has been boiled more than once.
- Do not reheat bottle feeds more than once.

TODDLER FEEDING

WEANING

The Department of Health (DoH 2004a,b) identify the following recommendations for weaning:

- Solid food should not be introduced before the age of 6 months. After this time, the baby will need more iron and nutrients than can be provided by breast milk alone.
- Suitable first weaning foods to be given by spoon are non-wheat cereals, fruit, vegetables, potatoes.
- Diet should include good sources of vitamin C to aid iron absorption.
- Non-breastfed babies should only receive infant formula milk for the first year (they may be given follow-on, iron-rich formula milks from 6 months onwards).

- From 6 months onwards the child should gradually receive a mixed diet, totally free from added salt and, wherever possible, free from added sugar.
- Drinking from a cup is to be encouraged from 6 months.
- If there is doubt that dietary iron is adequate, consider the continued use of iron-enriched formula/follow-on milk.
- Cow's, goat's or sheep's milk must not be introduced before 12 months of age.
- Discourage bottle feeds from 12 months.
- Water should be the drink of choice when milk is not required.
- 1–5 years: vitamin A and D supplements should be given unless there is certainty that the child is receiving adequate quantities in the diet and moderate exposure to sunlight.
- Prevent dental caries: promote healthy dentition by avoiding sugared or fizzy drinks and fruit juices. Give only at meal times via cup, not bottle or pacifier.

Note: However adequate the dietary iron intake, it is useless without intake of substances such as vitamin C which enables the iron actually to be absorbed (Palmer 1993). In addition, other dietary substances (tea, egg yolk) can inhibit the absorption of iron (Palmer 1993).

Factors to note

Feeding is important to several areas of the toddler's development. Social, fine motor and perceptual development can be demonstrated, for example, by a 10-month-old boy attempting to grasp and manipulate the spoon with which he is being fed and his determination to try to feed himself (Bee 1997). Whilst it can be frustrating for child and carer to see him continually drop food just before he gets it to his mouth, it should not be discouraged. Neither should he be discouraged from handling food, as exploring texture teaches him about the surrounding world. However, it is important to distinguish between acceptable learning behaviour in comparison to what would constitute unacceptable social behaviour if allowed to become established. Allowing the child to

experience different textures of food aids the development of speech.

The use of high glycaemic index foodstuffs during weaning and starting weaning early have been indicated as important factors associated with the increase in childhood obesity. The eating habits of parents are also considered as influential (Postnote 2003, BUPA 2004).

FEEDING A TODDLER (APPROXIMATELY 9–24 MONTHS)

Equipment

- High chair
- Food of appropriate consistency according to age and level of development, e.g. will he require finger foods, can he tolerate lumpy foods?
- Bib
- Feeder beaker of water or diluted fruit juice; avoid fizzy drinks and sugary squashes.
- Spoons for feeding (the toddler will often want one to himself, even if he is unable to feed independently)
- Documentation to record food given if required.

Method

1. Wash the child's hands and utilise the opportunity to teach him about washing his own hands prior to meals.

2. Wash hands thoroughly and put on an apron (to prevent cross-infection).

3. Ensure that the toddler is strapped safely and securely into the high chair.

4. Allow him to hold a spoon of his own. He may accept help to put food onto his spoon.

5. Put a small amount of food onto the spoon. If he is managing well with his own spoon, let him carry on. Do not try to get him to take food from your spoon.

6. If he is having difficulty, intersperse his own efforts at feeding by placing your

spoon just into the front of his mouth. Never force the spoon into his mouth.

7. Constantly encourage him and praise him when he manages to put food into his mouth himself and when he accepts food from you.

8. As children learn to manipulate their mouth and tongue muscles, inevitably some food gets spat out accidentally. However, it will become clear if there is a particular food which he does not like. He will try to spit it out and may well purse his lips and refuse to take another mouthful. Offer that particular food once more. If he still refuses or spits it out again, try another item of food from the plate instead.

9. Encourage him to feed himself finger foods, e.g. carrot, bread, fruit. This teaches him independence, different textures of food (not purée) and enables him to experience the achievement of feeding himself.

10. Offer him a drink from his feeder cup once or twice during the meal, at the end of the savoury course and at the end of the meal. The last drink of the meal would ideally be water to help rinse his mouth and prevent dental caries.

11. Allow him to feel his food if he so wishes, but discourage him from throwing his plate or utensils. Be firm and consistent in what behaviour is allowed and what is not tolerated.

12. At the end of his meal, clear away the remains and clean his face and hands.

Observations and complications

Observations
Observe how the toddler reacts to being fed. Does he help himself, or is he very passive? This can tell you something about his level of development.

Establish the toddler's likes and dislikes in different foods and textures.

Relate your observations of how he feeds and what he does and does not like to the information given to you by his parents.

Observe how he behaves when fed by his parents. Useful information about how he and his parents interact can be gained from observing them during a meal time.

Complications
There are few complications associated with feeding a toddler. There could be a risk of him choking on a piece of food, in which case he should be given emergency treatment for choking, following resuscitation guidelines.

If the food he is given is too hot, there is a risk of him burning his mouth.

Do and do not

- Do check the temperature of his food before feeding him.
- Do praise and encourage him when he succeeds in feeding himself.
- Do allow him to help feed himself.
- Do let him touch and feel his food.
- Do be prepared for a messy meal time.
- Do not give him a lot to drink prior to a meal that would fill his stomach and make him less hungry.
- Do not ever force him to take food.

References

Bates J 1994 Reducing fasting times in paediatric day surgery. Child Health 90(48): 38–39

Bee H 1997 The developing child, 8th edn. Addison-Wesley, New York, ch 5, p 128–129

British Paediatric Association Standing Committee on Nutrition 1994 Is breastfeeding beneficial in the UK? Archives of Disease in Childhood 71: 376–380

BUPA 2004 Avoiding childhood obesity. BUPA'S Health Information Team Leaflet. February

Chadderton M, MacDonald A, Munn J et al 1997 A healthy start – infant feeding policy. South Birmingham Community Health Trust, Birmingham Children's Hospital NHS Trust, Birmingham, UK

Department of Health 1994 Report of working group on weaning diet of the committee of medical aspects of food policy. Weaning and the weaning diet. HMSO, London

Department of Health 2004a Breastfeeding. DH, London. Online. Available: www.dh.gov.uk/asset Root/04/08/44/52/04084452.pdf

Department of Health 2004b Birth to five: your complete guide to parenthood and the first five years of your child's life. DoH, London. Online. Available: www.dh.gov.uk/asset Root/04/08/41/26/04084126.pdf

Hale T 2004 Medications and mothers milk, 11th edn. Pharmasoft Publishing, Amarillo, Texas

Hamlyn B, Brooker S, Oleinkova K, Wands S 2002 Infant feeding 2000. A survey conducted on behalf of the Department of Health, The Scottish Executive, The National Assembly of Wales and the Department of Health, Social Services and Public Safety in Northern Ireland. TSO, London

Heinig M J, Dewey K G 1996 Health advantages of breastfeeding for infants: a critical review. Nutrition Research Reviews 9: 89–110

Heinig M J, Dewey K G 1997 Health effects of breastfeeding for mothers: a critical review. Nutrition Research Reviews 10: 35–36

Hornell A 1999 Breastfeeding patterns in exclusively breast fed infants: a longitudinal prospective study in Uppsala, Sweden. Acta Paediatrica 88: 203–211

Hull D, Johnston D I 1993 Essential paediatrics, 3rd edn. Churchill Livingstone, Edinburgh, ch 5, p 75–89

Palmer G 1993 Any old iron. Health Visitor 66(7): 248–249, 252

Postnote 2003 Childhood obesity. Parliamentary Office of Science and Technology, London. Postnote No. 205 September

Riordan J 2005 Breastfeeding and human lactation, 3rd edn. Jones and Bartlett, Boston, MA

Shore C 1995 The COMA report: nursing implications. Paediatric Nursing 7(3): 14–17

Shore C 1998 Good practice guidelines for breastfeeding in paediatric units. Paediatric Nursing 10(1): 29–24

UNICEF UK Baby Friendly Initiative 1997 Breastfeeding guidance for paediatric units. UNICEF, London. Online. Available: www.babyfriendly.org.uk/paedunits.asp

World Health Organization (WHO) 2003 Global strategy for infant and young child feeding. WHO, Geneva, Switzerland

Further Reading

Agnew T 1996 Battle of the breast in the classroom. Nursing Times 92(2): 15

Baby Friendly website: www.babyfriendly.org.uk

Coldicutt P 1994 Children's options. Nursing Times 90(13): 54–56

Elia I 1994 Adoptive breastfeeding. Nursing Standard 8(43): 20–21

Henshel D, Inch S 1996 Breastfeeding: a guide for midwives. Books for Midwives Press, Hale, UK

Payne D 1995 A lot of bottle. Nursing Times 91(17): 20–21

Royal College of Midwives 1991 Successful breastfeeding. Churchill Livingstone, Edinburgh

Part 2: Enteral feeding

Christopher Bunford

Introduction

Enteral feeding is an artificial method of supplying the child with nutrition via a nasogastric tube or gastrostomy.

Learning outcomes

By the end of this section you should:
- be able to identify some typical situations in which a child may require enteral feeding
- be able to describe the techniques of providing enteral nutrition and hydration to the child who is unable to feed orally
- understand the possible risks and side-effects associated with some feeding techniques.

Rationale for enteral feeding

A children's nurse should be able to undertake enteral feeding, teach children and their families the different techniques and be aware of possible positive and negative effects of enteral feeding.

Factors to note

See Factors to note in Part 1 of this section.

Hambridge et al (1995) give reasons why some children are unable to feed orally:

- The child has cancer and the treatment causes anorexia and vomiting.
- The child is unable to take in sufficient nutrition for growth and development in an acute or chronic illness, e.g. severe bronchiolitis, gross reflux, renal failure or liver disease, particularly when the child has increased calorific and nutrient requirements.
- The child is unable to absorb the food, e.g. short bowel syndrome and severe, acute diarrhoea.
- The premature infant may not yet have developed a swallowing reflex.

These children can be fed enterally via nasogastric (NG) tube or gastrostomy (Hambridge et al 1995).

The multidisciplinary team is essential when a sick child has special dietary requirements:

- A children's dietitian and/or paediatrician may be required to prescribe a feed or extra calories (Maxijul) or additives, e.g. a thickening agent (Nestargel).

- A doctor may need to prescribe drugs, e.g. antireflux treatment, electrolyte supplements or intestinal motility regulators (domperidone, loperamide).

● Nutritional care nurse specialists may be available in some hospitals to help advise on practical aspects of feeding children.

● It is essential that a speech therapist conduct an assessment of the child's oral motor function if long-term NG feeding is required, and is a source of valuable advice with regard to the child's developmental needs associated with feeding (Langley 1994, NHS QIS 2003).

● Testing for acidity of gastric secretions to ensure correct positioning of NG tubes is essential to ensure safety. Gastric and respiratory secretions are both acidic to a degree (pH <7.0). Blue litmus paper will turn pink whenever the secretion being tested has a pH <7.0 and is not therefore sufficiently sensitive to distinguish between the pH of gastric and respiratory secretions when determining if a NG tube is correctly positioned. Indicator paper that measures pH range 0–4 should always be used when performing an aspirate test to check positioning of a NG tube (NHS QIS 2003, Medical Devices Agency 2004, NPSA 2005).

● The use of pH indicator paper in neonates has been questioned by practitioners as their gastric secretions may not be sufficiently acidic to entail a change. Similarly, gastric acid pH response may be altered when infants/children are taking antacids. In these chidren the pH reference range for testing with pH paper may be altered. Refer to local guidelines regarding type of pH paper and acceptable readings (Nutritional Care 2004, NPSA 2005). If there is any doubt that the tube may not be correctly positioned it should not be used until its correct position in the stomach has been confirmed by senior nursing/medical staff.

● It used to be common practice to check the position of a NG tube by listening with a stethoscope for the sound of air injected into the stomach via the NG tube. Research has shown this to be an inaccurate and dangerous practice and should no longer be used (Hendry et al 1986, Metheny et al 1990, NPSA 2005).

Nasogastric tubes

There are two main types of NG tube commonly used: a polyvinylchloride (PVC) tube, e.g. Portex, and polyurethane tubes. Polyurethane tubes are sometimes known as 'silk' tubes. They are single-use only and the PVC tube is primarily for short-term feeding, i.e. of less than 3 months' duration. The polyurethane tubes for longer-term feeding can remain in situ for up to a month.

The tubes are sized according to the width of their internal lumen; 6, 8 and very occasionally 10 French gauge (Fg) are most commonly used in children. If a thickening agent has been added to the child's feed, the small 6 Fg diameter tube may be too narrow to facilitate instillation of the feed. Tubes commonly come in two lengths, 50 and 100 cm for 'silk' tubes. The length used will depend on how big the child is. The tube must be long enough to cover the length from the outer edge of the child's face, through the nasopharynx and down into the stomach (see Fig. 10.11).

PVC tubes should be changed every 5–7 days and polyurethane tubes monthly to prevent increased risk of bacterial contamination and the material of the tube being eroded by gastric juices (Taylor & Goodison-McLaren 1992, Skipper et al 2003).

Gastrostomy tubes are made of silicone. There are three main types: skin-level 'button' or 'key' devices, percutaneous endoscopic tubes and surgically placed tubes, e.g. Foley catheter (see Fig. 10.12).

Once healed, the skin around a gastrostomy site should be washed daily to prevent the skin around the site becoming sore (Coldicutt 1994). Frequency and timing of tube changes vary according to the device used and the child's condition. The gastrostomy button is a device in which the exterior of the tube sits flush with the skin and, when not in use, resembles a button on the surface of the skin (see Fig. 10.12a). It is usually changed once every 3–6 months.

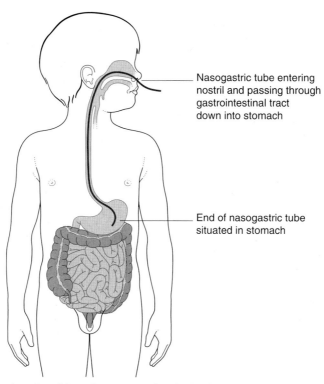

Figure 10.11 The length and position of a nasogastric tube in situ.

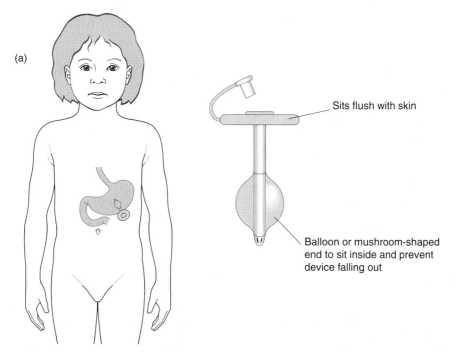

Figure 10.12 Types of gastrostomy tube: (a) Skin-level 'button' or 'key' device; sits a coin's depth (2 mm) above the skin.

Continued

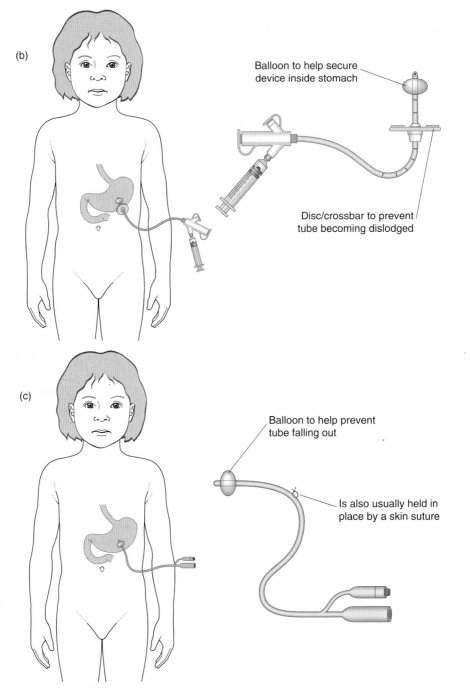

Figure 10.12 (b) Percutaneous endoscopic tube; disc/crossbar to prevent tube becoming dislodged and migration of tube past stomach into duodenum. (c) Surgically placed tube, e.g. Foley catheter; held in place by suture depending on type of tube and surgeon's preference.

However, in some areas, when the gastrostomy tract has been formed via a Stamm procedure (full surgical procedure), tubes are placed directly.

The percutaneous endoscopic tube (PEG) is a gastrostomy tube that is inserted through the skin into the stomach under endoscopic control, therefore avoiding the need for a full, laparoscopic surgical procedure (Booth 1991). It can stay in situ usually for up to 2 years.

A surgically placed tube such as a Foley catheter is usually much shorter term in use and should only be changed by a surgeon or nurse who has received training in the procedure. If it becomes displaced in the first 2 weeks postoperatively, before the tract has properly formed, it must be re-inserted as a matter of urgency or the skin and tissues will close over. Gastrostomy tubes are most commonly sized between 9 and 15 Fg, although smaller or larger tubes may be used in small babies or older children (Bowling 2003).

Research–based practice relating to the risks of enteral feeding

Research has highlighted the risks of nasogastric feeding, in particular the risk of aspiration of feed because of misplaced tubes, blocked tubes, infection transmission and the excessive vacuum pressure caused by using smaller-volume syringes (Taylor Goodison-McLaren 1992, Lord 1997, Anderton & Nivgough 1991, Skipper et al 2003).

Maintaining patency of nasogastric and gastrostomy tubes

NG and gastrostomy tubes must be flushed before and after a feed. During continuous feeding, or when not in use, NG tubes should be flushed regularly to maintain patency, e.g. every 4 hours during the daytime (Lifshitz et al 1991, Paul et al 1993). Gastrostomy tubes must also be flushed regularly, before and after use and every 3 hours when not in use to maintain patency (Lifshitz et al 1991, Paul et al 1994, Skipper et al 2003).

Preventing infection transmission via enteral feeding

Whenever an NG or gastrostomy tube is flushed, it should be done with cooled, boiled water, or sterile water, whatever the age of the child (Coldicutt 1994, Anderton 1995, Paul et al 1994, Skipper et al 2003).

In addition, feeds should be prepared only on surfaces which have been cleaned thoroughly with soap and water, dried and then wiped with 70% isopropyl alcohol-impregnated wipes (Anderton & Nivgough 1991). Any feed delivery systems should be single-use only, and feed containers (the visible external part of NG and gastrostomy tubes) should also be cleaned with alcohol-impregnated wipes prior to use (Paul et al 1994, Anderton 1995, Skipper et al 2003).

Size of syringe used when administering feed/flush via nasogastric tube

A polyurethane tube (e.g. silk tube or gastrostomy tube) is softer and more prone to damage. The smaller the syringe, the smaller is the bore (the hole in the middle) and the greater the pressure created when injecting with it; 1–5 ml syringes produce the highest pressure for a given force. Using a larger-sized syringe – 50 or 100 ml – reduces the pressure on the tube, thus minimising the risk of damage (Taylor & Goodison-McLaren 1992, Paul et al 1993, Sidey 1995). This is also mentioned in the manufacturers' guidelines, e.g. for a Merck tube. Any sized syringe can be used to flush a gastrostomy tube.

Guidelines

Parents and older children should be encouraged to be involved with enteral feeding. This can include being involved in or even trained to pass the NG or gastrostomy tube if they so wish. Involvement can help them to feel in control of the procedure and help their acceptance of the problem (Holden et al 1997).

PASSING A NASOGASTRIC (NG) TUBE

Equipment

- Plastic apron
- Disposable latex-free gloves
- Cooled, boiled water or sterile water for flushing tube
- Two sterile gallipots

- pH paper/strips capable of indicating an acid range of pH 0–4 (Metheny et al 1993)
- Two syringes – 5/10 ml for PVC NG tube or 50/60 ml for polyurethane NG tube (Lord 1997, Skipper et al 2003)
- 70% isopropyl alcohol-impregnated wipes
- Tape to secure the tube to the child's cheek (check that the child is not allergic to the tape)
- Scissors
- If the child has especially sensitive skin, you may need a hydrocolloid dressing such as extra-thin Granuflex to provide a protective layer between the child's skin and the adhesive tape holding the tube in place
- Dummy if the child uses it
- Drink of water if the child is older.

Method

Note:. Generally two people are needed to pass a NG tube, one to comfort and support the child and one to pass the tube.

1. Wherever possible, the child and family should have had psychological preparation to reduce the distress caused by the procedure (Holden et al 1997).

2. Wash hands thoroughly, dry them and put on a plastic apron to prevent cross-infection (Anderton 1995).

3. Clean the work surface/trolley on which equipment is to be placed as local policy, and wipe with alcohol (Anderton 1995). Allow alcohol to dry (it sterilises as it dries).

4. If using a hydrocolloid dressing, cut a piece and place it within easy reach. It should be wide enough to be at least three times the diameter of the NG tube and long enough to cover at least two-thirds of the child's cheek from the side of the nostril towards the ear (see Fig. 10.13). Normally, a piece 1.5 × 5 cm would be adequate for most children except for a very tiny neonate who would need less.

5. Cut a piece of adhesive tape and place it in easy reach. It should be wide enough to cover the NG tube with overlap at each side sufficient to hold it securely in place, and long enough to secure at least 3 cm of tube. If a hydrocolloid dressing is used, the adhesive tape should not extend beyond the boundary of the hydrocolloid.

6. Draw up 2–5 ml of the water into one of the syringes. Place on one side, in easy reach.

7. Put approximately 10 ml of water into a gallipot in easy reach.

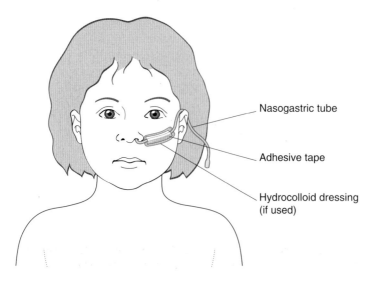

Figure 10.13 Size and position of tape securing nasogastric tube to cheek

Nasogastric tube

Adhesive tape

Hydrocolloid dressing (if used)

8. Open up the second syringe and place it in easy reach.

9. Take a strip of pH paper/strip and place it in the second gallipot.

10. Wash hands thoroughly, dry them and put on disposable gloves to prevent bacterial contamination of the tube (Anderton 1995).

11. Take the NG tube out of its sterile packaging. Ensure that it is not damaged in any way. If the tube has a guide wire, check that the wire is not bent and is correctly inserted down the middle of the tube. Measure what length of tube is to be passed. With the fingers of your dominant hand, hold the distal end of the tube (the end which will sit in the stomach) by the child's nostril. Measure the first length of tubing from the nostril to the edge of the cheek, by the ear (Fig. 10.14A). Then measure the second length of tubing from the edge of the ear down to the child's stomach and then two fingers below the xiphoid process (Fig. 10.14B). Mark this point on the tube by using a piece of surgi-

cal tape or a permanent marker pen (Nutritional Care 2004). Some tubes have black markings on the tubing at 10 cm intervals to give you a visual guide as to what length of tubing needs to be passed.

12. Ask the person assisting to position the child so that you can access the nostril. An older child should be encouraged to sit upright.

13. Maintain your hold on the proximal end of the tube (the end which will remain on the exterior) at the end of the pre-measured length. Lubricate the distal end of the NG tube by dipping it in the gallipot containing water.

14. Gently pass the distal end of the tube into the child's nostril. Angle it slightly upwards and gently guide it over the back of the nose and into the nasopharynx.

15. Continue to pass the tube downwards. As it gets to the back of the throat, the child will gag. To ease the passage of the tube encourage a baby to suck on a dummy and

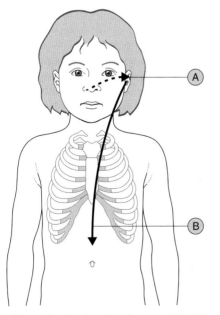

Figure 10.14 Measuring the length of nasogastric tube to be passed: **A**, holding the tip of the tube, measure from nose to ear; **B**, then measure from ear to stomach, aiming for two fingers below the xiphoid process.

try to persuade an older child to have a sip of water. Advance the tube as the child swallows. This will help ease discomfort and reduce the risk of the tube passing into the trachea, as the epiglottis will cover the trachea when swallowing.

16. Continue to advance the tube. You may have to pause in order for the tube to pass through the cardiac sphincter into the stomach. When the place you have marked on the tube is at the opening of the child's nostril, the distal end should now be in the stomach.

17. Ask the person holding the child, or the child personally, to place two fingers against the tube to prevent it slipping.

18. Check that the NG tube is in the correct position.

19. Connect a syringe (5/10 ml or 50/60 ml depending on type of tube) to the end of the NG tube and withdraw the plunger until fluid appears in the syringe – only a very small amount (0.5–1 ml) of fluid is required. Disconnect the syringe and close off the end of the tube.

20. Put the contents of the syringe onto the pH paper/strip and observe for an acid reaction (the aspirate must be in the pH range 0–4) indicating that the fluid originates from the stomach and the tube is correctly positioned.

    If no fluid was obtained, try changing the child's position and then aspirating the tube again. If still no fluid can be withdrawn and it is safe to do so, give the child a few millilitres (5 ml) of water, juice or milk orally and then aspirate the tube again.

    If it is still not possible to be sure that the tube is correctly placed, it may need to be withdrawn a little, or passed further, in order to obtain acidic aspirate. In exceptional circumstances it may be necessary to obtain an X-ray picture to determine whether the tube is correctly positioned.

21. Having established that it is correctly placed, gently flush the tube with 2–5 ml of water to ensure that it is patent. Remove

the guide wire if one has been used. Disconnect and close off the end of the tube.

22. Secure the tube to the child's cheek using the adhesive tape (and hydrocolloid if necessary).

FEEDING VIA A NASOGASTRIC OR GASTROSTOMY TUBE

Equipment

- Plastic apron
- Disposable latex-free gloves
- Cooled, boiled water or sterile water for flushing tube
- Two sterile gallipots
- pH paper/strips
- Two syringes – 5/10 ml for PVC NG tube or 50/60 ml for polyurethane NG tube
- 70% isopropyl alcohol-impregnated wipes
- Sterile feed – correct type and quantity at room temperature
- Bottle opener if required
- Documentation to record feed given.

For bolus feed
- Gravity feed delivery system with plunger if feed thickened or narrow bore (6 or 8 Fg)
- Separate clamp for gravity feed tube if roller clamp not integral to the system
- Dummy if appropriate (be aware that using a dummy may make establishing breast-feeding in the future more difficult)
- Toys related to feeding – plastic dishes, utensils, etc.

For continuous feed
- Enteral feeding pump with fully charged battery and lead to connect it to a mains electrical supply
- Continuous enteral feeding administration set and label to indicate when set changed.

Method

1. Clean the work surface/trolley on which feed is to be prepared and wipe it with alcohol-impregnated wipes (Anderton 1995). Allow alcohol to dry (it sterilises as it dries).

2. Check that the expiry date of the feed has not passed.
3. Wash and dry the bottle opener and separate clamp if used. Clean bottle opener and clamp (if used) and top of feed container by wiping with alcohol-impregnated wipes to prevent cross-infection (Anderton 1995).
4. Open the feed administration system and put all equipment on the work surface.
5. Wash hands thoroughly and put on disposable latex gloves to prevent bacterial contamination of feed (Anderton 1995).
6. Reassure the child and parent; explain what you are about to do.
7. Ensure that the child is comfortable and is positioned with the head above the level of the stomach to prevent aspiration, preferably sitting or nursed at an angle of about 30° (Lifshitz et al 1991). The neonate should be placed prone or on the right side (Taylor & Goodison-McLaren 1992).
8. Draw up 5–10 ml of sterile water (for flushing tube) into the appropriate-sized syringe for the type of tube. Smaller volumes will be used in neonates or children on fluid restrictions.
9. Check that the NG/gastrostomy tube is in the correct position and patent (see steps 19–21 for checking the placement of a NG tube). A gastrostomy tube should be allowed to free drain a small amount of fluid onto pH paper/strip placed in a gallipot or a small amount of fluid can be withdrawn using a syringe.
10. Prime the feed administration system. Apply a clamp to the tubing, fill the barrel/bag/burette with feed and then fill the tubing by gradually releasing the clamp. If necessary, run excess feed into the second gallipot. When the tubing is primed and all air removed, apply the clamp again.

Bolus feeding
11. Connect the feed administration set to the tube (Anderton 1995).
12. Slowly release the clamp and raise the barrel of the feed system to allow feed to flow into the tube by gravity. The higher the tube is raised, the faster the flow rate.

Administration of the feed should take the same length of time as it would take the child to have the same amount orally – usually 15–30 minutes.

If the feed is too thick, or the bore of the NG tube too narrow to allow feed to drip in by gravity, then the feed must be instilled using the plunger. *Gently* depress the plunger to deliver the feed at the same rate as if feeding by gravity. Never use force; this will make the child vomit.
13. Top up the barrel with the remaining feed as it begins to empty. Do not allow it to empty as far as the tubing until the feed is complete (to prevent instilling air into the tube, leading to discomfort and wind).
14. Whilst the feed is being given, encourage the child to suck (on a dummy) so that sucking is associated with the sensation of feeding. The older child can be tube fed at the dinner table to encourage normal socialisation associated with feeding. Similarly, the older child should be encouraged to play with feeding utensils whilst being tube fed.
15. When the feed is complete, remove the empty gravity feed system and close off the feeding tube before air can get into the tube.
16. Gently flush the feeding tube with the remaining 2–5 ml of sterile water in the appropriate size of syringe. Cap off the feeding tube.
17. Make the child comfortable and clear away equipment.
18. A gravity feed system must be discarded and a new system used after 24 hours to reduce the risk of bacterial contamination (Skipper et al 2003).

Continuous feeding
11. If the feed has preservatives and is sterile (e.g. a proprietary brand), the full amount of feed (up to 24 hours' worth) should be primed in the administration set to prevent the set being accessed frequently and therefore reduce the risk of bacterial contamination (Patchell et al 1998). If the feed does not have preservatives (e.g. it is made daily by a special feed kitchen), the set

should be primed with enough feed for 4 hours at a time (Skipper et al 2003).

12. Plug in and switch on the enteral pump. Test the alarm system on the pump. Load the administration set into the pump.

13. Set the pump to the correct rate (in ml/hour) to deliver the desired quantity in the required time period. If it is important that a limited, specific, quantity of feed is to be delivered use the appropriate function on the pump and set a total volume for delivery.

14. Connect the feed administration set to the tube.

15. Set the pump to run. The nurse should check the pump hourly and document the amount of feed that the pump has administered.

16. Aspirate the tube every 4 hours to test that it remains correctly in situ in the stomach.

17. The tube should be flushed with water every 4 hours to ensure patency.

18. If the set is to be topped up with feed 4-hourly, then a cleaned work surface/trolley should be used and apron and disposable gloves worn. The top of the feed container and the opening of the administration set are both wiped using alcohol wipes before feed is put into the system (Anderton 1995).

19. Change the feed administration set every 24 hours (Anderton 1995).

Observations and complications of enteral feeding

Observations

- Check when the tube was last changed and is due to be changed.
- Check the skin around a gastrostomy site for any signs of soreness caused by leakage from the stoma.
- Always check the position of the tube before using it. Be aware that pH paper/strips will not indicate the recommended acid reaction if the child is on antireflux treatment. An acid reaction of 0–4 using pH paper is the safest way to indicate an acidic aspirate, thus indicating that the

tube is correctly placed (Metheney et al 1993, NHS QIS 2003, Medical Devices Agency 2004, NPSA 2005).

- Whilst feeding, check that the child appears comfortable and is not showing signs of discomfort such as heaving or retching.
- Check the child's breathing and colour whilst administering the feed.

Complications

- Incorrect feed calculation could lead to too much or too little feed being given.
- The wrong feed or wrongly constituted feed could be given if not properly checked.
- The biggest risk of NG feeding is the tube being, or becoming, misplaced. This can cause feed to be delivered into the lungs, or feed to be aspirated. If at any time during a NG feed the child becomes blue or has difficulty breathing, the feed must be stopped immediately and the tube aspirated. The child may require suction.
- NG and gastrostomy tubes can also be misplaced in the wrong part of the gut. If either tube is in the small intestine rather than in the stomach, aspirate will be obtained, but will not be acidic. In this case, the tube should be repositioned and re-checked for correct position before use.
- Vomiting can occur if the feed is given too fast.
- Tubes may become blocked, but force should never be applied to try to unblock them as this could damage the tube and increase the risk of feed being instilled in the wrong place. If a tube remains blocked, it must be removed and a new one inserted if required.
- Rarely, a gastrostomy tube can migrate into the small intestine with the peristaltic action of the intestine. This can cause diarrhoea, vomiting and even intestinal obstruction and/or perforation, causing the child great discomfort and distress (Coldicutt 1994). Prevention is better than cure and the importance of correctly fitting and securing the tubes must be stressed.
- Bacterial contamination can lead to gastroenteritis.

- Prolonged absence of oral feeding can lead to developmental delay. Oral stimulation, sucking and swallowing can disappear and speech development can be affected (Evans Morris & Dunn Klein 1987, Taylor & Goodison-McLaren 1992). Manipulating food – chewing, swallowing, etc. – enables the child to learn the control of tongue and mouth muscles that is necessary to produce intelligible speech.

Without oral feeding, pleasant associations with oral stimulation such as gratification of hunger are lost and the child can become hypersensitised to touch and taste (Evans Morris & Dunn Klein 1987). This makes it increasingly difficult to reintroduce oral feeding after prolonged NG/gastrostomy feeding when the only associations with oral feeding are unpleasant sensations, e.g. vomiting and suction (Langley 1994). This can then lead to problems with social development as the child may not learn appropriate social behaviour associated with meal times.

All these aspects of development must be considered and action taken to try to mitigate the negative side-effects in children who are unable to feed orally.

COMMUNITY PERSPECTIVE

Many children who require enteral feeding are cared for by their families at home. It is therefore imperative that the carers are aware of all aspects of this care, including potential problems, how to deal with problems and who to contact.

Organisation of equipment is essential prior to discharge. This may include a feed pump and an ongoing supply of disposable equipment, nasogastric tubes, syringes, feed bags, gastrostomy button extension tubes, pH paper, etc. It can be frustrating if a child's discharge from hospital is delayed because of lack of supplies. Parents also need to know who to contact for further supplies, whether this is a company supplying the entire package, a local chemist, a community dietitian or the CCN. They must also be aware of local policy regarding the servicing of feed pumps. In smaller homes, the sheer volume of supplies needing to be stored can be a problem.

The role of the CCN is to support the carers, ensuring that they are not only competent in the techniques required but are also happy to undertake them. Whereas enteral feeding is a routine procedure in hospital, it is a major commitment for families at home, both physically and emotionally.

Concerns about altered body image may be problematic for parents, siblings and the child. The CCN will have the opportunity to recognise and address any concerns in the safe environment of the home and advise regarding referral for further psychological support if necessary.

Nasogastric feeding
Some parents are happy to undertake not only the technique of feeding but also replacing the tube. This is advantageous for carers and nursing staff, as tubes are frequently pulled out at the most inconvenient times, resulting either in parents having to travel back to hospital at short notice or community nurses having to reorganise their schedules to ensure that a child does not miss a feed.

Passing a nasogastric tube can be a frightening experience on the first few occasions and support for the carer at this time is vital. The opportunity to undertake the procedure in hospital prior to discharge is therefore most helpful and, on the first few occasions at home, the presence of a member of the CCN team is reassuring. There is the added advantage that the CCN can observe the carer's technique and check that they are confident and competent. Discussion can take place at this time on how to modify infection control measures, as the risk of cross-infection in the home is less, with the emphasis on handwashing techniques. The importance of including the tube-fed child at family meal times should not be overlooked. Parents should not be pressurised into taking on the responsibility of re-passing the nasogastric tube if they are reluctant. Often when they have gained confidence in managing feeds at home, they will feel ready to take on this skill.

Community Perspective continues

It is important to remember mouth care (see Hygiene, p. 198). Twice daily brushing of the teeth and the use of mouth washes (if appropriate) may improve the feel of the mouth as well as promoting good dental health.

A useful tip to stop the skin on the cheeks becoming sore is to apply a strip of Stomahesive or Granuflex/DuoDERM to the cheek (see above, p. 178), to which the tape is secured, rather than directly to the skin.

Gastrostomy feeding

Gastrostomy feeding is likely to be long term and, therefore, the child or the family will undertake the majority, if not all, of the care. The procedure should therefore fit in with the family's normal lifestyle and not dictate it. They should therefore be in a position to make decisions, in conjunction with medical, nursing and dietetic staff, relating to the type of device and the administration of the feed.

In addition to the points related to nasogastric feeding, the family need to be aware of the following:

- The stoma site should be cleaned with mild soap and warm water every day, care being taken to dry the area well.
- As part of this routine, the device must be turned daily. This helps form a healthy stoma and prevents the formation of adhesions (depends on make of tube).
- Treatment of overgranulation of gastrostomy site:
  - swab site for bacterial presence
  - excessive moisture can be controlled by using an absorptive dressing such as Lyofoam
  - a steroid-based, antibiotic, antifungal cream may be prescribed for application to the gastrostomy site
  - once a stoma site is fully healed, after 2–3 weeks, bathing and swimming are allowed (NHS QIS 2003).
- Balloon devices should be deflated and reinflated weekly to ensure that the correct amount of fluid remains in the balloon; however, this is dependent upon the make of the tube.
- When and how to change a balloon device – a replacement tube should be kept with the child (e.g. at school).
- Methods of unblocking tubes include instilling warm water or soda water.
- Manufacturers' recommended life of button extension sets, as these vary considerably.
- How to use a decompression tube if applicable.

The aim of the CCN is to ensure that families are empowered to give the recommended nutritional support to their child, whilst maintaining as relaxed a home environment as possible. This is best achieved by ensuring a smooth transition from hospital to home and providing ongoing support from the appropriate members of the multidisciplinary team without overwhelming families with professional input. Respite care should, if possible, be offered, either by nursing staff or by carers trained to undertake this care.

Do and do not

- Do always check that NG and gastrostomy tubes are correctly positioned before instilling anything into the tube.
- Do stop a NG feed immediately if the child experiences difficulty in breathing or develops cyanosis.
- Do aspirate and flush NG tubes 4-hourly to check position and maintain patency.
- Do secure a gastrostomy tube carefully to prevent peristalsis causing the tube to migrate into the wrong part of the intestine.
- Do encourage the child who is not fed orally to use the mouth in play – blowing, kissing, touching the mouth and putting fingers into the mouth.
- Do take all measures to prevent bacterial contamination of feed.
- Do make an early referral to a speech and language therapist for children requiring long-term feeding.
- Do not ever use a NG or gastrostomy tube if there is any doubt that it is correctly placed in the stomach.

References

Anderton A 1995 Reducing bacterial contamination in enteral tube feeds. British Journal of Nursing 4(7): 368–376

Anderton A, Nivgough C E 1991 Problems with the re-use of enteral feeding systems. A study of effectiveness of a range of cleaning and disinfection procedures. Journal of Human Nutrition and Dietetics 4: 25–32

Booth I W 1991 Enteral nutrition in childhood. British Journal of Hospital Medicine 46: 111–113

Bowling T 2003 Nutritional support for adults and children: a handbook for hospital practice. Radcliffe Medical Press, Oxford

Coldicutt P 1994 Children's options. Nursing Times 90(13): 54–56

Evans Morris S, Dunn Klein M 1987 Pre-feeding skills. A comprehensive resource for feeding development. Therapy Skill Builders, San Antonio, TX, p 320, 352

Hambridge K M, Sokol R J, Krebs N F 1995 Enteral and parenteral alimentation. In: Roy C, Silverman A, Alagille D (eds) Paediatric clinical gastroenterology, 4th edn. Mosby, St Louis, MO, ch 37, p 1030

Hendry P J, Akyurekli M D, McIntyre R, Quarrington A, Keon W J 1986 Bronchopulmonary complications of nasogastric feeding tubes. Critical Care Medicine 14(10): 892–894

Holden C E, McDonald A, Ward M et al 1997 Psychological preparation for nasogastric feeding in children. British Journal of Nursing 6(7): 376–381, 384–385

Langley P 1994 From tube to table. Nursing Times 90(48): 43–46

Lifshitz F, Finch N M, Lifshitz J Z 1991 Children's nutrition. Jones & Bartlett, Boston, MA, ch 27, p 518

Lord L M 1997 Enteral access devices. Nursing Clinics of North America 32(4): 700

Medical Devices Agency 2004 Enteral feeding tubes (nasogastric). Medical Devices Section of the Medicines and Healthcare Products Regulatory Agency. Online. Available: www.medical-devices.gov.uk

Merck. Tube manufacturer's guidelines. Merck Biomaterial, Alton, Hampshire, UK

Metheney N, Reed L, Wiersema L, McSweeney M, Wehrle M, Clark J 1993 Effectiveness of pH measurements in predicting tube placement: an update. Nursing Research 42(6): 324–331

Metheny N, McSweeney M, Wehrle M A, Wiersema L 1990 Effectiveness of the auscultatory method in predicting feeding tube location. Nursing Research 39(5): 14

NHS QIS 2003 Nasogastric and gastrostomy feeding for children being cared for in the community. Best Practice Statement. Nursing and Midwifery Practice Development Unit (now part of NHS Quality Improvement Scotland), Edinburgh

NPSA 2005 National Patient Safety Agency Alert 09. Reducing the harm caused by nasal and orogastric feeding tubes in babies under the care of neonatal units. NPSA, London

Nutritional Care 2004 Best practice guidelines for confirmation of nasogastric tube placement safety. Birmingham Children's Hospital NHS Trust, Birmingham, UK

Patchell C, Anderton A, Holden C et al 1998 Reducing bacterial contamination of enteral feeds. Archives of Disease in Childhood 78: 166–168

Paul L A, Holden C, Smith A et al 1993 Tube feeding and you. Birmingham Children's Hospital NHS Trust, Birmingham, UK

Paul L A, Holden C, Smith A et al 1994 Gastrostomy feeding and you. Birmingham Children's Hospital NHS Trust, Birmingham, UK

Sidey A 1995 Enteral feeding in community settings. Paediatric Nursing 7(6): 21–24

Skipper L, Cuffling J, Pratelli N 2003 Enteral feeding infection control guidelines. Infection Control Nurses Association, London

Taylor S, Goodison-McLaren 1992 Nutritional support – a team approach. Wolfe Publishing, London, ch 15, p 258, 273

Further Reading

Booklets produced by the manufacturers of the devices.

Patchell C J, Anderton A, MacDonald A, George R H, Booth I W 1994 Bacterial contamination of enteral feeds. Archives of Disease in Childhood 70: 327–330

Sidey A, Torbet S 1995 Enteral feeding in community settings. Paediatric Nursing 7(6): 21–23

Hygiene

Catherine Furze, Beryl Pearson

INTRODUCTION AND RATIONALE

Meeting the child's hygiene needs is an essential and integral aspect of nursing care, enhancing comfort, promoting self-esteem and preventing infection. Personal hygiene is an essential component in maximising physical well-being and is vital for a healthy future. As the child grows physically and becomes more independent, their needs change.

This section will introduce general principles of care practices for the baby or child who is unwell, and being cared for either at home or in hospital. It will then address specific care in relation to developmental age groups. More specific care of problems common in sick children can be found in other sections.

Learning outcomes

By the end of this section you should be able to explain:

- generic principles of hygiene practice for the healthy child

- prevention of cross-infection through good hygiene practice and awareness of the nurse's role in the maintenance and use of universal precautions
- the specific needs related to the developmental stage and abilities of the child
- adaptation of techniques to meet the specific needs of the ill child
- specific aspects of hygiene management for the infant, child and adolescent.

General factors to note

Safe practice
To maintain safe practice in any environment the nurse undertaking the activity must be aware of local policy guidelines, which must be followed as for any nursing procedure.

- The environment and safety of both the child and nurse when performing any aspect of hygiene care.

- Any baby and child should never be left unattended in a bath or with water.

- Hold and closely supervise the baby who is unable to sit unsupported and, where used, place a slip mat in the bath.

- The ambient temperature of the environment needs to be maintained between 22 and 25°C to reduce heat loss during hygiene care (Bailey & Rose 2000).

- The water temperature should be maintained, appropriate to the needs/size/age of the child; however, there is no evidence of a specific recommendation and therefore assessment is needed on an individual basis. The Child Accident Prevention Trust (CAPT) advocate that water should come out of bath taps at no more than 46°C to prevent the risk of serious scalding (CAPT 2002). In a clinical situation all water temperature should be thermostatically controlled.

Risk assessment

Consent and participation (see also concepts, p. 8)
The consent of the child and family needs to be sought in all circumstances, and family-centred care needs to be considered an integral aspect of the care of children in any environment (Smith 1999). Basic hygiene needs are considered fundamental to the child receiving nursing care; however, consent still needs to be sought from the child and family irrespective of the expectation that it may be provided as a basic requirement. Prior to the activity the nurse needs to negotiate with the child and the family the level of their interaction and participation during the personal care time (Coleman 2003). Full explanations of what actions are being taken should be given, and these should be reinforced during the interaction.

In general, the preparation and consent of children decreases their anxiety, promotes their cooperation, supports their coping skills and may foster a sense of achievement, independence and empowerment (Wong et al 1999).

Family inclusion
The child and family need to be fully involved throughout the child's care and encouraged to be partners in care (Casey 1988, Smith et al 2002). Education of the child and family and the sharing of information are important areas that are the nurse's responsibility (NMC 2002a). This involves the promotion of partnership and informed consent to develop the empowerment of the child and family in any given situation.

Family/carer presence and their involvement in the child's care will increase feelings of security, and decrease the anxieties of the child. Encouragement will need to be given to the family to promote their active inclusion in even the most basic of care activities. Their level of participation needs to be assessed early on, and then reassessed frequently to ensure opportunities are given for their involvement in the child's care. Nurses need to help them find specific ways in which they can support their child (NMC 2004).

The child needs to be encouraged to develop their independence and positive feelings of control by being able to choose the desired level of activity and participation. The nurse needs to be aware of all aspects of communication, including the use and observation of verbal and non-verbal body language during the activity

(Bannister 1997). Active communication may help the nurse, child and family to develop a rapport and provide assessment opportunities (Thomas 1996). Active communication is also combined with the use of play and humour during stressful situations (Wong et al 1999) (see also Appendix 1, p. 457).

Documentation and safe practice

All care should be documented in the nursing notes, in accordance with the Nursing and Midwifery Council *Guidelines for Records and Record-keeping* (NMC 2002b). Any changes resulting from assessment and reassessment should be noted and reported.

Prevention of cross-infection

Good hygiene represents an important defence against infection. A child's ability to fight infection will depend on their age, health and immunological status. The overprotection of children from contact with microorganisms may render them unable to develop a natural immunity, but allowing children to develop preventable illness because of poor hygiene practice and infection control is unacceptable.

Universal precautions to prevent infection should be taken (see also Control of Infection, p. 21). Hands should be washed thoroughly before and after handling any baby or child, in the home or in hospital (Lawson 2001). When handling any body fluids, and especially before any procedure requiring intimate contact, such as feeding or bathing, the nurse should wear gloves and other protective clothing (e.g. an apron) appropriate to the level of contact.

Handwashing is important for all carers and siblings. It may be especially important in hospital due to potential contact with unusual or highly infectious diseases and prevent cross-infection or spread of disease. Therefore the use of universal precautions and good hand-washing techniques are essential to reduce cross-contamination (Lawson 2001, RCN 2004a). Older sibling children should be told to wash their hands after using the toilet, and before and after meals, especially if they want to hold or touch the baby, or share toys. Younger children should be encouraged to wash their hands aided by an adult.

Developmental needs

- Each child is a unique individual with their own routine, temperament and personality.
- Guidelines of developmental age and ability are helpful but each child must be respected as an individual. This can be acknowledged by calling the child by their name.
- Care and support given should provide the child with encouragement and confidence to retain their level of independence in self-care activities.
- Personal hygiene forms an important element of the healthy child's normal everyday routine.

These routines and practices should be maintained as much as possible while the child is sick, either in hospital or at home, and details should be recorded in the nursing notes or health records. Keeping to established routine provides comfort and reassurance to the child and family, especially during periods of stress.

Privacy and dignity

The nurse should respect the child's changing needs for privacy at different stages of development and well-being. In the older child or adolescent, a need for privacy emerges as sexual awareness develops. Illness and disability require that intimate tasks, which would normally be performed by the child or young person, may need to be performed by nurses and parents. Assessment of the usual practices for intimate and personal care should be established, and care should then be negotiated between the nurse, parent/carer and child. It is vital that the child is consulted at all stages of the interaction and that their needs and requests become paramount in the achievement and maintenance of personal hygiene (Needham 1997). The nurse should involve parents, where appropriate, and same-sex nurses and carers should be allocated if possible (RCN 2003).

Cultural needs

Nurses need to be aware of the individual family cultural background. Consideration must be given to family lifestyle and specific cultural values and norms, including cultural rituals and/or rites of passage – especially related to health and personal care. Nurses should also be sensitive to the need for 'same gender' care delivery for all children regardless of age, sex, ethnic background or culture.

> The intimate nature of many nursing interventions, if not practised in a sensitive and respectful manner, could lead to misinterpretation. Care should be negotiated between the nurse, parent/carer and child. Assessment is the key to ensuring effective nursing care. Usual practices for intimate, personal care should be established and form the basis for care.
>
> Royal College of Nursing (2003)

Health promotion

The provision of personal care and the maintenance of hygiene provide an ideal opportunity for health education and promotion. The child and family may have concerns regarding their health and choose these times to raise concerns or discuss current/preventative practice. Aspects such as tooth cleaning, weight management, exercise, smoking and contraception are just some of the topics that may be discussed (Sutton 2001).

Play

Personal care time and the maintenance of hygiene are ideal times to utilise age-appropriate play strategies. Play has a number of specific functions; as well as promoting learning and development, it can also be a coping strategy and distraction for the child (Crawford & Raven 2002).

Observation

Performing hygiene tasks for a baby or child gives the nurse an ideal opportunity to observe and monitor the health and general well-being of a child. As each element of hygiene care is performed, there is an opportunity for detailed assessment of the condition of a particular area (e.g. ears or eyes). The nurse may observe, for example:

- signs of malnutrition
- chest recession in a child with respiratory distress
- bruises or bite marks on a child who may have been abused
- skin infections such as impetigo or ringworm.

Guidelines

Before commencing any hygiene task, consider:

- Is the task really necessary? Children who are sick, or babies who are premature, should be left in peace with minimal disturbance unless there is a good reason to do otherwise. The clustering of care may be considered to be of benefit and limit the negative effects of continuous interaction (Young 1996).
- Could any other aspect of care be combined with hygiene needs? Examples include observations of vital signs, topical drug administration and specimen collection.
- Consider family-centred care: Could the parents be involved or undertake the task with supervision, or would they prefer the nurse to do it?
- What can the child do independently? Or what can the child begin to learn to do on their own? If a child is able to learn a basic skill or develop their independence, for example hair brushing, tooth cleaning or dressing, it may encourage a sense of achievement and a feeling that something positive has occurred.
- The developmental stage of the child and the appropriate level of activity and interaction.
- How can you make the experience fun? Can you introduce play or toys into the experience?
- Have you collected all necessary equipment together?

SPECIFIC HYGIENE NEEDS OF THE BABY

Birth is a traumatic, exhausting experience for mother, father and baby. The newborn baby is covered with both a protective substance called vernix caseosa, white grease that protects the skin in utero from the amniotic fluid that surrounds the infant, and blood from the mother. The adaptation of the skin from intrauterine life, where the skin has been surrounded by amniotic fluid, to the predominately dry cool extrauterine life takes about 14 days. At birth the mean pH of skin is 6.34, which decreases to 4.95 by 4 days as the skin colonises with normal flora. The acidic quality of newborn skin provides a defence against harmful microorganisms (Medves & O'Brien 2001). After birth excess moisture is wiped away and the infant is placed naked on the mother's abdomen or breast, covered perhaps by a clean towel to maintain warmth. Positive skin to skin contact at this stage can provide an ideal opportunity for the mother, father and child to familiarise themselves and bond. However, babies can lose heat rapidly and therefore specific attention needs to be paid to the ambient temperature in the room (Bailey & Rose 2000).

A full-term healthy infant may be bathed within a few hours of birth, once the body temperature has stabilised (Trotter 2002). Newborn babies do not get especially dirty, and daily bathing of newborn babies is unnecessary as frequent bathing may disrupt the natural pH of the skin. It may also be unwise if the umbilical cord is still in situ (Skale 1992, Guala et al 2003). For the first 2–4 weeks baths should be carried out using only plain water and cotton wool for cleansing, then gradually introduce tiny amounts of baby bath product. These should be of a neutral pH, contain minimal dyes and perfumes, and be used only two to three times a week (Trotter 2002).

For any baby, bathing is not only for skin cleansing, but is also a time for contact and interaction. The timing of hygiene activities should be planned for when the baby will enjoy them, when awake and content.

Maintaining a clean environment for the baby is an equally important part of their hygiene care. Newborn babies have very little defence against microorganisms; once the placental transference of immunity has worn off at 3 months, or if breastfeeding has stopped, babies must develop their own defences (Lawson 2001). Likely sources of contaminants are feeds, feeding bottles or pacifiers. If formula feeds are to be used, they must be made up under sterile conditions. Feeding bottles and pacifiers should be sterilised after each use. Weaning foods must be prepared using food hygiene guidance (see also Feeding, p. 166).

Once the child is older and can reach for toys and put them in their mouth (usually at about 3 months), toys should be kept 'socially' clean, though sterilising them is not necessary.

Reinforcing and teaching handwashing techniques before and after contact with the baby are important for all carers and siblings. For older children this is especially important when sharing the baby's toys.

The environment around a baby whether at home, in a hospital cubicle or ward, should be clean and as free as possible from excessive build-up of dust and dirt. Once a child is crawling, the floor and other surfaces should be kept 'socially' clean.

Staff and visitors who have coughs or colds or other infections should not have close contact with a baby.

Any causation of ill health can interrupt the family bonding processes. Hygiene activities can form a useful way for the mother or father and baby to bond. They give an opportunity for face-to-face contact, touch and 'talking'. For example, if the newborn baby is in a neonatal intensive care unit, inviting the family to help with these activities can encourage bonding when they can no longer fulfil other caring functions (see also Complementary Therapies, p. 465).

BABY BATH

There are two ways of bathing a baby – to 'top and tail' or to give a baby bath. Babies, as mentioned above, do not need bathing daily unless they are sick or have very dirty nappies. Older babies who are more active, for example crawling, may require a daily bath. A baby bath may be too stressful for a sick child, for example a child with breathing difficulties or neurological disturbance. If this is the case, a top and tail can be performed instead.

TOP AND TAIL WASH

Topping and tailing is a useful alternative to bathing. Top and tail is to wash the baby's face, hands and their nappy area. A bowl of clean water is required for both the top and the tail (bottom).

Equipment

- A small dish of warm clean sterile water for the baby's eyes
- A bowl of warm clean water for the face
- A bowl of warm clean water for the nappy area
- Non-sterile swabs for eye care (or at home a clean soft cloth)
- Cotton wool balls/wash wipes/clean soft flannel for the rest of the baby's body
- A clean nappy
- Disposal bag or bucket for soiled nappy and clothes
- Soft baby hairbrush
- Clean clothes
- Clean warmed towels.

Method

1. Ensure that the environment is warm and comfortable, with no cool draughts.
2. Place the baby, dressed, on the towel.
3. Clean the baby's eyes. Clean the corners and outside the eye; do not attempt to clean under the lids. Use a different swab for each eye and discard after each use to prevent cross-infection.
4. Gently wash the rest of the face and around the mouth and nose with a clean cloth or swabs, and gently pat dry.
5. Do not attempt to clean inside any orifice, be it nose, eye, ear or mouth. All body orifices clean themselves naturally by production and secretion of mucus or fluid.
6. Wash the baby's hands with a wet washcloth, and dry. If nails are long, snip very carefully with blunt-ended baby scissors (preferably baby's own to maintain individual use and prevent cross-infection).
7. Gently brush the baby's scalp and hair with a soft baby brush to help prevent the occurrence of cradle cap.
8. Undress the baby so that the nappy area is accessible. With most babies' clothing this is possible without undressing the baby fully.
9. Take off the nappy. If the baby is wet, just clean with warm water. If the baby is soiled, wipe excess faeces away with cotton wool balls, the nappy or wipes. Observe for nappy rash. Always clean from front to back, thus avoiding contaminating the urethra with faeces. Wash the baby's bottom with a washcloth and dry.
10. Only the visible surface of genitalia should be cleaned: *Do not retract a boy's foreskin (which will not fully retract until the boy is 18 months to 2 years) or clean inside the labia in a girl.*
11. Ensure that all creases of skin and crevices are dry to prevent the development of a rash or infection.
12. Put on a clean nappy (underneath the umbilicus if the cord is still attached) and dress the baby in clean clothes.

Specific factors to note

- Before and after carrying out any baby care it is important to wash hands thoroughly.
- Cotton wool balls should not be used for eye care as, if small cotton strands enter underneath the eyelid, they can damage the cornea (Marsden & Shaw 2003) (see also Eye Care, p. 200).
- The internal aspect of the ears and nose should not be cleaned unless really necessary and the use of cotton buds should be avoided.
- Alkali soaps should not be used as they can potentially damage the 'acid mantle' of the skin and the skin's barrier function (Garcia-Gonzalez & Riviera-Rueda 1998). The 'acid mantle' is the skin's protector that takes between 2 and 8 weeks to develop, depending on gestational age (Trotter 2002).
- Many parents use talcum powder, but the hygiene benefits of this are unclear. Powder tends to cling and cake to moist areas, can cause skin irritation and can be inhaled by the baby (Skale 1992, Campbell & Glasper 1995).

- Baby soap or baby bath solution is not necessary unless the baby's nappy area is very soiled (Brennan 1996). Use cleansing solutions that are mild and free from alcohol and perfume.
- If the baby is changed regularly, nappy creams are not necessary under normal circumstances (Brennan 1996). However, if a baby is prone to nappy rash, a protective barrier cream may be useful to reduce friction, wetting and contact with urine and faeces (Atherton 2004).

BATHING A BABY

Equipment

As for top and tail, plus a baby bath and stand.

Method

1. The baby bath itself should be prepared, adding cold water first, and then warm, to reduce the risk of the water not mixing properly and hotter water remaining at the base of the tub. The water temperature should be comfortable and appropriate to the size, age, health and preference of the child. The Child Accident Prevention Trust (2002) advocate that water should come out of bath taps at *no more than 46°C* to prevent the risk of serious scalding.
2. It is essential that the temperature of the water is tested at intervals as a scald can occur if the water is too hot. The traditional method of assessing the temperature of the bath is to dip one's elbow into the water. The water should be no deeper than 10 cm (4 inches) and should feel just warmer than tepid.
3. Water thermometers are available – but should be for individual use.
4. Make sure that the bath is placed at a comfortable height, preferably on a stand. Kneel or sit, whichever is easier. Stooping while holding the baby can lead to back problems, and will mean that the person bathing the baby will not relax and enjoy the occasion.
5. Undress the baby. If the nappy area is very soiled, clean off the faeces with cotton wool balls, the nappy or wipes. Wrap the baby securely in a towel.
6. Before commencing, clean the baby's eyes, face and mouth with a clean cloth or swabs. Start with the eyes and use a different swab for each eye to prevent cross-infection (see Eye care, p. 200, for technique).
7. Whilst the baby is still wrapped in the towel, hold their head over the bath and gently wash water over the hair, avoiding the eyes. Although not necessary, a mild shampoo or a small quantity of baby bath solution can be used. Use a corner of the towel to dry the hair.
8. Unwrap the towel. Hold the baby securely, with one hand grasping the farthest upper arm, and the baby's neck and shoulders supported on the forearm (see Fig. 11.1).
9. Place the baby gently in the water, allowing them a little time to get used to the sensation. If the baby is learning to sit, support

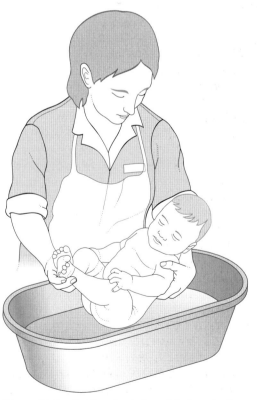

Figure 11.1 Holding the baby safely for a bath.

them sitting in the water with a hand around their back, but never leave a baby unsupported. It can only take a moment for a baby to topple over. This may put the baby off baths for some time or, in the worst scenario, the baby may drown. A non-slip mat or seat cradle should be used to prevent an accidental slip.

10. If bathing an active baby in an adult-size bath, make sure they cannot accidentally touch the hot tap.

11. Gently wash the baby with the free hand, under the arms, back and the nappy area. Pay particular attention to skin creases. Allow the baby to kick and splash, exploring the weightless sensation. This should be fun for both carer and baby, but if the baby is clearly distressed, bring them out of the bath as soon as possible.

12. Do not let the baby become cold. Wrap the baby in the towel. When dry, dress in clean dry clothes. The room should be warm enough for older babies to play naked for a while, to kick and wriggle, free from the constraints of a nappy.

13. Ensure that all creases of skin and crevices are dry to prevent the development of a rash or infection.

NAPPY AREA CARE

Nappy rash – irritant diaper dermatitis (IDD) – is frequently seen in babies and younger children. It is caused by prolonged and repetitive contact with an irritant, primarily urine and/or faeces, but *Candida* infections also cause excoriation of the nappy area. Underlying skins conditions, medical conditions and medication may be contributory factors (Turnball 2001). IDD is unusual before 3 weeks of age, usually developing between 3 weeks and 2 years (Atherton 2004), and could be linked with decreased nappy area changes, increased mobility or dietary changes. Any factor which changes the acidity of urine and faeces can cause IDD and consequent associated discomfort (Scowen 1995).

Nappies should be changed immediately after defaecating, and at reasonably frequent intervals to prevent IDD (Atherton 2004). Tim-

ing will depend on circumstances such as the developmental age of the baby, and therefore the volume of urine passed. On balance, changing a nappy immediately before a feed is preferable, though it can be frustrating for the baby, who may be crying with hunger. Changing the nappy immediately after a feed may either make the baby vomit or interrupt the progression to a sleep or resting time. If the baby has defaecated during feeding, the nappy should be changed.

When changing nappies, a cotton washcloth, mild soap and warm water are adequate to clean the area. Parents may prefer to use wash wipes, and there is some evidence to suggest that the modern types (gentle and non-alcohol based) may be gentler on both unbroken and broken skin (Odio et al 2001). Wipes should be avoided for babies less than 2–4 weeks old, as there may be potential to harm the 'acid mantle' in the skin of a newborn (Trotter 2002).

UMBILICAL CORD CARE

In the newborn the umbilical cord should normally separate within 2 weeks of birth, and usual recommendations are to allow the cord itself to naturally air dry, and not to apply or use any special treatment (Lund et al 1999); however, there is ongoing debate regarding definitive practice recommendations (Guala et al 2003). Care of the cord should be undertaken according to local policy guidelines.

The umbilical area must be observed for infection and swabbed for microbiological culture if any signs of infection are present (raised temperature, generally unwell, redness, inflammation, swelling of umbilicus or surrounding skin). If there is evidence of infection this must be reported immediately.

If an umbilical catheter is in situ, care should be as for an intravenous or arterial line: the line must be secured carefully and the entry site kept clean and dry and aseptic technique should be used if handling is necessary.

NAIL CARE

Babies have fingernails and toenails that are usually soft and flexible but that can cause injury. Nails that are 'ragged' or extend beyond the tip of the finger can cause scratches to the face and possibly eyes.

Clean the baby's hands and nails during regular bathing. Nails should be carefully trimmed using only baby's own baby nail scissors that have blunt rounded tips, and specially made baby clippers are now available. Baby's nails grow quickly and should be inspected regularly.

SPECIFIC HYGIENE NEEDS OF THE TODDLER AND PRESCHOOL CHILD

Due to the developmental and play experiences of this age group a daily bath or shower will become essential. Frequent washes of face and hands before, after and between meals will also be necessary.

Children being toilet trained should be taught and encouraged to wash their hands following toileting, as routine experience. Nappies where still worn should be changed every few hours.

Even if a child is ill, make hygiene activities fun and develop a comforting routine; encourage the child's independence and learning. Most toddlers and preschool children enjoy a bath, and will happily play in the water; either a soapy bath solution or soap can be used, though soap in the eyes can sting badly. If the child has any skin condition such as eczema, then special bath solutions and creams may be necessary. Some children will dislike baths and may prefer spraying themselves with the showerhead or having a sponge bath. At this stage of development toys and the environment should be kept socially clean. Attention will also need to be paid to hair, teeth and nails, continuing routines that should start as a baby.

Safety is paramount and small children must not be left alone in the bath even for a moment. They should be warned not to touch the hot tap, and the temperature of the hot water should be controlled so it cannot scald if turned on accidentally. Water temperatures above 46°C can cause injury, and at 60°C can cause second-degree burns in 3 seconds and third-degree burns in 5 seconds (CAPT 2002). Water temperature in clinical settings is thermostatically controlled, but in other areas a risk assessment may need to be made. The Health and Safety Executive (2003) recommend that:

> . . . water is delivered to the bath/shower outlet at no more than 44°C; or water is prevented from being discharged at >44°C from taps, which may be accessible to vulnerable service users, especially in areas where there is the potential for whole body immersion.

SPECIFIC HYGIENE NEEDS OF OLDER SCHOOL CHILDREN AND YOUNG PEOPLE

As school children grow older they become more independent. Hygiene needs alter as the body changes in adolescence: problems with acne, greasy hair or body odour may emerge; the menarche will occur as well as other sexual changes of puberty. Such changes can be disturbing even for the best-prepared teenager, especially when they manifest themselves outside the safety and reassurance of home or school. Teenagers can be very embarrassed if they cannot manage their own hygiene needs independently (Atmarow et al 1993). Sensitivity is needed if the adolescent requires assistance with hygiene activities in hospital (Horne 1999). When work is of a personal or intimate nature all nurses and healthcare staff, whether male or female, should follow the principles of good practice as outlined by the Royal College of Nursing (2003):

> Some children, particularly adolescent girls and those from non-Christian backgrounds, are likely to prefer a female carer. This reflects social, religious and cultural preferences, and should be respected and accommodated.

For both the toddler and older child a bed bath is usually given only when a child for whatever reason is too sick or disabled to get into a proper bath, and when a 'top and tail' wash is insufficient. Critically ill or unconscious children, children who have high temperatures and are sweating profusely, or children in traction after orthopaedic surgery may all need bed baths.

Parental involvement in bed bathing should be discussed with both the child and parent. Some children and parents prefer the nurse to perform the bed bath. For example, for some parents of chronically ill children it can be a welcome relief to have someone take over this aspect of care, whereas to parents of children who are acutely ill, continuing to care for their child's hygiene needs can be a way of maintaining control and feeling useful. The child may much prefer the parents to give the care, and their views and competence should be respected (Kristensson-Hallstrom 2000); however, as children get older their wishes and expectations may, at times, conflict with those of their parents (DoH 2003).

BED BATH

All children require similar basic equipment whether requiring a bath, a top and tail wash or a bed bath.

The basic principles of a bed bath are as follows:

- Ensure the time for the bath/bed bath is appropriate to the individual needs of the child.
- Gathering the equipment together and being well organised will save time and effort.
- Prepare the environment ensuring privacy and that it is safe, draught free and warm.
- Prepare the child.
- Consider other care interventions that can or may need to be planned into this activity, for example specimen collection, wound care, pain assessment and management.

The child may have their own individual preferences as to choice for personal cleaning lotions and materials.

Allow the child as much independence as is safe to do so and, if the child wishes, involve the parents/carers. Their safety must also be considered – for example if they are using hospital-based equipment.

Many children prefer the option of a shower, if available, and possible.

Equipment

- Washbowl with warm water
- Flannels or washcloths: at least two, one for the face and one for the genital area

- Soap or bath solution
- Hairbrush or comb
- Toothbrush and toothpaste
- Nail scissors
- Clean towel
- Clean clothes or nightclothes
- Clean bed linen
- Appropriate bags/receptacles for equipment disposal.

Method

1. Discuss the need for a bed bath with the child and parents and explain what will occur.
2. Other preparation may be necessary, e.g. toileting.
3. Prepare the environment: clear a surface, either a trolley or bedside table, for washing equipment.
4. Ensure that the water remains hot enough; it may need changing.
5. Raise the bed to a comfortable working height. Ensure that you are comfortable and safe; you may need assistance from colleagues or parents with turning or lifting. Use manual handling aids where possible. Do not stretch over the bed, but walk around to the other side if necessary.
6. Strip the bed and bed area of any non-essential items or bedclothes.
7. Undress the child and leave covered with a sheet and/or gown.
8. Wash the child's eyes, using a different corner of the washcloth for each eye. Use more specific eye care if indicated (see Eye care, p. 200).
9. Wash the child's face, paying special attention to mouth and ears (see Ear care, p. 201).
10. Help the child to clean their teeth.
11. Before washing each body part, place a dry towel beneath it to prevent water dripping onto the sheets.
12. Cover the upper body with a sheet or towel, but leave the arms exposed. Using soap and water, or bath solution or special lotion, wash the child's hands, and trim and clean the nails if necessary. Wash each

arm, paying particular attention to hands and nails, and the underarm area. Rinse the flannel and rinse off the soap. Rinsing may need to be repeated.

13. Gently remove the cover from the upper body, leaving genitalia covered, and wash and rinse the chest and abdomen.

14. Cover the upper body again, and wash the front of the legs and feet. Check for pressure sores on heels or ankles (see Pressure Area Care, p. 321).

15. With a different washcloth or flannel, wash the 'front' genitalia and rinse. Where possible children and young people may prefer to do this for themselves. *Note*: For postpubertal boys, the foreskin should be pulled back and the penis washed underneath (Campbell & Glasper 1995).

16. With assistance, turn the patient onto one side.

17. Wash back, legs and finally buttocks, and dry.

18. Position the patient comfortably.

19. Brush or comb the hair, and check behind the head for skin lesions or sores. If hair washing is necessary and the child can tolerate the procedure, wash the hair by holding the child's head over the end of the bed (help will be needed) over a washbowl, using a jug to rinse. Equipment may be available to assist with water collection.

20. Dress the patient in clean clothes as appropriate.

21. Tidy away the bowl of water and wash things.

22. Ensure the child is comfortable and any equipment moved is returned.

At the same time as doing a bed bath there may be an opportunity to:

- slide in a clean sheet to replace the old bottom sheet; change top sheet and pillowslips
- change the position of leads from monitoring equipment, or of catheters or tubes taped to the skin, to avoid skin irritation or damage due to prolonged adhesion or pressure (some units will have their own local policies on frequency of repositioning); clean off any remaining adhesive with a gentle adhesive remover
- perform passive limb exercises if indicated
- perform other nursing care, e.g. observations, topical skin treatments
- talk with the child; this may be an opportunity for the child to express their fears and thoughts about their illness, or just to have a good chat
- use play and make the bed bath fun. The more alert child will enjoy toys and games appropriate for their age; if the child has learning or sensory disabilities they may enjoy the touch, smell and feel of the experience.

TOILETING

Ensure privacy. All children should have access to handwashing facilities after using the toilet, and this should be proactively encouraged for all children. This practice should be maintained when a child is confined to bed.

Ensure the toileting facilities are to an acceptable standard, and that toilet paper, handwashing and drying equipment are accessible.

HAIR CARE

- Children's shampoo should be used and, where appropriate, hair conditioner.
- With ingenuity hair washing can be made fun and painless.
- Help children to brush or comb their hair at least once daily; they may require help to keep their usual style.
- Babies should have their hair washed when having a bath. For older children, follow their usual routine but they may require hair washing more frequently than usual. Babies may develop cradle cap, characterised by yellow scales on the scalp.
- Use the child's own hair toiletries, unless any specific prescribed care is required.
- If the child is unable to have their hair washed when bathing, then it may be necessary to wash this in their bed. This requires additional protection and equipment.
- Seek specific guidance from the child and their family regarding needs and preferences.
- Provide specific hair care for children with particular religious observances.

- Provide specific hair care for children who have kinky hair and require the use of special combs with wide teeth, and application of necessary hair products and toiletries.
- For children with long hair who are confined to bed, braiding or plaiting can help reduce knots or matting in their hair.
- Hair should not be cut without parental permission, although shaving of an area may be required for insertion of an intravenous cannula.

Head lice

Anyone can catch head lice, but preschool children, primary school children and their families are most at risk.

There are three forms of head lice:

1. Nits are head lice eggs. The oval, yellowy-white eggs are hard to see and may be confused with dandruff. They attach themselves to the hair shaft and take about a week to hatch. The eggs remain after hatching and many nits are empty egg cases.
2. Nymphs hatch from the nits. The baby lice look like the adults, but are smaller. They take about 7 days to mature to adults and feed on blood to survive.
3. Adults are about the size of a sesame seed. They have six legs and are tan to greyish-white. The legs have hook-like claws used to hold onto the hair. Adults can live up to 30 days and feed on blood.

Head lice cannot jump, hop or swim and are transmitted through direct, prolonged head-to-head contact with an infested person. This is especially common during play or sport at school and with close contacts at home. Transmission is possible through infected clothes, combs, brushes or towels, but extremely unlikely. The lifespan of a louse is very short once detached from the hair so fumigation is not necessary.

If head lice are found then medical advice should be sought for the appropriate current method of treatment (Health Protection Agency 1999).

ORAL AND DENTAL CARE

It is important to promote dental and oral hygiene to preserve the development of healthy teeth and gums. Studies show that levels of tooth decay are a good predictor of oral health in later life (Powell 1998). Dental hygiene should begin as the primary teeth erupt. Parents/carers should ensure children develop good dental habits from an early age.

Babies are obviously not able to clean their own teeth. For the baby it is often easier to use a foam sponge. As more teeth appear, use a baby toothbrush. For the younger child (under 7 years), effective positioning should facilitate carers' access to the child's mouth. One way of doing this is to stand with the child's back towards the adult, using one hand to cup the chin and the other to brush the teeth. In the case of an ill child, find a position that is most comfortable and reassuring. Good practice is to clean teeth at least twice a day, preferably after meals (British Dental Association 2003). The more frequently and the longer teeth are cleaned the greater the probability of effective plaque removal. Children often have their own preferred type of toothpaste, and many now use electric toothbrushes (these have been shown to achieve a modest reduction in plaque and gingivitis compared to manual tooth brushing). Advice from local health visitors should be sought about whether additional fluoride is necessary as the benefits of fluoride toothpastes are firmly established. Even when the child is not eating, such as when they are unconscious, regular and thorough mouth care is vital. There are occasions when an optimum oral hygiene regimen may be sacrificed for patient comfort.

In ill health, children may become more prone to dental and gum diseases, and medication may affect oral status. Children may also become susceptible to oral infections such as oral *Candida* (thrush), which can cause pain and discomfort in the mouth, and this in turn may affect eating and drinking. Children receiving chemotherapy or radiotherapy may experience specific problems. In addition to normal oral care, these children may require the use of antifungal agents and/or an antibacterial mouthwash.

Younger children will require encouragement and supervision, and this is an ideal opportunity for health education such as avoiding giving prolonged bottled feeds of milk or juice, prevention of injury, avoidance of sugary foodstuffs and other dietary needs, e.g. calcium intake.

Nurses should perform mouth care for children who, for whatever reason, are unable to do so for themselves. Encourage children to visit the dentist from an early age. Regular dental checks should include prophylactic teeth cleaning.

General conditions that may compromise oral well-being include the following:

- Cerebral palsy
- Epidermolysis bullosa
- HIV
- Combined immune deficiency
- Metabolic disorders requiring high intake of oral carbohydrates
- Glycoprotein storage disease (some types)
- Downs syndrome and other mentally handicapping conditions
- Measles
- Anorexia
- Dehydration
- Chronic constipation
- Effects of chemo/radiotherapy
- Post-cytotoxic therapy
- Fever
- Grinding of teeth
- Thumb sucking
- Habitual licking or biting of lips
- Accidents or other illness causing:
  - neurological damage
  - unconsciousness
  - loss of a limb
  - maxillofacial injury
- Restricted oral access due to:
  - orthodontic or maxillofacial surgery
  - enlarged, protruding tongue
  - respiratory problems
  - restricted movement of tongue due to surgery or pain
  - cleft palate (may have a prosthesis)

- Medication, e.g.:
  - antibiotics
  - antihistamine
  - atropine
  - diuretics
  - insulin
  - iron supplements
  - long term, high sucrose content medication, e.g. lactulose
  - morphine.

EYE CARE

Visual/structural problems for children range from the minor to the profound. It is essential that any nursing care ensures the child's comfort and does not cause problems that may worsen the child's eyesight.

Ensuring that the eyes are clean is part of the general care of any child. Equally, the nurse may see serious eye conditions where good eye care is part of the essential treatment. These may include common infections of the newborn, including, for example, *Chlamydia* infection, tear duct abnormalities and postoperative care.

Eye problems in children (McQuaid et al 1996)

- *Infection* – may be caused by a variety of organisms, including some of the sexually transmitted diseases in neonates (*Chlamydia trachomatis, Neisseria gonorrhoeae*), as well as the commonly found *Staphylococcus aureus* and *Streptococcus*.
- *Cataract* – opacity of the lens, causing loss of vision. This may occur as a result of rubella infection in the first trimester of pregnancy. Corneal transplants are now used to treat this condition.
- *Squint* – this refers to an inaccurate alignment of the axis of the eye. It may be congenital or acquired. Treatment includes corrective exercises, spectacles and surgery.
- *Retrolental fibroplasia* – the retina detaches and the area behind the lens becomes opaque, causing blindness. It is caused by rapidly raised or lowered blood oxygen levels in premature infants.

- *Retinoblastoma* – congenital tumour seen in babies and young children.
- *Ptosis* – the eyelid loses muscular control and droops over the eye. This can be characteristic of the neurological disease myasthenia gravis.
- *Congenital glaucoma* – fluid does not drain from the eye normally, causing increasing intraocular pressures. Treatment is by drops or surgery.

The following groups of children will be particularly at risk of complications, which may include corneal damage, and infection:

- unconscious children, especially those receiving muscle-relaxing drugs
- children whose eyes are not properly shut (*Note*: Incomplete eye closure of 1–2 mm can go undetected but may still result in exposure keratitis.)
- immunosuppressed children
- low-birth-weight infants, who are at increased risk of retinopathy of prematurity (Fleming et al 1996)
- newborn babies under 6 weeks old, who do not produce tears, which contain a natural antibiotic agent, lysozyme (McQuaid et al 1996)
- children undergoing eye surgery
- children who cannot blink.

General hygiene and eye care

In the well child it is unlikely that invasive eye care is required due to the natural self-regulation processes in the eye, which include the production of tears and the blinking mechanism (Rhee & Pyfer 1999). However, as with all nursing procedures, assessment is the vital first step. Early detection of eye problems can prevent further damage.

Eye care may be a distressing experience for any child. Explaining what will happen and building it into games, for example with dolls, may help the child to cooperate. Eye care may be performed by the parent or carer, or the children themselves, if they are happy to do so and have been taught any special techniques.

As eye care can require specialist knowledge, links with specialist ophthalmology colleagues should be developed by any children's unit.

Frequency of eye care

This will be variable. Healthy children may only need the area of skin around their eyes cleaned once or twice a day as part of their general hygiene routine; a sick or vulnerable child may need more frequent specific care. In other circumstances, for example if a child's eyes are discharging, they may require hourly treatment.

Purpose of eye care

- To maintain cleanliness of the eyes, thereby promoting comfort and preventing cross-infection
- To keep the mucosa moist
- To treat existing infection
- To administer medication.

Equipment

- Warm sterile saline/water
- Sterile gauze swabs. Cotton wool balls or material should not be used, as wisps of cotton may scratch the cornea (Laight 1996, Marsden & Shaw 2003)
- Eye swab if infection is suspected and cause unknown
- Gloves (preferably sterile)
- Disposal bag.

Technique and assessment

- Prior to any intervention the nurse should undertake a thorough handwash and wear gloves to reduce the possibility of cross-contamination (RCN 2004a).
- Observe the eyes for redness, inflammation and swelling, and the presence of any discharge, foreign body or eyelash defect. Each eye should be assessed independently (Marsden & Shaw 2003).
- If there is any concern that the eye is infected, swab the eye using an appropriate swab.
- In the well child, a clean face flannel or wash wipe can be used, and the eyes cleaned first with a different section of the flannel. Wipe

from the external inside aspect to the outside aspect of the eye. Do not use soap, which is unpleasant if it gets into the child's eyes.

- If the eye is infected, or the child particularly vulnerable to infection, use sterile swabs and sterile water/saline. To avoid cross-infection, clean the non-infected eye first, then the infected eye. Always wipe from the inside aspect to the outside aspect, and use a different swab for each eye (see also Administration of Medicines, p. 62).
- In a child who is at risk of corneal drying and ulceration, eyes should be kept moist using approved, prescribed artificial tear drops (e.g. hypromellose).
- Eye protection may be useful in such children if they are unconscious. This may be a simple eye dressing or a gelatine-based product such as Geliperm (Laight 1996).

EAR CARE

Caring for the ear should be part of routine hygiene care for all children. Occasionally the child will require clinical care of the external or middle ear; however, specialist knowledge is required to treat these conditions.

The ear has two important functions: hearing and balance. If either of these functions is disturbed, the child's normal sensations and perceptions can be altered, causing anxiety and confusion. Ear infections can also cause severe pain in children and attention should be paid to pain-relieving methods (RCN 2004a).

Ear problems experienced by children include:

- deafness
- otitis media or externa
- foreign bodies
- wax or 'glue'
- perforated eardrum
- conditions requiring surgery.

General hygiene and ear care

The external ear is covered by skin and needs daily care. Children often forget to clean behind their ears; however, daily ear cleansing should form part of the child's personal care

routines. As with other areas of skin, the ear can become itchy, dry or eczematous; in this case, skin creams, drops or ointments may be needed (Wong et al 1999, RCN 2004a) (see also Administration of Medicines, p. 61).

Never insert anything into the ear canal other than an auriscope or tympanic thermometer (and even in these cases, care must be taken). Cotton buds, hairgrips and fingers all have been known to cause inner ear damage (Martin 1994, Wong et al 1999).

The outer aspects of the ear (pinna) and the area behind the ear can be washed with warm water.

Special attention needs to be paid to the drying of the ear, but avoid the use of talcum powders due to the drying, allergic and other potential problems associated with this product.

Observation and examination of the ear

The nurse or parent should observe the outer ear during general hygiene care of the child.

If the nurse observes inflammation, this may indicate infection. Ear infections may be extremely painful, therefore close observation of the child's behaviour may aid in the assessment and treatment. Small children especially may be distressed, clearly in pain. Some may be able to locate the pain to the ear; others may try to rub their ear or rub it against something to gain relief.

It is quite normal for a small amount of wax (cerumen) to be seen at the entrance to the ear canal (RCN 2004a). Cerumen is normally honey coloured, becoming darker as it is exposed to air. However if the exudate is clear, this could indicate cerebrospinal fluid leakage, which may indicate a serious condition, for example head injury. If the exudate is green and/or offensive, this could indicate infection. The presence of blood may indicate haemorrhage, for example after surgery or trauma.

Foreign bodies

Foreign bodies, such as buttons, small toys, ends of cotton buds, even batteries, are not uncommon reasons for children to attend accident and emergency departments. The presence of a foreign body will sometimes go unnoticed for some time, but may be indicated by signs of infection, hearing loss, bleeding, otorrhoea (discharge) or pain.

Removal of a foreign body must only be undertaken by an experienced practitioner. The use of syringing, speculums and aural clamps may be attempted in a specialist department but surgery may be necessary in order to remove the item and observe for signs of damage or infection (RCN 2004b).

In rare instances, an insect will enter the ear canal, and may still be alive, causing an incessant buzzing and tickling of the ear. If a light is shone into the ear, the insect may be drawn out. Alternatively, a small amount of oil can be inserted into the ear to drown the insect, which is then syringed away.

Do and do not

- Do assess the child's eyes carefully, especially if they fall into one of the risk groups.
- Do not confuse eye care as part of general hygiene with clinical eye care. This can over-hospitalise the child. Most children will just need a clean wet flannel.
- Do not attempt to insert anything into a child's ear.
- Do not attempt to undertake any task for which you have not received training.

COMMUNITY PERSPECTIVE

The hygiene of the sick child who is at home will, as a general rule, be undertaken by the family. There may be occasions when they require help with this care and this gives the CCN the opportunity to assess the child in an informal but effective manner. It is important not to be judgemental about the family's standards of hygiene unless this raises concerns about the child's well-being.

References

Atherton D J 2004 A review of the pathophysiology, prevention and treatment of irritant diaper dermatitis. Current Medical Research and Opinion 20(5): 645–649

Atmarow G, Blomfield J, Brady S 1993 The clean gang: the health education teaching package designed for schoolchildren. Nursing Times 89(45): 30–32

Bailey J, Rose P 2000 Temperature measurement in the preterm infant: a literature review. Journal of Neonatal Nursing 6(1): 28–32

Bannister A 1997 Listening to children. Wiley, Chichester, UK

Brennan G 1996 Opinion: care of the new born baby's skin. Midwives 109(1303): 240

British Dental Association 2003 Frequently asked questions: children's teeth. Online. Available: www.dentalhealth.org.uk/faqs/leafletdetail.php?LeafletID=2-faq44

Campbell S, Glasper E A (eds) 1995 Whaley and Wong's children's nursing. Mosby, London

Casey A 1988 A partnership with child and family. Senior Nurse 8(4): 8–9

Child Accident Prevention Trust (CAPT) 2002 Scarred for life. Preventing bath water scalds in the home. Discussion paper. CAPT Fact sheet. CAPT, London

Coleman V 2003 Enhancing consumer participation using the practice continuum tool for family-centred care. Paediatric Nursing 15(8): 28–31

Crawford C, Raven K 2002 Play preparation for children with special needs. Paediatric Nursing 14(8): 27–29

Department of Health 2003 Getting the right start. National Service Framework for children: standard for hospital services. DoH, London

Fleming P J, Speidal B D, Marlow N, Dunn P M 1996 A neonatal vade-mecum, 2nd edn. Arnold, London

Garcia-Gonzalez E, Riviera-Rueda M 1998 Neonatal dermatology: skin care guidelines. Dermatology Nursing 10(4): 274–275

Guala A, Pastore G, Garipoli V, Agosti M, Vitali M, Bona G 2003 The time of umbilical cord separation in healthy full-term newborns: a controlled clinical trial of different cord care practices. European Journal of Pediatrics 162(5): 350–351

Health and Safety Executive 2003 Scalding risks from hot water in health and social care: local authority circular. Health and Safety Executive, Caerphilly, UK

Health Protection Agency 1999 Fact sheet for schools – wired for health. Online. Available: www.hpa.org.uk/infections/topics_az/wfhfactsheets/WFHheadlice.htm

Horne S 1999 Phenomenology: understanding the life experience of long-term ventilated adolescents. Paediatric Nursing 11(6): 37–39

Kristensson-Hallstrom I 2000 Parental participation in pediatric surgical care. AORN Journal 71(5): 1021–1029

Laight S 1996 The efficacy of eye care for ventilated patients: outline of an experimental research pilot study. Intensive and Critical Care Nursing 12(1): 16–26

Lawson L G 2001 Handwashing: a neonatal perspective. Journal of Neonatal Nursing 7(2): 42–46

Lund C, Lane A, Raines D 1999 Neonatal skin care: the scientific basis for practice. Neonatal Network 18(4): 15–27

Marsden J, Shaw M 2003 Correct administration of topical eye treatment. Nursing Standard 17(30): 42–44

Martin R L 1994 Nuts and bolts: how to care for the external ear. Hearing Journal 47(2): 43–44

McQuaid L, Huband S, Parker E 1996 Children's nursing. Churchill Livingstone, Edinburgh

Medves J, O'Brien B 2001 Does bathing newborns remove potentially harmful pathogens from the skin? Birth 28(3): 161–165

Needham J 1997 Teenage quality circles: not just a paper exercise. Paediatric Nursing 9(7): 15–17

Nursing and Midwifery Council (NMC) 2002a Code of professional conduct. NMC, London

Nursing and Midwifery Council (NMC) 2002b Guidelines for records and record-keeping. NMC, London

Nursing and Midwifery Council (NMC) 2004 Using a chaperone in clinical practice. NMC, London

Odio M, Streicher-Scott J, Hamsen R 2001 Disposable baby wipes: efficacy and skin mildness. Dermatology Nursing 13(2): 107–121

Powell L 1998 Caries prediction: a review of the literature. Community Dental and Oral Epidemiology 26: 361–371

Rhee D, Pyfer M 1999 The Wills eye manual. Williams and Wilkins, Philadelphia

Royal College of Nursing (RCN) 2003 Protection of nurses working with children and young people. RCN, London

Royal College of Nursing (RCN) 2004a Good practice in infection control. RCN, London

Royal College of Nursing ENT/Maxillofacial Nursing Forum 2004b Action on ENT: guidance on ear care. RCN, London. Online. Available for members of RCN only: http://www.rcn.org.uk/members/yourspecialty/newsletter-plus/ent-max/rl1_guidance_on_ear_care.php3

Scowen P 1995 Skin care and nappy rash. Professional Care of Mother and Child 5(5): 138

Skale N 1992 Manual of paediatric nursing procedures. J B Lippincott, Pennsylvania, PA

Smith L 1999 Family centred decision-making: a model for parent participation. Journal of Neonatal Nursing 5(6): 31–33

Smith L, Coleman V, Bradshaw M 2002 Family-centred care: concept, theory and practice. Palgrave, Basingstoke, UK

Sutton H 2001 Sexual health promotion: reducing the rate of teenage pregnancy. Paediatric Nursing 13(3): 33–37

Thomas D O 1996 Assessing children – it's different. RN 59(4): 38–45

Trotter S 2002 Skincare for the newborn: exploring the potential harm of manufactured products. RCM Midwives Journal 5(11): 376–378

Turnball R 2001 Treatment approaches to some childhood skin conditions. Community Nurse 6(12): 15–16

Wong D L, Hockenberry M, Wilson D et al 1999 Whaley and Wong's nursing care of infants and children, 6th edn. Mosby Year Book, St Louis, MO

Young J 1996 Developmental care of the premature baby. Baillière Tindall, London

Incubator care

Susan Alexander

Introduction

The maintenance of a neutral thermal environment is of the utmost importance when nursing the preterm, ill or cold infant. A neutral thermal environment is one which balances heat production and heat conservation and dissipation, thus enabling the infant to maintain a normal core temperature with minimal oxygen requirements and calorie expenditure (Amlung 1998).

The neutral thermal environment can be maintained in four main ways:

- by the use of an open crib with blankets and clothing: the dressed infant covered with blankets has the ability to maintain body temperature within a wide range of environmental temperatures; however, observation is greatly diminished
- by the use of a heated water-filled mattress – this has become a useful adjunct to care for the healthy preterm infant in the nursery, making access easier than closed incubators (Gray & Flenady 2003)

- by using radiant heaters, e.g. Baby Therms – infants can be nursed naked allowing for improved observation of the ill infant
- by using an incubator, where infants can be nursed naked (Fig. 12.1); however, the environment is enclosed.

This section discusses the care of the infant nursed in an incubator.

Learning outcomes

By the end of this section you should:

- have developed an understanding of thermoregulation in the term and preterm infant
- be able to identify the infant who requires to be nursed in an incubator
- be able to prepare an incubator to receive an ill infant
- be able to demonstrate an understanding of temperature regulation devices used in the incubator
- be able to provide safe and effective care to the infant nursed in the incubator.

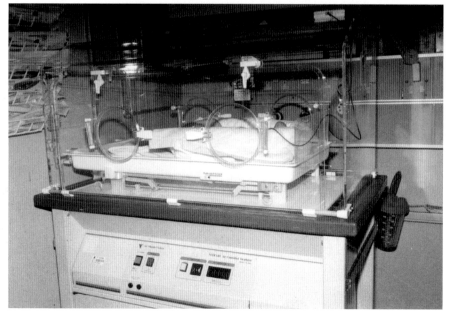

Figure 12.1   Infant being nursed in an incubator

Rationale

Both term and preterm infants have difficulty in maintaining body temperature owing to an inability to control their heat loss. Prevention of heat loss in ill and distressed infants is crucial to their survival; thus the provision of a neutral thermal environment, when nursing the infant, is of the utmost importance (Amlung 1998). Environmental temperature, which maintains the infant's skin temperature between 36.5 and 37.5°C (rectal 37°C) is known to promote minimal metabolic rate and oxygen consumption (Merenstein & Gardiner 2002). This is defined as the neutral thermal environment.

Factors to note

Infants are at risk of poor temperature control caused by an immature hypothalamus resulting in poor control of heat loss and heat production (see Temperature Control, p. 392). This is more marked in the preterm infant.

Preterm infants lack glycogen and stored fats, particularly brown fat which is important both as an energy source and for heat produc-tion. Brown fat is laid down in a variety of locations in the body between 26 and 28 weeks of gestation; infants born before this time may lack the ability to generate their own heat. Infants who do have brown fat have the ability to generate heat from birth. Brown fat in infants differs from that in adults in that it has a higher number of mitochondria and an abundant sympathetic nerve supply. Brown fat accounts for 10% of the term infant's total adipose tissue (Flaherty 1996).

Infants have a thin subcutaneous fat layer resulting in poor insulation (England 2003).

Term and preterm infants do not have the ability to shiver to produce heat in response to cold and their metabolic response is limited. Changes in peripheral vascular tone, with constriction of skin vessels, occur in an attempt to reduce heat loss, thus keeping the blood in the central circulation. Non-shivering thermogenesis may occur where heat production is achieved from brown fat (Fellows 2001).

Heat loss in the infant is nearly four times greater, per unit of body weight, than in adults. This is primarily due to the higher ratio of surface area to body weight in infants (Lyon 2004).

Infants lose heat in four ways:

- *by conduction* – occurring when the infant comes into direct contact with a cooler surface, thus losing heat to that surface (Fellows 2001)
- *by convection* – when warmth is lost to the surrounding air or water; this necessitates the maintenance of room temperature between 24 and 26°C (Fellows 2001)
- *by radiation* – heat loss from the infant to a surface nearby without direct contact; this may occur if the infant is placed near cold external walls (Lyon 2004)
- *by evaporation* – caused by the evaporation of surface body water; this water is converted into vapour and is of particular significance in the newborn (Lyon 2004).

Exposed to extremes of temperature, infants will suffer from decreased lung surfactant, hypoglycaemia, increased oxygen consumption and decreased blood coagulability in cold conditions, and increased fluid loss, hypernatraemia and recurrent apnoea in heat. Both extremes of temperature may result in death (Roberton 1993).

Equipment

- Incubator
- Temperature monitor
- Servo control skin probe (if required)
- Sterile water (if required).

Method

Incubators can be used to maintain a neutral thermal environment in two ways: skin servo control and air (non-servo) control. Skin servo control involves attaching a skin probe to the abdomen of the infant, normally over the liver. If the infant's temperature falls, additional heat is provided until the target temperature is reached. Recent incubators have a skin sensor detach alarm to prevent overheating in case the probe becomes dislodged (Lyon 2004). In the air (non-servo) control mode the air temperature of the incubator is raised or lowered depending on the measured temperature of the infant (Lyon 2004).

For detailed guidance on the use of individual incubators the nurse should refer to the manufacturer's operating guidelines.

- Position the incubator in an area of the ward away from direct sunlight and draughts. Direct sunlight will cause the incubator to overheat.
- Fill the water reservoir with sterile water if additional humidity is required. Ensure that the temperature of the incubator is maintained at a constant level, not in excess of the humidity, to prevent additional heat loss caused by evaporation.
- The room temperature should be maintained between 24 and 26°C (England 2003). This helps prevent heat loss through the incubator wall.
- The incubator heater should be switched on and temperature limits set (see Table 12.1). The incubator should be warmed to between these temperature limits before the infant is transferred into it.
- Attach the servo control probe to the infant's abdomen, if required, and adjust temperature limits for skin temperature (as per local policy).
- Prevent heat loss from the incubator by keeping the portholes closed when the infant is not being attended to.
- Minimal handling and coordination of care to prevent constant disruption (clustered care) will not only allow the infant to rest but will also reduce heat loss.
- Warm your hands before touching the infant.
- Warm additional equipment before putting it into the incubator.

Table 12.1   Neutral thermal environmental temperatures determined by age and weight

Weight (g)	Incubator temperature (°C)		
	Day 1	Days 2–7	1–2 weeks
<1000	35 ± 0.5	34 ± 0.5	33 ± 0.5
1000–1500	34 ± 0.5	33.5 ± 0.5	32 ± 0.5
1500–2500	33 ± 0.5	32 ± 0.5	30 ± 1

After Beischer et al 1997.

- Ensure that the infant is kept as dry as possible to reduce evaporative heat loss.
- Significant heat loss from the infant's head can be reduced by the use of a hat (Amlung 1998).
- Clean the incubator in accordance with the manufacturer's instructions.
- Change the incubator as per local policy.

Observations and complications

- The infant's temperature should be checked on a regular basis, if not continuously monitored. Bailey and Rose (2000) recommend the use of the axilla for monitoring neonatal temperature.
- Routine care should be clustered to reduce heat loss from the incubator.
- The incubator temperature limits should be set to ensure that the infant does not overheat or become hypothermic.
- Incubator temperature should be monitored continually and maintained within set limits.
- Replace the water in the reservoir fully every 24 hours to reduce infection risk.
- Porthole access may be problematic if the infant is unstable. Under these conditions the infant should be transferred to a radiant warmer.

TRANSITION FROM INCUBATOR TO OPEN COT

Weaning from an incubator to an open cot is an important step in the discharge preparation of an infant. Practice will differ between units, with some units having detailed policies. These policies may be based on a combination of the following:

- The infant's condition should be stable.
- The weight of the infant.
- Steady weight gain demonstrated by the infant.

- The temperature of the incubator being gradually reduced. This may be reduced over a 24-hour period; however, the incubator should never be turned off as this will result in air not being circulated.
- Monitoring the infant's temperature is important to ensure that they are maintaining their temperature.
- The infant should be placed in a cot, in a draught-free position in the ward.
- The infant should be clothed and wrapped. Special attention should be paid to the wearing of a hat because of the increased heat loss from the head. Clothing and wrapping may be commenced when the infant is in the incubator, with suggestions regarding clothing being the first stage of incubator weaning rather than decreasing incubator temperature (Medoff-Cooper 1994).

Do and do not

- Do ensure that the care is clustered to decrease disturbance of the infant.
- Do encourage parents in the care of their infant. This will help enhance the parent–infant relationship.
- Do ensure that the infant is wrapped well and that the head is covered if the infant is being removed from the incubator for feeding or cuddling.
- Do ensure that sheets etc. are warmed before putting them into the incubator.
- Do ensure that the sterile water in the reservoir, if used, is fully changed every 24 hours.
- Do not leave the incubator in direct sunlight or draughts.
- Do not leave portholes or incubator doors open unnecessarily.
- Do not allow the infant's head to be covered by the Perspex heat shield as this may cause hypoxia (Fraser & Cooper 2003).
- Do not turn off the incubator while the infant is inside.

References

Amlung S R 1998 Neonatal thermoregulation. In: Kenner C, Lott J W, Flandermeyer A A (eds) Comprehensive neonatal nursing: a physiologic perspective, 2nd edn. W B Saunders, Philadelphia, PA, ch 16

Bailey J, Rose P 2000 Temperature measurement in the preterm infant. Journal of Neonatal Nursing 6(1): 28–32

Beischer N A, Mackay E V, Colditz P B 1997 Obstetrics and the newborn, 3rd edn. W B Saunders, London

England C 2003 The healthy low birth weight baby. In: Fraser D, Cooper A (eds) Myles textbook for midwives, 14th edn. Churchill Livingstone, Edinburgh

Fellows P 2001 Management of thermal stability. In: Boxwell G (ed.) Neonatal intensive care nursing. Routledge, London, ch 4

Flaherty L 1996 Neonates and premature infants: overview of differences and ED management. Journal of Emergency Nursing 22(2): 120–124

Fraser D, Cooper A (eds) 2003 Myles textbook for midwives, 14th edn. Churchill Livingstone, Edinburgh

Gray P H, Flenady V 2003 Cot-nursing versus incubator care for preterm infants. The Cochrane Library, Oxford

Lyon A 2004 Applied physiology: temperature control in the newborn infant. Current Paediatrics 14: 137–144

Medoff-Cooper B 1994 Transition of the preterm infant to an open crib. Journal of Obstetric, Gynaecological and Neonatal Nursing 23(4): 329–335

Merenstein G B, Gardiner S L 2002 Handbook of neonatal intensive care, 5th edn. Mosby, St Louis, MO

Roberton N R C 1993 A manual of neonatal intensive care. Edward Arnold, London

Further Reading

Lyon A J, Pikaar M E, Badger P, McIntosh N 1997 Temperature control in very low birthweight infants during first five days of life. Archives of Disease in Childhood 76(1): 47–50

Moore J 2003 From birth to neonatal unit: a cold journey. Journal of Neonatal Nursing 9(4): 4 page insert

Short M A 1998 A comparison of temperature in VLBW infants swaddled versus unswaddled in a double-walled incubator in skin control mode. Neonatal Network 17(3): 25–31

Practice **13**

Intravenous therapy

Nan McIntosh

Introduction

Intravenous infusions for fluid replacement and drug administration are commonplace in the paediatric ward, whereas blood transfusion, platelet administration and total parenteral nutrition (TPN) are seen more commonly in haematology, intensive care and neonatal units. The use of home TPN has also increased to enable children with a variety of congenital and acquired gastrointestinal conditions to be cared for at home. Maintaining optimal function of intravenous infusions is of primary importance in children's nursing as fluid overload and electrolyte imbalance are potentially life threatening and the frequent resiting of intravenous cannulae is stressful to the child and family (Fitzsimons 2001).

Learning outcomes

By the end of this section and following additional reading and practise you should be able to:

- understand the differences between a child's and an adult's body fluids distribution
- recognise the need for intravenous fluid therapy
- ensure the safe administration of intravenous fluid therapy
- identify children who may require blood or blood products

- safely administer blood and blood products
- act appropriately should the child have a reaction to the treatment
- understand the need for total parenteral nutrition
- identify children who may require total parenteral nutrition
- safely administer total parenteral nutrition.

Factors to note

- Body surface area differs in children and adults, with the infant and child having a proportionally greater body surface area than the adult. There is also a different distribution, e.g. the head constitutes 20% of the infant's body surface area compared with 7–9% of the adult's (Davenport 1996, Willock & Jewkes 2000).

- The proportion of body weight that consists of water is greater in the infant and child; 75–80% of the newborn's body weight is attributed to fluid compared with approximately 60–70% in adolescents. This reduces to between 50 and 60% in the adult, with females having slightly more body fluid (Hazinski 1988, Livesley 1996, Hiu Lam 1998).

- Body fluids are distributed between the intracellular and extracellular compartments. In adults, intracellular body fluid normally constitutes around two-thirds (67%) of total body fluid. The extracellular compartment constitutes the remaining third (33%). The extracellular fluid consists of plasma, lymph, interstitial fluid, bone water and connective tissue water. In infants and children the majority of body fluid is found in the extracellular compartment; approximately one-half of this is exchanged daily to maintain homeostasis (Hazinski 1992, Livesley 1996).

- As a result of this distribution, dehydration will occur more quickly in the infant/child.

- Care should be taken when siting an intravenous cannula to be used for infusion of fluids to ensure that the child's dominant hand is not used.

- A suitable size of intravenous cannula should be selected that not only reflects the size of the child's vascular access but also the intended use.

- Intravenous administration sets may or may not have an 'in-line' burette. It is preferential to use a set with an 'in-line' burette for both neonates and toddlers, as this will minimise the amount of fluid that the child receives should there be free flow of fluid (Hazinski 1992).

As there are numerous types of infusion pump available, the nurse must be educated and competent in the use of the device and have regular updates when new pumps are introduced into the workplace. (NPSA 2004).

INTRAVENOUS INFUSIONS

The delivery of intravenous fluids is common within acute paediatric settings. Normally used to maintain hydrational status, intravenous infusions can also be used to administer drugs. Selection of the intravenous cannula site is important (see Venepuncture and Cannulation, p. 434); sites should be chosen that present the best calibre vein and that can also be suitably immobilised. Once the intravenous cannula is inserted and secured, the intravenous infusion can be commenced.

Equipment

- Intravenous fluid for administration
- Intravenous administration set
- In-line burette (if required)
- Air inlet (if required)
- Intravenous infusion pump
- Splint to immobilise limb
- Surgical tape and/or bandage to secure splint to limb and prevent intravenous line trailing.

Method

1. Explain the need for the infusion and the procedure to the child and parent/carer.
2. Ensure that hands are clean and dry.

3. Intravenous fluid should be checked by two members of the registered nursing staff (or as per local policy) against the medical prescription chart.

4. The expiry date and the batch number on the bag should be recorded on an intravenous infusion recording sheet or as per local policy.

5. Priming of the intravenous administration set is an aseptic procedure and care must be taken to avoid touching the spike or contaminating the system.

6. Remove the intravenous administration set from the sterile packaging.

7. Remove the in-line burette (if required) from the sterile packaging.

8. Insert the intravenous spike of the administration set into the exit line on the sterile burette.

9. Close all roller clamps attached to the burette and administration set.

10. Insert the spike of the burette into the appropriate port of the intravenous fluid bag. *Note:* If the intravenous fluid is in a bottle, the spike should be inserted into the appropriate place in the rubber stopper and an air inlet inserted. Clean the rubber stopper with 70% isopropyl alcohol (e.g. Mediwipes) and allow to dry prior to insertion of the spike and air inlet.

11. Fill the burette (if used) with around 20–30 ml of fluid by opening the roller clamp; then close the clamp.

12. Half fill the in-line bubble of the administration set with fluid by gently squeezing the bubble to expel air into the burette.

13. Open the clamp and allow fluid to flow into the administration set, thus expelling the remaining air. Once fluid has reached the end of the administration set, close the clamps and ensure that all air has been expelled.

14. Place the administration set into the intravenous infusion pump as per manufacturer's instructions.

15. Check patency of the child's intravenous cannula.

16. Attach the administration set to the child's intravenous cannula and secure with surgical tape.
    Note: Non-sterile tape should not be placed directly over the insertion site (see Venepuncture and Cannulation, p. 439).

17. Immobilise the child's limb if necessary with a splint, ensuring that the intravenous cannulation site can be easily observed.

18. Set the rate of infusion, as prescribed, on the infusion pump. Open all clamps and commence the infusion. Record time of commencement on appropriate chart.

Observations and complications

- Check the intravenous cannula insertion site, venous pressure (read from some computerised infusion pumps), volume infused, rate at which the fluid is infused and type of infusate hourly.
- Observe the intravenous cannula insertion site for signs of redness and swelling. The area approximately 2.5 cm (1 inch) above and below the insertion site should be easily observed.
- If the child complains of pain or there are signs of intravenous infiltration, stop the infusion immediately and report to medical staff. Infiltration can be graded, indicating the degree of possible damage to tissues (see Table 13.1).
- Record the volume infused and the rate on a fluid balance chart.
- A running total of fluid infused should be maintained. This provides an accurate hourly fluid intake.

Do and do not

- Do check the site on an hourly basis.
- Do ensure that the child's limb is immobilised.
- Do stop the infusion if the child complains of pain. Inform the medical staff/nurse practitioner.
- Do stop the infusion if there are any signs of extravasation.
- Do refer to local extravasation policy.

Table 13.1   Grading for intravenous infiltration

Grade	Manifestations
I	Painful intravenous site. No signs of swelling or redness
II	Painful site. Slight swelling. Good pulse and capillary refill below infiltration site. No blanching evident
III	Painful site. Marked swelling with blanching and skin cool to touch. Good pulse below infiltration site with brisk capillary refill
IV	Painful site. Very marked swelling with blanching of skin. Skin cool to touch, pulses absent below infiltration with slow capillary refill (>4 seconds). Skin breakdown or necrosis may be present; however, this may be delayed

After Flemmer & Chan 1993.
Infiltration may not traverse through all stages. Infiltration at Grade IV is possible on first detection.

- Do not obscure the intravenous cannula insertion site.
- Do not bandage fully the arm on which a cannula is sited.
- Do not put the bandage on too tightly.

BLOOD TRANSFUSIONS

Transfusion of blood or blood products is performed in children for a variety of reasons, including anaemia, acute haemorrhage, haematological disease, following surgery and in other acute and chronic conditions.

Advances in both surgery and medicine have been made possible partly through the availability of blood and blood products (McClelland 2001). The Serious Hazards of Transfusion Reporting scheme is a confidential, anonymous reporting system for transfusion errors and severe transfusion reactions. The report emphasises the vital role of correct checking of component and patient details at every step in the transfusion process. It deals with the main practical aspects of blood and blood components (fresh frozen plasma, platelets, cryoprecipitate) with particular emphasis on a safe approach to the confirmation of component and patient identity. The aim is to ensure that the *right blood* is given to the *right patient* at the *right time*, every time (SHOT 1999). The recommendations are in keeping with the *Guidelines for the Administration of Blood and Blood Components and the Management of Transfused Patients* drawn up by the Blood Transfusion Task Force.

Factors to note

- Erythrocytes (red blood cells) are formed in the red bone marrow from haemocytoblasts. As the red blood cell matures it loses its nucleus and caves in on both sides, giving the characteristic biconcave disc shape.

- The usual life span of a red blood cell is 120 days. Once the cells grow old, their membranes become fragile and rupture, the contents being phagocytosed by the macrophages in the spleen, liver and bone marrow.

- The balance of production and destruction is equal under normal homeostasis.

- The main function of red blood cells is to transport oxygen, bound to haemoglobin, to all cells of the body. Other functions include the transport of waste carbon dioxide and the maintenance of blood pH.

- Fetal haemoglobin has a greater affinity for oxygen than adult haemoglobin, which is suitable for the fetal environment. Towards the later stages of pregnancy, the fetus begins to develop adult haemoglobin. The neonatal haemoglobin level is higher than that of children.

- Whole blood transfusion will replenish the volume, red blood cells and oxygen-carrying capacity of the blood. Packed red blood cells, referred to as packed cells, consist of blood in which some 80% of plasma has been removed. A packed cell transfusion aims at replenishing red blood cell mass and thus the oxygen-carrying capacity of the blood; however, a packed cell transfusion will not replenish volume (Fitzpatrick & Fitzpatrick 1997, Place 1998, BCSH 1999).

- Whole blood transfusion is normally reserved for exchange transfusion for rhesus incompatibility, severe haemorrhage with depletion of coagulation factors and situations where more appropriate blood products are not readily available (Hazinski 1992).

- Washed red cells have had the plasma proteins, leucocytes and platelets removed by rinsing with a special solution; this decreases the chance of transfusion reaction. This type of prepared blood may be used in children who have frequent blood transfusions (Abernathy et al 1994, Campbell & Glasper 1995).

- Following bone marrow transplant, children require to have blood products irradiated.

- Blood should be stored at 4°C; therefore it must be refrigerated in a specialised blood refrigerator. Blood can be stored for up to 36 days, after which it will have to be discarded (Contreras 1990, BCSH 1999).

- The blood transfusion should be commenced within 30 minutes following the arrival of blood from the blood bank (McConnell 1997, McClelland 2001).

- There are no clear guidelines for the use of blood warmers and the decision is the responsibility of the consultant on each individual patient. This decision may be influenced by the temperature of the patient receiving the transfusion (i.e. hypothermic), the amount of blood being transfused, the duration of the transfusion, or patients with an antibody in their plasma which causes haemolysis when the temperature lowers (e.g. cryoglobulinaemia) (Iserson & Huestis 1991). A blood warmer actively warms the transfusion during administration by using tubing coils in a water bath. This may be performed during exchange transfusions or to prevent air embolism (Smith 2001, RCN 2003).

- Blood should be transfused over 4 hours. Transfusions exceeding this time may become contaminated with bacteria. If the volume of blood cannot be transfused within 4 hours, it should be divided into smaller volumes (paedipacks) and stored accordingly in the blood bank until required (Abernathy et al 1994, Campbell & Glasper 1995).

- Blood is obtained from people who are between the ages of 18 and 65 years. Frequency of donations is normally two to three times per year.

- Since 1985, all donor blood has been tested for human immunodeficiency virus (HIV 1 and 2 antibody). Testing for hepatitis (A, B and C), syphilis and *Treponema pallidum* antibody are routine (Blood Transfusion Service 1996). Selective testing for specific agents may be considered when administering blood to susceptible recipients, e.g. the testing for cytomegalovirus in immunosuppressed children. All donated blood has serologic tests performed to determine blood group (A, B, AB and O) as well as rhesus factor (Rh D +ve or -ve) (Contreras 1990, Campbell & Glasper 1995).

- Children with blood group AB can be transfused with blood groups AB, A, B and O. Children with blood group A can be transfused with groups A and O, and those with blood group B can be transfused with groups B and O. Those children with blood group O can only be transfused with blood group O (see Table 13.2). However, the blood that a child is transfused with must be rhesus compatible, i.e. -ve must have -ve, but +ve can have +ve or -ve. Blood group O is regarded as the universal donor whereas blood group AB is the universal recipient (BCSH 1999).

- Religious and cultural beliefs of the child and family must be taken into account when considering a blood transfusion. Families

Table 13.2 ABO group of blood products to be transfused

Patient's ABO group	Red cells	Platelets	Plasma
O	O	O, A, B	O, A, B, AB
A	A, O	A	A, AB
B	B, O	B, A	B, AB
AB	AB, A, B, O	A, B	AB, A

who are Jehovah's Witnesses may not agree to blood transfusions and substitutes may have to be considered. In cases where volume expansion is necessary, colloidal fluids may be as effective; however, if blood is a necessity, a court order may have to be obtained if the family do not give consent.

Equipment

Requirements are as for intravenous infusion. The following extra items are required:

- Blood or blood component administration set (this must be appropriate for the pump if one is being used), pack of blood or blood component
- Blood bank issue slip (supplied with the first unit of the batch sent from the blood bank. This includes details of each pack in the batch to be transfused); this should be readily available throughout the transfusion, located with the fluid administration chart at the child's bedside
- Blood components/products prescription
- Child's case notes, to enable checking of each unit administered
- 0.9% saline to prime the giving set
- In-line burette (if required)
- Infusion pump (e.g. Ivac pump).

Leucodepletion

Since 1999 all blood components have been leucodepleted ($<5 \times 10^6$/unit) at point of manufacture. This move was prompted by theoretical concerns about variant Creutzfeldt–Jakob disease (vCJD) transmission. Following this move the use of bedside leucodepletion filters has become redundant.

Blood must be transfused through a blood giving set with an integral mesh filter (170–200 micron pore size). Platelets, fresh frozen plasma and cryoprecipitate must be administered through a normal blood administration set or through a platelet/cryoprecipitate giving set. Plasma protein solutions (4.5% albumin or 20% albumin) do not require to be infused through a giving set with a filter. A standard infusion set as used for crystalloids or synthetic colloids is suitable.

Filters

Each giving set designed for the administration of blood or blood components contains an integral 170–200 micron pore size mesh filter to remove macroaggregate or particulate matter. For the vast majority of transfusions, no additional filter is required.

Microaggregate filters

There are several filters available designed to hold back particles down to 20–40 micron size (e.g. Pall Ultipore). There are few clinical indications, if any, for the use of these filters and their use for routine transfusions is unnecessary and expensive.

Method

1. Explain the procedure to the child and parent/carer and ensure that consent has been obtained. (This may be verbal or written depending on local policy.)

2. Wash and dry your hands.

3. Assemble the equipment and prime the administration set with 0.9% saline (see 'Intravenous infusions', above). Check the

blood for administration against the medical prescription and haematology/blood bank information. The child's name, date of birth, hospital identification number, blood group, rhesus factor status, blood bag number and expiry date should be checked using the identification label attached to the bag of blood, the haematology/blood bank information slip, the child's hospital notes and the child's identification band. Remember the final check must take place at the child's bedside (BCSH 1999).

4. If the child is known to have any special transfusion needs (e.g. irradiated components) the prescription form must state this and pack labelling should be checked to ensure that these requirements have been met.

5. Check the bag of blood for abnormal colour, gas bubbles, clumping or any extraneous material. This may give an indication of bacterial contamination (Abernathy et al 1994).

6. Attach the blood bag and prime the administration set with blood (if the child is not to receive the saline within the system, as may be the case if the child is fluid restricted) and attach to the child's cannula. Secure the child's limb as necessary (see 'Intravenous infusions', above).

7. Monitor and record the transfusion as per intravenous infusions.

8. Once the transfusion is complete, flush the administration set with 0.9% saline and proceed as per medical instruction.

Observations and complications

- *Prior* to commencing the transfusion *of each unit*, record the child's temperature, pulse and blood pressure on the appropriate chart (baseline recording). The child should be observed regularly (15-minute intervals) during the initial hour of the transfusion. Additional recordings are at the discretion of each area (recommendations are at least hourly) but are essential if the child is unstable or if they appear to be experiencing an adverse reaction.

- The child is observed during the transfusion of blood and blood components to detect any adverse event as early as possible in order that potentially life-saving action may be taken. Adverse reactions may be seen with all blood components and monitoring is therefore required even for patients receiving only fresh frozen plasma (FFP), platelets or cryoprecipitate. Severe reactions most commonly present during the first 15 minutes of a transfusion and the patient should be observed most closely during this period. These reactions can be categorised as haemolytic reactions, febrile reactions, allergic reactions and circulatory overload (see Table 13.3). If a reaction occurs, stop the transfusion and inform medical staff immediately.

- Prior to commencing the infusion briefly explain the procedure to the patient/carer and advise them to notify staff immediately if they become aware of any reaction such as shivering, flushing, urticarial rash, pain or shortness of breath.

- Wherever possible transfusions should be given in areas where the patient can be readily observed by the clinical staff and during day-time hours.

- When the transfusion is commenced, record the relevant information on the appropriate charts.

- Adjust the flow-rate to achieve infusion over the prescribed time period.

- Throughout the transfusion observe the patient for any sign or symptom of incompatibility or adverse reaction, e.g. flushing, urticaria, vomiting, diarrhoea, fever, itching, headache, haemoglobinuria, rigor, severe backache, collapse or circulatory failure. Should any of these be observed the transfusion must be stopped immediately and the doctor informed. Keep the IV line open with a slow infusion of 0.9% saline.

- The transfusion of a single pack of red cells should be complete within 4–5 hours of removal from the blood fridge. Platelets and FFP are generally infused over 30–60 minutes.

Table 13.3 Reactions to blood transfusions

Reaction	Manifestations	Management
Haemolytic reaction (Cause: incompatible blood. Rare)	Chills, fever, shaking, pain at IV site and along venous tract, breathlessness, abnormal bleeding, haematuria, progress to shock and renal failure	Stop transfusion Inform medical staff Retain sample of donor blood Obtain sample of child's blood Medical treatment to reverse shock
Febrile reactions (Cause: leucocyte, platelet or plasma protein antibodies)	Fever or chills	Stop transfusion Inform medical staff Administer prescribed antipyretic
Allergic reactions (Cause: allergens in donor's blood)	Urticaric rash, wheeze, breathlessness, laryngeal oedema	Stop transfusion Inform medical staff Epinephrine/steroid therapy may be used to counteract reaction Prophylactic antihistamines may be used in children who have a known reaction
Circulatory overload (Cause: rapid infusion)	Chest pain, cyanosis, noisy respirations, dysponea, distended neck veins	Stop transfusion Inform medical staff Place child in upright position Use diuretics to diminish fluid overload in children who can pass urine

FFP must be infused within 4 hours once thawed.

- Any suspected transfusion reaction or incompatibility should be investigated and the blood bank informed. The blood pack and any empty packs should be returned to the blood bank (if requested by blood bank staff) in an appropriate, sealed polythene bag. Further investigation may be required.

Discontinuation
- Record the volume of blood transfused on the fluid balance chart (or 24-hour chart).
- In the event of blood transfusion being followed by other intravenous fluids, a change of giving set is required. It is not necessary to give a 0.9% saline 'flush' on completion of transfusion.
- When all units to be transfused have been administered, file the blood bank issue slip in the case sheet.

Disposal
If observation of the child at completion of the transfusion reveals no evidence of an adverse reaction, the bags may be placed in the standard 'clinical waste' bags (yellow) for disposal. The giving set should be disposed of in an appropriate sharps container.

Do and do not

- Do reassure parents regarding the testing of blood and blood products.
- Do check with the parents whether the child has had a previous reaction to blood or blood products. Report promptly to medical staff.
- Do ensure that the blood is thoroughly checked prior to administration.
- Do stop the transfusion if there is any indication of a reaction.
- Do keep emergency equipment at hand in case of a severe haemolytic or anaphylactic reaction.
- Do report any errors/reactions to your local transfusion committee who will in turn inform SHOT.
- Do not, in the case of reaction, restart a transfusion until the child's condition has been fully medically evaluated.

- Do not administer any other medication intravenously using the same cannula during the transfusion.
- Do not give intravenous dextrose immediately before or after transfusion as haemolysis and clotting may occur within the administration set (Brunner & Suddarth 1991).

PLATELET TRANSFUSION

Platelets can be administered both prophylactically and therapeutically to children with thrombocytopenia, leukaemia or those undergoing chemotherapy (Abernathy et al 1994). These children are at risk of bleeding, which can be fatal in some instances.

Factors to note

- Platelets are formed from cells within the bone marrow. They are disc-shaped cells and there are between 50 000 and 400 000 per cubic millimetre of blood (Arnett 1998, Place 1998, Tortora & Grabowski 2002).

- The normal life span of platelets is approximately 5–7 days; the life span of transfused platelets is 4 days (Hazinski 1992).

- Platelets arrest bleeding through platelet plug formation, wherein the platelets adhere to the damaged blood vessel. This adhesion changes the characteristics of the platelets by activating a series of reactions within them. This reaction forms a platelet plug which prevents blood loss in small vessels. Although initially loose, the plug eventually becomes tight by being reinforced with fibrin threads during coagulation (Tortora & Grabowski 2002).

- Ideally, platelets are matched according to their ABO and rhesus factors; however, in emergency situations compatible (or even incompatible) platelet concentrates can be used (Contreras 1990).

- Platelet transfusion may not increase platelet count in children with idiopathic thrombocytopenic purpura, disseminated intravascular coagulation or antibody reac-

tions, because such conditions destroy platelets. However, platelet transfusion is of use in the treatment of severe haemorrhage in such children (Abernathy et al 1994).

- Platelets are stored in the blood bank at 22°C and must *never* be refrigerated. Platelets are issued as single donations of matched platelets in a single pack obtained from one donor by apheresis or pools of four random donors. The total volume is stated on the pack. Ideally, this product should be infused over not more than 60 minutes. Packs which have been refrigerated inadvertently *must not be used* but should be returned to the blood bank.

- Platelets must be transfused immediately on arrival to the ward/theatre. Specific areas have facilities to enable packs to be constantly agitated for periods prior to transfusion, but this is not necessary during the transfusion period.

- Platelets will usually be group O or group A. As there will be a small amount of contaminating red cells, the appropriate Rhesus D group will be issued to avoid Rhesus D sensitisation in female children.

Equipment

- Platelets for infusion
- Platelet administration set containing an integral 170–200 micron pore size mesh filter to remove macroaggregate or particulate matter
- Appropriate infusion pump (if used).

Method

1. Explain the procedure to the child and parent/carer.
2. Wash and dry your hands.
3. Check the platelets for infusion using the same criteria as those for blood (see 'Blood transfusions', above).
4. Prime the administration set (see 'Intravenous infusions', above).
5. Place the administration set into the pump as per the manufacturer's instructions.
6. Attach the administration set to the child's intravenous cannula and secure.

7. Administer the platelets as instructed by the medical staff. Platelets are normally administered rapidly in 20–40 minutes (Hazinski 1992).
8. Once administration is complete, disconnect the platelet administration set and discard it according to hospital policy. Record the volume of platelets infused on the appropriate chart.

Observations and complications

- As the platelets are administered relatively rapidly, it is important that the child is constantly observed to monitor any adverse reactions and for the infusion being completed.
- Observe the child for signs of fever, chills or rash, as reaction to platelets can occur. Reactions to platelets are normally treated with antihistamine drug therapy. Report any reactions to the medical staff and stop the infusion until the child has been evaluated.

Do and do not

- Do ensure that the platelets are agitated until they are to be transfused. This prevents them from clumping.
- Do administer the platelets rapidly.
- Do not administer platelets using a pump that is not designed for platelet infusion (refer to manufacturer's instructions).

TOTAL PARENTERAL NUTRITION

The development of total parenteral nutrition (TPN) some 30 years ago has enabled children with a variety of congenital and acquired gastrointestinal conditions to survive (Bilodeau 1995). Parenteral feeding is considered when a child cannot tolerate or absorb adequate nutrition orally or enterally. Parenteral nutrition is administered intravenously and refers to a nutrient solution which comprises dextrose, amino acids, fat, electrolytes, vitamins, micronutrients and water (Abernathy et al 1994, Gaedeke Norris & Steinhorn 1994, Galica 1997).

Factors to note

- TPN is used therapeutically for conditions such as short bowel syndrome, intestinal obstruction, bowel fistulae, chronic persistent severe diarrhoea and extensive burns or in children receiving chemotherapy (Bilodeau 1995, Campbell & Glasper 1995).

- TPN can be administered through a central venous catheter, e.g. a Hickman line, or a peripheral cannula. The route of administration will be determined by the length of time that the child is to receive parenteral nutrition and the concentration of dextrose that is to be used. A concentration of dextrose and amino acids of 20–30% may cause vein sclerosis or burns if extravasation occurs; hence for this concentration a central venous catheter is used. For dextrose concentrations below 10% a peripheral cannula can be used. The use of peripheral veins in the acutely ill is becoming more common (Hazinski 1992, Campbell & Glasper 1995, Carter & Dearmun 1995).

- Parenteral nutrition can be administered continuously throughout the day, as is often the case in the acutely ill, or can be administered overnight. Overnight administration would be considered for the child who is to receive long-term parenteral nutrition as it allows for more freedom of movement during the day.

- Parenteral nutrition is prepared on a daily basis and stored in a temperature-controlled refrigerator. If the child is acutely ill, electrolytes are altered in accordance with the child's own biochemistry. Children who are to receive their nutrition for a longer period of time and who are stabilised may not require daily alterations to their nutrition (Bilodeau 1995, Carter & Dearmun 1995).

- Dextrose is primarily used as a source of calories; amino acids are a source of nitrogen for protein synthesis. Electrolytes, minerals, trace elements and vitamins are added to meet the child's known nutritional requirements. Fat emulsions provide a major source of calories as well as preventing essential fatty acid deficiency states (Hazinski 1992, Galica 1997).

- Fat solution, e.g. Intralipid, is administered separately, as mixing it with dextrose solution may cause denaturing of the fat solution (Poskitt 1988). However, the same cannula/central line can be used for administration. Fat and dextrose solution are infused into the same central line using a three-way tap or a Y extension.

- The dextrose constituent of the TPN renders the child more prone to infection. An aseptic technique must therefore be used when changing bags of solution, and handling or changing intravenous lines (Hazinski 1992).

- Bags of nutrition should be stored in the refrigerator and removed around 30 minutes prior to the commencement of administration. This allows the solution to warm to room temperature.

Equipment

- Dextrose solution with additives
- Fat emulsion solution
- Amino acid solution, e.g. Vamin
- Intravenous administration set
- Intravenous infusion pump, e.g. Ivac pump
- Sterile drapes or dressing pack
- Sterile latex-free gloves
- 70% isopropyl alcohol
- Three-way tap or Y extension (if required).

Method

1. Explain the procedure to the child and parent/carer.
2. Wash and dry your hands.
3. Open all equipment and place on a sterile drape.
4. Two registered nurses (or as per local policy) should check the parenteral nutrition solution against the medical prescription. Check the solution for clarity, turbidity and particles. Check the expiry date.

5. Wearing sterile gloves, prime the intravenous administration set as described for intravenous infusions (p. 213); however, care should be taken to maintain asepsis.
6. Clean the child's central line with alcohol solution 2.5 cm (1 inch) from the tip. If the child has an existing administration set attached, clean 2.5 cm (1 inch) on either side of the join. Allow the alcohol to dry.
7. Attach the administration set and thread the line through the infusion pump.
8. Commence the infusion.
9. Monitor and record the infusion as per intravenous infusions (p. 213).

Observations and complications

- Monitor fluid and electrolyte balance closely.
- Protect the bag of dextrose solution from sunlight, if necessary. Some additives degrade in sunlight; hence the solution bag may have to be covered, e.g. with a bag made out of paper or dark plastic. Coloured infusion sets can also be used. Guidance should be sought from the pharmacy department.
- Monitor and record the child's temperature 4-hourly. Pyrexia (temperature $>38.5°C$) may indicate sepsis and blood cultures should be obtained (Hazinski 1992).
- Monitor and record blood glucose 4-hourly. The frequency of monitoring can be gradually reduced in accordance with the child's condition, but the test should be performed at least daily. Urine may also be tested for glucose as per local policy.
- Monitor weight daily. Height should be measured, but the frequency of measurement need not be the same as for weight (Gaedeke Norris & Steinhorn 1994).
- Observe for any signs of oedema.
- Change the intravenous infusion set every 24 hours (or as per local policy).
- To prevent oral dryness, perform oral hygiene frequently.
- If a central line is used, change the dressing in accordance with local policy.
- Sepsis, abnormalities in liver function, hyperglycaemia and hypocalcaemia are some complications of this therapy (Abernathy et al 1994, Bilodeau 1995).

COMMUNITY PERSPECTIVE

There are many issues surrounding these procedures when undertaken in the home; however, providing these are addressed, with safety being paramount, home intravenous therapy may be implemented. The responsibility for instigating such treatment must be given due consideration and, should the CCN feel insufficiently experienced or trained, accountability in practice must be considered. Specialist team input may be required, for example for the administration of TPN and immunoglobulin infusions (RCN 2003).

There will be situations where the CCN administers the infusion and others where the carers undertake the role.

The suitability of the home environment should be assessed before any suggestion is made to the family. Not every environment will be suitable and the presence of boisterous siblings and pets, for example, must be taken into account. Even in the most motivated families, a moment's inattention to a toddler intent on grabbing an intravenous line could be disastrous. These issues need to be discussed with the family before any decision is made. It may be possible to recruit the help of a neighbour or friend in arranging a 'special outing' for the sibling(s) to coincide with a crucial period in the treatment.

There are advantages for some families in that the child is likely to be more relaxed in the home environment and able to maintain a more normal lifestyle. The responsibility of undertaking this type of treatment, however, may be too overwhelming for some families, even with skilled teaching input and support from the CCN. This must be assessed, ensuring that carers are not left with feelings of guilt should they decide not to participate in this area of care. Other families may welcome the opportunity to be involved.

The carers will need an intensive teaching programme and issues such as cross-infection should be discussed. The CCN must feel confident in the ability of the carers to cope safely with the procedures.

It is important that carers have access to a telephone. Support for paying telephone bills may be available with advice from social services.

General principles

It is necessary to ascertain whether clinical responsibility rests with the hospital paediatrician or with the GP.

The CCN will be responsible for ensuring that carers are fully informed about the therapy to be given, including side-effects and possible complications. They will need to be competent in the use of any pumps or syringe drivers which may be required and be able to recognise signs of infection, either local or systemic.

Where an intravenous pump is to be used, this should be capable of running on its own batteries for some hours, in case of power failure.

Anaphylaxis kits should be provided and carers given the guidelines and information concerning dosages and usage.

Whenever possible, home intravenous therapy should be checked by two people; this will include dose, drug, dilution and expiry date, and always with the prescription sheet which will be written in line with local policy (see Administration of Medicines, p. 45).

Carers must know who to contact at any time during the treatment and, if the CCN is unavailable, be given a link to the ward.

Consideration should be given as to which intravenous system will be simplest for the families to use. This may not be the cheapest, and the CCN may need to convince the budget holder of the importance of this.

Commercial sharps boxes must be provided for safe disposal of ampoules, needles and syringes and disposed of as local policy dictates. This may entail making an arrangement with the council refuse department.

Specific considerations

Blood and blood products are only likely to be given in the community to enable a terminally ill child to remain at home. Should a child have had previous severe reactions then transfusion should not take place in the community (RCN 2001).

The GP must be aware that the procedure is taking place and ensure that they or a member of the paediatric medical team is immediately contactable if necessary.

Community Perspective continues

The CCN will need to remain in the home for the duration of the transfusion and for 30 minutes afterwards, monitoring vital signs throughout.

Kits for dealing with any spillage should be available (RCN 2003).

Home parenteral nutrition

Close links need to be developed between hospital and community-based staff, specialist pharmacists, dietitians and specialist commercial homecare companies.

A home TPN information document containing procedures and troubleshooting guidelines should be provided.

It should always be remembered that parents are shouldering a tremendous responsibility and, however competent they become, will need ongoing support.

Do and do not

- Do ensure that asepsis is maintained and manipulation of the line is kept to a minimum.
- Do ensure that the intravenous administration infusion set is changed every 24 hours.
- Do ensure, where necessary, that the bag of solution is protected from sunlight.
- Do ensure that parents are involved in care.
- Do not change intravenous lines without using aseptic technique.
- Do not use the same lumen of a central line or peripheral cannula for other drug or fluid administration whilst TPN is in progress.

References

Abernathy T L, Beck M L, Becker S I et al 1994 Handbook of therapeutic interventions. Springhouse, Pennsylvania, PA

Arnett C 1998 Thrombocytopenia in the newborn. Neonatal Network 17(8): 27–32

Bilodeau J A 1995 A home parenteral nutrition program for infants. Journal of Obstetrics, Gynaecology and Neonatal Nursing 24(1): 72–76

Blood Transfusion Service 1996 Handbook of transfusion medicine, 2nd edn. The Blood Transfusion Service of the United Kingdom. HMSO, London

British Committee for Standards in Haematology (BCSH) Blood Transfusion Task Force 1999 Guidelines for the administration of blood and blood components and the management of transfused patients. BCSH, London

Brunner L S, Suddarth D S 1991 The Lippincott manual of paediatric nursing, 3rd edn. Chapman and Hall, London

Campbell S, Glasper E A (eds) 1995 Whaley and Wong's children's nursing. Mosby, London

Carter B, Dearmun A K 1995 Child health care nursing. Blackwell Science, Oxford

Contreras M C 1990 ABC of transfusion. BMJ Books, London

Davenport M 1996 Paediatric fluid balance. Care of the Critically Ill 12(1): 26–31

Fitzsimons R 2001 Intravenous cannulation. Paediatric Nursing 13(3): 21–23

Fitzpatrick L, Fitzpatrick T 1997 Blood transfusion. Keeping your patient safe. Nursing 27(8): 34–42

Flemmer L, Chan J S L 1993 A pediatric protocol for management of extravasation injuries. Pediatric Nursing 19(4): 345–348

Gaedeke Norris M K, Steinhorn D M 1994 Nutritional management during critical illness in infants and children. AACN Clinical Issues 5(4): 485–492

Galica L A 1997 Parenteral nutrition. Nursing Clinics of North America 32(4): 705–717

Hazinski M F 1988 Understanding fluid balance in the seriously ill child. Pediatric Nursing 14(3): 231–236

Hazinski M F 1992 Nursing care of the critically ill child, 2nd edn. Mosby, St Louis, MO

Hiu Lam W 1998 Fluids in paediatric patients. Care of the Critically Ill 14(3): 93–96

Iserson K V, Huestis D W 1991 Blood warming: current applications and techniques. Transfusion 31(5): 558–569

Livesley J 1996 Peripheral IV therapy in children. Paediatric Nursing 8(6): 29–33

McClelland D B L 2001 Handbook of transfusion medicine, 3rd edn. TSO, London

McConnell E A 1997 Clinical do's and don'ts. Safely administering a blood transfusion. Nursing 27(6): 30

NPSA 2004 Standardising and centralising infusion devices – a project to develop safety solutions for NHS trusts. NPSA, London

Place B 1998 The transfusion of blood and its products. Nursing Times 94(34): 48–50

Poskitt E M E 1988 Practical paediatric nutrition. Butterworth, London

Royal College of Nursing (RCN) 2001 Administering intravenous therapy to children in the community setting: guidance for nursing staff, 3rd edn. Royal College of Nursing, London

Royal College of Nursing (RCN) 2003 Standards for infusion therapy, RCN IV therapy Forum. RCN, London

Serious Hazards of Transfusion Reporting Scheme (SHOT) 1999. Online. Available: www.shotuk.org

Smith C E 2001 Principles of fluid warming in trauma. In: Smith C E, Rosenberg A D, Grande C M (eds) Massive transfusion and control of haemorrhage in the trauma patient. Seminars in Anaesthesia, Perioperative Medicine and Pain 20: 51–59

Tortora G J, Grabowski S R 2002 Principles of anatomy and physiology, 10th edn. Harper Collins, New York

Willock J, Jewkes F 2000 Making sense of fluid balance in children. Paediatric Nursing 12(7): 37–42

fusion Service of the United Kingdom. HMSO, London

British Committee for Standards in Haematology (BCSH) guidelines. Online. Available: www.bcshguidelines.com

Dodsworth H 1995 Making sense of the use of blood and blood products. Nursing Times 91(1): 25–27

Glover G, Powell F 1995 Blood transfusions. Nursing Standard 9(33): 31–37

Laboratory Services Users' Handbook

Scottish Intercollegiate Guidelines Network (SIGN) Guideline on perioperative transfusion. Online. Available: www.sign.ac.uk/guidelines

SHOT Guidelines – Annual Report (*Serious Hazards of Transfusion*). Available within each hospital/trust

SNBTS Compendium of Product Information 1999

UK Blood Transfusion and Tissue Transplantation Guidelines: handbook of transfusion medicine. Online. Available: www.transfusionguidelines.org.uk

Further Reading

Blood Transfusion Service 2001 Handbook of transfusion medicine, 3rd edn. The Blood Trans-

Practice 14

Isolation nursing

Rachel Sales

Introduction

Microorganisms, as discussed in Control of Infection (p. 21), can cause a variety of infections within children. Adherence to basic hygiene principles, standard precautions, wearing appropriate personal protective clothing, a clean environment and segregation of the child where necessary will minimise the risk of cross-infection or colonisation by pathogenic organisms by interrupting the chain of transmission (May 2000, Curran 2001).

Wilson (2001) describes four factors that influence the necessity for isolation precautions:

- Ease of transmission
- Route of transmission
- Epidemiological significance, e.g. antibiotic resistance
- Presence of susceptible individuals.

The isolation of a child in hospital will be either to protect them from infection (*protective isolation*, e.g. if they are immunosuppressed) or to protect other patients from infection (*source isolation*, e.g. diarrhoeal illness).

The principal objective of isolating a patient is to minimise the risk of transmission of microorganisms. Wilson (2001) reminds us that it is important to remember that it is the microorganism that is being isolated rather than the patient.

Learning outcomes

By the end of this section you should understand:

- the principles of isolation nursing
- the importance of compliance to universal precautions
- the need for additional transmission precautions
- the effects that isolation nursing can have on the child and family

and be able to:

- prevent the spread of infection whilst caring for the child and family

- plan safe individualised care for the child and family
- alleviate any anxiety or stress felt by the child and/or family while the child is nursed apart from others.

Factors to note

Microorganisms cause a variety of infections and the incubation period and mode of transmission will vary according to the site of the infection and the microorganism involved (Benenson 1995).

Global and local epidemiological patterns of infection should be taken into account. For example, multiple antibiotic-resistant organisms such as meticillin-resistant *Staphylococcus aureus* (MRSA), vancomycin-resistant enterococcus (VRE) and aminoglycoside-resistant Gram-negative bacteria such as Klebsiellae are an increasing problem worldwide (Goldmann & Huskins 1997).

DEVELOPMENTAL AND FAMILY CONSIDERATIONS

Evidence suggests that isolation can be stressful for patients and relatives (Gammon 1999, Davies & Rees 2000, Rees et al 2000). Therefore careful explanation must be given to the child and parents as to why there is a need for segregation from others. The child needs to be made aware that the isolation is not a form of punishment for anything they have done wrong. Details of the mode of transmission, the need for protective clothing and appropriate precautions to take should also be given. Consideration of the cultural and social implications some infectious diseases may have for the individual and family, such as tuberculosis, measles or human immunodeficiency virus (HIV), must be taken into account (Helman 2000). Rees et al's (2000) study reinforces the importance of addressing the emotional, communication and information needs for patients in isolation.

General principles

The isolation of any patient should be undertaken in a systematic way following risk assessment (May 2000) and in compliance with local policy.

- Does the patient require isolation in a single room (such as protective isolation) or has an outbreak occurred which needs cohort isolation (nursing children together who have the same infection) such as a diarrhoeal illness or respiratory syncytial virus (RSV).
- Consider the environmental need for special high-efficiency particulate air filters (HEPA) for the child who is or may become severely immunosuppressed (a compromised host) and needs protection from opportunistic infections.
- The area should be uncluttered and thoroughly cleaned at least daily in accordance with local policy and national standards (NHS 2001).
- Special attention should be paid to the child's toys as these can be a source of infection (Avila-Aguero et al 2004). Whilst in isolation the child should have their own toys and not be sharing toys with other children or patients. All available toys need to be washable.
- Communal toilets should be avoided where the risk of transmitting the infection is increased, such as when the child has diarrhoea or vomiting.
- If en suite toilet facilities are available, they must be flushed after use, cleaned when visibly soiled and cleaned at least daily. Disposable toilet seats are not necessary.
- In the home setting, maintain standards of hygiene and cleanliness. Do not use communal washing/bathing equipment such as towels, flannels or toothbrushes as these may be a source of cross-contamination.
- Assess the need for a single room or for cohortion and how best to implement the appropriate transmission precautions. Consider whether the likely organism is transmitted via the airborne, droplet or contact route and whether the door of the room should be open or closed.
- Respect the need for privacy for the child and family by providing curtains/blinds for the bed area and knocking on the door before entry.

- Consider the precautions to be taken when visiting other departments such as the operating theatre or X-ray department. It may be advisable to place the child last on the operating list or to go to the X-ray department when the least number of children are there, such as at the end of the day.
- It is important that all children who are segregated from others receive the same care and time allocation as others.
- If there is a history of communicable disease in the family (e.g. chickenpox or blood-borne viruses) or signs of infection such as diarrhoea and vomiting, rash, cough or pyrexia, initiate appropriate microbiological investigation (see Specimen Collection, p. 363) and precautions as soon as possible.
- Check the need for prophylactic antibiotics for the family with diseases such as *Neisseria meningitidis* – meningococcal disease (PHLS 2000, Purcell et al 2004). Check whether relevant exposure of healthcare workers to the disease warrants prophylaxis. Healthcare workers should seek advice from the occupational health department or infection control team.
- Discuss with the medical staff whether the infection is a disease notifiable (to local authority proper officers) under the Public Health (Infectious Diseases) Regulations 1988.

Equipment for isolation nursing

- A notice on the door of the cubicle or area to indicate to staff and visitors:
  - the need for separation and the risk of cross-infection
  - the need to discuss entry to the area and visiting arrangements where individuals are non-immune to the infection, e.g. chickenpox
  - the necessity to comply with handwashing and the wearing of protective clothing
- Handwashing equipment – disposable hand towels, liquid soap or antiseptic solution, alcoholic hand-rub; basins should have lever-operated mixer taps or automated controls

- Protective clothing such as disposable gloves, plastic aprons, facial protection (mask, goggles, visor) as per local policy
- Foot-operated pedal bin with appropriately coloured, labelled disposable clinical waste bag with ties
- Sharps bin, if necessary
- Individual examination equipment such as a stethoscope, auriscope with earpieces, tape measure, tongue depressors, ophthalmoscope, patella hammer, sphygmomanometer with disposable or washable cuff, disposable thermometer
- Suction and oxygen equipment; easy access to resuscitation equipment
- Scales
- Scissors
- Pens, ruler, chart holder, calculator
- Disposable equipment according to the needs of the child such as suction catheters, sticky tape, sterile packs, syringes and disposable hypodermic needles, equipment for intravascular cannulation
- A clock with a second hand should be easily visible
- Equipment for summoning attention such as a call bell or intercommunication system
- Non-communal play equipment, television, radio and reading material, according to the needs of the child
- If last offices are to be performed, consider the requirements for protective body bags (see Bereavement Care, p. 104).

Hand hygiene

Handwashing is widely acknowledged to be the single most important activity for reducing the spread of disease (NICE 2003, Picheansathian 2004, RCN 2005). The need for and frequency of handwashing should be determined by actions and not routines.

Hands must be washed and thoroughly dried:

- when dirty
- before entry to the cubicle or cohorting area
- before and after caring for the child
- before aseptic procedures
- before handling food

- after dirty tasks such as toileting
- after removal of protective clothing including gloves
- after handling specimens
- on exit of the single room or cohorting area.

Handwashing facilities with appropriate liquid soap, antiseptic solution, alcohol handrub and disposable paper towels (Gould 1994) must be available inside the room, immediately outside it or in the cohorting area. Nurses also need to empower the child, family and visitors with the knowledge for safe handwashing and disinfection (Ward 2003).

Personal protective clothing

Have available inside and outside the room or cohorting area disposable gloves, aprons and facial protection (visors, goggles and masks as per local policy). Assess the risk of procedures which may contaminate the healthcare worker. If there is a risk of aerosols (fine sprays) or splattering of body fluid into the face or mucosal surfaces, facial protection must be worn. Additional protective clothing may be required if there is extensive bleeding or explosive diarrhoea or vomiting and the risk of contamination to the healthcare worker and the environment is high.

- Non-latex and/or powder-free gloves should be available for healthcare workers who are allergic to latex or starch powder (Booth 1995).
- The need for parents, siblings or visitors to wear protective clothing should be assessed individually and discussed with the child and parents.

Specimen collection

All specimens must be regarded as potentially infectious. Plan the need for appropriate specimens to be taken in consultation with the medical staff before explaining to the child and family. This aids better continuity of care and reduces the likelihood of unnecessary and repeated specimens. Document specimens taken.

- Wear protective clothing such as gloves when obtaining or handling specimens and remember to wash your hands before and after collection.
- Ensure that containers are adequately sealed and not leaking. Do not contaminate the outside of the container.
- Ensure that all specimens and laboratory forms are correctly labelled, safely packed and dispatched to the appropriate laboratory as per local policy as soon as possible.
- Do not store specimens in food or drug refrigerators.

If disposable potties, bedpans or urinals are used, they must be covered during transport to the dirty utility area and placed in a well-maintained macerator for disposal. The supporting frame should be washed in hot water and detergent and dried before storage. If non-disposable utensils are used, they must be covered during transport and placed in a heat disinfector/bedpan washer which reaches a temperature of at least 80°C for at least 1 minute (Ayliffe et al 1992). Where the above equipment is not available, any excreta should be disposed of down the toilet, the utensil rinsed and washed in hot water and detergent and dried. Gloves should be worn for handling and cleaning the utensil.

In the home setting, faeces from nappies or colostomy bags should be put down the toilet and the nappy or bag wrapped in newspaper or biodegradable polythene and disposed of in the dustbin.

Clinical waste

- The waste that is created during the care of a child in isolation may be contaminated and therefore requires safe disposal as per local policy. Ensure that waste is segregated at source, such as by the bedside, into clinical and non-clinical waste.
- Sharps bins may be a source of infection and should be removed and disposed of frequently, or when two-thirds full, and on discharge of the child.
- Use foot-operated pedal bins with lids for all clinical and non-clinical waste and laundry.

Hands will become contaminated if used for opening lids.

- Follow local infection control policies for decontamination of the environment on discharge of the child.
- Ensure that the waste bins are cleaned regularly, and on discharge of the child, with hot water and detergent and dried to prevent the risk of cross-infection. It is unnecessary to double bag clinical waste (Maki et al 1986).
- Infected clinical waste, including sharps, generated in the home may be collected by special arrangement organised by the primary health care team.

Linen/laundry

Under the Health and Safety at Work Act, health authorities have an obligation to prevent risk of infection to staff handling and laundering linen. Therefore local policy for the safe handling of linen must be adhered to (NHS Executive 1995).

Linen should be categorised as either used (soiled and foul) or infected and placed in an appropriately colour-coded container (see Control of Infection, p. 29). Infected laundry should be placed immediately into a water-soluble bag or soluble stitched bag within an outer bag, secured with a tie and labelled as to its origin before it is removed from an area (NHS Executive 1995).

Well-maintained domestic washing machines on a hot wash cycle may be used to decontaminate laundry in the home setting. This includes infections such as those causing diarrhoeal illness and blood-borne viruses.

Cleaning/decontamination

Curtains should be laundered frequently and changed if visibly dirty. If shedding of pathogenic organisms such as staphylococci is extensive, as on the skin scales of a child with eczema, then curtains should also be changed on discharge.

Mop heads should be laundered daily in a washing machine and stored dry. They should not be left soaking in disinfectants as this increases the risk of contamination with organ-isms such as *Pseudomonas*. The same mop should not be used in other communal areas or kitchens because of the risk of cross-infection.

Cleaning cloths should be disposable or laundered daily.

Documentation and planning of care

- Plan and document all care around the family and child, taking into consideration their cultural, spiritual, psychosocial and physical needs.
- Care should be individualised according to the risk of acquiring or spreading infection. Take into account the age of the child and their ability and understanding of the required isolation precautions.
- Assess the risk of infection to the child and staff (Macqueen 1996) and implement the wearing of appropriate protective clothing such as gloves, aprons, masks, visors or goggles. A careful explanation to the child and family must be given to avoid feelings of alienation. The wearing of protective clothing by family members will depend on the type of infection.
- Do discuss with parents and the child all precautions to be taken whilst the child is in hospital. Ensure that there is a means of communication if the child is in a single room, for example a bell, two-way intercommunication apparatus or telephone. Include the need to extend precautions in the home, at school or nursery. Seek help from the infection control team if parents require further explanations.
- Assess the risk of infection to the family, siblings and other visitors. Consider the precautions they should take whilst visiting in hospital. For example, have the family members had chickenpox or are they incubating it? If they have had the disease they can visit, but if not, do they pose a risk to others on the ward? Should visiting be restricted?
- Assess daily the need for all the precautions.
- Report any changes or deterioration in the child's condition or any signs or symptoms of infection in the family.

- Inform the infection control team, primary health care team or transferring hospital/unit of any actual or potential infections. Report to the infection control nurse/doctor any suspicions of secondary cases such as other people with diarrhoea, rashes or chest infections.
- Obtain written information for parents and children about the infection and the need for restricted precautions.
- Medical/nursing notes should be kept safely outside the room where possible to avoid unnecessary entry to the isolation area.
- Consider the need for health education for the child and family.
- If the child has an infection which could be transmitted through sexual contact, such as human immunodeficiency virus (HIV), then this should be discussed with the parents through the multidisciplinary healthcare team. Sex education, where necessary, should be given in accordance with government guidelines (DfEE 2000).
- Alleviate stress and anxiety felt by the child whilst separated from others through increased play activity, schooling (DfES 2001), television/videos and, where necessary, plan visiting as appropriate. Consider the need for voluntary workers.
- To prevent cross-infection occurring in nursery or primary schools, follow good housekeeping and hygiene principles (Ross 1993, Niffenegger 1997).

Do and do not

- Do remember that handwashing is the single most important point in controlling cross-infection.
- Do keep all cuts and abrasions covered with a waterproof plaster. If inoculation of mucosal or non-intact skin contamination with blood or body fluids occurs, act immediately and report to your manager and the occupational health department as soon as possible.
- Dispose of laundry bags when two-thirds full.
- Do not use laundry or waste bins with swing lids as this may cause aerosols and increases the risk of hand contamination.
- Do wear appropriate personal protective clothing.
- Do maintain confidentiality for both children and staff who have an infection or communicable disease.
- Do set an example as a role model for others to follow in basic hygiene principles.
- Do not make the child and family feel responsible, guilty or alienated.
- Do ensure that local infection control guidelines are easily available to both staff and parents.
- Do know how to contact the local infection control nurse/doctor for advice.

References

Avila-Aguero M L, German G, Paris M, Herrera J 2004 Toys in a pediatric hospital: are they a bacteria source? American Journal of Infection Control 32(5): 287–290

Ayliffe G A J, Lowbury E J L, Geddes A M, Williams J D 1992 Control of hospital infection, 3rd edn. Chapman and Hall Medical, London

Benenson A S 1995 Control of communicable diseases manual, 16th edn. American Public Health Association, Washington, DC

Booth B 1995 No time for kid gloves. Nursing Times 91(46): 43–46

Curran E 2001 Reducing the risk of healthcare-acquired infection. Nursing Standard 16(1): 45–52

Davies H, Rees J 2000 Psychological effects of isolation nursing (1): mood disturbance. Nursing Standard 14 (28): 35–38

Department for Education and Employment (DfEE) 2000 Sex and relationship education guidance. TSO, London

Department for Education and Skill (DfES) 2001 Access to education for children and young people with medical needs. TSO, London

Gammon J 1999 The psychological consequences of source isolation: a review of the literature. Journal of Clinical Nursing 8(1): 13–21

Goldmann D A, Huskins W C 1997 Control of nosocomial antimicrobial-resistant bacteria: a strategic priority for hospitals worldwide. Clinical Infectious Diseases 24(Suppl 1): S139–145

Gould D 1994 The significance of hand-drying in the prevention of infection. Nursing Times 90(47): 33–35

Helman C 2000 Culture, health and illness, 4th edn. Butterworth-Heinemann, Oxford

Macqueen S 1996 Think globally – act locally: germ invasion and risk analysis. Journal of Neonatal Nursing 2(1): 20–25

Maki D G, Alvarado C, Hassemer C 1986 Double bagging of items from isolation rooms is unnecessary as an infection control measure: a comparative study of surface contamination with single and double bagging. Infection Control 7: 535–537

May D 2000 Infection control. Nursing Standard 14(28): 51–57

National Institute for Clinical Excellence (NICE) 2003 Infection control. Prevention of healthcare-associated infection in primary and community care. No. 1: Standard principles. NICE, London

NHS 2001 National Standards of Cleanliness for the NHS. TSO, London. Online. Available: www.nhsestates.gov.uk/download/publications_guidance/es_NHS_cleaning_standards.pdf

NHS Executive 1995 health service guidelines: hospital laundry arrangements for used and infected linen. HSG (95)18. NHS Executive, London

Niffenegger J P 1997 Proper handwashing promotes wellness in child care. Journal of Pediatric Health Care 11: 26–31

PHLS 2000 Guidelines for public health management of meningococcal disease in the UK. Communicable Disease and Public Health 5(3): 197–204

Picheansathian W 2004 A systematic review on the effectiveness of alcohol-based solutions for hand hygiene. International Journal of Nursing Practice 10: 3–9

Purcell B, Samuelsson S, Hahne S J M et al 2004 Effectiveness of antibiotics in preventing meningococcal disease after a case: systematic review. British Medical Journal 328(7452): 1339–1343. Online. Available: http://bmj.bmjjournals.com/cgi/content/full/328/7452/1339

RCN 2005 Good practice in infection prevention and control. RCN, London

Rees J, Davies H, Birchall C, Price J 2000 Psychological effects of source isolation nursing (2): patient satisfaction. Nursing Standard 14(29): 32–36

Ross S 1993 Creche course in hygiene. Journal of Infection Control Nursing, Nursing Times 89(29): 59–60, 62, 64

Ward D 2003 Improving patient hand hygiene. Nursing Standard 17(35): 39–42

Wilson J 2001 Infection control in clinical practice, 2nd edn. Baillière Tindall, London

Further Reading

Edmond M 1997 Isolation. Infection Control and Hospital Epidemiology 18: 58–64

Lumbar puncture

Liz Gough

Introduction

Lumbar puncture is an invasive procedure in which a spinal needle is inserted into the subarachnoid space of the lumbar spine for diagnostic or therapeutic purposes. Small amounts of cerebrospinal fluid are analysed for red and white blood cells, protein, glucose and the presence of bacteria, viruses or fungi, or abnormal cells. In children, this procedure may be required as a planned procedure, for example, in an oncology patient. This could be diagnostic, as above, and/or therapeutic, when medications are injected directly into the spinal fluid. It can also be required in acutely ill child – for example, in a child with suspected meningitis. When planning and delivering care, the urgency of the procedure and the condition of the child should be key considerations.

Learning outcomes

By the end of this section you should be able to:

- give a rationale for lumbar puncture
- give a rationale for the preparatory care of a child and family
- understand and assess the risks and complications associated with the procedure and give a rationale for post-procedure care
- understand the role of the nurse in assisting with a lumbar puncture.

Rationale for lumbar puncture

Lumbar puncture is performed to:

- obtain a specimen of cerebrospinal fluid (CSF) for diagnostic purposes
- measure the pressure of the lumbar CSF
- instil therapeutic drugs
- instil contrast media during radiological investigations.

Factors to note

Lumbar puncture is an invasive procedure and therefore should be performed aseptically. Effective preparation facilitates a smooth procedure which is safe and minimises unnecessary distress for child, family and healthcare professionals. It requires the assistance of two nurses in addition to the doctor.

Administration of intrathecal drugs

Intrathecal drug administration (giving drugs directly into the spinal fluid during lumbar puncture) is a frequently used method of delivering cytotoxic agents, especially in the treatment of children with leukaemia. However, administration of the wrong drug intrathecally, and especially drugs of the vinca alkaloid family (also commonly used for treatment of leukaemia, but should only be administered intravenously), can cause the child to become paralysed or even to die (DoH 2003, SEHD 2004). Following incidences of vinca alkaloid drugs being accidentally instilled intrathecally causing patient paralysis and death, the Department of Health and the Scottish Executive Health Department (SEHD) have produced strict guidelines for the storage, preparation, collection, checking and administration of intrathecal drugs (DoH 2003). Therefore, whenever drugs are to be given intrathecally, national and local policy must be followed. For example, intrathecal drugs may only be given unsupervised by a consultant, specialist registrar or career grade doctor who is on the hospital's intrathecal register (SEHD 2004). Similarly, prior to administration, intrathecal drugs can only be checked by a professional who is a registered nurse, consultant, specialist registrar or career grade doctor who is on the hospital's intrathecal register. Individuals on the intrathecal register must be trained, assessed and certified as competent to an agreed standard of intrathecal drug administration.

Preparing the child and family

- A well-prepared child and family are necessary to ensure a clear understanding of how and why a lumbar puncture should be performed. This will minimise potential distress and anxiety and ensure cooperation and safety for all involved. This may not always be easy to achieve, particularly in the acute situation where attention to detail is paramount.

- A full explanation of the reasons for lumbar puncture, what the procedure entails and the potential risks and complications must be given, in the correct context, by the doctor to the family. An age-appropriate explanation should also be given to the child. The nurse's role is to ensure that the child and family understand what is involved and that any concerns, or questions, have been adequately addressed. This can be supported by written information sheets (Patient Information Group GOSH 2002).

- Consent should be gained by the doctor and options for analgesia and sedation discussed with the child and family, appropriate to the clinical situation.

- Parents may wish to stay with their child during the procedure, and may help to reassure the child by talking and/or holding a hand or head stroking. This is appropriate where the child is conscious and before and after any general anaesthesia.

- Allowing a child to prepare for the procedure through the use of play is a useful part of the preparation process, for example with dolls/soft toys/action figures, art (drawing/painting) and stories. This is beneficial where time and the child's condition allow. It is particularly helpful for those children who have to undergo repeated procedures, for example in cancer patients, especially acute leukaemia (Broome et al 1990, Klein 1992, Ellis & Spanos 1994).

- Generally, a child who requires routine and repeated lumbar puncture will be given the option of having the procedure performed under general anaesthesia or conscious sedation with local anaesthesia (Crock et al 2003). General anaesthetic via a face mask has many advantages, particularly in children with cancer (Crock et al 2003). It is likely that the procedure will be quicker and less likely to fail because of poor compliance. It is a safer procedure, as the child is fasted and would usually have a higher level of monitoring. It minimises the level of pain and distress caused and therefore the need for restraint. This will improve the child's and parents' experience of the procedure.

- For children with acute lymphoblastic leukaemia, initial lumbar punctures may ideally be performed under short-acting general anaesthesia to ensure that the child is still. This may reduce the possibility of a traumatic lumbar puncture which could lead to transfer of peripheral blast cells into the CSF (Gajjar et al 2000).

- Conscious sedation with local anaesthesia may, however, be a quicker and more convenient method in many situations without the need for fasting (Crock et al 2003). Some children may prefer psychological or behavioural techniques, with or without local anaesthesia, further minimising the need for sedation (Crock et al 2003).

- Local anaesthesia may be preferred in the acute situation, when meningitis is suspected. It is important to perform the lumbar puncture, as part of the diagnosis, in a timely and safe manner. If the child's condition allows, a topical local anaesthetic may be applied first, followed by injected local anaesthetic.

- Other effective methods of pain relief and sedation for pre-planned lumbar puncture include nitrous oxide (Kanagasundaram et al 2001) and bupivacaine for spinal anaesthesia in older children (Kokki & Hendolin 2000). Propofol anaesthesia has also been found to be an effective option in oncology patients in the paediatric intensive care setting (Hertzog et al 2000).

To conclude, therefore, no one technique will suit all clinical situations. It is important to remember that there can be a significant disparity between the perception of healthcare professionals and families with respect to how children cope with painful procedures. The child's and parents' experience should, therefore, be a significant focus when planning pain relief and sedation (Crock et al 2003).

Risks and complications

An understanding of the risks and potential complications of the procedure provides a basis for the nursing care of a child prior to, during and after a lumbar puncture. Most risks associated with the procedure can be minimised by good preparation and by following the correct procedural and post-procedural care (Wojner & Malkoff 2001).

Pain, discomfort and anxiety

Pain, discomfort and anxiety may vary between children and must be treated individually. These effects can be reduced by encouraging parents/carers to provide age-appropriate reassurances to the child and distraction by quiet play, e.g. reading or listening to stories, music or television, as the child's pre-existing condition allows. This may be helpful beforehand, to reduce anxiety anticipating the procedure, and afterward, providing distraction (The Children's Hospital at Westmead 2000). Many things may cause anxiety:

- being separated from parents during the procedure
- being held in an unfamiliar position
- unfamiliar sensations during the procedure
- previous experience of procedures.

Where possible, it is helpful for the nurse to determine potential issues for that child and family, addressing them practically and with information and clarification appropriate for the child's age and cognitive ability. With support from nursing staff, parents may feel able to be present during the procedure, to comfort their child, rather than to hold them.

Postdural puncture headache (PDPH)

Postdural puncture headache can occur after lumbar puncture. The pathophysiology is unclear, although it is thought to be related to the loss of CSF, the brain's protective buffer (Connolly 1999). Pain is exacerbated by standing, coughing or shaking of the head.

Studies in children suggest that PDPH occurs in 5–17% of patients, with higher rates generally in teenage children (Burt et al 1998, Kokki et al 1998). Although of a similar incidence, the duration and severity of PDPH do not appear to be as severe as in adults (Kokki et al 1998). PDPH is self-limiting and usually lasts no more than 1–2 days. Although bed rest may not prevent PDPH (Allan 1989), a plan of bed rest, hydration, analgesia (e.g. paracetamol) and antiemetics (for nausea) provide good symptomatic relief (Connolly 1999). Unfortunately, there is no evidence in the use of epidural blood patches which are reported to be of benefit in adults (Connolly 1999). Similarly, there is little evidence of any link between the gauge of needle and the incidence of PDPH (Burt et al 1998, Wojner & Malkoff 2001).

Lower back discomfort and haematoma

Lower back discomfort and haematoma swelling may occur at the puncture site after the procedure. The doctor should be informed and the site monitored. Lower back discomfort at the site should be assessed and treated with analgesia as appropriate, e.g. paracetamol (GOSH Trust 2002).

Infection

Infection is a risk of any invasive procedure and should be minimised by the use of an aseptic technique and covering the puncture site afterwards with an occlusive dressing, e.g. plaster or spray. The child must be observed for signs of meningitis (if previously well). These include pyrexia, headache, photophobia, neck stiffness and/or pain, vomiting, general malaise and drowsiness in the older child, and pyrexia, vomiting, drowsiness and irritability in the infant (Hazinski 1992). These symptoms must be reported to medical staff and treatment for infection commenced promptly. The site should also be checked for signs of local infection including redness, heat or oozing. Inform medical staff if present. Some degree of tenderness will be present because of the trauma of inserting a needle.

CSF leakage

CSF leakage can occasionally occur from the lumbar puncture site after the procedure, although it is not common. If CSF leakage occurs, the site should be covered with a sterile gauze pad, pressure should be applied and the child should be laid flat in the supine position, although it is unclear whether laying flat prone, or supine, is more effective to close the dura (Wojner & Malkoff 2001). Dressings or plasters can usually be removed after 24 hours, provided the wound has healed over. If leakage continues it is probably due to non-closure of the dura (Wojner & Malkoff 2001) and the medical staff should be informed promptly. Pressure should be reapplied and the child laid flat until the leakage has stopped.

Herniation of the brain stem

Herniation of the brain stem, also known as coning, is a rare occurrence in which the brain stem herniates through the foramen magnum, leading to death (Hazinski 1992). The reason why this occurs is unknown and controversy exists as to whether lumbar puncture itself is a causal factor in its precipitation (Turner 2003). Herniation is known to occur in patients with raised intracranial pressure (Turner 2003) resulting from a number of causes, including brain haemorrhage and meningitis. The decline in the number of lumbar puncture procedures over the last 20 years appears to be partly due to the fear of precipitating cerebral herniation which may be unfounded (Kneen et al 2002). Lumbar puncture must not be performed when there is possible incipient herniation, episodes of abnormal posturing, including tonic seizures, and obvious meningococcal disease (Kneen et al 2002) or if the child is in shock (Advanced Life Support Group 2001) (see Box 15.1).

The signs of herniation of the brain stem include cardiorespiratory and neurological deterioration and neck stiffness. A slow pulse, raised blood pressure and irregular respiration leading to apnoea are seen in the terminal stages (Advanced Life Support Group 2001).

It should be remembered that lumbar puncture in the majority of patients is a safe procedure in which the many benefits far outweigh the potential side-effects (Kneen et al 2002, Riordan & Cant 2002).

Box 15.1   Relative contraindications to lumbar puncture

- Prolonged or focal seizures
- Focal neurological signs, e.g. asymmetry of limb movement and reflexes, ocular palsies
- A widespread purpuric rash in an ill child
- Glasgow Coma Scale score of less than 13
- Pupillary dilatation
- Impaired occulocephalic reflexes (doll's eyes reflexes)

- Abnormal posture or movement – decerebrate or decorticate posturing or cycling movements of the limbs
- Inappropriately low pulse, elevated blood pressure and irregular respirations
- Coagulation disorder
- Papilloedema
- Hypertension

After Advanced Life Support Group 2001 (p. 134).

Restricted activities

Children are advised not to do sports activities for a week after the test (Patient Information Group GOSH 2002).

The nurse's role

The role of the nurse is to prepare and comfort the child and family before, during and after the lumbar puncture procedure which is usually performed by a doctor. Assisting the doctor by ensuring the correct positioning and holding of the child safely during the procedure is a crucial factor in obtaining a successful outcome. The correct posture, as described below, widens the intervertebral spaces and facilitates easier access for the spinal needle (Lang 1993). It is the role of the nurse to make sure that the procedure is performed in an appropriate environment and that the safety of the child is of paramount importance. It is crucial that the child is held securely to prevent sudden movement, which could result in the needle moving and damaging nerve roots when in the subarachnoid space (Allan 1989) (see Fig. 15.1).

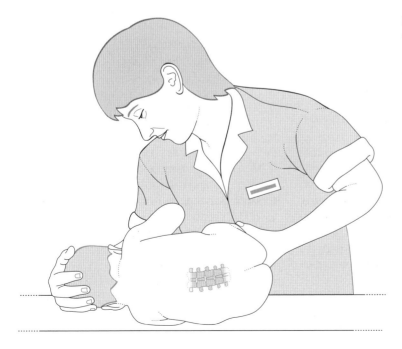

Figure 15.1 Positioning the child for a lumbar puncture

Continual visual observation of the child's respiratory, cardiovascular and neurological status is necessary to ensure prompt identification of serious and potentially life-threatening events, as described above. Should such events occur, the procedure should be abandoned and appropriate action taken (Advanced Life Support Group 2001). Patient observation can be supplemented by the use of monitoring equipment, e.g. an oxygen saturation monitor.

PERFORMING A LUMBAR PUNCTURE

(The procedure is adaptable for either planned or acute lumbar puncture, with general anaesthesia or conscious sedation.)

The procedure should be undertaken in an appropriate setting depending on the child's condition, equipped with emergency equipment (see 'Equipment', below). This may be in a quiet treatment room, in theatre or in a bedspace if the child cannot be moved. The procedure should take place at an acceptable working height to ensure safe handling of the child, both for the healthcare professional and the child. The risks of manual handling of the child must be assessed prior to commencing and an appropriate plan devised. Key risks and principles of movement are as follows:

1. Moving the child from bed to treatment couch should be preformed by the use of a hard sliding board, or slide sheet, if manual handling is required (National Back Pain Association/RCN 1998).

2. Positioning and holding the child in a fixed position for a period of time will be required. The healthcare professional should, therefore, be working with height-adjustable equipment (National Back Pain Association/RCN 1998) to prevent stooping or reaching, for both the nurse holding and the doctor carrying out the procedure. Both healthcare professionals must maintain good posture, aiming to keep the spine in as neutral a position as possible (Sales & Utting 2002), thereby avoiding 'rounding shoulders', 'slumping forward' or twisting. The centre of gravity should be over the base of the support (Sales & Utting 2002). This means the nurse should be holding as close as possible to the child, with feet under the treatment couch, set apart for stability. This may be done from a standing or a sitting position.

3. The child should be still and not struggling. This is not only potentially dangerous in terms of the procedure, i.e. the needle may move into an incorrect position and cause trauma, but will also be distressing to all. A struggling child would also increase the physical strain on the nurse who is holding. Sedation and general anaesthetic are, therefore, preferable options as previously described, depending on the clinical situation, child and family preferences and the service provision available.

Equipment

- Emergency equipment, e.g. oxygen, suction and age-appropriate airway adjuncts (oropharyngeal airways, bag–valve–mask equipment) and emergency drugs (Advanced Life Support Group 2001)
- Patient monitoring equipment, e.g. oxygen saturation monitor
- Dressing trolley (for aseptic technique)
- Topical local anaesthetic and cover dressing, to be applied allowing time for effect.

Note: Some hospital sterile services departments provide a lumbar puncture pack which contains most of the equipment listed below (excluding drugs and dressings):

- Dressing pack to provide sterile field
- Two spinal needles (one spare) (see Table 15.1)
- Sterile latex-free gloves
- Sterile drape with hole in middle
- Skin cleansing solution, e.g. chlorhexidine 0.5%
- 2 ml syringe and two needles (one 21 French gauge (Fg) for drawing up local anaesthetic and one 23 Fg (child) or 25 Fg (infant) for administering it) if local anaesthetic is to be used
- Local anaesthetic if required, e.g. 1% lidocaine

Table 15.1 Sizes of spinal needles commonly used (the doctor will decide the size to use)

	Age and size of child		
	Infants under 1 year	Children over 1 year	Adult-sized or over 40 kg
Gauge of needle	22 Fg	22 Fg	18–20 Fg
Length of needle	1–1^1/$_2$ inches 25–40 mm	2^1/$_2$ inches 60–65 mm	2^1/$_2$–3 inches 60–90 mm

- Manometer tube and three-way tap if CSF pressure is to be monitored
- Specimen collection pots as required (three separate samples for microscopy culture and sensitivity and a sample for CSF glucose content are common; pots should be labelled 1, 2 and 3)
- Waterproof plaster or other suitable waterproof covering, e.g. Opsite spray
- Rubbish bag
- Bravery certificate.

Method

Under ideal circumstances two nurses should be available to assist the doctor with the procedure. In this description, the first nurse will assist the doctor to draw up the local anaesthetic, and collect and label the specimens. The second nurse will care directly for the child.

1. Having prepared the child and family for the procedure, the second nurse, caring for the child, should continue to offer reassurance in a calm, warm and confident manner. This helps to promote feelings of security at an anxious time and facilitates cooperation. This is important even if the child has undergone the procedure before (Broome et al 1990). The child should have an empty bladder or have a clean nappy before beginning.

2. The child should be positioned on their side, at the very edge of the treatment couch or bed, with knees drawn up towards the chest and the head flexed forward, curled into a ball and held in this position by the nurse. The lumbar area is exposed and this flexing widens the intervertebral spaces to enable better access to the spinal fluid (see Fig. 15.1). Care should be taken not to compress the trachea or compromise lung expansion when positioning and holding, particularly in the infant with a softer airway (Smith 1995). Hypoxaemia can be pre-empted by preoxygenation in neonates (Fiser et al 1993). The spine should be kept parallel to the edge of the bed. This posture is very uncomfortable, particularly if the child has meningism, so do not position them until you are completely ready (Bacon & Lamb 1988) and then perform the procedure in as short a time as possible without compromising safety.

3. The second nurse should talk to and reassure the child throughout the procedure, promoting calm, reassurance and as much comfort as possible in a difficult situation. Instructions and explanations should be clear, simple and age/cognitive ability appropriate and should forewarn the child of the next move. Physical reassurance by a parent or nurse can be of great benefit by holding a hand/finger or stroking the child's head. This can be positive for both child and parents.

4. Handwashing and drying using the technique illustrated in Table 2 (see Control of Infection, p. 26) should be used and an aseptic technique followed and sterile gloves put on. The area of skin over the lumbar region is cleansed with antiseptic and sterile drapes placed around the exposed lumbar area.

5. A local anaesthetic (e.g. 1% lidocaine) is drawn up by the first nurse, and is checked

with and injected by the doctor into the tissue over the lumbar space to be accessed. A few minutes is allowed for the local anaesthetic to take effect whilst the doctor prepares the needles and the effect of the anaesthetic is ensured.

6. The needle is inserted into the lumbar space between either the third and fourth or the fourth and fifth lumbar vertebrae (Bacon & Lamb 1988). This point of entry is selected to avoid damage to the spinal cord, which terminates higher up at the level of the first lumbar vertebra (Hazinski 1992). Once the needle is in place, the stylet which blocks its core is removed and CSF can be observed to drip from the end of the needle; the stylet is replaced to prevent unnecessary loss of CSF. CSF is normally clear but can be cloudy with/without visible blood staining. If the needle catches a blood vessel, or the lumbar puncture is traumatic, blood staining will occur.

7. If CSF pressure is to be measured, it is performed prior to any CSF sample being removed. The manometer, with an attached three-way tap, is placed onto the end of the needle and a measurement taken.

8. CSF samples are obtained by removing the stylet (or manometer if it has been used) and allowing the CSF to drip into the labelled specimen bottle, held underneath by the first nurse. Between taking samples (usually 5–10 drops of CSF per sample bottle), the stylet should always be replaced to prevent excess CSF being lost and to prevent cross-infection. Three samples are commonly taken in case the first sample gets contaminated by blood as the needle is introduced (this is why samples are labelled 1, 2 and 3 in the order that they are obtained).

9. If drugs are to be administered, an equivalent volume of CSF is first removed to prevent increased pressure. To finish the procedure, the doctor removes the needle, immediately applying firm pressure on the lumbar puncture site with a gauze pad for about 30 seconds to prevent CSF leakage (Lang 1993).

10. A plaster, or waterproof dressing, is then placed over the site by the doctor or first nurse.

11. Time is provided for the child to recover from the procedure in a position comfortable and safe for the child. This could be on their back, or side, but preferably lying down, which may reduce the occurrence of headache following the procedure. If parents have not been present, they can then be encouraged to be with their child, giving comfort, support and praise. This can be reinforced from both, or one, of the nurses and the doctor involved. Rewards may be in the form of bravery certificates, stickers or other treats determined by staff and parents.

12. The first nurse should ensure that the equipment is disposed of correctly and safely to prevent injury and cross-infection. Correctly labelled samples are then sent to the laboratory, which may need notifying if results are required urgently.

Summary of possible complications
- Pain and anxiety
- Lower back discomfort and haematoma
- Postdural puncture headache
- Infection
- Leakage of CSF
- Respiratory distress
- Damage to nerve roots
- Herniation of the brain stem into the spinal canal.

Do and do not

- Do ensure that the child and family are prepared for the procedure.
- Do ensure that the child is adequately positioned and held during the procedure.
- Do observe the child carefully during and after the procedure for any indication of respiratory, cardiovascular or neurological deterioration and act appropriately.

- Do not allow a lumbar puncture to proceed when there is possible incipient herniation, episodes of abnormal posturing (including tonic seizures), obvious meningococcal disease or if the child is in shock (Advanced Life Support Group 2001). A lumbar puncture undertaken in these circumstances could result in herniation of the brain stem into the spinal canal via the foramen magnum. This can be fatal.

References

Advanced Life Support Group 2001 Advanced paediatric life support – the practical approach, 3rd edn. BMJ Publications, London, p 133–134, 136

Allan D 1989 Making sense of lumbar puncture. Nursing Times 85(49): 39–41

Bacon C J, Lamb W H 1988 Diagnosing and treating paediatric emergencies. Heinemann Medical Books, Oxford, p 268–270

Broome M E, Bates T A, Lillis P P, Wilson-McGahee T 1990 Children's medical fears, coping behaviours and pain perceptions during a lumbar puncture. Oncology Nursing Forum 17(3): 361–367

Burt N, Dorman B H, Reeves S T et al 1998 Postdural puncture headache in paediatric oncology patients. Canadian Journal of Anaesthesia 45(8): 741–745

Connolly M 1999 Postdural puncture headache American Journal of Nursing 99(11): 48–49

Crock C, Olsson C, Phillips R et al 2003 General anaesthesia or conscious sedation for painful procedures in childhood cancer: a family's perspective. Archives of Disease in Childhood 88: 253–257

Department of Health 2003 Updated national guidance on the safe administration of intrathecal chemotherapy. Health Service Circular 2003/010. DoH, London

Ellis J A, Spanos N P 1994 Cognitive–behavioural interventions for children's distress during bone marrow aspirations and lumbar punctures: a critical review. Journal of Pain and Symptom Management 9(2): 96–108

Fiser D H, Gober G A, Smith C E et al 1993 Prevention of hypoxemia during lumbar puncture in infancy with preoxygenation. Pediatric Emergency Care 9: 81–83

Gajjar A, Harrison P L, Sandlund J T et al 2000 Traumatic lumbar punctures at diagnosis adversely affects outcome in childhood lymphoblastic leukemia. Blood 96: 3381–3384

Great Ormond Street Hospital for Children NHS Trust Patient Information Group 2002 Lumbar puncture information for families. Online. Available: www.goshfamilies.nhs.uk

Hazinski M F 1992 Nursing care of the critically ill child, 2nd edn. Mosby Year Book, St Louis, MO, p 619

Hertzog J H, Dalton H J, Anderson B D et al 2000 Prospective evaluation of propofol anesthesia in the pediatric intensive care unit for elective oncology procedures in ambulatory and hospitalized children. Pediatrics 106(4): 742–747

Kanagasundaram S A, Lane L J, Cavalletto B P et al 2001 Efficacy and safety of nitrous oxide in alleviating pain and anxiety during painful procedures. Archives of Disease in Childhood 84: 492–495

Klein E R 1992 Premedicating children for painful medical procedures. Journal of Pediatric Oncology Nursing 9(4): 170–179

Kneen R, Solomon T, Appleton R 2002 The role of lumbar puncture in suspected CNS infection – a disappearing skill? Archives of Disease in Childhood 87: 181–183

Kokki H, Hendolin H 2000 Hyperbaric bupivacaine for spinal anaesthesia in 7–18 year old children: comparison of bupivacaine 5 mg ml^{-1} in 0.9% and 0.8% glucose solutions. British Journal of Anaesthesia 84(1): 59–62

Kokki H, Hendolin H, Turunen M 1998 Postdural puncture headache and transient neurological symptoms in children after spinal anaesthesia using cutting and pencil point paediatric spinal needles. Acta Anaethesiologica Scandinavica 42: 1076–1082

Lang S 1993 Procedures involving the neurological system. In: Barnardo L M, Bove M (eds) Pediatric emergency nursing procedures, 2nd edn. Jones and Bartlett, Boston, MA, ch 8, p 152–156

National Back Pain Association in collaboration with the Royal College of Nursing 1998 The guide to the handling of patients: introducing a safer handling policy, revised 4th edn. National Back Pain Association, London, p 182–184, 199

Patient Information Group. Great Ormond Street Hospital for Children NHS Trust 2002 London. Online. Available: www.goshfamilies.nhs.uk

Riordan F A I, Cant A J 2002 When to do a lumbar puncture. Archives of Disease in Childhood 87: 235–237

Sales R, Utting J 2002 Manual handling and nursing children. Paediatric Nursing 14(2): 36–42

SEHD 2004 Guidance on the safe administration of intrathecal cytotoxic chemotherapy. SEHD, Edinburgh

Smith C 1995 How to do it in paediatrics 2: the lumbar puncture. British Journal of Hospital Medicine 53(6): 273–274

The Children's Hospital at Westmead 2000 Westmead and Sydney Children's Hospital Randwick. Fact sheet – lumbar puncture. Online. Available: www.chw.edu.au/parents/factsheets/ptlumbaj.htm

Turner T 2003 Risk of cerebral herniation due to lumbar puncture in children with suspected meningitis. The Centre for Clinical Effectiveness, Clayton, Australia. Online. Available: www.med.monash.edu.au/healthservice/cce

Wojner A W, Malkoff M 2001 Lumbar puncture (perform). In: Lynn-McHale D J, Carlson K K (eds) ACCN procedure manual for critical care, 4th edn. W B Saunders, Philadelphia, p 602–606

Practice **16**

Neurological observations and coma scales

Alison Warren

Introduction

Neurological observations enable the nurse to assess the neurological status of infants and children. A coma scale is a tool that instructs the assessor to perform and record a series of prescribed neurological and haemodynamic observations on a scaled chart. Results are plotted on each level of the scale and a corresponding number allotted. The numbers for the different observations are totalled to give an overall figure known as the coma scale rating, with a maximum score of 15 and a minimum score of 3. The lower the rating, the poorer the child's neurological status (James & Trauner 1985).

Learning outcomes

By the end of this section you should:

- understand the importance of accurate neurological assessment
- be able to list the different elements of neurological assessment
- be able to explain the significance of changes in the child's neurological status

- understand how, when and why coma scales are utilised and appreciate their limitations.

Rationale

Deterioration in the level of consciousness can occur rapidly with devastating, sometimes fatal consequences which may only be averted with prompt action and treatment. The ability to accurately assess the child's neurological status and interpret the results in order to detect promptly any alteration in conscious level is a vital skill for a children's nurse.

Factors to note

Rapid assessment

Initial management of an infant or child with a decreased conscious level is to support airway*, breathing and circulation (* immobilise cervical spine if trauma is suspected). More recently a score has been introduced for rapid assessment of disability, particularly pre-hospital and in emergency departments. The score assesses neurological status as *alert* (A), responds to *voice* (V), responds to *pain* (P), or *unresponsive* (U) (Advanced Life Support Group 2001). This scoring system, entitled the AVPU score, is simple to use and requires little training (Mackay et al 2000), allowing the observer to swiftly evaluate priorities of care without the need for additional charts or equipment. It does not, however, replace more accurate coma scales that are essential for serial assessment and evaluation of the patient's level of consciousness.

Coma scales

Coma scales were introduced in the early 1970s in a successful attempt to standardise nursing and medical approaches to neurological assessment (Teasdale & Jennett 1974). Coma scales cover the following five main assessment criteria:

- Eye opening
- Verbal response
- Motor response
- Equality, size and reaction of pupils to light
- Strength and spontaneity of limb movement.

The most commonly used coma scale is the Glasgow Coma Scale (GCS). Devised by Teasdale and Jennett (1974), this is an adult scale that has also been adapted for children in recognition of the fact that verbal and motor responses must be related to the child's age (Campbell & Glasper 1995).

There are various paediatric adaptations of the GCS, for example that of James and Trauner (1985), and its subsequent revision as the Birmingham Children's Hospital (BCH) model, as demonstrated in Table 16.1.

Another adapted GCS scale is known as the Paediatric Glasgow Coma Scale (PGCS) or Adelaide scale. Physicians at Adelaide Children's Hospital first adapted it for use in paediatrics and their adaptations were to the verbal and motor responses. These were developed to correlate with expected developmental milestones of children of different ages. The adaptations themselves were minor. They expected nurses to be trained to use the tool and to be able to apply knowledge of normal development when assessing the verbal and motor components of

the scale. Table 16.2 demonstrates how a nurse would be expected to interpret a score against normal, verbal developmental milestones.

The Advanced Life Support Group (1997) developed a simplified version of a children's coma scale for use in children under 4 years (see Table 16.3).

Which scale to use is a matter of local choice according to the wishes of the multidisciplinary team. However, the nurse using the tool must have been given suitable tuition in how to use the tool and interpret the results, and be aware of the limitations of each scale.

In addition, it must be remembered that the normal responses of a child who is developmentally delayed, or has an existing neurological deficit, may not fall within the specified age range, i.e. 'child over 5 years' and 'child under 5 years'. It has been suggested that age-related scales should be replaced with criteria that reflect patients' 'usual ability' to allow for infants/children who have not achieved recognised developmental milestones (Warren 2000).

Applying a painful stimulus during neurological assessment

In a child who has a decreased conscious level, it is often necessary to apply a painful stimulus to evoke a response. The methods used to evoke a response differ according to trust/hospital policies, personal preferences and expertise.

Moreover, with a deteriorating conscious level, the necessity to accurately interpret a deficit in neurological status is of paramount importance so that the appropriate intervention can ensue. It is also essential that the choice of stimuli used, either peripheral or central, reflects the condition of the patient.

Frawley (1990) described the potential of damage to the nailbed following repetitive assessments, thus advocating the use of side finger pressure. Following this article, many healthcare professionals adopted side finger pressure to avoid potential trauma, assuming peripheral pressure is advocated.

However, many different modes of stimulus are regularly used in the paediatric setting, including squeezing the ear lobe, rubbing the

Table 16.1   BCH model, adapted from James & Trauner (1985) paediatric adaptation of Glasgow Coma Scale

	Adult/child according to usual ability	Child/infant according to usual ability	Score
Eyes open	● Spontaneously – without stimulation	● Spontaneously	4
	● To verbal stimuli – when spoken to, not necessarily on command		3
	● To pain – in response to any painful stimulus	● To pain	2
	● None – no eye opening at all		1
	● Eyes closed due to swelling/bandage		C
Best verbal response	● Oriented – able to give name and address in response to verbal question	● Usual ability – alert, uses sentences if previously able; recognisable words if not yet able to make sentences; babbles and coos for child not yet able to make words	5
	● Confused – able to converse but not oriented in person	● Less than usual ability, confused or no longer able to talk in sentences/ spontaneous irritable cry	4
	● Inappropriate – recognisable words but not in an exchange	● Cries to pain – cries only in response to painful stimuli	3
	● Incomprehensible – grunts, groans, incomprehensible sounds	● Only moans – but does not cry in response to painful stimuli	2
	● None – no verbal response even to painful stimuli	● None – no vocalisation, even to painful stimuli	1
Best motor response	● Obeys commands – obeys verbal commands	● Normal – normal play or voluntary or spontaneous movements	6
	● Localises – hands move above chin in response to supraorbital pressure painful stimulus	● Localises – as for adult/child or withdraws to painful stimulus	5
	● Withdraws – movement of limb away from painful stimulus	● Withdraws – as for adult/child	4
	● Flexion abnormal – decorticate flexion at wrist and elbow, and abduction at shoulder to painful stimulus	● Flexion abnormal – as for adult/child	3
	● Extension abnormal – decerebrate extension to painful stimulus	● Extension abnormal – as for adult/child	2
	● None	● None	1

C, closed.

sternum, pinching flesh under the arm, squeezing the shoulder and supraorbital pressure, with the most common being either nailbed or side finger pressure. No method of painful stimulus is regarded as a gold standard in the assessment of infants and children and few of the above techniques have been validated in paediatric practice.

Side finger pressure is performed by placing the child's finger (third and fourth fingers

Table 16.2   Paediatric Glasgow Coma Scale

	>1 year	<1 year	Score
Eye opening	● Spontaneously	● Spontaneously	4
	● To verbal command	● To shout	3
	● To pain	● To pain	2
	● No response	● No response	1
Best motor response	● Obeys commands		5
	● Localises pain	● Localises pain	4
	● Flexion to pain	● Flexion to pain	3
	● Extension to pain	● Extension to pain	2
	● No response	● No response	1

	>5 years	2–5 years	0–2 years	
Best verbal response	● Orientated and converses	● Appropriate words and phrases	● Smiles and cries appropriately	5
	● Disorientated and converses	● Inappropriate words	● Cries	4
	● Inappropriate words	● Cries	● Inappropriate crying	3
	● Incomprehensible sounds	● Grunting	● Grunting	2
	● No response	● No response	● No response	1

Reproduced from Lloyd-Thomas 1990 by kind permission of the BMJ Publishing Group.

are most sensitive) between the nurse's thumb and a pen or pencil and gradually increasing pressure until a response is obtained (see Fig. 16.1).

Applying pressure to the nailbed is achieved in a similar way to that of side finger pressure but is contraindicated in patients with poor perfusion or reported coagulopathy. Moreover, nurses should also be aware of the limitations of 'peripheral' stimuli when assessing deeply comatosed patients.

Supraorbital pressure, or 'central stimuli', is regarded as a more accurate method of evoking response in patients in deep coma. It is particularly painful and should only be performed by staff aware of the contraindications of the procedure and who are competent and confident to do so safely. The advantage of this painful stimulus over 'peripheral' methods is to avoid eliciting reflex responses, particularly in the lower limbs, which could mislead the observer.

There are two factors of paramount importance when evoking a pain response in children with a diminished level of consciousness:

● That the mode of stimulus used is consistent as variations can cause assessment anomalies. This can only be achieved by performing a full set of coma score observations at the bedside handover.
● That the assessing nurse is confident that the mode of painful stimulus used is sufficient to evoke a response. If there is any doubt, a senior nurse or doctor should be consulted.

Neonates

Neonates are notoriously difficult to assess neurologically and certainly most existing coma scales, even those that are adapted for infants and children, are not sufficiently accurate when assessing a child under 6 months of age (Allan 1994). Tatman et al (1997) devised and tested a grimace score for infants and children unable to

Table 16.3   Advanced Life Support Group children's coma scale: <4 years

Response	Score
Eyes	
● Open spontaneously	4
● React to speech	3
● React to pain	2
● No response	1
Best motor response	
● Spontaneous or obeys verbal command	6
Reaction to painful stimulus	
● Localises pain	5
● Withdraws in response to pain	4
● Abnormal flexion to pain (decorticate posture)	3
● Abnormal extension to pain (decerebrate posture)	2
● No response	1
Best verbal response	
● Smiles, orientates to sounds, follows objects, interacts	5

Crying	*Interacts*	
● Consolable	Inappropriate	4
● Inconsistently consolable	Moaning	3
● Inconsolable	Irritable	2
● No response	No response	1

Reproduced from Lawton 1995 by kind permission.

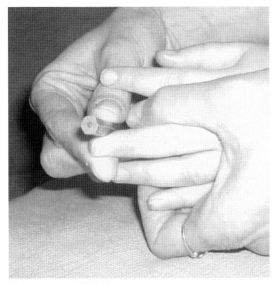

Figure 16.1   Side finger pressure

Table 16.4   Grimace score

Orofacial response	Score
Spontaneous normal facial/oromotor activity, e.g. sucks tube, coughs	5
Less than usual spontaneous ability or only responds to touch	4
Vigorous grimace to pain	3
Mild grimace or some change in facial expression to pain	2
No response to pain	1

After Tatman et al 1997.

vocalise. It is an assessment of orofacial movement as opposed to a vocal response and has five elements (see Table 16.4). Primarily aimed at intubated children in an intensive care unit, it has also proved effective for neonates and infants. Hazinski (1999) highlights the need to evaluate the baby's alertness and response to the environment, and Reeves (1989) highlights the importance of referring to the child's parents who are most cognisant of their child's normal behaviour. Palpation of the fontanelles is also beneficial when assessing for signs of elevated intracranial pressure (ICP) or volume status in an infant. The anterior fontanelle should feel firm and flat; however, it will bulge if pressure in the superior vena cava increases (a physiological sign of raised ICP or congenital heart failure). A sunken fontanelle is a sign of volume depletion and dehydration (Hazinski 1999). Measurement of head circumference and observing the shape of the skull can also be of significant value when assessing a neonate.

Sick children

A decreased level of consciousness can be associated with a number of causes with the end result being alterations in cerebral blood flow causing hypoxia, ischaemia, cerebral oedema and raised ICP. Common causes of these conditions are listed in Box 16.1.

It is worth noting that comatosed children require and respond to stimulation, both verbal and touch (Hendrickson 1987, Hobdell et al 1989).

In a review of major research studies, Chudley (1994) describes how some nursing interventions can cause an increase in ICP in patients with previously raised ICP. Suctioning of an endotracheal tube, repositioning/turning, moving the neck from the midline, clustering of care activities and invasive procedures, e.g. passing a nasogastric tube, are all mentioned. This highlights the importance of planning care to ensure minimal handling, with periods of rest to allow the ICP to stabilise or return to a baseline between care episodes, for any child with an actual or suspected raised ICP. However, decisions about timing of care must always be carefully balanced with the need to monitor closely in order to determine and act swiftly on any detrimental changes in the child's condition.

Box 16.1   Possible causes of decreased conscious level in children

- Reduced cerebral blood flow caused by:
  - respiratory insufficiency
  - hypovolaemia
  - gross anaemia
  - poor cardiac output state
- Cerebral oedema caused by:
  - fluid overload
  - multisystem failure
  - seizures
  - hyperpyrexia
  - electrolyte imbalance
- Raised intracranial pressure due to:
  - hydrocephalus
  - space-occupying lesion
  - intracerebral bleeding (traumatic or spontaneous)
  - meningitis
  - trauma/head injury
  - arterial blood gas abnormality, e.g. raised PCO_2
- Encephalopathy due to:
  - infection, e.g. chickenpox, herpes
  - sepsis
  - liver disease
  - renal disease
  - ingestion of toxins
  - hypo/hyperglycaemia
- Blood clots or air emboli caused by intravenous therapy and/or invasive monitoring extracorporeal techniques

Guidelines

The important role which parents play in the neurological assessment of a child must be further stressed. A frightened child is unlikely to cooperate, particularly if asked by a stranger to obey commands whether or not the child is physically able to do so. However, they may respond to requests made by their parents, rather than a nurse.

Hazinski (1999) describes phrasing questions to the child around people and things that are familiar to them, for example using a popular children's television character. This information will of course be gained from the initial history taken from the child (if able) or family (see Assessment, p. 83).

It is also of value to remember that head injury in a child, or baby, could be non-accidental, therefore child protection procedures should be instigated according to local policy and the interactions between the child and parents monitored closely.

Equipment

- Thermometer
- Blood pressure monitor
- Pen or pencil
- Pen torch or ophthalmoscope
- Colourful and noisy toys if appropriate
- Paediatric neurological observation assessment tool/recording chart.

Method

Initial observations

Always ensure the child's airway (± cervical spine*), breathing and circulation are stable.

- *Airway* – check the patency and maintenance of the airway (* if cervical spine injury is suspected, ensure immobilisation)
- *Breathing* – evaluate respiratory rate, air entry, work of breathing and colour
- *Circulation* – evaluate heart rate, peripheral and central pulses, skin perfusion and blood pressure (Resuscitation Council (UK) 2004) (see also Cardiopulmonary Resuscitation, p. 127).

Appropriate emergency equipment should be available to monitor and support ABC before (D) disability (neurological status) is assessed.

1. Collect equipment together and approach the child, and try to gain their confidence. Remember a child may not be cooperative, particularly if they are frightened or in pain.

2. Before undertaking physical observations, assess the child's clinical signs and behaviour generally, taking into account pre-existing conditions, previous hospital admissions, past medical history and the knowledge gained from the initial history-taking assessment.

   a. Is the child asleep or awake, settled and peaceful or irritable and unhappy?

   b. Note their general colour – is there evidence of pallor, redness, mottling or cyanosis? All over or in specific areas?

   c. Do they appear bothered by bright lights (photophobia)?

   d. Do they seem reluctant to move their head or cry out if their legs are straightened?

   e. Is the child sleeping or unusually quiet? Note their effort and efficacy of breathing – is it regular and easy, or shallow, laboured or irregular? Are there any audible respiratory noises, e.g. wheeze, grunting, stridor, etc.?

   f. Observe the eyes – is there evidence of bulging, deviation, drooping of the eyelids or 'sun setting' (the sclera being visible above the iris)? Is there any discolouration of the sclera or pupils?

   g. Smell their breath – can the odour of alcohol, solvents or ketones be detected?

   h. Are there any rashes, skin lesions and/or discolouration? A purpuric rash (purple/red spots) which does not blanch white if the skin is rubbed/depressed with a finger could be suggestive of meningococcal infection; café au lait spots (coffee-coloured patches on the skin) is an indicator of neurofibromatosis; jaundice is a sign of hepatic dysfunction and possible encephalopathy.

i. Is there evidence of seizure activity? If so, observe carefully, ensuring airway maintenance, record and report (see Seizures, p. 347).

j. If the child is awake and conscious, utilise normal play to assess conscious level, in particular, eye, motor and verbal responses in accordance with coma score documentation.

k. Does the child respond appropriately, both verbally and physically, according to age and expected developmental milestones? Remember that the effects of hospitalisation can cause psychological upset (Fletcher 1981), therefore behavioural changes could be associated with the fact that the child is in an unfamiliar and often frightening environment.

3. What sort of positioning has the child adopted? If mobilising, observe posture and gait – are the limbs flaccid or rigid when moved? In neonates and infants a typical sign of cerebral irritation is back arching and muscle rigidity – opisthotonos – accompanied by a high-pitched cry.

4. Summarise the initial assessment. Is there any cause for concern such as unusual, unexplained irritability? Severe agitation in a child, or baby, can be a sign of cerebral irritation and deterioration of conscious level.

5. If any anomalies have been detected inform a senior nurse or doctor immediately and proceed with the coma score assessment to ascertain if there is any further evidence of neurological deficit.

Assessment

It is advocated that a full coma score assessment is performed at every nursing handover to reduce the potential discrepancy between observers.

Before commencing, always check if the child/infant is on medication or has a pre-existing condition that could affect 'normal' parameters or behaviour. Information should be gained from the parents/primary carer in regard to the child's normal behaviour and whether or not they have reached developmental milestones (access to the child's 'Red Book' may be helpful).

1. Explain to the child, if applicable, and parents what you are about to do. Stress that the observations will not hurt.
2. Assess and record any observations which do not require physical intervention, e.g. respirations (see Assessment, p. 83).
3. Then proceed to recordings of temperature, pulse and blood pressure (see Assessment, p. 83).

    a. Temperature: Observe for swings in temperature; hyperpyrexia can be indicative of raised ICP due to pressure on the hypothalamus disrupting thermoregulation (Sherman 1990). Hyperpyrexia also increases cerebral metabolic rate, cerebral blood flow and cerebral oxygen consumption which further increases ICP (Hall 1997). Hypothermia can affect haemodynamic values (cardiac arrhythmias are not uncommon) and conscious level due to decreased cerebral metabolism and cerebral blood flow (Dennis & Mayer 2001).

    b. Pulse rate: Severe, raised ICP can be indicated by bradycardia caused by excessive pressure on the medulla; however, this is a late 'pre-terminal' sign in children and emergency assistance should be sought (Sherburne & Curtis 1990). Tachycardia could be attributed to a number of things including pain, infection, medications or blood loss.

    c. Blood pressure: Hypertension again can be a late sign of raised ICP in children due to pressure on the medulla, particularly when associated with bradycardia; this is a life-threatening event requiring immediate intervention (Hazinski 1999). Increases in systolic arterial pressure also occur if ICP is high; this is a physiological response to maintain cerebral perfusion – a phenomenon called autoregulation (Hazinski 1999). Other causes such as pain and anxiety should also be taken into account if the blood pressure is elevated. The phenomenon described as Cushing's triad – hypertension, bradycardia and respiratory depression – is a very late sign of severe, acute, irreversible brain damage with a high risk of mortality (Sherburne & Curtis 1990).

d. Respiratory rate: An abnormal respiratory rate can be attributed to a number of factors, for example anxiety, pain, infection, pyrexia or hypovolaemia. However, with suspected raised ICP, pressure on the medulla depresses the respiratory centre; therefore respiratory insufficiency can be a sign of brain stem compression (Hazinski 1999).

4. Eye opening, verbal/grimace and motor responses should be assessed simultaneously; all scores should be recorded in the appropriate section of the assessment chart.

a. If the infant/child has their eyes open and is responding to the environment, is vocalising and moving all limbs, then they would score the maximum – 15 (see Tables 16.1–16.3).

b. If the child is non-vocal or intubated then a grimace score is advocated (to maintain a maximum score of 15). In some cases neonates/infants are easier to score using this system as facial expression or grimace can ensure accuracy of neurological assessment (see Point 7 below).

5. Pupil reactions: Pupils should be of equal size and react briskly and equally to light. Any inequality of pupil size or reaction is indicative of a problem on the same side of the brain as the abnormal reaction. Fixed dilated pupils can be an ominous sign indicating brain stem herniation (coning). However, hypothermia and some drugs (e.g. large doses of atropine, some ophthalmic drugs) can cause dilated pupils. Similarly, certain pharmacological agents can cause pinpoint pupils.

a. It is important to assess and record the size and equality of the child's pupils *before* shining light into them.

b. Is there any evidence of a squint or deviation which was previously unreported?

c. If the child is asleep, try and rouse them first. If they cannot open their eyes, it may be necessary for the nurse to lift the eyelids. It is important that both lids are lifted simultaneously, this may require two people.

d. Ideally, pupil reactions should be tested by turning off the main overhead lights and shining a bright, narrow beam directly onto the pupil.

e. Note the size of the pupil and observe whether the pupil reacts to light. Does it contract briskly (+), is it sluggish (S) or non-reactive (–)?

f. A child who has been deeply asleep or sedated may be reluctant to open their eyes and, likewise, pupils may be a little sluggish to react at first.

g. With a child unwilling to cooperate, give them the torch to play with and observe what happens from a short distance away; flick the lights on and off until you observe pupillary response.

h. Be aware that pupil reactions can be affected by pre-existing conditions and pharmacological agents.

6. Verbal response: (for verbal scores in the child/infant, see Tables 16.1–16.3).

a. Is the child alert, vocalising and able to concentrate on what is being said to them? Listen – are they chatting apparently normally, aware of their surroundings and parents?

b. Is a baby babbling or cooing?

c. Is the toddler making words and noises which are normal for them? (check with parents). They may appear confused due to unfamiliarity with the surroundings.

d. Is any crying appropriate and can it be consoled by parents or with distraction techniques? Is it associated with pain, fear or hunger?

e. If an infant is crying, does it sound particularly high pitched? An abnormally high-pitched cry in a baby can be due to raised ICP or cerebral irritation.

f. Grunting noises in any child/infant are a sign that something is seriously wrong.

g. The child who makes no noise or facial expression could be deeply unconscious.

7. Grimace score: As previously mentioned, the grimace score is recommended as a verbal score alternative and is commonly used in the assessment of children/infants who have an endotracheal or tracheostomy tube in situ (in the absence of muscle relaxants) (Tatman et al 1997). However, this score has proved to be useful and less susceptible to observer error in neonates and infants where definition of vocal response can be misleading, particularly to a novice. Moreover, anecdotal evidence demonstrates that children who are uncooperative, postictal, receiving sedation/analgesia, have docu-

mented learning or sensory disability or are experiencing a language barrier have been neurologically evaluated with greater reliability using this scoring method.

The grimace score is a 5-point scale that corresponds to the verbal score, but reflects cerebral function by the assessment of oromotor or facial responses (see Fig. 16.2 and Table 16.4).

8. Motor response: Assess the child's movements (for motor response scores in the child/infant, see Tables 16.1–16.3). A decreasing conscious level can be determined by abnormalities in motor response.

a. Is the child playing with toys or feeding from a bottle using both hands?

b. Can they grasp your fingers equally in strength with both hands? Can they push your hand away?

c. Do the legs move normally – kicking or reacting if their feet are tickled?

d. If the child is not moving, can a response be elicited by asking them to move, e.g. 'Can you lift your arm for me?' Are the movements equal? What about symmetry of movement?

e. Does the infant reach towards a noisy toy or move lower limbs if tickled?

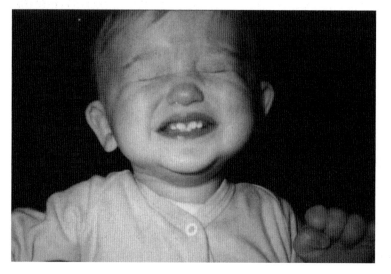

Figure 16.2 Vigorous grimace to pain

f. Pay particular attention to the muscle tone – are the limbs stiff (hypertonia) or flaccid/floppy (hypotonia)?

g. Decorticate posturing (abnormal flexion) is an indication of neurological deterioration. The child displays involuntary flexion of the limbs with adduction to the midline (Fig. 16.3a). If deterioration continues, decerebrate posturing (abnormal extension) ensues, the limbs increase in tone, straighten and are abducted away from the midline (see Fig. 16.3b). A child can alternate between decorticate and decerebrate posturing as a result of fluctuating cerebral blood flow to the brain stem and cerebral hemispheres. Opisthotonos is a sign of cerebral/meningeal irritation in neonates and infants.

h. If there is no movement, a sufficient painful stimulus must be used to evoke a response.

i. For a child to localise they must physically try to remove the person or object causing the pain, for example, grasping or pushing away the assessor's hand. Babies cannot localise but should withdraw the limb from the painful stimuli.

j. If the child is old enough/developmentally capable, ask them to close their eyes and touch their nose with the tip of their finger; this tests proprioception, the awareness of parts of the body in space without looking.

9. Strength and spontaneity of limb movement: Limb strength/power should be recorded for both the right and the left side of the body. Any notable inequality of the two sides can indicate a problem occurring in one side of the brain. If hypo- or hypertonia is present, is it evident in all limbs equally or just affect one side of the body?

a. Is one or more of the limbs weaker than the others?

b. Observe the conscious child at play – are all limbs being used equally?

c. Is the child sitting straight or showing a tendency to lean to one side?

d. In an infant, check their grasp – do they reach for toys, kick their legs?

e. Request the older child to wiggle their fingers and toes, kick with their legs and wave their arms.

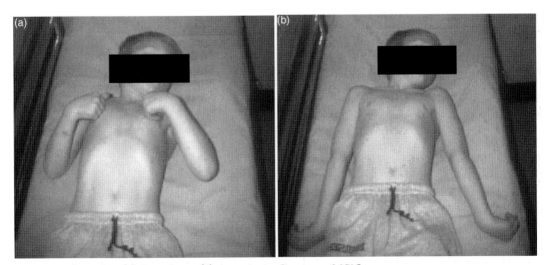

Figure 16.3 Posturing: (a) decorticate; (b) decerebrate. Courtesy of APLS.

The spontaneity of movements should be recorded independently to the strength/power. A child may display involuntary spontaneous movements but show no reaction to command or painful stimuli; this is a significant neurological indicator requiring documentation and reporting.

Summary

● All observations must be recorded on coma scale/neurological chart documentation (a modified paediatric coma scale is preferable but not essential).

● Total the score for all observations (maximum 15, minimum 3). Interpret, compare with previous observations (if recorded), evaluate and report findings.

● Is the child improving or deteriorating? Are there any observations which cause concern?

● Assess when subsequent observations should be performed. Generally, in the acutely unstable child/infant, a repeat set should be carried out within 15 minutes. As the condition stabilises, observations can be reduced; however, assessments used to determine deterioration in neurological status should not be performed any greater than hourly.

● Some paediatric centres have additional documentation to record 'significant events' and 'special instructions' that are facilitated to record additional information pertinent to the patient's neurological status and management, thus assisting in the evaluation of coma score and neurological status in children and infants (Warren 2000).

● For the intensive care child, if muscle relaxants are infusing, pupillary reaction is the only definitive observation that can be performed, although there are other indicators that can assist with neurological assessment. However, once paralysing agents are discontinued, regular observations should be recommenced. Accepting that sedation and analgesia will alter conscious level, the child should respond to tactile or painful stimuli and much can be gained from 30-minute to 1-hourly monitoring of pupil, grimace and motor responses.

Complications

There are no procedural complications associated with neurological assessment. However hazards lie in user error:

● the inexperienced practitioner inaccurately undertaking observations without adequate supervision/training
● misinterpretation of observational results: if a nurse is unsure of the implications of the neurological observation results, the advice of a senior colleague or doctor should be sought.

COMMUNITY PERSPECTIVE

Neurological assessment is a procedure that would not often be undertaken in the home. However, there will be occasions when carers and professionals involved in the child's care will need to be aware of altering levels of consciousness, for example in a child with a life-limiting condition or needing palliative care. It is unlikely that formal recording of observations will be appropriate and admission to hospital should be an option if the carers are concerned or unable to cope at home.

The role of the CCN would be to raise the awareness of the carers without causing apprehension, showing them how to undertake any monitoring required. During visits routine assessment of the child's neurological status should be performed and compared to the carers' observations. Findings will then be documented and liaison maintained with medical staff as necessary.

Do and do not

- Do ensure that airway, breathing and circulation are stable and maintained.
- Do remember that a child's neurological status can deteriorate rapidly; be alert for signs of raised intracranial pressure.
- Do remember to gain as much information about the child's/infant's usual activities and capabilities: observe movements, vocal ability and reaction to the surroundings prior to neurological assessment.
- Do remember that the child's parents are invaluable when trying to ascertain what is normal or abnormal for their child; this information will aid evaluation of neurological status.

- Do report any abnormalities, however trivial as they could be a sign that the child's condition is altering.
- Do ensure that painful stimuli are adequate to evoke a response. If in doubt, consult a senior nurse/doctor.
- Do be aware of the limitations and contraindications of peripheral stimuli and be knowledgeable of other methods of evoking a pain response.
- Do perform a bedside handover to reduce the risk of misinterpretation of the same physical signs.
- Do not omit neurological observations. If the child/infant is sleeping, a sleeping child could be comatosed.

References

Advanced Life Support Group 1997 Advanced paediatric life support: the practical approach, 2nd edn. BMJ Publications, London, p 119

Advanced Life Support Group 2001 Advanced paediatric life support -the practical approach, 3rd edn, BMJ Publications, London, p 17

Allan D 1994 Paediatric coma scale. Surgical Nurse 7(3): 14–16

Campbell S, Glasper E A (eds) 1995 Whaley and Wong's children's nursing, UK edn. Mosby/Times Mirror International, London, ch 31, p 660–679

Chudley S 1994 The effect of nursing activities on intracranial pressure. British Journal of Nursing 3(9): 454–459

Dennis L J, Mayer S A 2001 Diagnosis and management of increased intracranial pressure. Neurology India 49(Suppl 1): S37–50

Fletcher B 1981 Psychological upset in posthospitalized children: a review of the literature. Maternal Child Nursing Journal 10: 185–195

Frawley P 1990 Neurological observations. Nursing Times 86(35): 29–34

Hall C A 1997 Patient management in head injury care: a nursing perspective. Intensive and Critical Care Nursing 13: 329–337

Hazinski M F 1999 Manual of pediatric critical care. Mosby Year Book, St Louis, MO

Hendrickson S L 1987 Intracranial pressure changes and family presence. Journal of Neuroscience Nursing 19(1): 14–17

Hobdell E F, Adams F, Caruso J, Dihoff R, Neverling E, Roncoli M 1989 The effect of nursing activities on the intracranial pressure of children. Critical Care Nurse 9(6): 75–79

James H E, Trauner D A 1985 The Glasgow Coma Scale. In: James H E, Anas N G, Perkin R M (eds) Brain insults in infants and children. Grune and Stratton, Orlando, FL p 179–182

Lawton L 1995 Paediatric trauma – the care of Anthony. Accident and Emergency Nursing 3: 172–176

Lloyd-Thomas A R 1990 Primary survey and resuscitation – II. British Medical Journal 301: 380–382

Mackay C A, Burke D P, Burke J A, Porter K M, Bowden D, Gorman D 2000 Association between the assessment of conscious level using the AVPU system and the Glasgow coma scale. Pre-hospital Immediate Care 4: 17–19

Reeves K 1989 Assessment of pediatric head injury. Journal of Emergency Nursing 15(4): 329–332

Resuscitation Council (UK) 2004 European paediatric life support course, provider manual. Resuscitation Council (UK), London

Sherburne D, Curtis B 1990 Disorders of brain function. In: Porth C (ed.) Pathophysiology: concepts of altered health states. Lippincott, New York, p 929–968

Sherman D 1990 Managing acute head injury. Nursing 90: 47–52

Tatman A, Warren A, Williams A, Powell J E, Whitehouse W 1997 Development of a paediatric coma scale in intensive care clinical practice. Archives of Disease in Childhood 77(6): 519–521

Teasdale G, Jennett W B 1974 Assessment of coma and impaired consciousness. A practical scale. Lancet 2: 81–84

Warren A 2000 Paediatric coma scoring researched and benchmarked. Paediatric Nursing 12(3): 14–17

Further Reading

National Institute for Clinical Excellence (NICE) 2003 Head injury. Triage, assessment and early management of head injury in infants, children and adults. NICE, London. Online. Available: www.nice.org.uk

Scottish Intercollegiate Guidelines Network (SIGN) 2000 Early management of patients with a head injury. Publication 46. SIGN, Edinburgh. Online. Available: www.sign.ac.uk

Westbrook A 1997 The use of a paediatric coma scale for monitoring infants and young children with head injuries. Nursing in Critical Care 2(2): 72–75

Practice **17**

Oxygen therapy

Rebecca Giles

Introduction

Adequate oxygenation is vital to prevent tissue damage. Prolonged hypoxia (a decreased availability of oxygen to the tissues) can result in cell death if allowed to persist, which ultimately leads to brain damage and multiorgan failure; 100% oxygen is therefore the first drug given in an emergency/resuscitation situation (Resuscitation Council (UK) 2000). Oxygen requirements can vary between individuals but are more significant in children as they have a lower pulmonary reserve and a higher metabolic rate than adults and can therefore decompensate more quickly if supplementary oxygen is not provided (Advanced Paediatric Life Support Group 2001). Administering oxygen to children can be difficult as they do not tolerate oxygen masks well, but nasal cannulae and headboxes are often effective. Oxygen can also be administered via an incubator but is not without problems (see Incubator Care, p. 205). Accuracy of the amount delivered can also be problematic as will be discussed later within this chapter.

Learning outcomes

By the end of this section you should be able to:

- assess the most appropriate delivery device for each child according to age, size, development and condition
- assess whether or not the oxygen delivery system requires humidification
- prepare the equipment necessary to deliver oxygen (humidified where necessary) by both headbox and nasal cannula
- state possible complications of oxygen administration.

Rationale for oxygen administration

Administration of oxygen is a life-saving intervention commonly used in children's nursing and an important skill for a children's nurse to acquire.

Factors to note

Oxygen should be regarded as a drug and planned delivery of oxygen therapy should always be prescribed by a doctor (Chandler 2001, BMA 2005). As with any drug there can be adverse effects. Therefore, in any patient, oxygen should be delivered at the lowest concentration possible and for the shortest time possible (Tasker 1995, Chandler 2001, Wong et al 2002). Administration of oxygen to children is usually undertaken using one of three methods: via oxygen mask, which is well covered in other literature (Chandler 2001, Wong et al 2002, Frey & Shann 2003), nasal cannula or headbox. How much oxygen is delivered to the child is expressed as the fractional inspired oxygen concentration (FiO_2) – literally, the percentage concentration of oxygen the child is breathing in.

Headbox or body/trunk box

The advantages of these types of device are that they give effective oxygen delivery, it is possible to monitor the FiO_2 and they are totally non-invasive. Disadvantages are that carbon dioxide rebreathing will occur at low oxygen flow rates, <4 litres/minute (Frey & Shann 2003), removal of the box quickly dilutes the oxygen delivered and a cold gas supply will quickly cool an infant. Therefore, it is important that the gas supply should be warmed. It is also desirable to humidify when prolonged oxygen therapy is required (Chandler 2001, Frey & Shann 2003, Pilkington 2004). Normally, inspired gas is warmed and humidified in the nasopharynx and reaches the upper trachea with a relative humidity of about 90% and a temperature of 32–36°C; it has reached a temperature of 37°C by the time it reaches the alveoli (Hazinski 1998). Mucociliary transport is impaired when relative humidity falls below 75% at 37°C (BCH 1993, Pilkington 2004).

Nasal cannula

Advantages of nasal cannulae are that they are reasonably well tolerated by children (particularly in comparison with a face mask) and carbon dioxide rebreathing does not occur (Chandler 2001). Humidification is not necessary as the gas is entering via the nasal passages where it is warmed and moistened in the normal way (Frey & Shann 2003). Disadvantages

are that nasal cannulae are only suitable for use with a low flow of oxygen, i.e. maximum 2 litres/minute (Bower et al 1996, Chandler 2001). Higher flows may be uncomfortable and dry the nasal mucosa. In addition, a child who mouth breathes will dilute the FiO_2 with air.

Healthy children

Healthy children should have an arterial oxygen saturation level of 95–98% (Sims 1996). Some children who have underlying heart conditions may have an oxygen saturation level well below this, even when otherwise healthy. It is therefore essential for nurses to be aware of the child's 'norm' and parents are a vital source of such information.

Neonates

Administration of continuous oxygen therapy to neonates must be monitored very carefully. High inspired oxygen concentrations have been clearly linked to the development of retinopathy of prematurity, although there is more recent speculation that wide swings in oxygen saturations may be more to blame than simply too high concentrations of oxygen (Kotecha & Allen 2002). Prolonged exposure to high oxygen tensions may also cause pulmonary oxygen toxicity and permanent lung damage, e.g. bronchopulmonary dysplasia (George & Gordon 1995, Kotecha & Allen 2002).

Sick children

Children with respiratory problems may benefit from being nursed upright, well supported with pillows. An infant may benefit from being placed in a baby chair for periods of up to 4 hours or longer if absolutely necessary. Any child should have a change of position 4-hourly if possible, to relieve pressure areas. If the child is too ill to sit up, consider tilting up the head of the bed or cot.

Recent studies have demonstrated that a child with chronic lung disease can and should have oxygen saturations maintained above 92% and within a target range of 94–96% to provide a buffer zone against desaturation during sleeping and feeding (Kotecha & Allen 2002). These targets aim to reduce complications from pulmonary artery hypertension and promote growth (Kotecha & Allen 2002). However, in a small number of children with chronic lung disease, e.g. some children with cystic fibrosis, the dependence of respiratory drive on CO_2 and bicarbonate concentration is lost. In these children inflammatory changes in the lungs result in increased alveolar CO_2 tension, which ultimately leads to a gross saturation of the chemoreceptors, making them dysfunctional (Ashurst 1995). Administering high concentrations of oxygen to these children can cause carbon dioxide narcosis leading to unconsciousness (Chandler 2001). The BMA (2005) states that any patient with a chronic chest condition should not be administered more than 28% concentration of oxygen alongside repeated blood gas measurements.

Guidelines

Careful explanation to parents and child (if age and cognitive development allow) about the need for oxygen therapy will help to maximise cooperation. Careful explanation of all the equipment involved is important to minimise anxiety by reducing fear of the unknown.

Parents can be taught how to perform oral care to help maintain a moist, clean mouth if oxygen therapy is causing drying of the mucosa (see Hygiene, p. 198).

Equipment for headbox and body/trunk box delivery

- Oxygen supply (even if supply is piped, consider the need for a spare portable cylinder in case of emergencies, e.g. loss or failure of supply)
- Humidifier: preferably a warmed, water bath humidifier such as Aquapak; some humidifiers have temperature controls to enable the water to be heated to different temperatures
- Nipple to connect humidifier to oxygen supply
- Apparatus to connect humidifier, water and oxygen together (usually supplied as a complete, sterile unit for once-only use, e.g. Aquapak)
- Sterile water for humidification; tap water must not be used as it increases the risk of contamination with *Legionella pneumophila* (Stevenson 1992)
- Elephant tubing
- Oxygen analyser
- Headbox of a size sufficient to enclose the baby's head whilst sitting over the baby's neck (see Fig. 17.1) or Manchester/Derbyshire chair
- Oxygen saturation monitor and probe.

Equipment for nasal cannula delivery

- Oxygen supply
- Nasal cannula
- Oxygen saturation monitor and probe

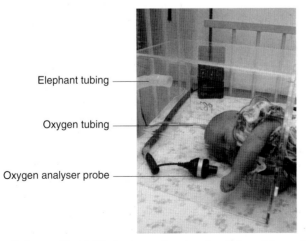

Elephant tubing

Oxygen tubing

Oxygen analyser probe

Figure 17.1   Delivery of humidified oxygen via a headbox (viewed from above)

- Tape for fastening the cannula in place
- Low-flow oxygen meter if required.

Method for headbox delivery

1. Explain the procedure to the parents to reduce fear of the unknown and aid compliance with the therapy.

2. If using a portable oxygen supply, ensure that the cylinder is full or nearly full. Determine how many hours' supply will be provided by the cylinder.

3. Set up the humidification system according to the manufacturer's instructions.

4. Test the alarm and set upper and lower alarm limits on the oxygen analyser. Calibrate the analyser to air and to 100% oxygen to ensure accuracy of monitoring. Put the probe of the oxygen analyser into the headbox via the purpose-built (smaller) hole.

5. Position the baby on their back or side in the cot and attach the oxygen saturation monitor probe. Turn on the saturation monitor. Set the upper and lower limit alarms for oxygen saturation and pulse rate (according to medical staff instructions) and record the child's oxygen saturation and pulse rate.

6. Place the headbox carefully on top of the baby's head, preferably with the shoulders outside. Sometimes the shoulders have to go inside the box as well, particularly in a smaller infant. Ensure that the box does not exert undue pressure anywhere on the baby's body. Do not block the gap around the infant's shoulders as this will cause carbon dioxide retention within the headbox.

7. Position the elephant tubing so that it delivers the oxygen through the purpose-built, larger hole and is behind the head or to one side of the baby's face.

8. Position the oxygen analyser probe so that it is at the opposite side of the box to the point at which the oxygen is being delivered, near to the baby's face.

9. From the prescription sheet, determine the percentage oxygen to be delivered and turn on the oxygen to flow at 4.5 litres/minute minimum. The dial on the humidifier equipment will tell you how many litres of oxygen are needed for specific concentrations of oxygen.

10. Read the oxygen analyser and regulate the flow of oxygen until the prescribed percentage of oxygen is attained.

11. Monitor the effect on the baby's saturation level and record frequently (every 1–4 hours depending on the child's condition). Report to medical staff if the prescribed percentage of oxygen does not maintain the baby's saturations at a level predetermined by the doctor. Report to medical staff if the saturations are decreasing despite prescribed oxygen flow.

12. Monitor the baby's respiratory rate and effort.

13. Monitor the amount of oxygen remaining in a portable oxygen cylinder at least hourly. Ensure that a replacement cylinder is available before the one in use empties.

14. Monitor the level of water in the humidifier bottle.

Method for nasal cannula delivery

1–2. Follow steps 1 and 2 of headbox delivery.

3. Ensure that the child's nose is cleaned of any dried mucus. Take the nasal cannula and place it over the child's head. Position it so that the prongs slant towards the child's face and each of the two prongs sits in a nostril (see Fig. 17.2).

4. Tighten the cannula to fit closely by sliding up the movable sheath at the back of the tubing.

5. If necessary, fasten the cannula in place by taping the tubes onto the child's cheeks. Ensure that the child is not allergic to the tape. If the skin is particularly delicate or sore, consider using a protective barrier such as a piece of extra-thin hydrocolloid sheet (e.g. Granuflex).

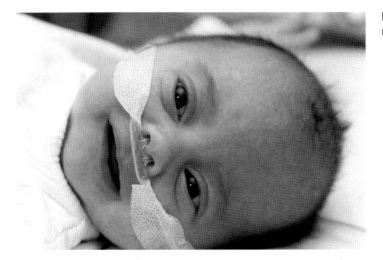

Figure 17.2   Delivery of oxygen via nasal cannula: nasal prongs in situ

6. Attach the oxygen saturation monitor probe. Turn on the saturation monitor. Set the upper and lower limit alarms for oxygen saturation and pulse rate (according to medical staff instructions) and record the child's oxygen saturation and pulse rate.

7. Attach the end of the nasal cannula tubing to the oxygen supply.

8. From the prescription sheet, determine the oxygen flow rate to be delivered and turn on the oxygen accordingly.

9–10. Follow steps 11 and 12 of headbox delivery.

Observations and complications

A child requiring oxygen therapy should always be monitored carefully. Oxygen saturations should be monitored continuously while oxygen is being delivered, using a pulse oximeter. Pulse oximetry will detect hypoxia long before clinical signs become apparent (Hanna 1995). The child's oxygen saturation level, respiratory rate and effort and percentage/flow rate of oxygen delivered should be monitored and recorded regularly, between 1- and 4-hourly depending on the stability of the child's condition. If using headbox oxygen, for accuracy it is important to read the concentration of oxygen from the analyser which should be placed near the baby's mouth and not from the delivery system. Report any decrease in saturations and increase in respiratory rate and/or effort. If using a portable supply, check the cylinder regularly to ensure that sufficient oxygen remains in it. Even if piped oxygen is supplied, it may still be prudent to have a spare, portable cylinder close by in case of emergencies/loss of supply. Remember to change the humidifier water bottle at least once every 24 hours or in accordance with the manufacturer's instructions to prevent infection (Mehtar 1992, Pilkington 2004).

Humidifiers are a common source of Gram-negative bacilli and viruses associated with the respiratory system (Mehtar 1992, Pilkington 2004). The highest incidence of hospital-acquired pneumonia occurs amongst patients who have had respiratory therapy, and bacterial contamination is a particular problem when gases are mixed with water as in humidifiers (Wilson 1995, Chiumello et al 2003). Check the humidifier regularly (4-hourly) to ensure that it has not emptied. Ensure that the nostrils remain free from dried mucus; they may need gentle cleansing with warm water. Remember that some infants will not tolerate being removed from the headbox for washing, feeding, etc. They may require a source of oxygen close to their face during the time that they are removed from the headbox.

Risks of oxygen therapy

- There is a risk of eye damage associated with PO_2 above 15 kPa (see Factors to note, p. 258).
- There is a risk of lung damage associated with prolonged, continuous administration of

COMMUNITY PERSPECTIVE

Prior to discharge

- Ensure that the parents are aware of all the constraints and problems that caring for a baby/child on long-term oxygen therapy can pose and consent to take on this role.
- Initiate a teaching programme for parents. This will need to cover:
  - recognising normal and abnormal respiratory patterns in their child, including signs of desaturation
  - knowing what action to take in the event of problems occurring
  - training in resuscitation
  - familiarisation with the use of the oxygen delivery system (e.g. oxygen cylinders, oxygen concentrator, liquid oxygen)
  - knowing what action to take should there be problems with the equipment. They will also need the telephone number of the oxygen supplier and an engineer in case of emergencies
  - training in order to gain competence in caring for their baby/child with nasal prongs in situ and being able to change the prongs when necessary
  - familiarisation with the use of an apnoea monitor if one is in use
  - information on the need to inform their insurance companies and the local fire station that they will be storing oxygen at home, and may carry cylinders in their car
  - ensuring that they recognise the need for no smoking and are prepared to enforce this
  - having the contact numbers of the CCN and the children's ward readily available.
- A home visit by the CCN or special care baby unit (SCBU) liaison nurse will need to be arranged to check the suitability of the home and discuss the positioning and storage of the oxygen delivery system.
- The parents will need to have a telephone and arrangements should be made to install one if necessary.
- The medical practitioner responsible for prescribing the oxygen delivery system may vary locally between hospital and community.
- Each child should have an individual management plan with information relating to

clinical signs and symptoms. It should include:
  - oxygen prescription
  - amount of oxygen required (litres/minute)
  - sliding scale of parameters or variables with indication of when to seek advice
  - mode of delivery (e.g. face mask, nasal cannulae)
  - delivery system required
  - equipment to be used (e.g. humidifier, pulse oximeter, apnoea monitor).
- Discharge planning is essential, as is the transfer of information to all relevant professionals between hospital and community.

Equipment required

- Apnoea monitor and possibly baby alarm
- Nebuliser/nebuhaler if necessary
- Portable oxygen cylinder
- Low-flow head compatible with the cylinder and a carrying bag
- Spare nasal prongs and tape
- Humidifying device if necessary
- Prescribed drugs including saline nasal drops as required
- Equipment to measure oxygen saturation and heart rate if the child needs monitoring overnight.

The family will need to be in touch with the social worker to claim any benefits to which they are entitled, e.g. payment of telephone and electricity bills. They will be entitled to a disability living allowance, but may require help to complete the appropriate forms.

They may find it helpful to be given the name of a family in a similar situation (Golder 1993).

Initially the family will need frequent home visits as they often feel very isolated at home and may experience a delayed reaction to their baby's admission to a SCBU (Golder 1993).

Ongoing support is essential to enable the parents to cope with the oxygen-dependent baby or child. As they become more proficient and the child more stable, the CCN can advise the parents on future management to enable them to be more mobile.

high-pressure oxygen therapy (see Factors to note, p. 259).

- There is a risk of respiratory depression in children who have chronic obstructive respiratory disease (see Factors to note, p. 259).
- Whenever oxygen therapy is administered, remember that there is an increased risk of fire as oxygen is highly flammable.

Do and do not

- Do ensure that the oxygen is prescribed.
- Do remember to check whether or not humidity is required.
- Do check whether the child has any chronic lung disease which could affect the normal

functioning of the respiratory centre and therefore the child's response to oxygen therapy.

- Do monitor the duration and concentration of oxygen therapy at all times.
- Do not administer high concentrations of oxygen over prolonged periods without discussion with senior medical staff (particularly to the neonate or premature infant).
- Do not administer more than 6 litres/minute of oxygen via a nasal cannula, or more than 2 litres/minute in neonates and infants <6 months (Bower et al 1996).

References

Advanced Paediatric Life Support Group 2001 Advanced paediatric life support – the practical approach. BMJ Publishing, London

Ashurst S 1995 Oxygen therapy. British Journal of Nursing 4(9): 508–515

BCH 1993 Oxygen administration within children's services unit. Birmingham Children's Hospital Procedure Manual. BCH, Birmingham, p 132–137

Bower L, Barnhant S L, Betit P 1996 Selection of an oxygen delivery device for neonatal and pediatric patients. American Association of Respiratory Care, Clinical Practice Guideline. Respiratory Care 41(7): 637–646

British Medical Association (BMA) 2005 British National Formulary 49. British Medical Association and The Royal Pharmaceutical Society of Great Britain. The Pharmaceutical Press, Oxon. Online. Available: www.bnf.org

Chandler T 2001 Oxygen administration. Paediatric Nursing 13(8): 37–43

Chiumello D, Bottino N, Pelosi P 2003 Conditioning of medical gases during spontaneous breathing. In: Vincent J (ed.) Yearbook of intensive care and emergency medicine. Springer-Verlag, Berlin, Germany, p 255–263

Frey B, Shann F 2003 Oxygen administration in infants. Archives of Disease in Childhood 88(2): F84–F88

Golder S 1993 Parents support group. Paediatric Nursing 5(3): 14

George C D, Gordon I 1995 Imaging the paediatric chest. In: Prasad S A, Hussey J (eds) Paediatric respiratory care. Chapman and Hall, London, ch 3, p 34–35

Hanna D 1995 Guidelines for pulse oximetry use in pediatrics. Journal of Pediatric Nursing 10(2): 124–126

Hazinski M F 1998 Manual of pediatric critical care. Mosby, St Louis, MO

Kotecha S, Allen J 2002 Oxygen therapy for infants with chronic lung disease. Archives of Disease in Childhood 87(1): F11–F14

Mehtar S 1992 Hospital infection control. Oxford University Press, Oxford, ch 5, p 121–123

Pilkington F 2004 Humidification for oxygen therapy for non-ventilated patients. British Journal of Nursing 13(2): 111–115

Resuscitation Council (UK) 2000 Paediatric advanced life support. Resuscitation Guidelines. Resuscitation Council (UK), London. Online. Available: www.resus.org.uk/pages/pals.htm

Sims J 1996 Making sense of pulse oximetry and oxygen dissociation curve. Nursing Times 92(1): 34–35

Stevenson G 1992 Infection risks in respiratory therapy. Nursing Standard 6(18): 32–33

Tasker R 1995 Management of the acutely ill child in respiratory failure. In: Prasad S A, Hussey J (eds) Paediatric respiratory care. Chapman and Hall, London, ch 4, p 43–45

Wilson J 1995 Infection control in clinical practice. Baillière Tindall, London, ch 5, p 235–238

Wong D L, Hockenberry M, Wilson D et al 2002 Whaley and Wong's nursing care of infants and children, 7th edn. Mosby Year Book, St Louis, MO

Practice **18**

Pain management

Sue Pickup, Susan Aitkenhead

Introduction

Pain is a subjective experience which is inherently difficult to assess, particularly in children, who often lack the verbal or cognitive ability to express their feelings of pain (Gaffney et al 2003). However, pain assessment is essential, not only to detect pain but to evaluate the effectiveness of our pain management interventions if we are to provide optimal pain control.

Learning outcomes

By the end of this section you should:

- be aware of the myths surrounding pain in children
- recognise how your own feelings and beliefs may affect your assessment of pain in children
- have developed an awareness of the different types of assessment tools and the factors affecting their application
- understand the importance of routine pain assessment and documentation, involving the parent and, more importantly, the child where possible
- be aware of the commonly used analgesic drugs and the different routes of administration
- understand the importance of administering balanced analgesia
- have an insight into the assessment and treatment of chronic and recurrent pain in children
- understand the need for sedation and have an insight into the principles of good sedation practice.

Rationale

The treatment and alleviation of pain is a basic human right that exists regardless of age (Schechter et al 2003). The consequences of untreated pain include a delay in mobilisation, psychological trauma, an increase in the risk of infections, slower recovery and a delay in discharge from hospital. The undertreatment of pain in children is evident in the literature (Wilson & Doyle 1996, Nikanne et al 1999); however, over recent years, the problems of managing pain in children are beginning to be addressed. In 1993, in a publication entitled *Children First: A Study of Hospital Services*, the Audit Commission identified pain relief as an indicator for measuring quality of care for children in hospital. More recently, the *National Service Framework for Children* has outlined standards for managing pain in hospital (DoH 2003). Assessment of a child's pain is problematic but it is essential if we are to provide effective management and therefore it must be an integral part of our nursing care.

ASSESSMENT OF PAIN

Guidelines

The family has an important role to play in ensuring that a child's pain is managed effectively (Liossi 2002). Where the situation permits, this involves determining a child's past pain experiences and whether these were good or bad. Children may use a variety of words to describe pain and these should be identified prior to potentially painful experiences (RCN 1999). A description of the child's behaviour which would normally indicate the presence of pain should be sought from the parents. The family may already employ certain coping strategies; these, along with analgesics used at home, should be discussed. Parents can also be helpful in identifying the pain assessment scale that may be appropriate for their child. Parents can be a particularly valuable resource with children with complex needs. Some pain assessment tools are available to help guide the professional to assess the pain in this group of children (RCN 2001, Voepel-Lewis et al 2002). These children may be unable to articulate or express their pain verbally or behaviourally. Carter et al (2002) found that parents used various strategies to identify their child's pain

based on their in-depth knowledge of their child. The identification of this skill is also supported by findings from a study by Stallard et al (2001).

Pain is difficult to measure accurately and reliably in children. There are several pain scales available for paediatric use; however, development of verbal skills and cognitive ability show wide variation in children and this must be taken into account. Sociocultural and environmental factors must also be noted. In addition to selecting the appropriate scale for an individual child, the nurse must consider several issues:

- the period of time that is available to teach the child how to use the assessment scale
- whether the child is able to grasp the function of the scale, enabling the nurse to achieve an accurate assessment
- whether the child is comfortable with using the scale; it is important that the nurse obtains the child's commitment to working with it
- if the child has a choice of pain scales, the nurse must abide by the choice and preference of the child.

It is vital that the nurse is completely familiar with the use of the pain assessment scale. A problem identified by Harrison (1991) is the need to differentiate between inaccuracy and bias when assessing pain. Harrison (1991) suggests that to overcome this problem nurses and observers should be trained to use assessment techniques more skilfully, thus helping to increase their sensitivity to pain cues. This is particularly important with children who are too sick to use self-reporting scales, neonates/infants and children with special needs. Pain assessment should be part of a holistic approach to the child. The nurse should be able to take the information provided by the child and interpret it with skill. For example, a report of pain described in a particular manner may indicate a full bladder and urinary retention rather than wound pain. This should be treated in a different way and it is important, therefore, that the information given is channelled correctly.

It is also vital that children who can comprehend the pain scale and self-report are made aware that if they are in pain the treatment of that pain is patient friendly.

Harrison (1991) also concluded that children are capable of providing an accurate pain assessment but that the consequences of doing so may prevent them.

It is widely recognised that self-reporting pain scales are the most accurate when children can describe their pain in an appropriate manner and relevant language for their age and development (Broome & Huth 2003). However, for certain patients this will not be possible.

Factors to note

Sick children

A very sick child may be too ill to comprehend instructions regarding the use of a pain scale. A child in an intensive care setting, who is perhaps ventilated, sedated or paralysed, will be unable to use a self-reporting scale that would normally be used for their age and development. With these patients, physiological and behavioural factors should be considered jointly to enable the nurse to judge whether the child is distressed by pain. The child may also become distressed by the requirement for suction, position change or oral hygiene and this should be taken into consideration. As the nurse develops a relationship with the patient they will be able to differentiate between distress and pain and the pain scale will be an aid to this nursing skill.

Culture

It is accepted that culture can influence an individual's perception and response to pain (Bates 1987). However, over the years most of the studies looking at culture have been in relation to adults (Bernstein & Pachter 2003). Recommendations have been made which suggest we should recognise the importance of cultural factors which affect the assessment of pain in children (RCN 1999). It is important that, whilst being aware of cultural differences in pain expression, we should try to avoid stereotyping (Bernstein & Pachter 2003).

Neonates

Neonates cannot communicate by verbal report so they are dependent on caregivers to recognise that they are in pain. Physiological and behavioural signs must be observed and interpreted as an indication of pain being present. A variety of scales have been made available for neonates, taking into consideration physiological and behavioural factors such as facial expression, crying, body position, body movement, colour, oxygen saturation (SaO_2), respiratory rate, blood pressure and heart rate (Hodgkinson et al 1994, Krechel & Bildner 1995). However, it should be noted that these observations can be affected by a variety of factors as well as pain, such as ventilatory support, drugs and the neonate's clinical condition. The scales that take this into consideration may be more accurate (Sparshott 1996).

Infants/toddlers

Similar problems occur with infants and toddlers regarding the use of pain scales. Again the nurse should be able to pick up pain cues from the infant/toddler by observing physiological and behavioural signs and then act appropriately. Toddlers may clutch at the site of the surgery. They may also display the characteristic signs of frustration and unhappiness that they cannot communicate verbally.

Children (preschool to 7 years)

Studies have shown that many 3 year olds can identify the presence and absence of pain and can report a pain intensity (Harbeck & Peterson 1992, Romsing et al 1996). It is recommended that the choice of pain intensity scores for this age group should be limited to around four choices. They can usually verbalise in appropriate language, to the nurse or their parents, a description of 'their hurting'. It is important to remember that younger children may choose extremes of measurement and some may even confuse the scales with measurements of happiness. Some children in this age group may experience behavioural disturbances due to the trauma of hospital admission. Regression to earlier stages in development, such as loss of speech, clinging to parents or a return to bed wetting, may be noticed. Aggression may be a form of identifying pain. Children may be in pain but unable or reluctant to indicate that it is present. Their behaviour becomes aggressive as a response to this pain. It is important that nursing staff can recognise this and educate parents to avoid a child being labelled as naughty.

Older children (7 years to adolescence)

Older children of a normal developmental level can usually self-report their pain and understand the use of visual analogue scales.

Although adolescents are developing quickly physically, emotional development can be at a different rate. It should be remembered that they will be anxious and often frightened about hospitalisation. They may be aware of peer group pressure and may not admit to pain because of fear of ridicule or comparison to another child. Fear of treatment may also be a problem. The nurse should ensure that adolescent patients have complete privacy and quiet to report any pain and that they are aware of the 'patient-friendly' treatments.

Conducting a pain assessment

History taking

It is vital that the nurse, on admitting a child to the ward or unit, takes a pain history from the parents or guardian. The nurse should record the child's reaction to pain, the usual method for reporting pain (if developmentally able) and what happens in response to pain at home. This information should be incorporated into the nursing care plan. The appropriate scale should be selected at this time, if possible taking into account:

- age
- mechanical interventions that may be necessary
- special needs
- clinical condition
- type of pain, i.e. acute, chronic or recurrent.

Documentation of pain assessments should occur and guidelines recommend that they be recorded on the routine observation chart (Royal College of Surgeons and the College of Anaesthetists 1990). This is important because there is evidence to suggest that accurate documentation increases the assessment of pain and the administration of analgesia (Savedra et al 1993, Goddard & Pickup 1996). For postoperative pain, for example, a pain scale should be used to assess a child's pain with the routine postoperative observations, decreasing in frequency as the observations decrease but more regularly if a child is complaining of pain or analgesia has been administered.

Pain assessment scales usually incorporate one or more of the following:

- behavioural assessment
- physiological assessment
- self-report techniques.

Behavioural assessment

This involves looking at how a child behaves in response to pain.

Types of distress behaviour, e.g. facial expression, cry and body movements, have been associated with pain. However, difficulties include differentiating this behaviour from behaviour that results from anxiety or hunger (Gaffney et al 2003).

Several coding systems have been developed for infants; however, intense crying with high motor activity could indicate pain, whilst equally an infant that is withdrawn and quiet could also be in pain, highlighting the difficulties.

It must be remembered that behaviour can be affected by many things including drugs, splints, ventilation and prematurity.

Behavioural pain assessment has some advantages in that it is non-invasive, does not put any demands on the child and does not depend on their cognitive ability or language skills.

Assessment of behavioural signs could indicate the presence of pain and help determine the effect the pain is having on the child or infant.

Physiological assessment

Physiological signs vary greatly, particularly in premature infants (Stevens et al 1996).

Different parameters have been examined, including:

- pulse rate
- respiratory rate
- blood pressure
- neurochemical and neurohormonal activity
- palmar sweating
- SaO_2.

There is a debate surrounding the reliability of using physiological signs to determine the presence of pain (Carter 1994). There is in fact insufficient evidence to suggest that physiological signs are directly related to the pain experienced. Like behavioural responses, physiological responses can be affected by many things, resulting in problems of interpretation.

Self-report techniques

As pain is a subjective experience, self-reporting techniques are acknowledged as the most accurate indicators of pain (Broome & Huth 2003); however, they rely on children having the relevant language for their age and development and the ability to describe their pain in an appropriate manner. It must be remembered that a child's self-report of pain may be affected by contextual factors or concerns regarding the pain-relieving interventions that may be offered.

For many years there has been agreement that multidimensional assessment is essential. Ross and Ross (1988) suggested that the three pain assessment components – behavioural assessments, physiological assessments and self-report techniques – taking into account contextual factors, 'enable us to draw some conclusions about the child's pain'.

A well-established approach that takes these factors into account is QUESTT (Baker & Wong 1987):

Question the child
Use pain assessment scales
Evaluate behaviour and physiological signs
Secure the parents' involvement
Take the cause of pain into account
Take action and evaluate results

Some of the pain scales that are available for children are listed in Table 18.1. Other scales are:

- Poker Chip Tool (Beyer & Wells 1989)
- Oucher (Beyer & Wells 1989)
- Colour Scales (Beyer & Wells 1989)
- Coloured Vertical Analogue (McGrath et al 1996)
- Horizontal Linear Analogue (Beyer & Wells 1989)
- Adjectival Self Report (Morton 1993)
- Sheffield Children's Hospital Pain Assessment Tool (Goddard & Pickup 1996) (see Fig. 18.1).

MANAGEMENT OF PAIN

Pain has both physical and psychological components and as a result both physical and psychological methods of pain management can be employed.

NON-DRUG METHODS OF PAIN MANAGEMENT

Psychological techniques including distraction, using interactive toys and games, e.g. pop-up books, music books, blowing bubbles and guided imagery, where the child is encouraged to imagine something pleasant, e.g. a favourite holiday destination, have been shown to reduce pain (Duff 2003). These techniques can help distract and relax a child. Transcutaneous electrical nerve stimulation (TENS) machines can relieve pain and be useful in reducing conventional analgesic requirements (Merkel et al 1999).

Massage, aromatherapy and reflexology have a role to play in pain management. For further information on these methods, see 'Complementary Therapies', (p. 465).

DRUG METHODS OF PAIN CONTROL

Broadly speaking there are two types of analgesia: centrally acting and peripherally acting. These terms describe their specific sites of action in the nervous system: centrally acting drugs act on the opioid receptors in the brain and spinal cord; peripherally acting drugs inhibit the production of prostaglandins, which sensitise the nerve endings to pain.

Analgesics are generally described as either opiates or non-opiates.

Table 18.1   Children's pain scales

Scale	Age range	Comments
OPS (Broadman et al 1988)	Neonate to 7 years	Easy to use Follows pain over a period of time Accurate between assessors Cannot be used with intubated or paralysed patients
CRIES (Krechel & Bildner 1995)	Neonate	Easy to use Reliable down to 32 weeks gestational age Uses SaO_2 as a measure, which can be affected by many other factors
COMFORT (Ambuel et al 1992)	Neonate to 7 years	Complicated scale to use Cannot be used with intubated or paralysed patients
TIPPS (Tarbell et al 1992)	Infant/toddler	Correlates with nurse and parent assessment Pain scores follow the effects of the analgesia, i.e. decrease if analgesia satisfactory, increase when more is required
FACES (Beyer & Wells 1989)	Child 3–7 years	Younger children may choose extremes Some children may confuse with happiness measurements
CHEOPS (McGrath et al 1985)	Child 3–7 years	Complicated behavioural scale May not track postoperative pain adequately in children of this age who are experiencing behavioural disturbances due to trauma of hospital admission
NPS (Lawrence et al 1993)	Neonate	Cannot be used in intubated or paralysed patients Six categories but two of these very similar

Routes of analgesia administration

Oral

This tends to be the preferred route of analgesia administration in children because of their dislike of needles.

Rectal

This route is useful when children are experiencing nausea and vomiting or are nil by mouth.

Intravenous

Analgesia can be administered via this route as a bolus dose, a continuous infusion or as patient-controlled analgesia (PCA) (see 'Opiates', below).

Intramuscular

This is the least preferred route of analgesia administration, often causing pain and anxiety.

Subcutaneous

The subcutaneous route, through a subcutaneous cannula, can be used as an alternative to intramuscular injections. Analgesia can be administered continuously or as a bolus dose when required.

Topical

The use of a topical local anaesthetic cream, e.g. EMLA or Ametop, can reduce the pain and discomfort a child may experience during intravenous cannulation or blood sampling.

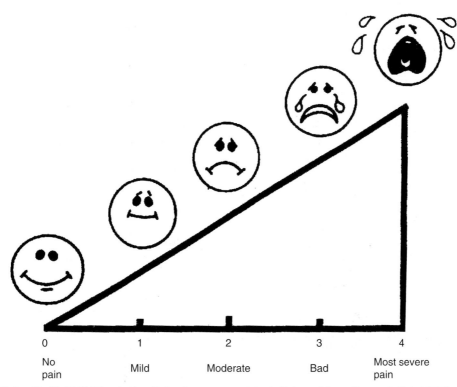

0   1   2   3   4

No pain   Mild   Moderate   Bad   Most severe pain

Figure 18.1   Sheffield Children's Hospital pain assessment tool. (Adapted from Brown & Fisk 1992.)

Local/regional

For postoperative analgesia, blocks – including femoral nerve blocks, lumbar plexus blocks, penile blocks and ilio-inguinal blocks – are performed by the anaesthetist whilst a child is anaesthetised. Wound infiltration with local anaesthetics is also used for postoperative pain and for procedures in the accident and emergency department.

Inhalation

Entonox, for example, is a self-administered inhaled gas that will provide analgesia for procedural pain of short duration (for further information, see Analgesia – Entonox, p. 275).

Intrathecal

This is the instillation of drugs into the subarachnoid space to produce an analgesic effect.

Epidural

This is the instillation of drugs into the epidural space (extradural space). A caudal block is an epidural block using a sacral approach (see Fig. 18.2).

Transdermal

This is where an analgesic drug is absorbed through the skin, creating a systemic effect. Fentanyl patches are an example of transdermal analgesia.

Transmucosal

Drugs are rapidly absorbed from the oral and nasal mucosa. The analgesic buprenorphine utilises this route.

Analgesia

EMLA and Ametop

These are topical local anaesthetics that are used to reduce the pain experienced during blood tests and venous cannulation. When using either EMLA or Ametop, they need to be applied to the skin and then covered with an

Epidural Pain Management

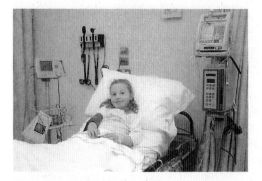

You have had your operation and wake up back in the ward.

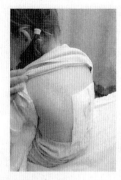

To stop you feeling sore you will have a special tube in your back. This tube will have been put in when you had your operation. Sticky tape stops this tube from falling out.

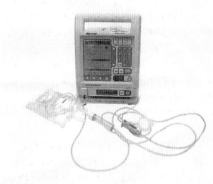

A machine will give you medicine through this tube to stop you feeling sore.

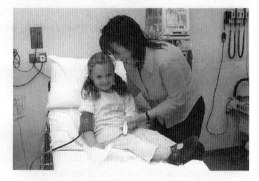

Sometimes this medicine can make your legs feel a bit wobbly but don't worry this won't last too long. **Remember – ask for help if you want to get out of bed.**

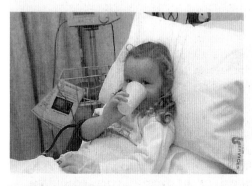

You are still able to sit up in your bed and eat and drink when your doctor says that you can......

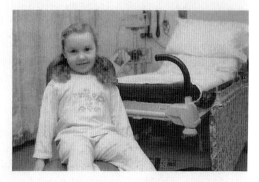

You will probably only need this tube for a couple of days.

Figure 18.2   Epidural pain management

occlusive dressing. EMLA needs to be applied at least 60 minutes before the procedure and can be used for children over 1 year of age. Ametop works more quickly, needing to be applied 30 minutes before blood taking and 45 minutes before venous cannulation. Ametop can be used with children and infants from 1 month of age upwards.

Paracetamol

Although paracetamol is highly toxic in overdose, it is a safe and effective analgesic when administered in therapeutic doses (Hanson et al 1999). It has antipyretic properties but no recognised anti-inflammatory effects.

Suboptimal doses of paracetamol have been shown not to provide analgesia postoperatively (Pickering et al 2002). *Medicines for Children* (RCPCH 2003) gives clear guidance on appropriate analgesic dosages. The guidance includes appropriate loading and maintenance dosages, highlighting the increased dosages required when paracetamol is administered rectally.

Ibuprofen and diclofenac

These are non-steroidal anti-inflammatory drugs (NSAIDs). They produce an analgesic, antipyretic and anti-inflammatory effect. NSAIDs should be administered with caution to children who are asthmatics. There is a theoretical risk of an allergic reaction to these types of drug. Extreme caution should be taken if a child has a coagulation defect, renal disease or any renal impairment.

Opiates

There are several methods of administering opiate analgesia, with the subcutaneous and intravenous routes currently increasing in popularity. Morphine remains the most widely used opiate in children.

Some children, although not requiring opiates continually to control pain, may still require one or two doses of opiate during the postoperative period. To avoid the use of intramuscular injections, a subcutaneous cannula can be sited in theatre or on the ward, after applying EMLA or Ametop. Nursing staff can then administer bolus doses of morphine as required. Morphine can also be administered continuously via this route. This method of analgesia administration should be used with caution in a child who has impaired peripheral circulation.

Patient-controlled analgesia (PCA) is a method of intravenous analgesia administration, usually of an opioid such as morphine sulphate. The child (usually aged 5 and over) controls their own analgesia by means of a hand-held button attached to a computerised pump. The child's developmental age should be appropriate for the chronological age and the child must understand cause and effect relationships in order to appreciate that pain relief will result from pressing the button.

The pump is set up with a suitable dose of analgesia calculated on the child's body weight and age. The pump permits the child to self-administer a small pre-set amount of analgesia by pressing the handset. A maximum dose per hour and a lockout interval is programmed into the pump so that the child cannot overdose, thus ensuring safety. The child is then able to titrate their own requirements of analgesia in an efficient and safe manner (see Fig. 18.3).

Some studies have found that the administration of a background (continuous) infusion for the first night following surgery gives the child a better sleep pattern (Doyle et al 1993). The child also has the handset available for breakthrough pain but this continuous infusion seems to 'take the edge off' the pain and lets them sleep comfortably (Fisher 2000).

It is important that all children and parents are given a clear explanation regarding the use of PCA. It should always be stressed that for safety reasons only the child presses the handset. Parents can encourage their child to press the button when they are sore and younger children need regular reinforcement of the idea to maintain optimal analgesia (Fisher 1999). Parents should never press the button for the child. If the child is unable to comprehend or physically press the handset, nurse-controlled analgesia should be considered.

For children in whom PCA is not appropriate, an intravenous infusion of opiate can be

P.C.A. Pain Management

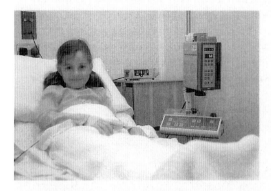

You have had your operation and wake up back in the ward.

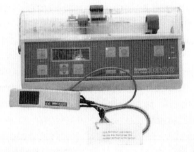

To stop you feeling sore you will have a special machine.

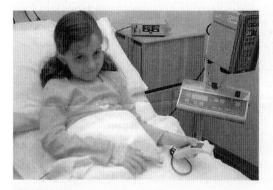

This machine also has a button – see the picture above.

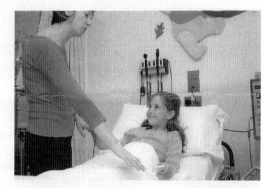

This button is for you to press only if you are sore – no one else must press this button – not even the doctors and nurses!!!

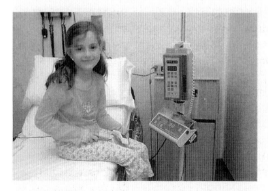

You can also press your button before you get out of bed......

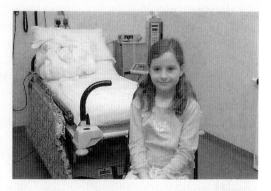

You will probably only need your machine for a couple of days.

Figure 18.3   PCA pain management

connected to run continuously. Nurse- or parent-controlled analgesia may also be an option, following specifically produced guidelines.

The aim of morphine administration is to achieve the optimum level of analgesia with minimal side-effects. Side-effects include excessive sedation, respiratory depression, nausea, vomiting, pruritus and urinary retention. A child's vital signs should be monitored for complications and the child observed for side-effects. Regular pain assessments are necessary to determine if the morphine is having the desired effect.

Codeine phosphate and dihydrocodeine are opiates most commonly administered orally.

Entonox

Entonox is an analgesic gas composed of 50% nitrous oxide and 50% oxygen. It is an effective inhalation method of managing procedural pain of short duration. The gas is self-administered through a demand apparatus. When the child starts to become drowsy their hand will fall away, thus safeguarding the child from overdose. The onset of analgesia is rapid, usually within 2–3 minutes and the effects wear off quickly. It can be used alone or with analgesics and has few side-effects and contraindications (British Oxygen Company 1995).

Entonox has been shown to be useful in several situations. It is effective in the accident and emergency department for fracture reduction (Wattenmaker et al 1990), chest drain removal (Bruce & Franck 2000) and the removal of orthopaedic wires and screws (Pickup & Pagdin 2000/2001).

Supervision of a child self-administering Entonox can be carried out by a nurse who has received appropriate training. Nursing staff should be aware of the indications for use, the side-effects and contraindications, the administration equipment, the need to scavenge waste gases and the benefits of Entonox for managing procedural pain.

Balanced analgesia

Pain control can be enhanced by using a combination of analgesic approaches. A child using a morphine PCA pump, for example, will have their pain more effectively managed if an NSAID and/or paracetamol are administered. This will reduce the child's opiate requirements and therefore the potential for side-effects, whilst attacking the pain both centrally and peripherally. Also, the use of local and regional analgesia techniques can significantly reduce the amount of analgesia required postoperatively.

Evaluation

Record keeping is a fundamental part of nursing practice (NMC 2004). It is necessary to evaluate and document the efficacy of any pain-relieving interventions regularly. It is also important to observe that the child is not experiencing side-effects as a result of analgesia administration. It must be remembered that other factors can increase the pain experienced by a child, for example anxiety and muscle tension, and this must be taken into account in planning pain-relieving interventions.

Sedation

Invasive procedures such as lumbar punctures or bone marrow aspirations, the administration of intrathecal drugs or urinary catheterisation, etc. can be extremely distressing for children. It is often suggested that to reduce the distress or anxiety caused by these procedures children should be sedated. Sedation is defined as 'a drug-induced depression of consciousness during which patients respond purposefully to verbal commands, either alone or accompanied by light tactile stimulation. No interventions are required to maintain a patent airway, and spontaneous ventilation is adequate' (SIGN 2002).

Drugs with sedative properties usually do not provide analgesia and the choice of technique or drug should be determined by considering if the procedure to be undertaken is painful or painless (SIGN 2002).

Studies indicate that few paediatric departments have protocols for the safe and effective sedation of children (Morton & Oomen 1998). The research suggests that available resources rather than scientific evidence influence practice. Non-pharmacological techniques are often not considered and the valuable resource of the play specialist not requested. All sedation techniques are considered to carry some sort of risk (Cote et al 2000). A Scottish guideline has therefore been developed to provide recommendations in the practice of sedation of children who are undergoing diagnostic and therapeutic procedures to minimise this risk (SIGN 2002). This guideline recommends the following principles of good sedation practice:

- A combination of non-pharmacological and pharmacological methods should be considered.
- Some children may be unsuitable for sedation and may require general anaesthesia.
- An individual approach should be taken for each child to minimise fear, anxiety, distress and pain.
- Sedation should only be undertaken in an environment where the facilities, equipment and personnel to manage paediatric emergency situations are immediately available.
- It is essential that informed consent be obtained prior to any procedures being undertaken with a clear explanation of the sedation technique proposed and possible adverse effects.
- Monitoring should be commenced from the time of administration of the sedative agent until predetermined recovery criteria are met.
- Discharge should not be initiated until all predetermined criteria are met.

The sedation of children should not be undertaken lightly. Cote et al (2000) found that children could suffer drug-related adverse outcomes after the administration of a variety of medicines and routes of administration. Every child undergoing sedation should receive an optimal standard of monitoring by experienced paediatric health professionals with facilities and equipment to manage paediatric emergency situations immediately available.

MANAGEMENT OF CHRONIC PAIN

Not all children experience pain continuously. Many children experience recurrent pains, the most common of which are abdominal pain, limb pain and headaches (Eccleston et al 2003).

Chronic or recurrent pain can be debilitating for both the child and family as it leads to a general reduction in activity, which in turn affects school attendance, participation in sports and leisure activities, resulting in loss of social contacts and isolation. The pain can result in lack of sleep, affecting concentration and schoolwork. All these factors eventually alter attitude and mood, creating a downward spiral of the child's confidence and self-esteem.

Chronic pain assessment should follow the same decision-making processes from the nurse as the assessment of acute pain. Few validated pain assessment tools are available for the assessment of chronic pain in children, although it has been recognised that the paediatric chronic pain management centres in the UK have developed local tools to aid the assessment process (Aitkenhead 2001).

History taking is vital and a thorough background report to the pain, including the following, should be undertaken:

- Pain details – when did the pain begin? Where is the pain? Is it present all the time? Can you get to sleep at night? Does the pain wake you up?
- Words to describe the pain (this is particularly helpful in the identification of neuropathic pain).
- How does the pain affect your life?
- What medications have helped or not helped (helpful in identifying non-opioid responsive pain).
- Is there anything else that helps the pain (non-pharmacological strategies)?
- Any trigger points?
- A drawing of the pain.

Whether or not an identifiable organic cause is found, children experiencing chronic or recurrent pain require specialised help and support to enable them to cope.

It has long been recognised that the management of chronic pain in adults benefits from a multidisciplinary approach, involving physiotherapy, psychological techniques and medication (Bonica 1953). This approach was first applied to the care of children experiencing chronic or recurrent pain in the late 1980s (Berde et al 1989). Unfortunately, in the UK there are still very few children's hospitals able to offer this approach.

Whether a child is an inpatient or is being seen as an outpatient, it is important that the professionals work collaboratively through the use of an interdisciplinary model. This is where the child sees the professionals together in both the assessment and treatment process rather than being sent from professional to professional.

Due to the complex nature of chronic pain, a variety of treatments are often required which may include the following.

Physiotherapy
- General exercise programmes, stretching, relaxation and massage as part of an individual programme
- Advice regarding 'pacing' and graduated regaining of functional activities
- Transcutaneous electrical nerve stimulation and other methods such as ultrasound therapy may be used.

Psychology
- Hypnosis/guided imagery and relaxation to control anxiety and help reduce pain
- Cognitive–behavioural techniques to modify pain-related attitude and behaviour patterns
- Individual or family therapy.

Medicines
- Various types of analgesia
- Sedatives

- Antidepressants
- Anticonvulsants
- Regional or local nerve blocks.

Children experiencing chronic or recurrent pain and their families often present with a variety of medical, social and psychological difficulties. It is this variety of problems that creates a challenge for the professionals, demonstrating the need for a multidisciplinary approach.

Summary of pain assessment complications

- There may not be consistent behavioural and physiological changes in all infants and children experiencing pain.
- Many factors, including distress, can affect both behaviour and the physiological signs used to assess pain.
- It is difficult to distinguish between stress and pain, particularly in the infant or neonate.
- The ability to self-report depends on the cognitive ability and language skills of a child and may be affected by clinical condition, drugs or mechanical interventions.
- Children may report lower pain intensity than they are experiencing for fear of the consequences.
- A child's pain can be affected by previous pain experiences, cultural and social expectations and levels of anxiety.
- As nurses, our own experiences of pain and our preconceived ideas about how much an injury or certain type of surgery should hurt may affect our interpretation of a situation.

COMMUNITY PERSPECTIVE

Parents are likely to be more 'tuned in' to their child in pain than professionals. However, there will be times when parents lose their objectivity about this, especially during terminal care. Denying the level of pain may be a coping strategy for a parent but this takes away the rights of the child.

The role of the CCN is to be aware of the dynamics within the family and sensitively to lead the parents to a more objective assessment. For this to be possible, the family must have developed trust in the CCN and, when appropriate, other members of the team. Once their cooperation has been gained in titrating analgesia and

Community Perspective continues

they are able to recognise that the child is more settled and possibly able to participate in family life, a hurdle will have been surmounted, the child's pain will be better managed and the relationship between family and nurses strengthened.

Each individual case will need consideration as to whether the use of pain scales will be helpful. Although it may be appropriate to use them in an acute pain situation, for example the child with a fractured femur, it may be less so for the terminally ill child. Ongoing assessment of pain, however, is essential, whether this is undertaken using pain scales or as an ongoing assessment as part and parcel of family life. The preference of the child must be valued.

For the child with communication difficulties, the parents are almost without exception those who recognise when their child is in pain. The role of the CCN here is to listen and learn from the parents and take action accordingly.

Do and do not

- Do involve the parents and, more importantly, the child.
- Do take into account the child's age, clinical condition, type of pain, and any special needs or mechanical interventions.
- Do use a multidimensional pain assessment scale where possible.
- Do evaluate any pain-relief strategies.
- Do consider the use of non-pharmacological pain-relieving strategies, either individually or in conjunction with pharmacological strategies.
- Do not let your own beliefs and values cloud your judgement when assessing pain.
- Do not let the common myths and misconceptions surrounding pain in children affect your assessment strategies. These include:
  - babies and infants do not feel pain
  - children do not remember pain
  - children who are playing or sleeping cannot be in pain
  - children always tell the truth about their pain.

Remember that pain is a subjective experience which is not solely dependent on the amount of tissue damage involved. It can be affected by many things which should be reflected in our assessment strategies and choice of assessment scales.

References

Aitkenhead S 2001 Managing chronic pain in children. Nursing Times 97(29): 34–35

Ambuel B, Hamlett K W, Marx C M, Plummer J L 1992 Assessing distress in pediatric intensive care environments. The COMFORT scale. Journal of Pediatric Psychology 17: 95–109

Audit Commission 1993 Children first: a study of hospital services. HMSO, London

Baker C, Wong D 1987 Q.U.E.S.T.T.: a process of pain assessment in children. Orthopaedic Nursing 6(1): 11–21

Bates M S 1987 Ethnicity and pain: a biocultural model. Social Science and Medicine 24(1): 47–50

Berde C B, Sethna N F, Maset B, Fosby M 1989 Paediatric pain clinics: recommendations for their development. Paediatrician 16: 94–102

Bernstein B A, Pachter L M 2003 Cultural considerations in children's pain. In: Schechter N L, Berde C B, Yaster M (eds) Pain in infants, children and adolescents, 2nd edn. Lippincott, Williams and Wilkins, Philadelphia

Beyer J E, Wells N 1989 The assessment of pain in children. Pediatric Clinics of North America 36: 837–853

Bonica J J 1953 The management of pain. Lea and Febiger, Philadelphia

British Oxygen Company 1995 Entonox Medical Gas Data Sheet G4042. BOC Gases, Guildford, UK

Broadman L M, Rice L H, Hannallah R S 1988 Testing the validity of an objective pain scale for infants and children. Anesthesiology 69: A770

Broome M E, Huth M M 2003 Nursing management of the child in pain. In: Schechter N L, Berde C B, Yester M (eds) Pain in infants, children and adolescents, 2nd edn. Lippincott, Williams and Wilkins, Philadelphia

Brown T C K, Fisk G C 1992 Anaesthesia for children, 2nd edn. Blackwell Scientific, Oxford, p 129

Bruce E, Franck L 2000 Self-administered nitrous oxide (Entonox) for the management of procedural pain. Paediatric Nursing 12(7): 15–19

Carter B 1994 Child and infant pain. Chapman and Hall, London

Carter B, McArthur E, Cunliffe M 2002 Dealing with uncertainty: parental assessment of pain in their children with profound special needs. Journal of Advanced Nursing 38(5): 449–457

Cote C J, Karl H W, Notterman D A, Weinberg J A, McCloskey C 2000 Adverse sedation events in pediatrics: analysis of medications used for sedation. Pediatrics 106: 633–644

Department of Health 2003 Getting the right start. National Service Framework for children: standard for hospital services. DoH, London

Doyle E, Robinson D, Morton N S 1993 Comparison of patient controlled analgesia with and without a background infusion after lower abdominal surgery in children. British Journal of Anaesthesia 71(5): 670–673

Duff A J A 2003 Incorporating psychological approaches into routine paediatric venepuncture. Archives of Disease in Childhood 88: 931–937

Eccleston C, Malleson P N, Clinch J, Connell H, Sourbut C 2003 Chronic pain in adolescents: evaluation of a programme of interdisciplinary cognitive behaviour therapy. Archives of Disease in Childhood 88: 881–885

Fisher S 1999 Small relief. Nursing Times 95(23): 52–53

Fisher S 2000 Postoperative pain management in paediatrics. British Journal of Perioperative Nursing 10(1): 80–84

Gaffney A, McGrath P J, Dick B 2003 Measuring pain in children: developmental and instrument issues. In: Schechter N L, Berde C B, Yaster M (eds) Pain in infants, children and adolescents, 2nd edn. Lippincott, Williams and Wilkins, Philadelphia

Goddard J M, Pickup S E 1996 Postoperative pain in children: combining audit and a nurse specialist to improve management. Anaesthesia 51: 588–590

Hanson T G, O'Brien K, Morton N S, Rasmussen S N 1999 Plasma paracetamol concentrations and pharmacokinetics following rectal administration in neonates and young infants. Acta Anaesthesiologica Scandinavica 43(8): 855–859

Harbeck C, Peterson L 1992 Elephants dancing in my head: a developmental approach to children's concepts of specific pains. Child Development 63(1): 138–149

Harrison A 1991 Assessing patients' pain: identifying reasons for error. Journal of Advanced Nursing 16: 1018–1025

Hodgkinson K, Bear M, Thorn J et al 1994 Measuring pain in neonates: evaluating an instrument and developing a common language. Australian Journal of Advanced Nursing 12: 17–22

Krechel S W, Bildner J 1995 CRIES: a new neonatal postoperative pain measurement score. Initial testing of validity and reliability. Paediatric Anaesthesia 5: 53–61

Lawrence J, Alcock D, McGrath P, Kay J, MacMurray S B, Dulberg C 1993 The development of a tool to assess neonatal pain. Neonatal Network 12: 59–65

Liossi C 2002 Procedure-related cancer pain in children. Radcliffe Medical Press, Abingdon, UK

McGrath P J, Johnson G, Goodman J T, Schillinger J, Dunn J, Chapman J A 1985 CHEOPS: a behavioural scale for rating postoperative pain in children. Advances in Pain Research and Therapy 9: 395–402

McGrath P A, Seifert C E, Speechley K N, Booth J C, Stitt L, Gibson M C 1996 A new analogue scale for assessing children's pain – an initial validation study. Pain 64: 435–443

Merkel S I, Gustein H B, Malviya S 1999 Use of transcutaneous electrical nerve stimulation in a young child with pain from open perineal lesions. Journal of Pain and Symptom Management 18(5): 376–381

Morton N S 1993 Development of a monitoring protocol for the safe use of opioids in children. Paediatric Anaesthesia 3: 179–184

Morton N S, Oomen G J 1998 Development of a selection and monitoring protocol for safe sedation of children. Paediatric Anaesthesia 8: 65–68

Nikanne E, Kokki H, Tuovinen K 1999 Postoperative pain after adenoidectomy in children. British Journal of Anaesthesia 82: 886–889

Nursing and Midwifery Council (NMC) 2004 Guidelines for records and record-keeping. NMC, London

Pickering A E, Bridge H S, Nolan J, Stoddart P A 2002 Double-blind, placebo controlled analgesic study of ibuprofen or rofecoxib in combination with paracetamol for tonsillectomy in children. British Journal of Anaesthesia 88(1): 72–77

Pickup S, Pagdin J 2000/2001 Procedural pain: Entonox can help. Paediatric Nursing 12(10): 33–36

Romsing J, Hertel S, Moller-Sonnergaard J, Rasmussen M 1996 Postoperative pain in children: comparison between ratings of children and nurses. Journal of Pain and Symptom Management 11(2): 42–46

Ross D M, Ross S A 1988 Assessment of pediatric pain. Issues in Comprehensive Pediatric Nursing 11: 73–91

Royal College of Nursing (RCN) 1999 Clinical practice guidelines. The recognition and assessment of acute pain in children: recommendations. RCN, London

Royal College of Nursing (RCN) 2001 Clinical practice guidelines. The recognition and assessment of acute pain in children: implementation guide. RCN, London

Royal College of Paediatrics and Child Health (RCPCH) 2003 Medicines for children. RCPCH Publications, London

Royal College of Surgeons and the College of Anaesthetists 1990 Commission on the provision of surgical services. Report of the working party on pain after surgery. Royal College of Surgeons, London

Savedra M C, Holzemer W L, Tesler M D, Wilkie D J 1993 Assessment of postoperation pain in children and adolescents using the adolescent pediatric pain tool. Nursing Research 42(1): 5–9

Schechter N L, Berde C B, Yaster M 2003 Pain in infants, children and adolescents, 2nd edn. Lippincott, Williams and Wilkins, Philadelphia

Scottish Intercollegiate Guidelines Network (SIGN) 2002 Safe sedation of children undergoing diagnostic and therapeutic procedures. SIGN, Edinburgh

Sparshott M 1996 The development of a clinical distress scale for ventilated infants: identification of pain and distress based on validated behavioural scores. Journal of Neonatal Nursing 2: 5–11

Stallard P, Williams L, Lenton S, Velleman R 2001 Pain in cognitively impaired, non-communicating children. Archives of Disease in Childhood 85(6): 460–462

Stevens B, Johnston C, Petryshen P et al 1996 Premature infant pain profile (PIPP): development and initial validation. Clinical Journal of Pain 12: 13–22

Tarbell S E, Cohen I T, Marsh J L 1992 The toddler–pre-school postoperative pain scale: an observational scale for measuring postoperative pain in children aged 1–5. Preliminary report. Pain 50: 273–280

Voepel-Lewis T, Merkel S, Tait A R, Trzcinka A, Malviya S 2002 The reliability and validity of the face, legs, activity, cry, consolability observational tool as a measure of pain in children with cognitive impairment. Anaesthesia and Analgesia 95(5): 1224–1229

Wattenmaker I, Kasser J R, McGravey A 1990 Self-administered nitrous oxide for fracture reduction in an emergency room setting. Journal of Orthopaedic Trauma 4(1): 35–38

Wilson G A M, Doyle E 1996 Validation of three paediatric pain scores for use by parents. Anaesthesia 51: 1005–1007

Further Reading

Aitkenhead S 2001 Managing chronic pain in children. Nursing Times 97(29): 34–35

Campo J V, Comer D M, Jansen-McWilliams L, Gardner W, Kelleher K J 2002 Recurrent pain, emotional distress, and health service use in childhood. Journal of Pediatrics 141(1): 76–83

Kashikar-Zuck S, Goldschneider K R, Powers S W, Vaught M H, Hershey A D 2001 Depression and functional disability in chronic pediatric pain. Clinical Journal of Pain 17(4): 341–349

Morton N S (ed.) 1998 Acute paediatric pain management: a practical guide. W B Saunders, London

Munro F J, Fisher S, Dickson U, Morton N 2002 The addition of antiemetics to the morphine solution in patient controlled analgesia syringes used by children after an appendicectomy does not reduce the incidence of postoperative nausea and vomiting. Paediatric Anaesthesia 12(7): 600–603

Sury M R, Hatch D J, Deeley T, Dicks-Mireaux C, Chong W K 1999 Development of a nurse-led sedation service for paediatric magnetic resonance imaging. Lancet 353: 1667–1671

Walters A S, Williamson G M 1999 The role of activity restriction in the association between pain and depression: a study of pediatric patients with chronic pain. Children's Health Care 28(1): 33–50

Practice **19**

Phototherapy

Susan Alexander

Introduction

Hyperbilirubinaemia, commonly referred to as jaundice, is a condition wherein the production of bilirubin is greater than its elimination (Boyd 2004). Management of this condition is dependent on the cause and can be either phototherapy or exchange transfusion. This chapter will review the use of phototherapy which consists of the application of fluorescent light to reduce the serum bilirubin level of an infant. This light is normally a mixture of blue and white radiant light and is not in the ultraviolet range (Metherall 2003).

Learning outcomes

By the end of this section you should be able to:

- identify the infant with a raised serum bilirubin level
- initiate phototherapy, as directed by medical staff, safely and appropriately
- understand the needs of the infant undergoing phototherapy
- recognise any adverse reactions
- explain the need for phototherapy to the parents/primary caregivers.

Rationale

The primary aim of phototherapy is to prevent kernicterus, i.e. mental retardation caused by persistent raised serum unconjugated bilirubin (Johnston & Bhutani 1998, Boyd 2004).

Factors to note

Normal red blood cell life in the adult human is approximately 120 days. In the neonate this is reduced to a lifespan of between 40 and 70 days (Boyd 2004).

Red blood cells are broken down in the spleen (by the reticuloendothelial system) and to a lesser extent in the liver. Bilirubin is one of the end-products of red blood cell breakdown, being derived from the haem part of haemoglobin (see Fig. 19.1). Bilirubin, unconjugated, is not water soluble and is toxic to the body at high levels. If not converted to the water-soluble (conjugated) bilirubin, the unconjugated bilirubin will be deposited in the brain cells, which will lead to a condition called kernicterus.

Unconjugated bilirubin is transported in the bloodstream bound to albumin, a plasma protein, to the liver where, following a complex

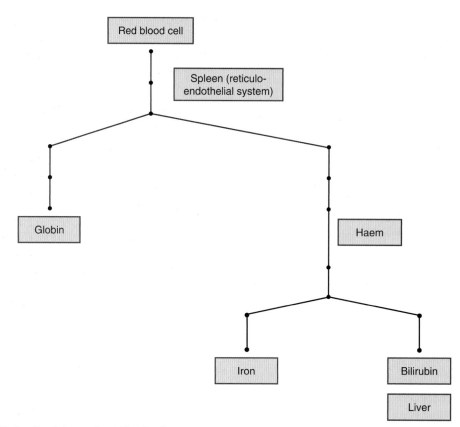

Figure 19.1 Breakdown of red blood cells

process of enzyme actions, it is converted to conjugated bilirubin.

Conjugated bilirubin is water soluble and is excreted by the liver via the biliary system into the intestine.

In the intestine the bilirubin is converted to urobilinogen, some of which is absorbed by the enterohepatic circulation and is eventually excreted in the urine. The majority of the urobilinogen is oxidised in the colon to a brown pigment, urobilin, which is excreted in the stool (Marshall 1995).

An increase in serum bilirubin causes jaundice, a yellow/amber discoloration of the skin, also seen in the sclera of the eyes and mucous membranes (American Academy of Pediatrics 2004). This is seen when the serum bilirubin rises above 80 micromoles per litre. Often the nurse who notices the infant's jaundice initi-

ates the checking of the serum bilirubin level (Truman 2003). In the majority of cases this is relatively benign; however, close monitoring of the serum bilirubin level is important because of the risk of kernicterus.

An early high level of serum bilirubin, normally within the first 24 hours of life, may indicate ABO or Rhesus incompatibility.

Persistent jaundice after the first week of life must be fully investigated to determine the cause. Biliary atresia is one condition where the prognosis is improved with an early diagnosis (Hussein et al 1991, Merenstein & Gardner 2002).

Breast milk jaundice is a benign condition, which may persist up to 3 months after birth and is thought to be caused by a factor within the breast milk which inhibits bilirubin conjugation (Shaw 1998, Percival 2003).

Estimations can be made using a transcutaneous bilirubin monitor; however, the serum level should always be obtained before phototherapy is commenced (Ruchala et al 1996).

Phototherapy is ineffective before the infant is jaundiced; hence it cannot be used prophylactically. However, early use in infants with known haemolytic disease is indicated as a means of control of the serum bilirubin level. Initiation of therapy is dependent not only on the serum bilirubin, but also the gestational age at birth of the infant (Percival 2003).

Preterm and sick infants are more prone to the complications of jaundice; hence phototherapy is initiated at lower serum bilirubin levels.

Equipment

- Open cot, Baby Therm or incubator
- Phototherapy unit(s)
- Eye shield/cover.

Method

Commencement of phototherapy is determined by the serum unconjugated bilirubin level (Metherall 2003, Truman 2003).

The following guidelines refer to the use of a phototherapy unit (Fig. 19.2). Some neonatal units, however, use fibreoptic blankets, known as 'bili blankets', which are wrapped around the infant (Hamlin & Seshia 1998, Mills & Tudehope 2004).

1. The infant is placed naked, with gonads protected, into an open cot, Baby Therm or incubator.
2. The phototherapy unit is placed over the infant, approximately 45 cm above the body. (*Note:* The units are normally fixed onto stands at this height.) More than one unit may be used.
3. The infant's eyes are covered to prevent retinal damage (Ostrowski et al 2000).
4. The phototherapy unit is switched on; treatment can be given continuously or intermittently.
5. The infant should be turned on a regular basis, every 2 hours, to ensure that all of the skin is exposed. However, it must be noted that some authors advocate that changing position frequently has no effect on the efficacy of phototherapy (Chen et al 2002, Shinwell et al 2002).
6. The phototherapy unit should be switched off when the infant is being fed or the eye shields are removed.

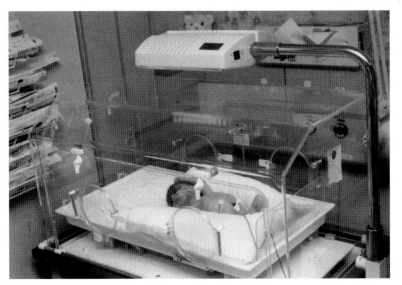

Figure 19.2 Infant under the phototherapy unit

7. The duration of treatment will be determined by the level of serum unconjugated bilirubin.
8. In some areas the nursing staff may be responsible for checking the serum bilirubin level by capillary heel stab.
9. Where the infant is being constantly observed, protective glasses should be available for staff use.
10. Care should be coordinated (clustered care) to ensure minimal disruption to the infant.

Observations and complications

- Check the infant's temperature regularly as infants are prone both to hypothermia (due to being naked) and to hyperthermia because of heat radiated from the phototherapy unit.
- Increase fluid intake by 25–30% (or as determined by local policy) to maintain hydration, as the infant's insensible losses are known to rise (Mathew 1995, Boyd 2004).
- Cover the gonads of the very and extremely low birthweight infants; this has to be balanced with maximum skin exposure. DNA mutations and breaks have been reported with the use of phototherapy (Edwards 1995). Theatre masks worn by the infant as bikini bottoms may be used.
- Check skin colour using daylight, as assessment of jaundice is often difficult under artificial light (Blackwell 2003).

- Loose green stools are common during treatment. Stools should be monitored, as fluid loss may increase as a result of frequent loose stools.
- Ensure that the infant's eyes remain closed when shields are in place, as corneal abrasions may occur. The shields should be removed and the eyes checked on a regular basis (Ostrowski et al 2000).
- The effect of phototherapy on the eyes is uncertain. However, animal studies indicate that retinal degeneration can occur if there is continuous exposure (Sisson 1970).
- The infant may become lethargic, irritable and develop poor feeding.
- Tanning and rashes are common. This is referred to as 'bronze baby syndrome'.

Do and do not

- Do encourage parents to be involved in care.
- Do ensure that care is clustered.
- Do encourage mothers to continue with breastfeeding.
- Do ensure that the position of the infant is changed to ensure maximum exposure.
- Do not use creams, lotions or oils on the infant's skin, as they may cause burning.
- Do not remove the eye shields while the phototherapy unit is in operation.

References

American Academy of Pediatrics 2004 Management of hyperbilirubinemia in the newborn infant of 35 or more weeks of gestation. Pediatrics 114: 297–316

Blackwell J T 2003 Management of hyperbilirubinaemia in the healthy term newborn. Journal of the American Academy of Nurse Practitioners 15(5): 194–198

Boyd S 2004 Treatment of physiological and pathological neonatal jaundice. Nursing Times 100: 40–43

Chen C M, Liu S H, Lai C C, Hwang C C, Hsu H H 2002 Changing position does not improve the efficacy of conventional phototherapy. Acta Paediatrica Taiwanica 43: 255–258

Edwards S 1995 Phototherapy and the neonate: providing safe and effective nursing care for jaundiced infants. Journal of Neonatal Nursing 1(5): 9–12

Hamelin K, Seshia M 1998 Home phototherapy for uncomplicated neonatal jaundice. The Canadian Nurse 94(1): 39–40

Hussein M, Howard E R, Mieli-Vergani G et al 1991 Jaundice at 14 days of age: exclude biliary atresia. Archives of Disease in Childhood 66(10): 1177–1179

Johnston L, Bhutani V K 1998 Guidelines for management of the jaundiced term and near-term infant. Clinics of Perinatology 25(3): 555–574

Marshall W 1995 Illustrated textbook of clinical chemistry, 3rd edn. Lippincott/Gower, London

Mathew R 1995 Nursing care of infants on phototherapy. Nursing Journal of India LXXXVI(9): 197–198

Merenstein G B, Gardner S L 2002 Handbook of intensive care, 5th edn. Mosby, St Louis, MO

Metherall J 2003 Phototherapy for neonatal hyper-bilirubinaemia: delivering an adequate dose. Journal of Neonatal Nursing 9(6): 182–186

Mills J F, Tudehope D 2004 Fibreoptic phototherapy for neonatal jaundice. Cochrane Database Systematic Reviews 4. Wiley, Chichester, UK

Ostrowski G, Pye S D, Laing I 2000 Do phototherapy hoods really protect the neonate? Acta Paediatrica 89: 874–877

Percival P 2003 Jaundice and infection. In: Fraser D, Cooper M (eds) Myles textbook for midwives, 14th edn. Churchill Livingstone, Edinburgh

Ruchala P L, Seibold L, Stremsterfer K 1996 Validating assessment of neonatal jaundice with transcutaneous bilirubin measurement. Neonatal Network 15(4): 33–37

Shaw N 1998 Assessment and management of hematological dysfunction. In: Kenner C, Lott J W, Flandermeyer A A (eds) Comprehensive neonatal nursing: a physiologic perspective. W B Saunders, Philadelphia, ch 28

Shinwell E S, Sciaky Y, Karplus M 2002 Effect of position on bilirubin levels during phototherapy. Journal of Perinatology 22(3): 226–229

Sisson T 1970 Retinal changes produced by phototherapy. Journal of Paediatrics 77: 251

Truman P 2003 Jaundice in the preterm infant. Journal of Neonatal Nursing 9(1): 22–26

Practice **20**

Plaster care

Lynne Chadburn

Introduction

Plaster casts are used to obtain complete immobilisation, protection and correction of bony or tissue damage or deformity.

Correct care is essential to prevent complications arising.

Learning outcomes

By the end of this section you should:

- understand the principles of plaster care
- develop an understanding of the factors which predispose to common complications
- be able to recognise common complications
- be able to explain nursing interventions required when complications arise
- be able to advise carers and their children on future plaster care.

Rationale

It is essential that children and carers are adequately prepared and understand the necessity for the application of the cast, its subsequent care and the recognition of possible complications. It is therefore necessary that the nurse has the required skills of cast application and knowledge of the principles involved, including possible complications which may arise (BOA 1998, RCN 1999).

Factors to note

Plaster materials

Plaster of Paris, fibreglass cast and polyurethane-based materials are the most commonly used materials today. Each has its own advantages and disadvantages for use (Miles et al 2000).

Plaster of Paris

This is a high-quality gypsum impregnated onto an open weave fabric material. It has been the most common choice for immobilisation for many years. It is relatively inexpensive, pliable and easy to mould, smoothing to conform almost exactly to the extremity (Dandy & Edwards 1998).

However, despite starting to set in 5–7 minutes, it may take up to 48 hours for the plaster cast to dry completely (Prior & Miles 1999a). During this time, the wet cast should be supported by a pillow and handled with the palms of the hands to prevent denting the cast (Prior & Miles 1999a). Walking on a cast before it is fully set will cause the same problem.

Fibreglass

A fibreglass cast is usually a knitted fibreglass fabric impregnated with a polyurethane resin which hardens on exposure to water in a matter of minutes. It only takes a few seconds in water to initiate the chemical reaction.

It comes in a variety of colours, is radiolucent, lightweight and is stronger than plaster of Paris (McRae & Esser 2002). However, it requires five to eight layers for weight-bearing casts and, although more resistant to damage, it can be brittle and crack from repetitive use and can leave a sharp edge, potentially causing excoriation of the skin.

It takes approximately 30 minutes to dry completely, making weight bearing and use of the casted limb possible much sooner (Prior & Miles 1999a). Fibreglass casting materials have water-resistant properties. However, the underlying padding can pose a problem if exposed to water and may result in excoriation of the skin or formation of a pressure sore.

The resilience of the material makes it more difficult to conform well to the extremity and, unlike plaster of Paris, it does not mould specifically. The extremity must be in the correct position before application; if not, wrinkles may develop which cannot be smoothed out and can result in pressure sores (Miles et al 2000).

The resin becomes tacky when in contact with water and may make the material resist coming off the roll. If pulled too hard on application, it may compromise the circulation. It is essential that casting personnel are familiar with the products they are using and read the manufacturers' advice and instructions for use (Miles et al 2000).

Fibreglass is more expensive than plaster of Paris and for this reason is often not the initial cast of choice following trauma or surgery, when removal may be necessary because of swelling or wound inspection. Fibreglass casts can leave sharp edges and, as noted by Prior and Miles (1999a), may cause breakdown of the skin.

Polyurethane-based materials

Polyurethane-based materials that incorporate a flexible polyester are used in some areas. It is radiolucent, lightweight, durable, flexible and conforms to the limb shape very easily and is more child friendly. Fewer layers are required for weight-bearing purposes. This material can sometimes be removed with a serrated scissor edge; however, it is more expensive and gloves are required for application.

All materials generate heat initially; therefore it is advisable to use cool or tepid water for dipping the tape, otherwise the patient may sustain a plaster burn (Prior & Miles 1999b).

Allergic skin reactions can sometimes be caused by certain paddings and casting materials. Parents and children should be advised on what to look for (Miles et al 2000).

Effects of application on the patient and family

The cast is most often applied following trauma. However, it can also be applied to correct bony or tissue deformities which may be present at birth, e.g. developmental dysplasia of the hip and congenital talipes equinovarus.

Irrespective of the reason for a cast being applied nurses must be aware that, although the procedure may be routine for them, it can be very stressful for both child and carers. This is why clear explanation of the reasons behind the application and its subsequent care are essential.

Very often carers are not prepared for the frustrations, fears and difficulties associated with the child's cast confinement (Prior & Miles 1999b). Preparation of the family for the reality of home care could help to make what may be a difficult recovery period more acceptable to all concerned. Problems may not be eliminated fully but prior warning enables the carers and child to deal with them in whatever way is convenient to their circumstances (Miles et al 2000). What makes these problems overwhelming is learning about them after discharge when lack of knowledge, equipment and support becomes apparent.

A simple explanation of what is normal and what is not can be very helpful, for example the psychological aspects of cast confinement may mean that a once independent child may now be totally dependent, causing insecurity, frustration, tantrums and demanding behaviour. Educating the family will help to eliminate this.

Casting can be used over a prolonged period. This is often age and disease related and may be for a number of years rather than weeks or months. This can cause major disruption to family life at home.

Written as well as verbal reinforcement of cast care is essential.

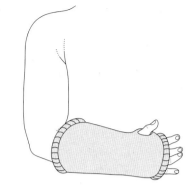

Figure 20.1   Below-elbow cast

Types of cast
There are many different types of cast which can be altered as dictated by the orthopaedic medical staff to meet the individual's needs.

The most common casts used in paediatrics are:

- below elbow – distal radius and ulna fractures (Fig. 20.1)
- above elbow – proximal radius and ulna fractures; supracondylar fractures (Fig. 20.2)
- scaphoid – scaphoid bone injuries (Fig. 20.3)
- below knee – fibula and tibial fractures, metatarsal fractures, ligament and tendon injuries (Fig. 20.4)
- above knee – fibula and tibial fractures, patella fractures, tendon and ligament injuries, talipes equinovarus (Fig. 20.5)
- cylinder – patella fractures, ligament and tendon injuries (Fig. 20.6)
- hip spica – femoral fractures, developmental dysplasia of the hip (Fig. 20.7)
- broomstick – developmental dysplasia of the hip (Fig. 20.8).

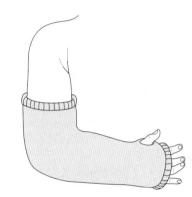

Figure 20.2   Above-elbow cast

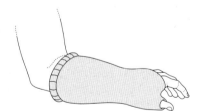

Figure 20.3   Scaphoid cast

The multidisciplinary team
The child in a cast may require input from various members of the multidisciplinary team whilst in the hospital and in the community.

Physiotherapists
Advice can be given to the carers on lifting techniques, sitting, turning and carrying of the child, especially those whose needs prevent them doing it themselves. Many carers experience low back pain as a result of not being taught how to lift correctly (Newman & Fawcett 1995).

Physiotherapists may also provide wheelchairs (reclining or ordinary), leg extensions and extra-wide pushchairs.

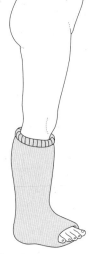

Figure 20.4   Below-knee cast

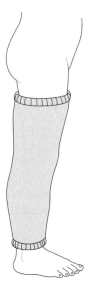

Figure 20.6   Cylinder cast

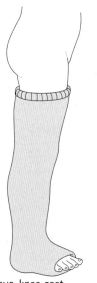

Figure 20.5   Above-knee cast

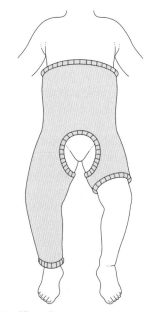

Figure 20.7   Hip spica cast

Teaching the correct method and use of crutches may also be carried out by physiotherapists.

Occupational therapists
Occupational therapists may be required to assess the home circumstances and provide various aids to caring for the child at home, e.g. a wheelchair ramp, plastic bedpans, etc.

APPLICATION OF THE CAST

Equipment

Whatever the type of cast or reason for application, there is usually little variation in the equipment used.

- Stockinette
- Lantor, a conforming undercast padding

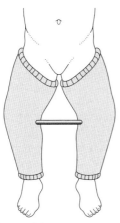

Figure 20.8 Broomstick cast

- Plaster of Paris or fibreglass/polyurethane-based material
- Disposable apron
- Disposable latex-free gloves
- Protective sheet
- Plaster bucket and stand
- Plaster sink
- Limb support
- Tepid/cool water.

Method

The nurse applying the cast needs to understand the medical prescription, identify the patient and the affected limb to be cast, inspect the child's skin and assess the necessity for appropriate prescribed analgesia prior to application, e.g. oral or inhalational (Entonox).

1. Prepare the child and carer for the procedure, explaining why the cast is being applied and what the equipment is for. This is to minimise anxiety and gain cooperation.

2. Ensure that any administered analgesia has taken effect. This is also to reduce anxiety and gain cooperation.

3. Ensure privacy and protect the child's and carer's clothes using a protective sheet.

4. Position the child comfortably, using a limb support, if necessary, to facilitate progress of the procedure.

5. Apply the stockinette first. Stockinette is supplied in different sizes; choose the one that when applied will be smooth and close fitting, avoiding any wrinkles or pleats. Apply a conforming undercast padding, a single layer application, 50% coverage on each turn. Do not protect bony prominences with extra padding as this creates space between cast and limb, allowing movement of the cast and potential plaster sore development. If concerned about bony prominences, use a suitable undercast felt. The undercast padding will protect the skin during the period of immobilisation, and from the plaster saw when the cast is being removed.

6. The nurse should wear a plastic apron to protect clothing and use disposable gloves, especially if a fibreglass cast is to be used as it may be an irritant to the skin.

7. Position the affected limb correctly or as directed by the orthopaedic medical staff. Persuade children to achieve the position themselves if possible. The application of above-elbow and lower limb casts should only be applied using a minimum of two members of staff to hold and maintain the position from the outset to the completion of the cast.

8. Unwind the cast bandage for approximately 10 cm before immersing it in the water. This prevents the end of the bandage becoming lost in the roll. If fibreglass is used, immerse totally in the water for 10–15 seconds to initiate the chemical reaction of the resin, allowing the material to be applied and to eventually become rigid (Barrett & Bryant 1990).

9. Withdraw the bandage from the water, gently compressing it to remove excess water. Do not wring out the bandage, especially if plaster of Paris is being used, as this will result in a loss of the plaster cream.

10. Apply the wet cast bandage with even pressure around the correctly positioned limb, taking care not to pull too tightly, as this may

compromise circulation. Apply the next cast bandage to the previous before it begins to dry. This will ensure good lamination between layers and an even finish. Warn the child that the bandage may feel warm and explain that it is the chemical reaction which will eventually harden the cast.

11. Turn back the ends of the stockinette and apply the casting material, allowing enough padding to remain visible at each edge. This will ensure patient comfort and reduce the risk of the cast rubbing against the skin and causing a sore. During application, cut the casting material around digits to ensure correct fit. Use undercast felt to protect the skin. Check the edges of the cast upon completion and trim if necessary.

12. When handling a wet cast, use the palms of the hands and not just the fingers. Supporting the cast thus will minimise the risk of indentations, which may cause pressure sores and the development of cracks in the cast, which will weaken the support it provides.

13. The limb should be elevated for the first 24–48 hours and circulation checks maintained. This will minimise swelling of the limb and aid early detection of any possible circulatory problems.

14. On discharge, all carers must be given written as well as verbal instructions about the cast to ensure continuity of care.

Observations and complications

Frequency of observations varies from centre to centre depending on the reason for the application of the cast and the severity of the injury.

Circulatory, motor and sensory checks are essential, as trauma to a limb can affect the circulation, muscles and nerves. These checks may be performed every 30 minutes to 1 hour initially for up to 24–48 hours, depending on the severity of the injury.

Circulation
Indication of a problem in the circulation to the limb is noted by a change in colour to a blue or pale appearance, a change in the temperature of the peripheries from warm to cool and by the absence of a distal pulse. (*Note:* It may not be possible to feel the distal pulse as it may be covered by the cast.)

Muscle
Damage to muscle following injury, if neglected, may be irreparable, especially if a condition known as compartment syndrome develops. (*Note:* Compartment syndrome is an orthopaedic emergency.) Observations to detect this are referred to as the five Ps:

1. **Pain** – increasing in nature and extreme pain, made worse on flexion of digits on the affected limb
2. **Pallor** – of the extremities with swelling
3. **Pulse** – diminished or absent
4. **Paraesthesia** – altered sensation, often tingling
5. **Power loss** – inability to move the associated extremities (Prior & Miles 1999b, Miles et al 2000).

Nerves
Damage to nerves is indicated by altered sensation, pins and needles or numbness.

- Any of the above changes must be reported immediately to the senior orthopaedic medical staff.
- If a compartment syndrome is suspected then the cast can be split through to the skin immediately and, if necessary, supported with a loosely applied crepe bandage. Do not wait for the orthopaedic medical staff to arrive.
- Do not elevate the limb as this could compromise the circulation further.

Swelling
Swelling usually peaks in 24–48 hours, which is why elevation is important during this period. This helps to prevent venous pooling and oedema (McConnell 1993).

Wound infection and pressure sore
Assess for the following signs and symptoms:

- drainage/seepage at the ends of the cast or over the wound site

- foul odour
- tingling or burning sensation under the cast
- pain under the cast, particularly over bony prominences or pins.

If wound infection or a pressure sore is suspected, a window may be cut out of the cast. If a sore or infection has developed, this enables dressings to be changed and the window can be replaced and held in position with tape or a bandage.

Too tight/loose

Too tight a cast will lead to circulatory problems. If it is too loose, it will not support the limb and may cause friction and potential cast sore development. In both circumstances the cast should be removed and replaced.

Skin

Inspect the skin regularly for signs of irritation or rubbing around the edges of the cast. To avoid this occurring ensure that adequate padding is used on application of the cast. If the cast is rubbing then it can be trimmed to below the affected area and protected with more padding (Prior & Miles 1999a).

Advice to carers

Hygiene and skin care

Information about keeping a cast clean, particularly around the perineal area for those in a hip spica, is very important. Excreta can seep inside the cast and cause skin and odour problems (Newman & Fawcett 1995).

Miles et al (2000) suggested using a smaller-sized nappy than usual, tucking it between the skin and the cast and ensuring that the plastic backing is next to the cast's inside surface. Observation of the area immediately under the cast is needed to ensure that the nappy is not causing any pressure sores. However, this very much depends on whether adequate space has been left around the perineal area to allow for this. Where possible, do not place the nappy over the cast as excreta will be absorbed into the cast causing odour and softening.

Also suggested by Miles et al (2000) is the use of a smaller nappy inside a larger nappy to absorb more urine, particularly at night. Carers are also advised to check and change the nappy more frequently and as necessary.

For the older child in a hip spica, the use of a bedpan and urinal is recommended. Carers need to be made aware that they will require these items before discharge home. Waterproof tape (sleek) can be placed around the edges of the cast and replaced as necessary.

A thorough wash from head to toe may replace normal bathing. Hairwashing may be a problem and require two people – one to hold the child's head over the sink/bath, the other to wash. An alternative is to use dry shampoo.

Positioning and safety

The affected limb should be positioned on cushions or pillows initially when at rest.

A hip spica cast often extends up to the diaphragm, so enabling the child to sit up requires special consideration. The use of pillows and cushions or a bean bag may assist in achieving this.

Turn the child from front to back several times a day to prevent pressure sores. The change in position also encourages different play activities.

Safety straps on pushchairs and highchairs, and side rails on cots/beds, will be required as children soon learn how to manoeuvre themselves. A car seat may require alterations to ensure safe transportation.

Eating and drinking

The extension of a hip spica cast may cause eating and drinking to be awkward, and the child may experience discomfort after meal times because of the restriction caused by the rigid cast. It is better to ask carers to give smaller, more frequent meals to avoid discomfort, than let them discover this through experience. If the cast reduces mobility, it may be necessary to increase the fibre content in the diet and give more fluids to prevent constipation.

A closed cup or the use of a flexible straw may be the best method for drinking to prevent too many accidents and spillages on to the cast.

Sleeping

Sleeping may be affected as a result of the effects of trauma and/or hospitalisation. Cramp can be caused by the inability of the child to turn over in bed so they need turning during the night. If itching occurs underneath the cast, due to the weight and heat from the bed covers, lift the bed clothes off the cast using extra pillows at the bottom of the bed. Faced with these difficulties the child may be restless and may only sleep for short periods.

Mobility

Balance may be affected by lower limb casts. If a weight-bearing cast has been applied crutches may be advised initially, but the child must not be discharged home until shown the correct use of crutches by an appropriately trained person, e.g. a physiotherapist.

The ability to get out of the house is important for both the carers and the child to prevent social isolation. Input from the physiotherapist and occupational therapist is necessary for the provision of ramps, wheelchairs, wide pushchairs, etc.

Transportation may be a problem, especially with hip spica casts. A hospital taxi or ambulance may be required for discharge and follow-up appointments. If the child cannot safely be strapped into a car seat, a seat belt extension may need to be obtained.

Clothing

Shirts, shorts, dresses and skirts can usually be worn normally. However, a larger size may be necessary for those in a spica cast. Underwear, trousers, etc. for lower limb casts, spica and broomstick casts can be split at a side seam and Velcro strips, poppers or zips inserted for ease of access.

Advice for parents is available from national associations such as Action for Sick Children, STEPS (National Association for Children with Lower Limb Abnormalities) and the Scoliosis Association.

REMOVAL OF A CAST

Equipment

Tools for removal of cast:

- plaster saw – used only for removing dry casts
- plaster shears – for removing wet casts
- plaster spreaders
- bandage scissors.

Method

1. Ensure that the equipment you require is available.
2. Explain to the child and carer what you will be doing, and give reassurance regarding the use of the saw and the noise it makes (Prior 1997). The blade oscillates, so an explanation is needed to reassure the child that the blade will not cut through the protective padding. Children should also be told that they may experience a vibrating or tickling sensation and slight warmth, especially during the removal of a large cast. This will help minimise anxiety and gain cooperation for the procedure to continue.
3. If necessary, mark the cast with a pen for exact lines to be cut avoiding bony prominences and fracture/wound sites. This will minimise the possibility of trauma. The cast should be bivalved, i.e. the cast is cut in two on both sides, lengthways to allow safe removal of the limb from the cast.
4. Position the child comfortably, enabling easy access to the cast on a secure and steady surface. Remove any clothing covering the cast and protect other clothing with an apron, or protective sheet, if necessary.
5. When applying the saw to the cast, support the neck of the saw with one hand to avoid too much pressure being exerted downwards. Each time the blade cuts through the cast it should be lifted out, and the procedure repeated so a series of small cuts are made. The blade should not be run up and down the length of the cast, as this causes a

great deal of heat to be generated by the blade because of friction (Miles 1997).

6. Avoid using the saw on the extreme edges of the cast. These areas should be cut with the plaster shears.

7. When cutting is complete, open the cast with care using the plaster spreaders, avoiding too much disturbance to the limb.

8. Use the bandage scissors to cut the padding.

9. Note any signs of pressure from the cast on the skin or damage from the saw. If any, notify the doctor.

10. *Note:*
  – lower limb plasters – the child should not weight bear until seen by a doctor
  – upper limb plasters – arms should be supported until seen by a doctor.

11. Carers and child should be advised that once the cast is removed it may take some time for life to return to normal. A rehabilitation period may be necessary as muscles and joints have been inactive for some time.

Adapting to mobilising in a cast, and losing the security of this immobilisation, can cause anxiety and discomfort for the child, as well as frustration at not being able to use the limb normally immediately (Cuddy 1986).

COMMUNITY PERSPECTIVE

The CCN will liaise with the family on the ward to ensure that they feel confident to take the child home.

Home visits may be arranged to advise on adaptations in the home, e.g. moving the child's bed downstairs.

Discharge planning should ensure that there is sufficient equipment at home, e.g. pillows, vacuum cushions, bedpans/urinals. Referral to the physiotherapist may be needed for advice about seating, mobilising and appropriate use of a buggy or wheelchair.

The family should be given information concerning the charity STEPS (National Association for Children with Lower Limb Abnormalities) which may be able to provide additional equipment such as pushchairs or a low table with attached seat for a child with a hip spica.

The CCN will need to visit to ensure that the parents are coping with the physical care as well as the frustrations of restricted mobility and changed pattern of family life. The CCN may be required to trim casts and apply sleek plaster to the edges.

Where there is a community play specialist, visits may be helpful in showing parents ways in which to occupy the child and the use of play techniques to relieve frustration and encourage normal development.

School-age children will need the involvement of the education department to supply a home tutor.

Results of findings by STEPS showed that 'high levels of emotional distress associated with diagnosis and treatment were often exacerbated by lack of information and equipment at the point of discharge' (Hinde 1996). The provision of equipment for children with hip spicas and splints was found to be both uncoordinated and patchy. Often the first problem for parents is that of safety in the car, which is likely to occur immediately on discharge. They require access to appropriate harness devices or car seats. The problems for children with hip spicas are ongoing, as there appears to be a national lack of suitable equipment. Even where families are able to acquire a suitable pushchair, there may be a problem of access to the home as adaptations such as ramps are not usually available because this is not a long-term need.

Do and do not

- Do carry out observations for complications.
- Do exercise extremities as well as joints proximal to the cast. This will encourage venous return and thus help to reduce swelling. It will also help to prevent muscle wasting and joint stiffness.
- Do use the palms of the hands when moving a newly casted limb for the first 24 hours if plaster of Paris is used, and for 30 minutes if fibreglass material is used.
- Do elevate the limb whenever possible, especially during the first 24–48 hours after application.
- Do instruct the patient and carers to return to the hospital if:
  - pain is experienced that is disproportionate to the injury
  - there is marked swelling or discoloration of the peripheries
  - there is altered sensation or inability to move fingers or toes
  - the cast cracks, becomes soft, loose or uncomfortable.
- Do inspect the skin around the edges of the cast.
- Do advise the patient to use the crutches as instructed.
- Do give written cast care instructions.
- Do not allow the patient to weight bear until the cast is completely dry, or as instructed by orthopaedic medical staff.
- Do not permit any writing on the cast until it is completely dry, and advise the use of felt tip pens only as ball point pens may cause cracks to develop in the cast.
- Do not allow the cast to get wet.
- Do not encourage anything to be poked down inside the cast such as pencils, knitting needles, etc., as sores may develop as a result.
- Do not allow the cast to become too hot, e.g. sitting too close to a fire or radiator. Once hot, the cast will take some time to cool down and may cause a burn beneath the cast.

References

Barrett J B, Bryant B H 1990 Fractures – types, treatment, perioperative implications. AORN Journal 52(4): 755–771

British Orthopaedic Association (BOA) 1998 The British Orthopaedic Association advisory book on consultant orthopaedic and training services. BOA, London

Cuddy C M 1986 Caring for the child in a spica cast: a parent's perspective. Orthopaedic Nursing 5(3): 17–21

Dandy D J, Edwards D J 1998 Essential orthopaedics and trauma, 3rd edn. Churchill Livingstone, Edinburgh

Hinde S 1996 Provision and availability of equipment for children in hip spicas and splints. STEPS, Lymm, Cheshire, UK

McConnell E A 1993 Providing cast care. Nursing 23(1): 19

McRae R, Esser M 2002 Practical fracture management, 4th edn. Churchill Livingstone, Edinburgh

Miles S 1997 The removal business: safely removing a cast. Journal of Orthopaedic Nursing 1: 195–197

Miles S and Members of the Royal College of Nursing and the Society of Orthopaedic Nursing 2000 A practical guide to casting, 2nd edn. BSN Medical, Hull, UK

Newman D, Fawcett J 1995 Caring for a young child in a body cast: impact on the care giver. Orthopaedic Nursing 14(1): 41–46

Prior M 1997 The sharp end of cast removal: safety and education issues. Journal of Orthopaedic Nursing 1: 111–113

Prior M A, Miles S 1999a Casting: part 2. Nursing Standard 13(29): 43–47

Prior M A, Miles S 1999b Casting: part 1. Nursing Standard 13(28): 49–53

Royal College of Nursing (RCN) 1999 Education and training in casting. RCN, London

Further Reading

Dandy D J, Edwards D J 1998 Essential orthopaedics and trauma, 3rd edn. Churchill Livingstone, Edinburgh

Jolleys J V Caring for a child in a cast. Presented by Orthopaedic Products, 3M Healthcare, Bracknell, UK

Kelly A, Miljesic S, Mant P, Ashton N 1996 Plaster checks by nurses: safe and efficient? Accident and Emergency Nursing 4(2): 76–77

McRae R, Esser M 2002 Practical fracture management, 4th edn. Churchill Livingstone, Edinburgh

Miles S and Members of the Royal College of Nursing and the Society of Orthopaedic Nursing 2000 A practical guide to casting, 2nd edn. BSN Medical, Hull, UK

Royal College of Nursing (RCN) 2000 A framework for casting standards. RCN, London

Williamson M J 1994 Paediatric forearm fracture. Orthopaedic Nursing 13(3): 65–68

Practice **21**

Positioning, handling and exercises

Susan Rideout

Introduction

Correct positioning is an integral part of the care of sick children, or those with a physical disability, and can be used to enhance their speed of recovery, promote normal development and prevent deterioration in their condition (Turrill 1992, Short et al 1996). Competent handling is a crucial part of holistic care, as is the provision of appropriate opportunities for exercise, both active and passive (Jones 1999).

Learning outcomes

By the end of this section you should:

- understand the benefits of correct positioning
- be able to assess the most appropriate positions and specific handling needs for children according to age, size, developmental level and condition
- recognise the dangers of incorrect positioning
- be able to determine whether specialised advice and equipment is necessary

- be aware of the need to assess the risk of lifting and handling
- be aware of the child's exercise requirements according to age, developmental level and condition.

Rationale

Any child with limited ability to move, whether because of age or condition, requires assistance to ensure appropriate and comfortable positions are achieved (Finnie 1997). This will maximise recovery and minimise deterioration. Some children have specific handling requirements, for example premature infants or those with certain conditions such as cerebral palsy. Others may require intervention by means of active, or passive, exercise.

Factors to note

Positioning

In order to practise good positioning it is necessary to understand how it is used and the benefits it affords. Variations in position will allow the child to be comfortable and ease the pressure exerted on any one area. Changing positions will help prevent the skin becoming sore or breaking down and the subsequent pain and limitation of movement which might result. Certain positions can be used to help facilitate play. Allowing the child to experience movement in a range of different positions encourages normal development (Bly 1994).

Specific positioning may be an important part of training a child to feed by ensuring correct head-on-body alignment. Positioning can assist the child with respiratory difficulties to drain secretions or reduce the work of breathing (Hough 1984, Badr et al 2002, Harcombe 2004). Positioning can have an influence on an infant's ability to lose heat and on the speed of gastric emptying (Hallsworth 1995). Children who have limited ability in movement need regular alterations to their positions in order to prevent the formation of muscle contractures and deformities (Dubowitz 1969, Goldspink et al 2002). It has also been shown that children with abnormal movement patterns and involuntary movements can have their problems reduced by correct positioning (Finnie 1997).

Normal infants

Extensive research by the Foundation for the Study of Infant Deaths (Epstein 1993) and the Department of Health (1993) has shown that the risk of sudden infant death syndrome is significantly reduced by ensuring that young babies are not positioned to sleep on their fronts. The risk is further reduced by ensuring that they are positioned on their backs. Recent guidelines also suggest that babies should be positioned with their feet close to the foot of the bed so that they cannot slide down under the covers.

Recent evidence has advised that all babies should be encouraged to have 'tummy time' when awake and being observed. The prone position will reduce the risk of positional occipital plagiocephaly, i.e. cranial moulding/flattening of the head, and will provide an opportunity for the baby to develop shoulder girdle strength (AAP 2000, Persing et al 2003).

The judicious and considered handling of children can bring many benefits to certain situations, helping to build trust and promote psychological well-being as well as, at times, being an integral part of their treatment.

Manual handling

The risks of musculoskeletal problems to which all who work with children are exposed should be recognised, whether they come from continual lifting, stooping or working at an awkward level (Alexander 1997). With the advent of the Manual Handling Operations Regulations (HMSO 1992), employees' responsibilities for their own safety are clearly set out. In summary these are:

- to avoid manual handling where there is risk of injury so far as is reasonably practicable
- to assess the risks in those operations that cannot be avoided
- to take action to reduce risks to the lowest level reasonably practicable.

In order to undertake risk assessment, there are many factors that must be taken into account. These can generally be classified into four categories as follows:

- the load (the child) – weight, age, muscle tone, compliance/comprehension, drips/drains, plasters/splints, wound site, pain level, required oxygen, mobility
- the task – frequency, duration, distance, posture, fatigue, individual capability
- the environment – space, floor surface, carer's uniform/footwear, patient's clothing, furniture (height and stability)
- the equipment available – hoists, transfer sliding boards/sheets (Chartered Society of Physiotherapy 1994).

It is important to note that this is only a brief guide to risk assessment and that each employer will have its own local code of practice with which its employees have a duty to cooperate (Royal College of Nursing 1993).

Exercise

Exercise is the practice or training of a movement (Larin 1998) and is a natural and essential part of development. It provides children with an outlet for energy (Montgomery et al 2003) and enables them to learn about themselves, their environment and others (Aarnion et al 2002).

Guidelines

Whenever possible all carers should be aware of the specific positioning, handling and exercise needs of their child, and careful explanation should be given at all times to the family to maximise their input and support.

Preterm babies

A full-term infant spends the last 4–6 weeks in utero in an increasingly compressed position. A preterm infant does not experience this time in flexion and so when born exhibits a floppy, extended posture. Babies who are born early, typically have low muscle tone and often require special life-supporting care. The above, together with immature development at birth, is likely to limit their ability to move against gravity and hence encourage them to lie in a flattened, frog-shaped posture (Fig. 21.1). Meanwhile, hypotonic neck muscles cause the head to rest flat on the side, resulting in narrow

elongated head shape moulding. The aim of positioning must therefore be to:

- stimulate active flexion of the trunk and limbs
- encourage midline orientation
- minimise facial moulding and ensure full range of active head rotation
- encourage a balance between extension and flexion
- allow more symmetrical postures and enable postural stability
- facilitate smooth antigravity limb movements (Updike et al 1986).

Preterm babies should be cared for in a variety of positions mimicking normal development. However, some babies may be given specific positions by a physiotherapist because of 'particular concerns following a birth history indicating abnormal factors that are likely to cause handicap' (Sweeney & Gutiernez 2002).

When a baby is first admitted to a neonatal intensive care unit, the primary goal of care is to achieve physiological stability. Commonly, the prone position is best able to facilitate this, leading to improved oxygen saturation, heart

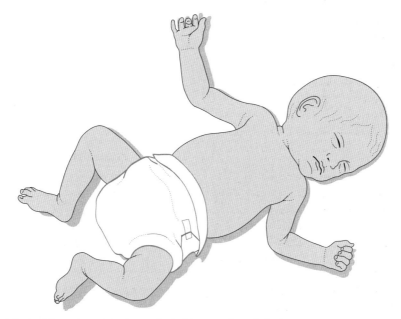

Figure 21.1   A typical frog-shaped posture adopted by a preterm infant

rate and pulmonary resistance, and also helping to prevent gastric reflux and aspiration. Energy expenditure and heat loss are less in the prone position and babies are found to sleep better and startle and cry less.

When positioning a baby prone, Turrill (1992) suggests that the arms should be placed close to the body with the hands symmetrically brought up close to the mouth; the head then needs to be turned to one side. To discourage asymmetrical development, ensure that the head is not always turned to the same side. The legs should be encouraged to flex, with the knees brought up towards the chest, raising the hips slightly. This position is best maintained by using a soft rolled blanket to make a boundary (Fig. 21.2).

There are times when sick, preterm babies will be nursed in a supine position, for example to enable necessary equipment to be placed on the baby, for medical procedures or to make observation easier. This position does nothing to assist with the acquisition of a flexed posture, and so should be avoided whenever possible. To minimise the detrimental effects of this position the baby should be 'nested', i.e. given adequate support using small fabric rolls (Fig. 21.3) or carefully swaddled (Short et al 1996). This will help to achieve the following desired position whilst giving the baby security and comfort:

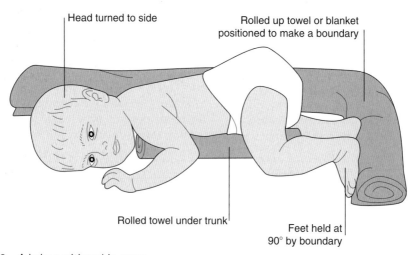

Head turned to side

Rolled up towel or blanket positioned to make a boundary

Rolled towel under trunk

Feet held at 90° by boundary

Figure 21.2 A baby positioned in prone

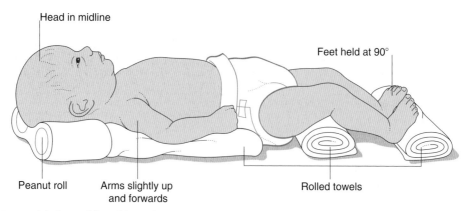

Head in midline

Feet held at 90°

Peanut roll

Arms slightly up and forwards

Rolled towels

Figure 21.3 A baby positioned in supine

- head in midline
- shoulders protracted
- hands to midline
- hips abducted and flexed (supported in neutral)
- knees flexed
- feet 'neutral' (Hallsworth 1995).

From this position the baby will be able to begin to develop head control, maintain a symmetrical posture, achieve normal flexor tone and establish visual skills (Sweeney & Gutiernez 2002). It will also encourage the baby to bring the hands together in the midline and to kick against gravity.

Side-lying is a valuable position that can be used to encourage flexion and symmetry in the preterm infant. It is important to ensure that the trunk is held perpendicular to the cot surface by the use of a roll along the baby's back (not touching the back of the head as the baby may be stimulated to push back into it). The legs should be flexed, and the upper leg supported in a neutral position by the use of a folded nappy or roll between the legs (Fig. 21.4). In this position, the head is already in the midline and the arms can be placed forwards and up towards the mouth. It is also suggested that a thin soft towel can be placed

for the baby to hold between the arms to give a stimulus to flex towards (Turrill 1992).

Note that 'the baby's position can affect the parents' perceptions. A comfortable curled baby with hands touching face looks far more appealing than a flat, extended baby' (Warren 1993).

When handling preterm babies, it is important to consider certain principles:

- Handling of sick, preterm babies should be kept to a minimum, as handling in any way will usually cause their condition to deteriorate, typically by making them hypoxic (Gagnon et al 1999).
- It is valuable to maintain positions of flexion during handling, either by lifting babies in a side-lying or prone position, with appropriate head support, or by swaddling them before they are lifted (Turrill 1992).
- Massage therapy has been found to be beneficial in terms of increased weight gain in certain medically stable preterm infants (Maimous 2002, Deiter et al 2003) (see Complementary Therapies, p. 465).

Acutely sick children

The positioning of an acutely sick child will often be a compromise in order to allow two or

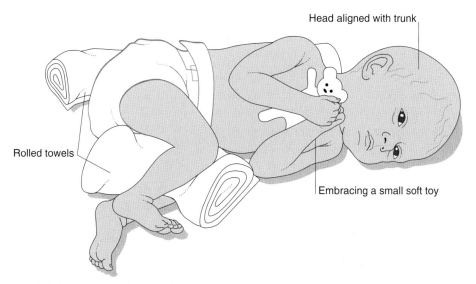

Figure 21.4   A baby positioned in side-lying

more body systems to be cared for simultaneously. However, it is important to understand the rationale for positioning for each of the different problems encountered.

Respiratory system

Drainage of secretions

The child is positioned to assist the drainage of secretions from specific areas of the lungs by means of gravity. The positions relate to the anatomy of the bronchial tree. A physiotherapist may choose to leave a child in a certain position, the relevance of which is indicated in Table 21.1. Babies should only be positioned head down following specific instructions by the physiotherapist, due to the high risk of reflux.

Improving gaseous exchange

- Lung volume can be increased by helping a child to sit upright rather than slumped, or by positioning in side-lying when the abdominal contents will fall forwards away from the diaphragm (Kim et al 2004).

- Adequate gaseous exchange is dependent on adequate ventilation and adequate perfusion. Inadequate ventilation can be caused by pneumonia, paralysed hemidiaphragm or pneumothorax. Inadequate perfusion can be caused by pulmonary vasoconstriction or pulmonary embolus. In unilateral disease (only one lung affected), gas exchange is optimum when the child is side-lying with the good lung uppermost

and the child should therefore be positioned thus.

Reducing the work of breathing

When in respiratory distress there are six relaxed positions a child could adopt: high side-lying; forward lean sitting; forward lean kneeling; relaxed sitting; forward lean standing; and relaxed standing (Davis 1983).

Central nervous system

Control of raised intracranial pressure

These children may be nursed in a head-up position with a 30 degree tilt, in order to reduce cerebral blood flow and with the head in midline, in order to prevent any compression of the cerebral vessels.

Skin

- The avoidance of breakdown of pressure areas demands frequent changes in position. Children who are at particular risk are those with reduced active movement, diminished sensation or poor circulation. Often a regular 30 degree turn is all that is necessary (see Pressure Area Care, p. 321).

- Following a burn, skin or joint contractures may develop. Collagen formation and contraction begin before the wound is healed and continue until the scars are fully mature. A child in pain will assume a position of comfort, generally a position of flexion (Sadowski 1992). Therapeutic positioning and exercises must be performed as soon as possible, and continued with regular monitoring

Table 21.1 Positions to aid postural lung drainage	
Area of lung to be drained	**Possible positions**
Right or left upper lobes	Sitting Supine lying – flat Three-quarters prone lying – flat
Right middle lobe	One-quarter left side-lying – head down 15 degrees
Lingula	One-quarter right side-lying – head down 15 degrees
Right or left lower lobes	Prone – head down 20 degrees Supine – head down 20 degrees Left or right side-lying – head down 20 degrees

throughout rehabilitation, to prevent the onset of contractures and subsequent disability. The use of splints and/or pressure garments may be necessary.

Chronically/long-term sick babies

Chronically sick babies often suffer from delayed development due to inadequate nutrition, recurrent illnesses and lack of stimulation. It is important to try to provide them with a position and environment from which they can get satisfaction in play with minimal effort. This should then increase their motivation to further explore their environment. Side-lying with a roll behind the back, to stop them falling back, helps to bring their hands together and position their head in midline, which is crucial in the development of coordination between the two sides of the body (Bly 1994). Sitting in a car seat, bouncy chair or tumble form chair enables them to see their surroundings and toys more easily, and will encourage them to try to reach out for them. Baby walkers are not recommended as they are considered dangerous and are thought to delay rather than facilitate walking (Siegal & Burton 1999, AAP 2001).

In addition, prolonged hospitalisation may interfere with parental bonding. The parents may be reluctant to be involved with the normal care of the child (cuddling, feeding, changing, playing, etc.). When medically stable, these babies should be exposed to as much handling and interaction during such activities as possible.

The floppy child

A child may be floppy for many reasons, for example:

- acute illness (infection, dehydration)
- paralysis
- neuromuscular diseases (muscular dystrophy, spinal muscular atrophy, neuropathies)
- other disorders of the central nervous system (some types of cerebral palsy, Down syndrome)
- metabolic disease.

When positioning these children, special consideration should be given to the prevention of deformities, which could eventually prove to be a greater disability than their weakness (Dubowitz 1969). They must, therefore, have regular changes of position throughout each day (sitting, prone, supine and side-lying) with an emphasis on providing enough support through the use of pillows, cushions or rolled towels to maintain a symmetrical posture. Floppy children, because of their inability to move against gravity, will find side-lying and sitting helpful positions to enable them to develop their skills.

In order to help prevent the development of contractures, active movement, coupled with passive movement of the joints through their full range, should be encouraged. Passive movements must only be carried out by an appropriately trained carer as the joints are very vulnerable to damage. Spinal braces or foot splints, where provided, must be worn.

When lifting a floppy child, remember that such children are likely to be unstable (owing to their lack of trunk control) and difficult to grasp (characteristically 'falling through' when lifted from under the arms). Special care should therefore be taken by the lifter to ensure that there is no accidental damage to the child's lax joints.

The neurologically impaired child

Disorders of the central nervous system are the result of either abnormal development of the central nervous system itself or an insult to the brain or spinal cord, commonly affecting the sensorimotor activities of the child (Bedford & McKinlay 1993). The largest group with these problems will be children diagnosed as having cerebral palsy. The principles of positioning and handling for these children can be extended to other children with neurological impairment such as head injury, cerebrovascular accident, cerebral tumour or other acute insults including meningitis and encephalitis.

The main feature of this type of disorder is abnormal movement which may be:

- limited, stiff and in stereotyped patterns due to spasticity
- floppy, feeling loose and with greater range than one would normally expect
- athetoid – almost continuous and unwanted movement which the child cannot control
- ataxic, jerky and uncoordinated.

Children with neurological impairment may have various combinations and distributions of any of these abnormal movements, and the first step towards effective handling and treatment calls for a full assessment of the child by a physiotherapist (Finnie 1997). Good positioning and handling are vital to help to:

- reduce abnormal movements
- break up and control stiffness
- maintain the improved muscle synergies achieved through active treatment.

Poor positioning will potentially worsen these children's problems (Appleton & Baldwin 1998).

A general guideline is to place and carry children in a different position from that which they assume naturally, but abnormally.

The extending child should not be left flat supine (Finnie 1997). In this position, the force of gravity pulls the body into an increasingly extended posture, making it more difficult for the child to move. Side-lying, with the inclusion of semi-flexion at the neck, hips and knees, the legs separated by a towel or pillow and the arms placed forwards, is helpful. In addition, sitting in a chair may be useful. It can provide support to ensure a position with 90 degree hip and knee flexion, trunk and head alignment in the midline, and the shoulders

prevented from being retracted. When carried, the child should first be moved into a more flexed and symmetrical position (e.g. sitting) and then held facing the lifter, with the legs apart and flexed at the hips and with the arms up and forwards on the lifter's shoulders.

In contrast, predominantly flexed children should be carried on their side or front in an extended position, with arms reaching up and legs held apart (Finnie 1994). It may also be appropriate for them to be positioned to sleep on their tummy, but it is important that they are fully assessed by a physiotherapist before this is attempted. The child should be monitored whilst in this position to ensure they have no problems (AAP 2000).

A child who is strongly asymmetrical and usually holds the head turned to one side is helped most if the bed, or seating, is positioned so that all stimulation is from the opposite side (Finnie 1997).

Both athetoid and ataxic children need stability when they are being lifted or carried, and so handling should be steady and firm; the child usually responds well to generally flexed positions.

Observations and complications

Having positioned any child, always stand back and observe the child in the new position:

- Have you achieved what you were aiming for?
- Is the child comfortable?
- If you are having difficulty making the child comfortable, contact a physiotherapist for advice at the earliest opportunity.

COMMUNITY PERSPECTIVE

Prior to the discharge of a child who has a specific problem of mobility, it must be ensured that the parents are aware of any special procedures and that they have been taught how to carry them out. Moving and handling techniques should be explained, demonstrated and assessed.

Consideration should be given to the fact that one parent is likely to be on their own for the majority of the time and that the average home is not designed to cater for carrying older children from one room to another, or up and down stairs. These factors may pose a considerable risk to both carer and child.

Community Perspective continues

An assessment should be made of the home, involving other members of the multidisciplinary team as necessary, for example the occupational therapist to advise on bath aids, hoists and possible adaptation/extension of the home.

Part of the role of the CCN is to monitor the impact that constant moving and handling is having on the carers and to act accordingly. The families may have no-one else who can help and the CCN may need to organise respite care or press for a speedy implementation of adaptations and provision of equipment.

Do and do not

- Do think before you start: 'What am I trying to achieve for the child?'
- Do keep the handling of acutely sick children to a minimum.
- Do remember to involve a physiotherapist.
- Do remember to assess any manual handling/lifting situation for risk.

- Do not put a baby to sleep on their front, unless advised by the medical staff or physiotherapist. The baby should be monitored closely during this time.
- Do not put a stiff extended child onto their back, unless advised by the physiotherapist or for medical reasons.

References

Aarnion M, Winter T, Kujala V, Kaprio J 2002 Association of health related behaviour, social relationships and health status with persistent physical activity and inactivity. A study of Finnish adolescent twins. British Journal of Sports Medicine 36: 360–364

Alexander P 1997 Handling babies and young children. In: The guide to the handling of patients, 4th edn. National Back Pain Association/Royal College of Nursing, London

American Academy of Pediatrics (AAP) 2000 Task Force on Infant Sleep Position and Sudden Infant Death Syndrome. Changing concepts of sudden infant death syndrome: implications for infant sleeping position. Paediatrics 105(3): 650–656

American Academy of Pediatrics (AAP) 2001 Committee on Injury and Poison Prevention. Injuries associated with infant walkers. Pediatrics 108(3): 790–792

Appleton R E, Baldwin T (eds) 1998 Management of brain-injured children. Oxford University Press, Oxford

Badr C, Elkins M, Ellis E R 2002 The effect of body position on maximal expiratory pressure and flow. Australian Journal of Physiotherapy 48(2): 95–102

Bedford S, McKinlay I 1993 Disorders of the central nervous system. In: Eckersley P M (ed) Elements of paediatric physiotherapy. Longman, London, p 115–155

Bly L 1994 Motor skills acquisition in the first year. Therapy Skill Builders, Tucson, AZ

Chartered Society of Physiotherapy 1994 Manual handling training. Factsheet 9. CSP, London

Davis A J 1983 Medical chest physiotherapy. In: Downie P A (ed) Cash's textbook of chest, heart and vascular disorders for physiotherapists. Faber and Faber, London, p 298–329

Deiter J N, Field T, Hernandez-Reif M, Emory E, Redzepi M 2003 Stable preterm infants gain more weight and sleep less after five days of massage therapy. Journal of Pediatric Psychology 28(6): 403–411

Department of Health 1993 Cot death. HMSO, London

Dubowitz V 1969 The floppy infant. Heinemann, London

Eckersley P M 1993 Elements of paediatric physiotherapy. Longman, London, p 343–375

Epstein J 1993 The Foundation for the Study of Infant Deaths campaign to reduce the risk of cot death. What is the research evidence? Maternal and Child Health 18(1): 6–8

Finnie N R 1994 Handling the young cerebral palsied child at home. Butterworth-Heinemann, Oxford

Finnie N R 1997 Handling the young child with cerebral palsy at home, 3rd edn. Butterworth-Heinemann, Oxford

Gagnon F E, Leung A, McNab A J 1999 Variation in regional cerebral blood volume in neonates associated with nursery care events. American Journal of Perinatology 16(1): 7–11

Goldspink G, Williams P, Simpson H 2002 Gene expression in response to muscle stretch. Clinical Orthopaedics and Related Research 1(403): S146–S152

Hallsworth M 1995 Positioning the preterm infant. Paediatric Nursing 7(1): 18–20

Harcombe C J 2004 Nursing patients with ARDS in the prone position. Nursing Standard 18(19): 33–39

HMSO 1992 Manual handling operations regulations and guidance on regulations L23. HMSO, London

Hough A 1984 The effect of posture on lung function. Physiotherapy 70(3): 101–104

Jones A 1999 Teamwork is vital for spasticity. Therapy Weekly May: 6

Kim H Y, Lee K S, Kang E H, Suh G Y, Kwon O J, Chung M J 2004 Acute respiratory distress syndrome: computed tomography findings and their applications to mechanical ventilation therapy. Journal of Computer Assisted Tomography 28(5): 686–696

Larin H M 1998 Motor learning: a practical framework for paediatric physiotherapy. Physiotherapy Theory and Practice 14: 33–47

Maimous R O 2002 Infant massage as a component of developmental care. Past, present and future. Holistic Nursing Practice 17(1): 1–7

Montgomery C, Jackson D, Kelly L, Reilly J, Grant S, Paton J 2003 Intensity of physical activity and its relationship with energy expenditure in young children. Obesity Research 11: 127

Persing J, James H, Swanson J, Kattwinkel J 2003 Prevention and management of positional skull deformities in infants. Pediatrics 112(1): 199–202

Royal College of Nursing (RCN) 1993 Code of practice for the handling of patients. RCN, London

Sadowski D A 1992 Care of the child with burns. In: Hazinski M F (ed) Nursing care of the critically ill child. Mosby, St Louis, MO, ch 13, p 875–927

Short M A, Brooks-Brunn J A, Reeves D S, Yeager J, Thorpe J A 1996 The effects of swaddling versus standard positioning on neuromuscular development in very low birth weight infants. Neonatal Network 15: 2–31

Siegal A C, Burton R V 1999 Effects of baby walkers on motor and mental development in human infants. Journal of Development and Behavioural Pediatrics 20(5): 355–361

Sweeney J, Gutiernez T 2002 Musculoskeletal implications of preterm positioning in the NICU. Journal of Perinatal and Neonatal Nursing 16(1): 58–70

Turrill S 1992 Supported positioning in intensive care. Paediatric Nursing 4(4): 24–27

Updike C, Schmidt R E, Macke C, Cahoon J, Miller M 1986 Positional support for premature infants. American Journal of Occupational Therapy 40(10): 712–715

Warren I 1993 How to place a baby. MIDIRS Midwifery Digest 3(4): 452–453

Postoperative care

Fiona Lynch, Sue Tulp

Introduction

Postoperative care commences as the child leaves the operating theatre and ends when they are discharged from the ward. However, in today's ever-changing national health service environment, hospital inpatient stays are reducing and more children are having surgery undertaken on a day case basis. Consequently, postoperative care may continue into the home care setting and be supported in part by community children's nurses (The Scottish Office 1994, O'Connor-Von 2000, Pfeil et al 2004).

Learning outcomes

By the end of this section you should:

- understand the three stages of postoperative care
- be able to understand fundamental postoperative care
- recognise the role of the child and family carer in the child's recovery

- recognise the involvement of the multidisciplinary team.

Rationale

Care of the child in the postoperative phase is aimed at preventing complications and ensuring as quick a recovery from the operation and anaesthetic as possible. Postoperative care covers many different surgical specialities; however, the fundamental principles of care can be applied to any surgical procedure. The care of the child continues after discharge (Pfeil et al 2004) and often requires further nursing input while they are at home.

Factors to note

There are three stages of postoperative care:

- the immediate recovery period
- the intermediate stage of dependency
- returning to normality (Lyon & Best 1994, Andersen et al 2000, Discolo & Hirose 2002).

These three stages are not perhaps thought of consciously but are planned for from the moment the child is admitted. Surgery can be planned, emergency or day case (see Preoperative Care, p. 316).

A good preoperative preparation can make a difference to the child and their family postoperatively (Tazbir & Cronin 1999).

If children are treated honestly with realistic values and expectations, they can begin to accept the surgery and the consequences of it.

THE IMMEDIATE RECOVERY PERIOD

Immediate recovery from anaesthesia should be in a fully equipped recovery unit with a one-to-one ratio of nursing personnel trained in children's nursing (Association of Anaesthetists of Great Britain and Ireland 2002). Recovery units may be known by a different name in some areas, such as reception or post-anaesthetic care units (PACU). The recovery unit is usually situated near the operating theatres. This enables easy access to the patients by the surgical and anaesthetic staff should an emergency arise.

Whilst the child has been in theatre and recovery, the bed/cot area should have been prepared for return to the ward. In some areas the bed may have been transferred to the recovery unit perioperatively to minimise pain and distress for the child postoperatively. All beds must have a tilt facility and must be able to be raised up and down. (The tilt facility is important if children are experiencing postoperative shock or vomiting as it allows the child's head to be lowered or raised according to need.)

It is imperative that the bed space has access to working oxygen and suction. It may also be necessary for the child to be moved nearer the nursing station for closer observation. Neonates may need to be transferred in an incubator or Baby Therm and the same principles apply to them. Equipment that may be required postoperatively such as infusion pumps and monitoring equipment should be tested and ready when the child is transferred back to the ward. During the perioperative phase of nursing, the theatre nurse is responsi-

ble for the child whilst under anaesthetic and serves as the patient's advocate.

Once the theatre nurse has handed the child over to the recovery unit, immediate postoperative management is the responsibility of the anaesthetist involved in the surgery and the unit staff (Andersen et al 2000). Handover should incorporate the condition of the child whilst under anaesthetic, any problems which may have occurred and any analgesia which has been administered.

Serious complications can occur during the initial stage after surgery; hence the child receives short-term intensive care nursing whilst in the recovery unit. The duration of a child's stay in the unit depends on the type of surgery undertaken and the child's reaction to anaesthesia. If the child's condition indicates further intensive nursing intervention, the child will be transferred to the high-dependency unit (HDU) or the intensive care unit (ICU) (Tazbir & Cronin 1999, Andersen et al 2000).

In the recovery unit the child is attached to a multifunctional monitor which tracks the following: heart rate, ECG, respiratory rate, oxygen saturation, non-invasive blood pressure and skin temperature. This kind of monitoring reduces disturbance to the child yet provides more detailed information for the nurse. Not all children will need all these facilities, as this depends on their condition and the type of surgery undertaken.

All vital signs, e.g. temperature, pulse, blood pressure, respirations and conscious level, are affected by the surgery and anaesthetic. On recovery from anaesthesia initially, the child will be supine with their head tilted; this ensures that the jaw is kept forward, positioning the tongue so that it does not obstruct the airway.

Airway management is one of the most important areas of recovering a child from anaesthesia and should only be undertaken by appropriately trained staff. The airway requires support and this usually entails the administration of oxygen via a facemask and continuous monitoring of oxygen saturation.

If the child has an airway in situ, the nurse waits for signs of returning consciousness before it is removed.

Anaesthesia-induced unconsciousness will mean normal reflexes are absent and respiration must be supported. During semi-consciousness the reflexes, e.g. breathing, coughing, swallowing and blinking, begin to return and finally the patient should be awake and orientated with the return of all normal reflexes.

The airway is usually removed when the patient coughs it out or tries to remove it. It should be stressed that monitoring is only an aid to continuous nursing observation. One of the most common surgical complications is haemorrhage, which can lead to shock. Any deterioration in condition is usually rapid and demands urgent attention. When shocked, the child will be pale, tachycardic and not responding as normal. In children, and especially neonates, it only takes a small amount of blood loss to make transfusion or rapid fluid replacement essential.

It is imperative that each bed/trolley space has working oxygen and suction, an emergency buzzer and easy access to the resuscitation trolley. The nurse should observe the colour of the child, and whether it is good for that particular patient. This type of information is often gained during the preoperative visit or from the ward's nursing documentation. Many children with special needs or those with cardiac/pulmonary problems can be pale or even cyanosed. Their oxygen saturations may also be lower than is normal. The promotion of safety and comfort is paramount and the use of cot sides is universal.

Although the child may feel alert and capable of moving, the remaining effects of the anaesthesia and sedation may mean that movements are uncoordinated. Special consideration should be given to children who have had spinal and epidural anaesthesia. Frequent assessment of the lower extremities should be made to determine the return of function. Temperature, colour and range of sensation and movement should be observed. In recovery, the relief of pain and encouragement to rest are also of high priority. The inclusion of parents in the recovery unit is a relatively new idea. The child has to be sufficiently recovered, e.g. fully conscious and maintaining their own airway, for the inclusion of the parent.

The presence of the parent affords reassurance and comfort and is effective in reducing postoperative distress and anxiety. However, the presence of parents who are themselves visibly distressed, or anxious, can have an adverse effect on the child's emotional condition. It must also be stressed that not all hospitals allow a parent into the recovery unit, although this is becoming more common.

Before the child is transferred back to the ward certain criteria must be fulfilled:

- the child is conscious (but may be asleep)
- the protective reflexes have returned
- the child is maintaining their own airway and respirations are satisfactory
- the child's colour is good for that particular patient
- postoperative observations have been stable
- the child is comfortable and pain is adequately controlled
- the child's temperature is above 36°C
- the child is clean and tidy.

THE INTERMEDIATE STAGE OF DEPENDENCY: RETURN TO THE WARD

Postoperative observations may include:

- temperature, pulse, respirations, blood pressure, colour and conscious level of the child
- observation and monitoring of the wound site
- maintenance of intravenous infusion
- monitoring of drains and urinary catheters

and will be dependent upon the type of surgery that the child has undergone. The frequency of routine postoperative observations may vary and is dependent on the child's condition (Andersen et al 2000). Observation of pulse and respirations is more frequent when intravenous opiate analgesia is in progress. One of the side-effects of opiates is respiratory depression, so the rate, depth and quality of respiration are monitored. Reduction in frequency of postoperative observation is based on the nurse's assessment of the child's condition.

Research has shown that the nurse often carries out more frequent observations than the patient's condition dictates, mistakenly believing that the regime had been prescribed by the hospital or by nursing policy (Botti & Hunt 1994).

Hydration

Normally, the reintroduction of oral fluids is left to the discretion of the nurse and is determined by the type of surgery undertaken. However, if the surgery requires that the child has no fluid, or dietary, intake for a long period of time, e.g. following bowel surgery, hydration needs will have to be met by intravenous means until the child can tolerate fluids orally (Andersen et al 2000). In this instance a fluid balance chart is crucial to monitor all input and output. Output includes urine, vomit, wound leakage, gastric aspirate and stool.

The nurse should also observe for signs of dehydration, e.g. decreased urine output, dark sunken eyes and dry mucous membranes.

Oral fluids should be reintroduced once the child is sufficiently awake. However, in more complex surgery it is common to wait until bowel sounds have returned, and fluids should be commenced as advised by the surgeons. Should it be anticipated that the child is going to be nil by mouth for some time, a nasogastric tube will be inserted for the purpose of draining the stomach of bile and secretions. These losses are replaced millilitre for millilitre with intravenous fluid to prevent the child from becoming dehydrated.

Enteral feeding is usually commenced within 24 hours of surgery unless contraindicated (Tazbir & Cronin 1999). For example, a child having undergone a fundoplication and/or gastrostomy may have to wait 48 hours prior to commencing enteral feeds to allow primary healing. Parenteral nutrition may be administered to children who have been poorly for some time and have no expectation of being able to tolerate diet and fluids normally within a few days. Again, bowel surgery is a good example of this.

Pain (see also pain management, p. 265)

Many hospitals have a pain management policy for children which focuses on pain prevention and, where possible, children should be involved in assessing their own pain level. Pain assessment tools rely on the child's understanding of numbers, colours and drawings, so a selection of pain assessment tools is helpful in finding the right one to suit the child's level of understanding (Twycross 1995).

Parents play an important role in communicating with the child and, for those who cannot communicate verbally, pain management is something that should be discussed preoperatively.

As well as pharmacological pain relief, alternative methods include distraction, massage and snoozelen therapy. Snoozelen therapy works with all the senses, using aids such as soft music, optic fibre lights and tactile toys.

Pain is not just a consideration in the immediate postoperative period. The nurse has to prepare the child and family for potentially painful procedures such as removing drains and mobilisation. On these occasions, the play specialist can provide distraction therapy during the procedure. It is important, where possible, to carry out such procedures away from the bedside as the bed should be seen as a safe haven and a place of comfort. Privacy and dignity should be maintained at all times.

Method

1. Establish baseline information. Record temperature, pulse, respirations and blood pressure. Vital signs should be monitored and recorded regularly to detect any complications such as haemorrhage or compromise of the airway. They may also indicate that the child is experiencing pain. Assess consciousness level. Report any changes or concerns.

2. Observe the pallor of the skin. If oxygen is to be administered, ensure that the mask is correctly positioned and that the oxygen is delivered at the prescribed rate. Mouth care is essential to ensure patient comfort (see Hygiene, p. 198).

3. Check wound sites and drains. Monitor wound sites at regular intervals for signs of leakage and mark as necessary; change

dressings or add additional padding as required. Report any excessive leakage. If drains are in situ, record output regularly and note the characteristics of the fluid, e.g. haemoserous fluid.

Note: Aim to observe the wound site at the same time as these observations to reduce disturbance to the child.

4. Commence fluid balance chart. If an intravenous infusion is in situ, maintain it at the prescribed rate and record the amount infused hourly. Check the access point for signs of extravasation or phlebitis and report immediately. Reintroduce oral fluids as advised and increase intake as tolerated. All intake and output should be recorded. In the absence of oral fluid intake, ensure that adequate mouth care is provided.

5. Observe for signs of dehydration. Look for decreased urine output, poor skin turgor, dark sunken eyes, sunken fontanelle (in babies), dry mucous membranes and prolonged episodes of vomiting. Inform the medical staff of concerns. If an intravenous infusion is not in progress, it may be necessary to site one. Antiemetics may help to reduce nausea and vomiting and need to be prescribed and monitored as to their effectiveness.

6. Assess pain. Use a pain tool relevant to the child's age and development to assess the need for analgesia. All analgesia should be given as prescribed and monitored for any adverse reactions and effectiveness. If intravenous analgesia is in progress, such as patient-controlled analgesia (PCA), maintain it at the prescribed rate and record pulse and respirations hourly, as some opiates may cause respiratory depression. Report any significant changes immediately. Liaise with the pain management team, if available, to regularly manage the child's pain safely and effectively.

7. Remember reduced mobility. Observe and relieve pressure areas at regular intervals. Encourage the child to move by themselves where possible, but nursing staff should be there to assist. Changing position can also help to relieve any pain or discomfort the child may be experiencing. If appropriate, and if parents feel confident, babies and young children can be nursed on a knee or in a pushchair.

Encourage older children to cough and deep breathe. It may be necessary to involve the physiotherapist to relieve any chest problems and help with mobilisation. This type of involvement is usually for those who have had more major surgery, e.g. appendicectomy, nephrectomy. It is usual to mobilise as soon as the child's condition allows.

Reduced mobility can also affect bowel movement. Monitor for signs of constipation and give aperients as prescribed if necessary. When diet and fluids have been re-established, encourage a good fluid intake and a diet which contains roughage. Depending on the type of surgery undertaken, for example following fundoplication, it may be advisable for the child to have smaller meals more frequently until normal dietary intake is re-established.

The family

Following the acute stage of surgical nursing care the priority is to encourage a safe return to normality.

It should be stressed to the parents and the family that the child still needs periods of rest. Sometimes this can be hard, especially when many paediatric wards and hospitals encourage an open visiting policy. Again it must be emphasised that not all wards will have this policy.

The paediatric nurse should always take account of the different ages of the children being cared for. Adolescents have specific needs and provision should be made to keep children of a similar age together where possible. Privacy and dignity should be maintained at all times.

DISCHARGE PLANNING

The nurse should begin planning for discharge from the time of admission whenever possible. Usually, the initial assessment will identify potential problems, such as transport home and referrals to community nurses. Effective discharge planning can reduce any delay once the decision has been made to allow the patient home. Many areas have pre-printed discharge plans, which form part of the nursing documentation, and these often extend to printed discharge advice leaflets. The discharge plan should include any supplies that may be required, e.g. dressings, catheter bags, etc. Drugs required on discharge and specific instructions are important. Examples of such information are when the child should resume school and physical exercise. Information should also be given regarding pain relief,

observation of the wound site and who to contact in an emergency.

Personal experience has shown that parents find it useful to have written instructions for reference, and contact numbers should be included for advice if they are having any problems.

If a child is a day case, it may be appropriate to arrange for a district nurse, probably a paediatric community nurse, to visit the child the following day to perform a postoperative check and ensure that the parents are happy with their child's recovery. Again it should be noted that this is not always the case; local policy may dictate this practice.

COMMUNITY PERSPECTIVE

The role of the CCN in postoperative care can vary, particularly in reference to day surgery, from maintaining telephone contact with the family to check that all is well, to regular visiting to help with nursing care and monitor progress, ensuring that recovery is at the expected rate. This can be reassuring for parents, should any unforeseen problems occur. In some areas this routine postoperative care may be undertaken by district nurses, who can refer cases to the CCNs if they feel this to be appropriate.

It may be necessary to visit to change dressings or remove sutures.

Do and do not

- Do encourage the parents to participate in their child's care.
- Do explain the planned care to the child and the family.
- Do explain the use of any equipment, e.g. infusion pumps, and also the purpose of any drains in situ.
- Do encourage the child to rest.
- Do explain discharge arrangements to the parents prior to discharge.
- Do outline the limitations, if any, when the child returns home, i.e. return to school and exercise.

- Do not allow the child to be discharged without arranging follow-up or community nurse input, if required.
- Do not forget that surgery is never routine for the child or the family.
- Do not assume that the parent or carer will want to participate in postoperative care. This should always be negotiated.
- Do not forget to give parents a contact number for advice should they have any problems.

References

Andersen D, DeVoll-Zabrocki A, Brown C, Inverson A, Larsen J 2000 Intestinal transplantation in pediatric patients: a nursing challenge. Part 2: Intestinal transplantation and the immediate postoperative period. Gastroenterology Nursing 23(5): 201–209

Association of Anaesthetists of Great Britain and Ireland 2002 Immediate post-anaesthetic recovery. AAGBI, London

Botti M A, Hunt J O 1994 The routine of post anaesthetic observations. Contemporary Nurse 3(2): 52–57

Discolo C M, Hirose K 2002 Pediatric cochlear implants. American Journal of Audiology 11: 114–118

Lyon M H, Best B J 1994 Immediate postoperative recovery: management and care. British Journal of Nursing 3(17): 866, 868–870

O'Connor-Von S 2000 Preparing children for surgery – an integrative research review. AORN 71(2): 334–343

Pfeil M, Mathur A, Lind J 2004 Early discharge following uncomplicated appendicectomy in children. Paediatric Nursing 16(7): 15–18

Tazbir J S, Cronin D C 1999 Indications, evaluations and post operative care of combined liver–heart transplant recipients. AACN Clinical Issues 10(2): 240–252

The Scottish Office 1994 Caring for sick children: a study of hospital services in Scotland. HMSO, Edinburgh

Twycross A 1995 Children's nursing in Canada. Paediatric Nursing 7(4): 8–10

Further Reading

Fairchild S 1996 Peri-operative nursing: principles and practise, 2nd ed. Little Brown, Boston, MA

Royal College of Nursing 2004 Sheet 3: day surgery information. Children/young people in day surgery. RCN, London

Smith F 1995 Children's nursing in practice – the Nottingham model. Blackwell Science, Oxford

Websites

www.aagbi.org

www.actionforsickchildren.org

Preoperative care

Fiona Lynch, Sue Tulp

Introduction

Effective preparation of children who are to undergo anaesthesia and surgical intervention is an important factor in reducing the anxiety experienced by the child and their family during hospital admission (RCN 2004). Children provide a unique challenge in that the education and preparation that they require must not only meet their needs, but also the needs of their parents/primary carers (Kelly & Adkins 2003).

Learning outcomes

By the end of this section you should:

- recognise the need for safe preparation for theatre
- understand the role of the parent in the preoperative phase
- be able to identify the needs of different age groups and their level of understanding
- recognise stressors affecting both parent and child
- be able to identify multidisciplinary involvement in preoperative care
- be able to assist in the safe preparation of a child for theatre
- consider the importance of preparing for discharge within the preoperative period.

Rationale

Children, regardless of age, need to be appropriately prepared for theatre. This involves both physical and psychological aspects of care. Children who are familiar with their surroundings, and who are informed of events associated with surgical procedures, are more likely to cope with the overall experience (Newman & Scott 1990, O'Connor-Von 2000).

Parents who are fully informed and involved are confident and capable partners in the hospitalisation and recovery process of their child and on discharge (Darbyshire 2003). Children who are informed will have a reduction in anxiety related to the procedure and also to the hospital environment (LeRoy et al 2003).

Factors to note

Planned surgery

- Planned, or elective, surgery lends itself very well to good preparation prior to the day of surgery (O'Connor-Von 2000, Sexton & Redfearn 2003). There is time to involve other disciplines who can make a contribution to the overall readiness of both the child and family for forthcoming surgery.

- Psychological preparation can begin at home well before the planned date of admission. There is a wide range of books and other visual aids available from libraries and bookshops which offer the opportunity to talk through the need for hospitalisation and what to expect. Schools and nurseries will often facilitate role-play which involves dressing up and acting out the nurse/doctor roles. These are all recognised as ways of allaying fears and anxieties of children and can help those parents who have little experience of hospitals themselves (LeRoy et al 2003). Preparation should include information on what will happen postoperatively including relevant information on wound care.

- The development of pre-admission programmes, such as Saturday morning clubs, facilitates interaction between hospital staff, children and parents and provides the opportunity to discuss pain control and the admission procedure. Efforts made at this stage of contact promote a feeling of well-being and aid in the speedy recovery of the child (LeRoy et al 2003, Sutherland 2003).

- On admission, there is the opportunity to involve play specialists and theatre staff. Action for Sick Children (1991) highlighted the value of play in hospital and this role has been further developed in paediatric areas. The benefit of the involvement of play specialists in overcoming operation anxiety, the use of photograph albums and visits made by recovery staff, all give a broader view of what the child will experience and the parents' role in the process (see Play, p. 457).

Emergency surgery

- Unplanned surgery often means that there is little time for the psychological preparation of the parent or child. Some children go to theatre directly from the accident and emergency department, and so there may be limited time for explanations or time for premedications. Sudden loss of contact with parents and siblings can cause additional stress to the child. The nurse should be aware of these factors and deal with them sensitively.

- When the child has been transferred to theatre it is usual for the parents to be taken to the admitting ward to wait for the surgery to be completed. It is during this time that additional information and emotional/psychological support are given.

- When a child is transferred to the ward only a short time prior to surgery, emphasis is mainly on physical preparation, with medical staff completing tasks such as obtaining consent and examination of the child. There may be an opportunity for the parents to speak with the anaesthetist or surgeon, but this is not always possible. Fuller explanations of procedures and planned care usually take place whilst the child is in theatre and upon return to the ward.

Day care surgery

- Day surgery has many advantages for both the child and family. The report *Caring for Children in the Health Service* (Action for Sick Children 1991) explored the benefits of paediatric day care from an economic viewpoint, and from the child's needs with regard to avoiding the necessity for overnight admission. This was reinforced by the Audit Commission report, *Children First* (1993), which encouraged the development of such facilities.

- Morton and Raine (1994) defined some of the benefits as absence of parental separation, less disruption to the family and an increase in the amount of parental involvement. All of these should be supported by care being available in the community for children following attendance at a day care facility.

- The National Association for the Welfare of Children in Hospital (NAWCH, now known as Action for Sick Children) produced advice and 12 quality standards for children admitted as day cases in a report entitled *Just for the Day* (Thornes 1991). This covered the need for pre-admission programmes, literature available outlining parental responsibilities and a friendly environment. Some hospitals may have a designated area for children within an adult setting. In these instances great care must be taken to provide adequate facilities suitable for both children and their families.

- To shorten the admission time it is preferable that routine preoperative investigations are completed during outpatient visits so that all necessary results are available on the day of admission. LeRoy et al (2003) suggest that younger children (age 3–5 years) should have the preparation as close to the day of surgery as possible, whereas older children (age 6–12 years) benefit more from earlier preparation, i.e. up to 1 week before.

- Written instructions for preoperative fasting should be given to the parents along with information about giving routine medications, e.g. inhalers. Parents should be encouraged to bring any medications with them on the day of admission.

- At some centres, children can travel to theatre on bicycles and in motorised cars which makes the journey much more acceptable and exciting. The wearing of their own clothes is becoming more widespread, but parents should be advised to bring a change of clothes as a precaution.

- Most areas now use topical anaesthetic creams such as EMLA or Ametop, and this can sometimes negate the need for oral premedications. The use of local anaesthesia (e.g. nerve blocks) during surgery was shown to reduce the complications of pain,

nausea and vomiting. In addition, the children were awake more rapidly following anaesthesia, allowing diet and fluids to be accepted (Cohen et al 1990). This enables discharge to occur earlier, therefore minimising the stay in hospital.

- It should be stressed to the parents that there may be the possibility of an overnight stay if events change. This enables the family to make further arrangements if necessary.

- Arrangements should be made in advance for transport home (according to local policy), a discharge letter to be sent to the GP and, in some instances, a postoperative home visit.

Children with disabilities

- The preparation of children with disabilities may place more emphasis on the parents' or carers' involvement depending on the degree of disability. However, the basic principles of preoperative care still apply and the methods by which the children are prepared for theatre may need only slight adjustment. For example, the preparation of a child with visual impairment will be verbal rather than visual, but although photograph albums are of little use to the child, they may be helpful to the parent or carer who in turn may help you to explain procedures in a language that the child can understand.

- Distraction therapy may be useful to reduce the anxiety of the child and involvement of play specialists is helpful in this instance (Honeyman 1994, Kelly & Adkins 2003) (see Play, p. 457).

- For those children who cannot communicate verbally, one of the most important discussions, which should take place prior to surgery is that of pain control. The non-verbal signs used by the child to convey pain, or discomfort, are more readily known by the parent; similarly they usually know what comforts the child, such as rocking, stroking or talking. Richardson (1992) highlighted the fact that professionals sometimes underestimate the amount of pain experienced by children; it is therefore desirable to secure parental involvement in pain control when possible.

General points

Parents within the anaesthetic room

Policies for allowing parents into the anaesthetic room vary from hospital to hospital. However, adequate preparation of the parents as to their role in the anaesthetic room should remove one of the main reasons for their exclusion (Hall 1995). Where parents are excluded, the role of the named nurse or primary nurse has great importance in reducing separation anxiety (Gahan & Rogers 1993).

Parents, who do accompany their child to theatre, are the responsibility of the ward nurse who will ensure that the parent is not becoming distressed and will take them back to the ward once the child is asleep.

Toys and comforters

Any toys or comforters with the child will either be given to the parent or taken to the recovery room in readiness for the child being received from theatre.

Preparation

Whenever possible, the child should have every opportunity to be prepared for theatre by both professionals and parents. Their involvement may affect the level of cooperation the child is willing to give, and will lessen the amount of anxiety and stress felt by the child and family alike.

Preoperative fasting

It is now widely acknowledged that excessive fasting prior to surgery is inappropriate for children (Doswell et al 2002, Winslow et al 2002, Meurling 2004). As early as 1990, Schreiner et al showed that clear fluids up to 2 hours before surgery for children of any age posed no additional risk of pulmonary aspiration during elective surgery. It is now accepted that children should not be fasted overnight prior to surgery/procedures and that a minimum fasting period of 2 hours may be sufficient (Meurling 2004). However, it is important for the nurse to be aware of hospital policy or protocol on fasting and, if unsure, to check with the appropriate anaesthetist.

Age-appropriate preparation

- Age-appropriate preparation is vital. Children have different attention spans and their ability to take in information and make sense of it may be limited. In these instances it is more appropriate to direct most of the educational efforts towards the parents.
- Older age groups are looking for answers; knowledge gives them a sense of control and the ability to cooperate. They are more able to contribute to their own care by becoming involved in the planning and negotiating of preoperative care (Slote 2002). Explanations of the planned surgery and the sensations they will experience are appropriate (Stinson 1996).
- In the physical preparation, involve the parents as much as possible whilst giving them the opportunity to opt out of any part of the process with which they do not feel comfortable.

Method

1. Introduce yourself to the child and family as the nurse designated for the child's care.
2. Familiarise the child and family with the ward environment and the child's allocated bed.
3. Complete the admission procedure including baseline observations and current weight. Assist the medical staff with any preoperative investigations, e.g. haemoglobin levels, if necessary.
4. Encourage the child to bathe if not already done and remove any nail varnish. The fingertip colour is a good indication of the level of oxygenation in the bloodstream and is observed during the operative stage.
5. Remove any jewellery, or tape it if it cannot be removed, and either give it to the parents for safekeeping or lock it in the hospital

safe. (Jewellery can act as a conductor of electricity and may result in contact burns if not managed appropriately.)

6. Encourage the child to empty their bladder or put on a clean nappy prior to giving any premedication.
7. Make a note of any loose teeth and inform the anaesthetist. If a tooth is very loose, the anaesthetist may suggest that they remove it when the child is asleep to safeguard accidental ingestion or inhalation during the operation. Remove any dentures or plates.
8. If the child has long hair, tie it up using a non-metallic device.
9. Remove any prosthesis, hearing aids or spectacles. The latter two may be removed in the anaesthetic room at the last moment.
10. Some hospitals may allow children to wear their own clothes. If this is the case, ensure that they do not restrict access to the operation site; otherwise make sure that a suitable theatre gown is available for the child to wear. Small babies and neonates may also need to wear a hat as they lose most of their body heat through the scalp.
11. Check that the child has been fasted for a specified time.
12. Check that the child's name and hospital number are correct and legible on the wristband as sometimes these can become unclear after bathing.

13. Ensure that the premedication has been given by the prescribed route and at the prescribed time. If there are any queries relating to the premedication, check with the anaesthetist.
14. Check that the case notes, X-rays (if applicable) and nursing documentation are available, and that the consent form has been completed correctly.
15. Ensure that the operation site, if previously marked by the medical staff, is still clearly visible.
16. Complete the theatre checklist, as per local policy, and await confirmation that theatre is ready to receive the child. (The checklist should be completed immediately prior to the child going to theatre.)
17. Where the child's surgery has been delayed on the day of theatre, it is important to keep the family/parents informed. The anaesthetist must be contacted where the child is being maintained nil by mouth for an extended period as a result of delay to avoid extensive fasting.
18. Accompany the child to theatre, having first checked the patient details with the theatre slip brought by the theatre porter. Some hospitals may check the details in theatre reception to confirm the identity of the child.

COMMUNITY PERSPECTIVE

Referral to the CCN team depends on the capacity and referral criteria of the team.

There are some cases where parents can be helped to organise specific equipment prior to admission, for example when a child is to have a hip spica plaster applied. It is always important to ensure that parents are well informed because any anxiety of the parent will be transmitted to the child.

Preoperative therapeutic play can be undertaken in the home environment by community play specialists, where these are available (Shipton 1997). In this way potentially traumatic situations can be defused by familiarising the child with medical equipment. Children with needle, or hospital, phobia may be referred prior to admission and, in the safe environment of the home, be helped to overcome their fears by various play techniques. In some centres the play specialist can meet the children in the hospital on admission and continue to work with them.

Children who are on the waiting list for a renal transplant can be prepared in advance in the home (Wilson 1992). This can be done by storytelling, playing with dolls and introducing medical equipment. In this way, children are helped to cope with some of their anxieties.

Do and do not

- Do involve the parents in the preparation if they wish.
- Do be honest in answering the child's questions.
- Do remember that this is not routine to the family and be aware of their fears and anxieties.

- Do give clear and concise information.
- Do not assume that children who have had previous operations are not in need of support.
- Do not devolve total responsibility to parents to enforce fasting. Sometimes this can be misunderstood as meaning food only.

References

Action for Sick Children 1991 Caring for children in the health service. Action for Sick Children, London

Audit Commission 1993 Children first: a study of hospital services. HMSO, London

Cohen M, Cameron C B, Duncan P G 1990 Pediatric anaesthesia morbidity and mortality in the perioperative period. Anaesthesia and Analgesia 70: 160–167

Darbyshire P 2003 Mothers' experiences of their child's recovery in hospital and at home: a qualitative investigation. Journal of Child Health Care 7(4): 291–312

Doswell W M, Jones M, O'Donnell J M 2002 One size may not fit all. American Journal of Nursing 102(6): 58, 61

Gahan B, Rogers M 1993 Recent advances in child health nursing. In: Glasper A, Tucker A (eds) Advances in child health nursing. Scutari, London, p 91–105

Hall P A 1995 Cited in British Medical Journal 310(6983): 871

Honeyman L 1994 Play for children with special needs. Paediatric Nursing 6(3): 18–19

Kelly M M, Adkins L 2003 Ingredients for a successful pediatric preoperative care process. AORN Journal 77(5): 1006–1011

LeRoy S, Elixson E M, O'Brein P et al 2003 Recommendations for preparing children and adolescents for invasive cardiac procedures. Circulation 108: 2550–2564. Online. Available: www.circulationaha.org

Meurling S 2004 Paediatric aspects: no fasting in children? Scandinavian Journal of Nutrition 48(2): 83

Morton N S, Raine P A M 1994 Paediatric day case surgery. Oxford Medical Publications, Oxford

Newman J, Scott G 1990 Preoperative care. In: Paediatric nursing. Springhouse Clinical Rotation Guides. Springhouse, Pennsylvania, p 219–224

O'Connor-Von S 2000 Preparing children for surgery – an integrative research review. AORN Journal 71(2): 334–343

Royal College of Nursing (RCN) 2004 Sheet 3: Day surgery information. Children/young people in day surgery. RCN, London

Richardson J 1992 Acute pain in childhood. Surgical Nurse 22

Sexton K, Redfearn M 2003 Preadmission testing in a children's facility. AORN Journal 78(4): 604, 606, 608–612, 614–615, 617

Schreiner M S, Treibwasser A, Keon T P et al 1990 Ingestion of liquids compared with pre-operative fasting in paediatric outpatients. Anaesthesiology 72(4): 593–597

Shipton H 1997 Play at home. Cascade. Action for Sick Children, London, p 8–9

Slote R J 2002 Psychological aspects of caring for the adolescent undergoing spinal fusion for scoliosis. Orthopaedic Nursing 21(6): 19–30

Stinson A 1996 Cochlear implantations in children. AORN Journal 64(4): 561–571

Sutherland T 2003 Comparison of hospital and home base preparation for cardiac surgery. Paediatric Nursing 15(5): 13–16

Thornes R 1991 Just for the day. Action for Sick Children, London

Wilson L 1992 The home visiting programme. Paediatric Nursing (July): 10–11

Winslow E H, Crenshaw J T, Warner M A 2002 Best practice shouldn't be optional. American Journal of Nursing 102(6): 59, 63

Further Reading

Action for Sick Children 2002 Setting standards for children undergoing surgery. Action for Sick Children, London

Department of Health 1996 Services for children and young people. DoH, London

Donnelly J 1998 RGN. Nursing Standard 12(42): 22–23

Heath S 1998 Perioperative care of the child. Quay Books, Salisbury, UK

Practice 24

Pressure area care

Louise Dyer, Bev Embling

Introduction

Historically, scant attention has been given to the reporting of pressure sores in the child population (Tooher et al 2003). Waterlow's (1997) study identified that children can develop pressure sores as a consequence of immobility, illness or hospitalisation, thus requiring the need for appropriate education, assessment and intervention. However, since then, the issue of research into the risk factors associated with the development of pressure sores appears to be very low on the research agenda, with very little new evidence to further support Waterlow's (1997) work.

Pressure sore risk assessment is now considered an essential element of care in adults as shown in the document *Essence of Care*; this focuses on quality of care and benchmarking to deliver evidenced-based practice (DoH 2001). Whilst this is a positive step forward, it does not specifically include the child population; there are essential elements of pressure sore risk assessment, care and management that can be applied in principle when caring for children and young people (Braden et al 1987, Bedi 1993, Waterlow 1997, DoH 2001, NICE 2003a,b).

Learning outcomes

By the end of this section, you should be able to understand and explain:

- the causes of pressure sores
- the principles of pressure risk assessment
- nursing care and pressure sore prevention
- policy-driven changes to improve pressure risk assessment and management.

RISK ASSESSMENT

Whilst there are various pressure risk assessment scoring methods in use within clinical and community healthcare practice, none was developed for the sole purpose of caring for children (Bedi 1993, Waterlow 1997). This suggests consideration should be employed when assessing risk factors for children. Bedi (1993) provided a template for scoring risk assessment

(Fig. 24.1) which can be modified for use in all aspects of children's nursing. All formal assessments of risk should be documented and accessible for other professionals within the multidisciplinary team. There is insufficient evidence to recommend one risk assessment scale as superior to another, or appropriate for use in all child healthcare settings (McGough 1999).

Risk factors to consider

Bedi (1993) and Waterlow (1997) identified factors which affect pressure sore risk as either extrinsic or intrinsic.

- Extrinsic factors include:
  - pressure: compression on a local point, due to reduced or lack of mobility
  - shearing: distortion of the skin beyond its ability to adapt, due to poor positioning
  - friction: the skin is in contact with the supporting surface, due to inappropriate manual handling techniques
  - moisture to the skin: delayed hygiene/elimination needs met.
- Intrinsic factors include:
  - nutritional status: obesity or lack of body mass
  - dehydration: skin turgor.

Consideration of these factors provides identification of children who may be at risk of pressure sore development. Waterlow (1997) recommends each child should be assessed using a questionnaire, along with use of body maps and documentation. Although this presents a challenge when assessing the unwell child with an altered level of consciousness, an acute illness or complete immobility, a full and thorough assessment of pressure risks is essential (RCN 2001). It is important therefore to consider the following aspects in the assessment.

Body weight
Children who are overweight, or have excess weight due to fluid retention as a consequence of the side-effects of medications, may also experience difficulty in mobilising. Special consideration should be given to neonates who have less body mass, and therefore may expe-

rience increased risk over bony prominences and high localised pressure (e.g. the back of the head) (Barnes 2004).

Elimination
The child who is experiencing continence problems is not only at risk of developing pressure sores but is also at increased risk of infection due to breakdown in skin integrity as a consequence of prolonged contact with urine and faecal matter (Waterlow 1997). Whilst infants may be considered as incontinent, it is prolonged contact with urine and/or faecal matter that will cause a break in skin integrity and not as a consequence of undue pressure (Waterlow 1997).

Skin integrity
Children with special needs may experience poor skin integrity due to reduced circulation, poor hydration and inactivity, and therefore have a tendency to have dry and fragile skin that excoriates easily. Conversely, these children may have a greasy or oily skin type which may become sore and chaffed due to excessive perspiration. Children with thermal injuries are at particular risk of further skin breakdown due to excessive fluid loss (Bosworth-Bousfield 2002). Neonates are also vulnerable because their skin is very translucent and delicate.

Mobility
The body's natural response to prolonged pressure discomfort in any part of the body is to try to change position spontaneously. In the child with reduced mobility due, for example, to altered conscious levels, the child with special or complex needs, the child in traction or the severely thermally injured child, the increased risk of pressure sore development due to immobility is even greater (Jones 1997). It is therefore essential that a high quality of nursing care be provided to prevent pressure sores developing. Equally, the child who has been in theatre for a prolonged period or the ventilated child in intensive care is also at risk from breakdown in skin integrity (Neidig et al 1989, Barnes 2004).

Nutrition and hydration
These are vital aspects in reducing and assessing pressure area risk. Malnutrition increases

PAEDIATRIC PRESSURE RISK ASSESSMENT SCORE CHART

Patient name: _____

Ward:_____

Date of birth: _____   Date of admission _____

Please assign a numerical value to each of the following

ASSESSMENT PERIOD DATE ⇨ TIME ⇨														
BUILD AND WEIGHT FOR AGE														
Average according to age	0													
Above average	1													
Overweight	2													
Below average	3													
SKIN CONDITION														
Healthy	0													
Ciammy (e.g. pyrexial)	1													
Cannulation/arterial access	1													
Dry skin, dehydrated, lack of turgor	2													
Oedematous or discoloured	2													
Broken skin	3													
MOBILITY														
Full, normal for age	0													
Restless, fidgety	1													
Moves with limited assistance	2													
Skeletal traction/POP/limb splinting	2													
Dependent on others/Special Needs Children	3													
APPETITE/NUTRITION														
Normal for child	0													
Insufficient to maintain weight, altered appetite + Requiring N/G feeding	2													
Poor, eats + drinks little, IV fluids	2													
Very poor, refuses food	3													
ELIMINATION/NAPPY AREA														
Completely continent for age/condition	0													
Occasionally incontinent/catheterised	1													
Frequently incontinent/nappy rash	2													
Fully incontinent, no control	3													
DRUGS														
IV antibiotics	1													
Continuous IV morphine/sedation	2													
Cytotoxic drug therapy	3													
High-dose steroids or high-dose NSAIDs	3													
THERMAL INJURIES														
Lower body <2% and/or upper body <8%	0													
General distribution 10–24%	1													
Lower body 3–24%	2													
Mainly upper body 25–35%	2													
Lower body >25% or general distribution >35%	3													
TOTAL RISK SCORE														
ASSESSOR'S INITIALS														

Patient's risk score:

Low risk (0–5) assess every 3–5 days
Medium risk (6–10) assess daily
High risk (11–14) assess 4-hourly/daily
Very high risk (>14)

Action:

Change patient's position regurlarly. Consider dietary intake
Consider position. Diet. Softform mattress/Airwave mattress
Consider position. Diet. Airwave mattress/Tissue viability nurse
2-Hourly pressure care. Diet. Hygiene. Airwave mattress

Figure 24.1   Paediatric pressure risk assessment score chart. (Adapted from Bedi 1993.)

the skin's vulnerability to pressure sore formation. It is essential that the child's dietary requirements are fully documented on admission and throughout the child's care. It is vital to liaise with other healthcare professionals such as the dietitian to ensure that essential nutritional elements are provided, for example:

- vitamin C – essential for collagen synthesis
- vitamin E – to reduce tissue damage
- protein – to encourage collagen synthesis and wound remodelling
- zinc – if deficient, delays wound healing (Olding & Patterson 1998).

Accurate nutritional and fluid assessment by the nurse is fundamental, as other nutritional deficits such as failure to thrive and eating disorders can become more complex in the critically ill child. Maintaining adequate fluid and nutrition aids skin suppleness and tissue perfusion, thereby increasing circulation and reducing the risk of skin breakdown (Dealey 1999). If the infant or child is dehydrated, the skin can become dry, scaly and fragile. Children that are oedematous can experience similar changes in skin integrity (Barnes 2004).

Medication
Some drug therapies cause skin to change, for example the use of long-term steroid therapy, anti-inflammatory and cytotoxic drugs. These pharmacological preparations can cause the skin to become fragile, dry and at increased risk of damage due to inhibition of the body's immune system. Some inotropes cause peripheral vasoconstriction. Sedation can also lead to

altered consciousness, where the child is less likely to alter their position to relieve pressure (Barnes 2004).

PRESSURE SORES

Pressure sores can occur anywhere, depending on the cause, but typical sites for pressure sores in children will include any bony prominences, including sacrum, buttocks, ear, heels and the back of the head. Waterlow (1997) particularly noted the additional risks of medical equipment such as tubing, leads or intravenous lines.

Several scales are in use in adult practice for grading the severity of pressure ulcers; an example is given in Box 24.1.

PREVENTION

It is essential to carry out pressure risk assessment as part of the normal admission and in the ongoing assessment of the child whilst they are in hospital. The purpose of assessment is to identify areas of potential risk and implement interventions to reduce the chances of skin breakdown occurring.

Consideration of the child's environment is essential; lying on something hard such as monitor leads, intravenous lines or a toy even for a short period can initiate pressure sore development.

These interventions may be the subject of local policy, which rationalises use of scarce or expensive pressure-relieving equipment. Waterlow (1997) and Cockett (2002) recognise

---

Box 24.1   The Stirling Pressure Sore Severity Scale (SPSSS)

Stage 0: No clinical evidence of a pressure sore. May be normal skin, or healed, scarred skin, or tissue is damaged but due to other causes
Stage 1: Discoloration of intact skin, light finger pressure to site does not alter discoloration. There may be some local heat
Stage 2: Partial-thickness skin loss or damage involving dermis or epidermis. Blister, abrasion, shallow ulcer

Stage 3: Full-thickness skin loss, damage or necrosis of subcutaneous tissue not extending to underlying structures (bone, tendon, joint capsule)
Stage 4: Full-thickness skin loss with extensive destruction and tissue necrosis extending to underlying structures

that pressure sores can occur even when preventive aids are used.

Developmental considerations

- Age can affect the area of the body where pressure damage can occur: older children tend to develop sacral sores (Willock et al 2000), whereas in the neonate or small child the back of the head is particularly at risk and often forgotten.
- Zollo et al (1996) revealed that children in intensive care units are at particular risk, requiring increased nursing awareness and management, such as regular turning. If this pressure-relieving action is not possible, then it is vital to employ other methods immediately.
- Assessment, identification and the correcting or avoiding of risk factors are the most important aspects of prevention and care. For example, malnutrition and dehydration can be corrected through nutritional and fluid management; for the child experiencing continence difficulties, the nurse's responsibility is to ensure effective hygiene care, which may include the management of continence.

EDUCATION

It is an essential component of pressure area risk assessment and management that parents and nursing staff are trained and competent in the use of pressure risk tools and equipment. This can be achieved through liaison with other health professionals such as the tissue viability or wound management specialist nurses. It is also important to carry out pressure area care utilising evidence-based practice to improve standards of care (DoH 2001).

Equipment

Use of guidelines in conjunction with local policy will assist with pressure relief (Southmead Health Service NHS Trust 1997, Waterlow 1997, RCN 2001). An in-depth assessment and accurate documentation of the child's needs is also vital.

- Children deemed to be at low risk could use a standard mattress.

- For medium-risk cases, use of a pressure-relieving mattress or overlays is advisable, depending on local/trust policy. Other aids such as silicone gel or foam pads may be beneficial.
- Children at high risk of skin breakdown, e.g. children having prolonged surgery, should have access to a soft conforming theatre table along with the use of other appropriate pressure-relieving aids. Use of airwave inflation systems, such as the dynamic flotation systems Nimbus and Pegasus, is essential.
- For the child with total restrictions on mobility, e.g. the child with complex wound management needs or the thermally injured child, specialist equipment such as Clinitron air-fluidised therapy and low-flow therapy beds will assist in their nursing care.

WOUND MANAGEMENT

Wound management should follow accepted principles of wound care (see Wound Care, p. 441).

Potential risks of inappropriate prevention and management of pressure sores

- *To the child and family*: pain, scarring and disfigurement, low self-esteem, risk of further complications, septicaemia and death.
- *To the nurse*: vulnerability to litigation for negligent practice; failure to fulfil obligations set out in the *Code of Professional Conduct* (NMC 2002); decreased job satisfaction.
- *To the organisation*: cost of litigation cases; increased costs for inpatient care, due to prolonged bed occupancy. There is also a need to question the quality of service provision, which could have a negative impact upon the trust in question.

Pressure risk and clinical governance

The prevention and management of pressure sores is a quality issue and therefore nurses have a responsibility to ensure that it forms part of the clinical governance agenda in their clinical area. Clinical governance in relation to pressure area care can be viewed under the following components:

- *Clinical risk management*: This is achieved through assessment, analysis and learning from actions seen and perceived.
- *Clinical effectiveness*: Pressure risk assessment and management is monitored and evaluated as to the effectiveness of care. This

includes evidence-based practice, clinical guidelines and clinical outcome measures (DoH 2001). Key aspects are education, information and critical appraisal.

- *Clinical audit*: Ensures high standards of patient care, measuring current practice against standards of best practice; audit will then lead to improving clinical practice (DoH 1998).

COMMUNITY PERSPECTIVE

Children with a variety of conditions who are cared for at home may be at risk of developing pressure sores.

The responsibility of the CCN is to ensure that carers are aware of all potential problems. The CCN will need to educate the carers on pressure-relieving methods, such as positioning and turning, and on fluid and dietary requirements. Some families may require the loan of specialist equipment, the use of which will need

to be demonstrated by the CCN. Some household equipment may need to be adapted to meet a specific need.

The CCN will need excellent knowledge of local resources in order to meet the needs of the family. Although some community nursing services have a good supply of equipment, the CCN may need to pursue and persist in order to obtain the optimum equipment for a particular child.

Do and do not

- Do assess each child individually, taking into account potential/actual extrinsic and intrinsic factors.
- Do not make assumptions that children do not get pressure sores.
- Do ensure all potential risks are documented accurately in the child's care record.
- Do utilise all available resources and literature to improve clinical practice and reduce potential risks of pressure development.

Conclusion

It is essential that assessment of every child is thoroughly implemented, taking into account all known and potential risk factors. Accurate documentation of the child's skin integrity status is vital to assist with effective tissue viability management; it should also be noted that collaboration with other significant members of the multidisciplinary team should be encouraged to ensure that a seamless service of care is provided.

References

Barnes S 2004 The use of a pressure ulcer risk assessment tool for children. Nursing Times 100(14): 56–58

Bedi A 1993 A tool to fill the gap: wound risk assessment for children. Professional Nurse 9(2): 112–120

Bosworth-Bousfield C 2002 Burn trauma: management and nursing care, 2nd edn. Whurr, London

Braden B, Bergstrom N, Laguzza A, Holman V 1987 The Braden scale for predicting pressure sore risk. Nursing Research 36(4): 205–210

Cockett A 2002 A research review to identify the factors contributing to the development of pressure ulcers in paediatric patients. Journal of Tissue Viability 12(1): 16–23

Dealey C 1999 The care of wounds: a guide for nurses. Blackwell Science, Oxford

Department of Health 1998 A first class service: quality in the new NHS. TSO, London

Department of Health 2001 Essence of care. Patient focused benchmarking for health care practitioners. TSO, London

Jones A 1997 Pressure sores in children with special needs: a neglected area. Journal of Tissue Viability 17(3): 82–83

McGough A J 1999 A systematic review of the effectiveness of risk assessment scales used in the prevention and management of pressure sores. MSc Thesis, University of York, York, UK

National Institute for Clinical Excellence (NICE) 2003a Pressure ulcer prevention. Clinical Guideline 7. NICE, London

National Institute for Clinical Excellence (NICE) 2003b The use of pressure relieving devices (beds, mattresses & overlays) for the prevention of pressure ulcers in primary and secondary care. NICE, London

Neidig J R, Kleiber C, Oppliger R A 1989 Risk factors associated with pressure ulcers in the pediatric patient following open heart surgery. Progress in Cardiovascular Nursing 4(3): 99–106

Nursing and Midwifery Council (NMC) 2002 Code of professional conduct. NMC, London

Olding L, Patterson J 1998 Growing concern. Nursing Times 93(38): 74–79

Royal College of Nursing (RCN) 2001 Pressure ulcer risk assessment and prevention. RCN, London

Southmead Health Services NHS Trust 1997 Guidelines for the prevention and management of pressure sores. Southmead Health Services NHS Trust, Bristol, UK

Tooher R, Middleton P, Babidge W 2003 Implementation of pressure ulcer guidelines: what constitutes a successful strategy? Journal of Wound Care 12(10): 373–382

Waterlow J 1997 Practical use of the Waterlow tool in the community. British Journal of Nursing 2(2): 283–286

Willock J, Hughes J, Tickle S et al 2000 Pressure sores in children: the acute hospital perspective. Journal of Tissue Viability 12(2): 59–62

Zollo M B, Schmidt J E, Gostisha M L, Berens R J, Weigle C G M 1996 Altered skin integrity in children admitted to a pediatric intensive care unit. Journal of Nursing Care Quality 11(2): 62–67

Further Reading

Chambers N, Jolly A 2002 Essence of care: making a difference. Nursing Standard 17(11): 40–44

European Pressure Ulcer Advisory Panel 1998 A policy statement on the prevention of pressure ulcers from the European Panel Advisory Panel. British Journal of Nursing 7(15): 888–890

Flanagan M 1997 Choosing pressure sore risk assessment tools. Professional Nurse 12(Suppl 6): 3–7

National Institute for Clinical Excellence 2001 Working together to prevent pressure ulcers: a guide for patients and carers. NICE, London

Quigley S M, Curley M A 1996 Skin integrity in the pediatric population: preventing and managing pressure ulcers. Journal of the Society of Pediatric Nurses 1(1): 7–18

Practice **25**

Radiography

Tricia Kleidon

Introduction

This section is written to help nurses understand their role in preparing children for radiological investigation and assisting the radiologist to perform radiological investigations on children. Some radiology departments may have a designated radiology nurse who is experienced in all aspects of the department and the procedures that are performed. When this facility is not available, the role will often fall on the ward nurse who accompanies the child to the radiology department. In some instances, even if there is a radiology department nurse available, it may be necessary for the nurse caring for the child to stay during the procedure to assist with holding, provide advice on the child's condition and utilise previously developed nurse–patient and parental rapport to gain optimal imaging. The role of the escort nurse will be primarily that of patient advocate but equally important will be the preparation of the child and carer, based on a thorough assessment of the child and knowledge of the examination required. The nurse may be involved in the preparation of equipment prior to the examination and will also be required to support the child and family. The nurse may also assist the radiographer in ensuring that the child remains in the correct position.

Learning outcomes

By the end of this section you should be able to:

● prepare a child and their family for X-ray examination
● identify ways to minimise radiation
● provide detailed explanation to child and family of what they will see, hear and feel throughout the radiological examination

- observe and adhere to IRMER (2000) guidelines
- explain the difference between ionising radiation and non-ionising radiation
- assist in performing a radiological examination safely with or without sedation
- describe the common types of radiological investigations.

Rationale

The need for an X-ray examination is usually for diagnostic purposes. The most common types of radiology modalities include plain film, ultrasound, computed tomography (CT), magnetic resonance imaging (MRI), interventional radiology/angiography and nuclear medicine. Interventional radiology is a rapidly growing subspecialty within radiology that is becoming increasingly popular and useful as both a diagnostic and treatment tool (Kaye 2000, Roebuck 2001). A child may also need to be supported during radiotherapy. If children are being treated in district general hospitals and require X-rays, in a department that mainly treats adults, the child's nurse will need to ensure that they are adequately prepared, taking into account the size and unfamiliarity of the equipment.

Factors to note

- All X-ray examinations must be requested either by a medical practitioner or by a nurse or other healthcare professional that has undergone the appropriate training and has been allowed by their trust/hospital to request certain radiology examinations. The benefits of radiological information that may aid in clinical diagnosis or treatment must be balanced against the potential hazards of the exposure to radiation (IRMER 2000).

- The X-ray examination is clinically directed by the radiologist or trained physicist.

- The radiographer normally directs and is responsible for the examination.

- All X-rays hold a potential risk.

- It is important to remember that although the risk to the individual child is insignificant, it is general philosophy that the dose to the general public from medical use of ionising radiation should be reduced.

- The dose to the child in diagnostic radiology is generally a very low or low dose. We are all exposed to background radiation on a daily basis and a child's chest X-ray is equivalent to 1 day of background radiation, therefore one could assume that a child undergoing a plain chest X-ray is one day older in radiation terms (Crawley 2002).

- The net gain should outweigh the risk; this is especially pertinent to children undergoing frequent X-ray examinations.

- Before any investigations are performed on any child the principles laid down in the Ionising Radiation (Medical Exposure) Regulations 2000 must be adhered to (IRMER 2000).

- Nurses should take responsibility and act as an advocate for the child, i.e. ensure there is no possibility of pregnancy in girls of child-bearing age.

- Nurses or mothers who are pregnant should not assist with X-ray examinations in order to protect the unborn child. It is the responsibility of the operator to determine whether or not the patient and/or their carers may be pregnant. It is suffice to ask the accompanying adult if there is any chance they may be pregnant. Determining possible pregnancy in children undergoing tests requires diplomacy and sensitivity. If the child is competent to answer the question independently, you must determine whether they have started having regular periods. For patients with regular periods undergoing low-dose tests, e.g. plain chest film, who are sure their period is not overdue, you should proceed with the examination. Patients requiring high-dose procedures, e.g. barium enemas, CT of abdomen and pelvis, interventional procedures involving direct exposure of the abdomen and pelvis, and nuclear medicine tests with high fetal dose investigations, should be asked when their last period started. If it was within 10 days of the start of their last period, the test may proceed. If the test is requested more than 10 days since the start of their last period, it must be determined if there is any chance they may be pregnant. The answer to the pregnancy question should be documented on the radiology request form (IRMER 2000). Staff that think they may be pregnant are asked not to accompany the child into the examination room, and all young females are asked if they have started their menstrual cycle; if so, the steps outlined above are actioned, otherwise no further action is taken.

GENERAL PRINCIPLES

General environment

Many radiology departments are largely adult focused, particularly in district general hospitals. It is important that consideration is given to the child in the environment of the X-ray department. The area should be child friendly with toys and games appropriate for different ages. Posters of current television favourites may be displayed. This helps to distract the child and may help in developing a relationship that will assist the radiographer. The *National Service Framework for Children* (DoH 2003) clearly states that children should be cared for in child-friendly hospitals and that hospitals should be safe and healthy places for children. Children should receive care based on their needs and the needs of their family. They should also be encouraged to participate in their care. Children often feel that the X-ray room is a controlled environment where they can have no say or choice about whether the procedure is performed (Fegley 1988). Children should be encouraged to bring one of their favourite toys into the department with them so that they can be X-rayed together. Depending on the type of test being carried out, it may be possible for children to listen to their favourite CD or watch a

video. These options should be discussed with the child prior to arriving at the radiology department and, if appropriate, the child can choose their entertainment or bring their own with them.

The X-ray room should be warm to avoid cooling of the child. Some clothing can be left in place, depending on the type of X-ray examination; if there is any doubt the nurse should check with the radiographer. It is advisable to remove any clothes with metal buttons or zippers beforehand. If it is anticipated that the procedure will be lengthy or if the patient is a neonate, a warming blanket should be placed on the bed. Children undergoing a MRI scan need to be checked more thoroughly by a trained person to ensure they have nothing on them that is incompatible with the MRI scanner. This includes any jewellery, body piercings and medical implants. Anything metallic that can be removed should be, and any surgical implants should be thoroughly investigated prior to the scan to ensure they are MRI compatible.

The stability of the child's condition must be assessed before considering a move to the radiology department. The use of portable X-ray machines within intensive care units and isolation cubicles is common practice. Children whose access to the department is difficult or whose condition might be compromised, e.g. children in balanced traction or immune-suppressed children being reverse barrier nursed (nursed in protective isolation), should also be considered for a portable X-ray machine.

Wall-mounted oxygen, suction and monitoring equipment should be available in every radiology room.

Full resuscitation equipment for all ages of children must be present within the department.

Preparation of the child and parent/carer

Preparation is one of the most important parts of any investigation in paediatric radiology. Parent participation is actively encouraged.

A full explanation of the procedure, equipment and process of events will help alleviate both the child's and the parent's anxiety. The provision of age-appropriate leaflets should be made available for the parent and child to take away with them to read at their leisure; this allows them the opportunity to think of any questions they may want answering prior to the planned procedure. A play specialist may also provide useful demonstrations using a favourite toy to show the child where they will be placed within the room and how close the X-ray equipment will come to them, but will not touch them. The explanation to the parents and the child should be provided before the child enters the investigation room. The language and depth of the explanation should be appropriate to the patient's age and understanding and will include any activity expected of the child, e.g. drinking the medication, holding their breath or micturating during the procedure. If the investigation requires the insertion of a cannula or catheterisation, the child and family will need to be given an indication of how and when this is likely to occur.

The child and parents need to know and understand that it is important for the child to remain still during the X-ray examination. If analgesia or sedation is to be used, this needs to be discussed with the parents as part of the preparation. There should also be a discussion on the most appropriate person to accompany the child to the department. This should be the person who is most able to comfort, calm, help restrain and offer reassurance to the child during the investigation.

An assessment of the child will be required as part of the admission process. If the child is an outpatient, an explanation of what will happen and reinforcement of the events during the procedure are necessary. Heiney (1991) promotes the development of a care plan for a child who is undergoing any procedure, particularly if there may be discomfort or pain, e.g. cannulation.

The child should be weighed to enable the correct doses of drugs and radiopaque dye to be administered.

There needs to be communication between the nurse and radiologist to arrange the most suitable time for the procedure and to enable

analgesia and sedation to be administered at the most appropriate time for it to be effective.

Always check the name and date of birth of the child against the radiology request form prior to undertaking any investigation.

Preparation books

Books and leaflets written for children can help in explaining the type of equipment that will be used and the procedures involved. These will give a simple explanation of the process during the procedures and explain that the X-ray machines are large, can be mobile, i.e. move around the child, and that sometimes a tube above them may move towards them but it will never actually touch them during the procedure. The examination table on which the child is lying may also move at various times throughout the procedure. If a detailed explanation, including pictures, is given to the child and their parent/carer beforehand, it may help to alleviate unnecessary anxiety and make the equipment appear less frightening. Some departments may have an album with photographs of the various members of staff that the child and parents will meet and the various pieces of equipment they may encounter.

Play therapy

Some hospitals are fortunate in having a play therapy department. Play therapists are trained to help prepare the child for a variety of procedures, through play (see Play, p. 457).

General care

Privacy

This is an important aspect of any procedure. All children should have their investigation in private and only people who are necessary for the investigation should remain in the X-ray room.

Protection

The nurse and/or parent must wear a lead apron and thyroid collar if assisting with the X-ray examination. Local protection for the child may be required, for example ovary/gonad pads.

When X-rays are being taken on the ward using portable equipment, a safe zone should be established, ensuring that no unnecessary personnel are present in the area and that those who are required are wearing protective clothing.

The nurse may be asked to help if the mother is pregnant and is unable to hold the child herself.

Positioning

The correct positioning of the child and the maintenance of the position during the X-ray examination is one of the most important aspects of the care. The radiographer will assist the nurse and/or parent in achieving the position that is required. The difficulty in positioning is greater with a child up to the age of 5 years (Gyll 1982) but does become easier as the child gets older. The radiographer may provide various adapted boxes or stools for the child to sit or lie on, to get the best picture/results first time.

It is the nurse's role to ensure that the child is not restrained against their will or for any great length of time and that appropriate explanation and reassurance are given (RCN 1999).

In the case of a wheelchair-bound or physically handicapped child it is always advisable to ask the child's usual carer how to lift the child without harming yourself or the child. It may not be possible to obtain particular X-rays on some physically handicapped children because of their inability to move or maintain a particular position. The nurse should remember that they are the child's advocate on these occasions. Local lifting and handling policies must be adhered to.

Praise and reward

At the end of any X-ray examination the child must be praised for their cooperation and, if appropriate, a bravery certificate, sticker or small present awarded.

Sedation and general anaesthetics

As imaging technology advances, the need to keep children absolutely still during some X-ray procedures, especially interventional, MRI and CT scans, is increasing. In younger children this may only be achieved by using either sedation or general anaesthesia. Local policy regarding fasting, preparation and monitoring during sedation and general anaesthesia must be adhered to. Invasive procedures require an appropriately trained nurse to remain with the patient, as any deterioration or distress may require intervention.

In very young babies, i.e. less than 6 weeks old, and/or those less than 5 kg, it is recommended that they be given their usual feed if this is not contraindicated, and then wrapping them snugly. Babies will often fall asleep as they usually would after their feed, thus avoiding the need for sedation.

If sedation is required, a doctor will prescribe it, the type and method of administration being adjusted according to the estimated length of the procedure. If children are attending as outpatients, sedation will normally be administered before they enter the examination room. If your radiology department does not have a day stay facility and, depending on local hospital policy, it is strongly recommended that a day bed be prearranged within the hospital so the child can recover fully before going home.

Children who have been given sedation should arrive in the department already asleep or drowsy. Monitoring of these children is the responsibility of the nurse present. A set of baseline observations should be taken, including colour, pulse, respiration and, if possible, pre-sedation oxygen saturation.

During the investigation the child should be constantly monitored for colour, O_2 saturation, pulse and respiration.

The child should be sent back to the ward after the investigation with a full set of observations and a complete handover should be given to the ward staff.

Recently some units have developed nurse-led sedation programmes which are finely tuned to meet the sedation requirements of their particular unit. Sury et al (1999) discovered that children require deep sedation to remain suitably still for successful completion of their MRI scan. This study showed that, with the appropriate training, a nurse-led sedation service can be safely used for MRI in children. They also found that sedating a child in the unit where the examination is to take place increases success of sedation, as opposed to transporting a drowsy child between departments. Great care must be exercised in adhering to the sedation policy of these units and ensuring that staff are appropriately trained.

A child with airway problems, raised intracranial pressure or difficult behavioural problems should be carefully reviewed prior to sedation. Sedation is not usually indicated under these circumstances and the child should receive a general anaesthetic. General anaesthesia is administered by an anaesthetist and anaesthetic nurse who will be responsible for all patient monitoring during and immediately after the procedure. The child should then be sufficiently recovered before returning to the ward (Sury et al 1999).

If the child requires a general anaesthetic, the ward nurse should accompany the patient with the parents into the anaesthetic area and check the patient's name, hospital number and date of birth with the anaesthetic nurse. A consent form should also be signed by the parents or carers prior to the investigation. In most anaesthetic areas one parent is usually allowed to stay until the child is asleep. Once asleep, the parent and ward nurse should leave the anaesthetic area unless the ward nurse is required to assist with the investigation.

Following the procedure and extubation, a recovery nurse should monitor the child until they are able to maintain their own airway and are rousable by speech. Once the child demonstrates they are able to maintain their own airway, they should be sent back to their ward or day stay unit until they have completely recovered and returned to their pre-anaesthetised state, before being discharged. Age-appropriate resuscitation equipment must be available in all areas where a child is sedated or given a general anaesthetic.

INVESTIGATIONS

The majority of radiological investigations require radiopaque dye to be administered, the method of administration usually involving an invasive procedure such as cannulation and sometimes catheterisation. These procedures should be carefully explained to the child and their parent prior to them arriving in the radiology department. Some children may have an allergic reaction to the contrast medium. Although the incidence of this is very rare, children or their carers should be questioned prior to administration to ensure they have not had any previous reaction to radiopaque dye or other iodine-based substance.

Some common investigations

Plain X-rays

These are usually X-rays of the chest, skeleton or abdomen. The radiographer should explain exactly what is to happen, before the child is positioned. The aim is to keep the child still and correctly positioned, e.g. not rotated for a chest X-ray, so that only the minimal number of exposures are taken. They are non-invasive and should not give any discomfort to the child.

Micturating cystogram

A micturating cystogram is one of the most common investigations performed on children with any indication of pelvic, ureteric or bladder obstruction or malformation and urinary reflux.

Radiopaque dye is instilled into the bladder via a catheter. In most hospitals the catheter is inserted by the medical staff or radiologist but it may also be performed by the nurse if proficient in this practice. The child is then encouraged to micturate and X-rays are taken. As the bladder contracts, malformations or abnormalities of the bladder or ureter may be demonstrated.

Barium study

Barium or contrast swallows, meals and follow-throughs are some of the most common upper gastrointestinal investigations performed in paediatric radiology. They are used to indicate the patency of the gastrointestinal tract and any abnormalities of anatomy or physiology within it. Barium swallow investigates the child's swallowing technique, the oropharynx, the oesophagus and the fundus of the stomach.

According to the child's underlying condition, the choice of contrast medium will be at the discretion of the radiologist.

The child's age must be taken into account when selecting the vessel from which to drink the medium. A small baby can be given a bottle, but the hole in the teat has to be made slightly larger to allow the barium through. A toddler will normally take a drink from a beaker. It may be advisable to use the child's own beaker as the familiarity may encourage drinking the barium. Older children can use a straw or ordinary cup. Flavouring the barium is also advised. This can be achieved with either milk shake flavourings or powders.

A barium meal follows on from the barium swallow and follows the gastrointestinal tract into the stomach, the duodenum and jejunum.

Barium meal and follow-through encompasses both of the above, but follows the entire intestinal tract to the terminal ileum and the ileocaecal junction.

A barium contrast enema is used to investigate the large bowel, its patency and any abnormalities. The contrast is administered by a rectal tube via the anus and rectum.

In some sick children, the risks involved in contrast enemas are high and include perforation of the gut and respiratory distress in a child who is obstructed. The procedure should therefore not be undertaken lightly and must be under the direct supervision of a radiologist following a request from a surgical colleague. Oxygen, suction and full resuscitation equipment should be available.

Air enema

Intussusception is a commonly occurring condition in infants, characterised by the bowel backing up into itself. Air is instilled under pressure via a Foley tube placed in the rectum. It is important that a good seal is achieved and the pressure under which the air is instilled is increased gradually. Not all intussusceptions are fully reducible using this method and in some instances reduction using air enema is contraindicated. If this is the case the child should be referred for surgical review (Bisset & Kirks 1988, Reijnen et al 1990).

Computed tomography (CT) imaging

A CT scan is a type of X-ray examination and refers to the way in which the equipment works.

X-rays, like radio waves, can pass through objects and be focused to create a picture. During an X-ray examination, the beam of rays goes through the body, where it is absorbed to differing degrees by tissues such as bone and muscle and by organs. When the rays emerge on the other side of the body, they create a pattern of light and dark on a film, the X-ray.

During a CT examination the child has to lie on a table which moves slowly through the CT scanner. The patient is alone in the room while the X-ray pictures are taken, but can hear the radiographer speaking. If the child cannot be left on their own, a nurse or parent may enter at the discretion of the radiographer, but must wear a lead apron and must not be pregnant (see p. 330).

The length of the CT scan is variable, depending on the type of scan required and the machinery. Generally CT scans take about 5–10 minutes. However, some departments have installed new multi-slice CT scanners which take a fraction of the time to complete the examination. The preparation required prior to CT examination depends on the area of the body being scanned.

It is often necessary for the child to have an injection of contrast dye into a vein in the arm via an intravenous cannula, which may have been inserted on the ward. This contrast allows better visualisation of some organs. It contains iodine which can make the child feel very warm whilst it is injected, but this feeling passes quickly and is quite normal. In some very rare cases a child may develop an allergic reaction to the contrast, and it is therefore imperative that any previous allergies are ascertained prior to the procedure. There are no long-term side-effects of this contrast as it passes quickly through the kidneys to the bladder.

Whilst the pictures are being taken, the child may sometimes be asked to breathe in and hold their breath. This should be practised beforehand. Children find it difficult to keep still, which is why a good explanation beforehand is vital.

Ultrasound

This is a type of scan which takes place in the radiology department. It uses sound waves, not X-rays, and is therefore safe. The sound waves pass through the body, giving back a signal and providing a black and white image which is produced on a television screen. This image is then interpreted by a radiographer or radiologist.

The preparation required will depend on the part of the body which is to be examined. When the pelvis is to be checked, it is useful if the bladder is full; however, this is not always practical in all age groups. A full bladder provides a 'window' to look through and see the other organs in the pelvis.

The child lies on a couch and uncovers the part of the body which is to be examined. Gel is squirted onto the skin to give good contact between the machine and the skin. The transducer, which looks like a microphone, is then moved gently over the skin.

The examination does not hurt at all; it tickles and the child may complain that the gel is cold. The child may be asked to breathe in and hold their breath whilst a clear picture is taken.

After the scan, the gel is wiped off and the child is free to go. As no X-rays are used, parents or nurses can accompany the child. The mother is often able to give the child a good explanation, as the procedure is similar to that used during pregnancy.

Magnetic resonance imaging (MRI)

MRI is a way of looking inside the body without using X-rays. MRI can produce two- or three-dimensional images using a very large magnet, radio waves and a computer. The magnet is large enough to surround a patient, which is why it is sometimes referred to as a tunnel. The magnetic fields used are not known to be harmful, which means that children can have someone with them, although expectant mothers are advised to remain outside the room.

There is no preparation required for an MRI scan, but everyone entering the magnetic area will be checked for metallic objects, which may not be taken into the room as they can damage the magnet or the patient if they become projectile. No one with metallic implants should enter the scan room.

Children do not have to undress as long as they are not wearing clothes with zips or other metal bits. They can come in pyjamas or zipperless jogging suits.

The child has to keep very still during the scan, as one movement can spoil all the images, unlike X-rays. This is because the images are built up from information collected during the whole of the scanning time. A child who is not able to keep still for about 30 minutes may have to be sedated. The child will be asked to lie on the table; they can be comforted and reassured and choose a video or music to play whilst they are being scanned. Before moving into the scanner, headphones should be placed over their ears so they can hear their chosen video or music clip and block out some of the noise made by the scanner.

MRI scanning can be frightening for a young child who may therefore need sedation. Children over the age of 5 years may find it quite interesting. They can take a favourite toy in with them, as long as there is no metal in it.

Once the child is in the magnet, the machine starts to make a whirring and thumping noise which can get very loud and this continues for the whole of the scan. The child can talk to the radiographer whilst in the magnet. The child also has a bell to press should they wish the examination to stop. In practice, many children go to sleep and have to be woken up when the scan is finished.

Occasionally it is necessary to inject a small amount of contrast, which does not contain iodine, into the arm. Allergic reactions are therefore rare.

No special care is required following a scan, provided the child has not received sedation.

Nuclear medicine

Nuclear medicine uses computers, detectors and radioactive pharmaceutical substances called radioisotopes to provide information about disease processes. The levels of radiation delivered in nuclear medicine studies are often less than, or comparable to, equivalent X-ray procedures, although they provide functional rather than anatomical images. The radiation risk received from nuclear medicine study is generally at a level considered negligible by the International Commission on Radiological Protection (ICRP 1977/1978). Nuclear medicine scans are useful for detecting tumours, bony infection, irregular or insufficient blood flow to organs, blood cell disorders and inadequate function of organs such as thyroid and pulmonary function. The radioisotopes are usually injected into the bloodstream via an intravenous cannula, therefore children will need to be prepared for the insertion of a cannula prior to attending the nuclear medicine department for their scan. It is essential the person injecting the radiopharmaceutical has undergone special training so they are aware of what they are injecting and the precautions required to contain the radiopharmaceutical and dispose of waste matter appropriately. Local policy should be followed when doing so.

Some of the more common nuclear medicine scans are as follows.

Bone scans

Bone scanning detects radiation from a radioactive substance that, when injected into the body, collects in bone tissue. The substance accumulates in areas of high metabolic activity, and so the image shows 'bright spots' of high activity and 'dark spots' of low activity. Bone scanning is useful for detecting tumours and infection, which generally have high metabolic activity (Sharp et al 1998).

^{99m}Tc Dimercaptosuccinic acid (DMSA) and ^{99m}Tc diethylenetriamine–pentaacetic acid (DTPA)

There are a number of radiopharmaceuticals available for demonstrating renal function and imaging of the urinary tract. The most appropriate radiopharmaceutical is chosen for the examination and is dependent upon whether the examination is to look at the kidney and its function or the drainage characteristics of the urinary tract.

A DMSA and DTPA renal scan are most commonly used. The radioisotope or tracer is administered intravenously and is observed through a special gamma camera.

- DMSA is bound to plasma proteins and is cleared from the blood by uptake by the renal tubules. The proximal convoluted tubular tissue takes up DMSA, accumulating in the renal cortex. Because of the high specificity of the uptake in the renal cortex, DMSA is of use for the visualisation of the renal parenchyma. Therefore these scans are useful for assessing the size, shape and position of the kidneys and to demonstrate if renal dysfunction is occurring in both kidneys. DMSA scan also demonstrates scarring and narrowing of the renal cortex in pyelonephritis.

- DTPA is commonly used for renal transplant studies. When injected intravenously, it is distributed throughout the extracellular space. As it is excreted rapidly from the body by glomerulofiltration, it gives a good correlation with the standard measurements of glomerular filtration rate. DTPA is useful for both assessment of individual kidney function, and the study of renal function and drainage in obstructive uropathy (Sharp et al 1998).

Interventional radiology

Interventional radiology is a medical specialty that uses image-guided, minimally invasive diagnostic and treatment techniques that are often an alternative to surgery. Interventional radiologists assist in diagnosis and treatment of diseases using small catheters or other devices guided by radiological imaging. Procedures performed by interventional radiologists are generally less costly and are less traumatic to the patient as they involve smaller incisions, less pain and shorter hospital stays.

Central venous access

As the demand for long-term central venous access increases, and with the recent publication of NICE guidelines (2002), many interventional radiology departments are now carrying out a large proportion of these procedures. These devices are increasingly used for the administration of antibiotics and chemotherapeutic drugs, for total parenteral nutrition, and for providing high-flow access for haemodialysis and plasmapheresis. Indwelling catheters also offer the ability to obtain frequent blood samples, which may be needed in some patients. Many children are reliant on lifelong central venous access for nutritional requirements and haemodialysis; repeated placement of such devices in these children proves challenging when traditional venous access sites are compromised by stenosis or occlusion of the central vessels. Placing central venous catheters in the interventional radiology department equipped with dedicated ultrasound and fluoroscopic machines allows the planned vascular access site to be evaluated prior to catheter placement. Ultrasonographic investigation of the neck prior to the procedure may alert the operator to small collateral vessels instead of a single large jugular vein. This is important as it may be indicative of a stenosis or occlusion of the main vein. In many instances, one of the collateral veins can be accessed under direct ultrasonographic visualisation or the large brachiocephalic vein may be easily identified and punctured with ultrasound guidance. Therefore, by using fluoroscopic guidance, contrast material, guidewires and catheters, an interventional radiologist can usually bypass these thrombosed or stenosed vessels and access the central circulation, allowing placement of a catheter via vessels that could not otherwise be used.

Venous access under ultrasonographic and fluoroscopic guidance has the added advantage of significantly decreasing the rate of immediate complications such as inadvertent arterial puncture, pneumothorax and catheter tip malpositioning (Calvert et al 2002, NICE 2002, Silberzweig et al 2000).

Central venous line (CVL) insertion

This is a procedure that involves placement of a soft infusion catheter into a centrally located vein using vascular interventional techniques. The most commonly placed lines include:

- peripherally inserted central venous catheter (PICC)
- Hickman lines (single and double lumens)
- venous port device
- temporary and permanent haemodialysis catheters.

Depending on the type of central venous access required, placement can be carried out under either local or general anaesthetic. For a PICC or other non-tunnelled central venous catheter, local anaesthetic with or without sedation is sufficient in the older child; however, for tunnelled catheter insertion such as a Hickman catheter which requires a large amount of compliance, a general anaesthetic is strongly recommended to ensure the procedure is carried out as safely and as pain free as practicable (Roebuck 2001, Calvert et al 2002) (see also Central Lines, p. 137).

A recent report from the National Institute for Clinical Excellence recommends ultrasound-guided placement of all central venous catheters into the internal jugular vein in adults and children in elective situations, and that ultrasound-guided placement should also be considered in emergency situations (NICE 2002).

Renal biopsy

Renal biopsy is undertaken to identify a specific disease process, determine extent of kidney damage, detect early transplant rejection and assess transplant failure (Roebuck 2001, Kessel & Robertson 2002). The kidney to be biopsied is visualised using ultrasound guidance, the intended biopsy tract is infiltrated with local anaesthetic and a thin needle is passed through the skin into the area of the kidney. Inside the needle is a sharp cutting edge that slices and removes small pieces of the kidney. In older children this procedure is successfully performed with sedation or demand-valve equimolar nitrous oxide (Entonox). If the child is young or not suitable for either sedation or Entonox, a general anaesthetic is recommended. As there is a small risk of postoperative bleeding, it is imperative that clotting results are obtained prior to the procedure and the operator is informed if the child is on medication that may interfere with clotting, for example children receiving aspirin for treatment of their underlying renal disease. Postoperative observations should include blood pressure monitoring for early detection of complications such as bleeding.

Angiography

Angiography is an X-ray examination of the arteries and veins to diagnose blockages and other blood vessel problems. Depending on the age and level of cooperation of the child, this procedure may be performed under local anaesthetic, sedation or general anaesthesia. The most common method for carrying out this procedure is with the child positioned supine; a small nick in the groin is made and the femoral artery is punctured. In small children it is advisable to use ultrasound guidance to obtain femoral arterial access as their arteries are smaller and not as easily palpable as those in older children, making access more difficult

(Roebuck 2001). Once arterial access is obtained, a guidewire is inserted and the access needle is exchanged for an arterial sheath; this allows the insertion of a guiding catheter which is advanced to the blood vessels of interest and an injection of contrast or dye gives the radiologist a clear picture of any abnormal vessels.

One of the most common reasons for angiography is to see if there is a blockage or narrowing in a blood vessel that may interfere with the normal flow of blood through the body. In many cases, the interventional radiologist can treat a blocked blood vessel without surgery at the same time as the angiogram is performed. Interventional radiologists treat blockages with techniques such as angioplasty where a balloon is guided to the site of narrowing and expanded to overcome narrowing; sometimes a small metal stent is inserted to aid in keeping the vessel open. Other conditions which may indicate an angiogram are arteriovenous malformations, trauma, vasculitis, renovascular hypertension and cerebral arteriovenous malformations (Roebuck 2001).

Postoperatively, bed rest is encouraged for at least 6 hours or according to local hospital policy to minimise risk of bleeding from the puncture site. Circulation of the limb used for arterial access should also be assessed during routine postoperative observations.

Do and do not

- Do ensure that the child and parents have received a full explanation of the procedure.
- Do maintain the child's privacy.
- Do remove jewellery or any metal fastenings.
- Do ensure resuscitation equipment is available for children of all ages.
- Do observe the child closely if any contrast medium containing iodine is used.
- Do ensure all radioactive material is disposed of correctly.
- Do ensure local radiation protection guidelines are available and adhered to by all staff members.
- Do not allow pregnant mothers/carers or nurses to be exposed to X-rays.

References

Bisset G S III, Kirks D R 1988 Intussusception in infants and children: diagnosis and therapy. Radiology 168(1): 141

Calvert N, Hind D, McWilliams R et al 2002 The effectiveness and cost effectiveness of ultrasound locating devices for central venous access. Anaesthesia 59(11): 1116–1120

Crawley T 2002 Ionising radiation safety: a handbook for nurses. York Publishing, York, UK

Department of Health 2003 National Service Framework for children. DoH, London

Fegley B 1988 Preparing children for radiological procedures. Research in Nursing and Health 11: 3–9

Gyll C 1982 Investigations into and a comparative study of techniques for basic radiography in children's hospitals. Radiography 48(573): 175–184

Heiney S 1991 Painful procedures. American Journal of Nursing 91: 20–24

International Commission on Radiological Protection (ICRP) 1997/1978 Recommendations of the International Commission on Radiological Protection. ICRP Publication 26, Annals of the ICRP 1977; 1: No. 3; Annals of the ICRP 1978; 2: No. 3

Ionising Radiation (Medical Exposure) Regulations (IRMER) 2000 DoH, London. Online. Available: www.opsi.gov.uk/si/si2000/20001059.htm

Kaye R 2000 Pediatric intervention: an update – Part II. Journal of Vascular Interventional Radiology 11: 807–822

Kessel D, Robertson I 2002 Interventional radiology – a survival guide. Churchill Livingstone, London

National Institute for Clinical Excellence (NICE) 2002 Guidance on the use of ultrasound locating devices for placing central venous catheters. Clinical Guidance 49. NICE, London

RCN 1999 Restraining, holding still and containing children. Guidance for good practice. RCN, London

Reijnen J A, Festen C, van Roosmalen R P 1990 Intussusception: factors related to treatment. Archives of Diseases in Childhood 65(8): 871–873

Roebuck D J 2001 Paediatric interventional radiology. Imaging 13: 302–320

Sharp P F, Gemmell H G, Smith F W 1998 Practical nuclear medicine, 2nd edn. Oxford University Press, New York

Silberzweig J, Sacks D, Khorsandi A S, Bakal C W 2000 Reporting standards for central venous access. Journal of Vascular Interventional Radiology 11: 391-400

Sury M R, Hatch D J, Deeley T, Dicks-Mireaux C, Chong W K 1999 Development of a nurse-led sedation service for paediatric magnetic resonance imaging. Lancet 353: 1667–1671

Further Reading

Chapman S, Nakielny R 1988 A guide to radiological procedures, 2nd edn. Baillière Tindall, London

Kandarpa K, Aruny J 2001 Handbook of interventional radiologic procedures, 3rd edn. Lippincott, Williams and Wilkins, Philadelphia

Milner A D, Hull D 1992 Hospital paediatrics, 2nd edn. Churchill Livingstone, Edinburgh

Removal of drains and packs

Fiona Lynch, Sue Tulp

Introduction

Surgical wound drains and packs are primarily used to promote effective wound healing. Removing excess fluid from a wound will reduce the risk of infection and skin breakdown, while simultaneously easing wound pain through reducing swelling (McConnell 2001). Removal of the drain or pack at a time specified by medical and nursing assessment will help further promote wound healing by enabling earlier mobility, well-being and ultimately recovery.

Learning outcomes

By the end of this section you should:

- be aware of the different types of wound drains and packs
- be aware of their uses in wound healing
- following observation, be able to remove, or assist in the removal of, wound drains or packs
- be aware of the initial follow-up care of the site.

Rationale

The aim of the drain or pack is to promote effective healing and therefore reduce the risk of complications. This in turn will lead to a quicker recovery and result in a shorter stay in hospital for the child.

Factors to note

Types of surgical wounds

- Clean wounds – where during surgery no infection is encountered and no organ is opened.
- Clean contaminated wounds – where during surgery an organ has been opened with little content leakage.
- Contaminated wounds – where during surgery an organ is opened and this is accompanied by extensive spillage of contents without pus. Also included in this category are fresh wounds occurring through trauma.
- Dirty wounds – where during surgery pus or perforation in an organ is found. Also

included in this category are old wounds caused by trauma. (i.e. >4 hours old).

Types of healing

Wound healing is a complex process comprising four main phases: haemostasis, inflammation, proliferation and maturation. These phases occur concurrently, but the length of time taken in each phase can vary considerably. Factors which can affect the rate of wound healing include malnutrition (Clancy & McVicar 2002), poor wound care, inquisitive fingers and sleep disturbances.

Normal healing occurs by either primary or secondary intention, both of which involve all four stages outlined above.

Primary intention

This occurs in wounds where there has been a clean cut, or incision, with little or no tissue loss. The edges can be brought together and held with sutures, tapes, etc., thus eliminating any space below the wound surface.

Secondary intention

This occurs when there has been substantial tissue loss and it is not possible to bring the edges together. These wounds heal from the base upwards by the formation of granulation tissue and wound contraction. Owing to the large amount of tissue involved, these wounds take considerably longer to heal (Zerbe et al 1996) (see also Wound Care, p. 441).

Types of packs

Packs are used to fill a resultant cavity when healing by secondary intention is the intended and preferred healing process. They include:

- Wicks – a variable length of ribbon gauze inserted into an open cavity after immersion in a suitable substance. Substances other than saline should be prescribed appropriately on the child's prescription sheet prior to use. An alternative to soaked ribbon gauze is an alginate-type dressing.
- Foam – a compound made from the mixing of a polymer and a base, which is poured into the cavity and expands to the contours

of the wound, allowing for granulation, e.g. Cavi-Care.

Availability of dressings is subject to pharmacy guidelines and hospital constraints. Although the use of ribbon gauze (wicks) continues to be seen in practice, its benefit when compared to other dressing materials has been questioned (Pulman 2004). Moore and Foster (2000) identified that an alternative hydrofibre dressing facilitated an earlier discharge when compared to ribbon gauze. Although the cost of the dressing was more prohibitive, the overall net effect was more beneficial when considering earlier discharge and more effective use of hospital beds was seen as being advantageous.

Types of wound drains

Drains are used when healing by primary intention is the intended healing process. The aims of drains are:

- to drain intra-abdominal collections of pus
- to drain any postoperative collections
- to re-route body fluids from a new suture line.

Types of drains include:

- suction or sump drains – a vacuum is present to exert a low suction to remove any wound exudate from a cavity (Zerbe et al 1996, McConnell 1999), e.g. Redivac drain, Monovac drain, Shirley Sump drain
- non-suction drains – these allow wound exudate to leave a cavity by a natural process, e.g. Penrose drain, Yates drain.

Note: The age and cooperation of the child should be taken into consideration by the surgeon when wound management is required.

All of these drains are removed when wound leakage has significantly reduced or stopped. Within adult patients the use of closed suction wound drains has been questioned. Chandratreya et al (1998) identified that there was no difference in terms of mobilisation, postoperative infection and length of hospitalisation in adult orthopaedic patients who had a wound drain in situ when compared to those who did not have a wound drain. Purushotham et al (2002) concurred with this and indicated that using sutured wound flaps resulted in shorter hospitals stays. However, no literature relating to children was identified to support these adult findings.

Analgesia

Effective analgesia and/or sedation must be taken into consideration and should be administered at least 30 minutes before the procedure is commenced to allow time for it to take effect. However, the recent introduction of Entonox as an acceptable form of analgesia for children gives an alternative and allows for effective pain control during difficult procedures (see Pain Management, p. 275).

Children are naturally inquisitive and may be more cooperative if they are able to participate in their own care. However, the nurse must continually assess the situation, and involvement by the play specialist can provide useful distraction during procedures. Some ways in which the child can participate are by loosening or removing tape, holding tubing or counting down to the removal of the drain. Not all children will be able to cooperate owing to their age or ability to understand; however, it is important to ensure that children are given information at a level that they are able to understand. In these instances it is helpful to have support from the parents to assist in providing comfort and security whilst the removal of the drain or pack is being carried out.

Equipment

- Dressing pack
- Sterile stitch cutter or scissors
- Cleansing agent
- Selection of sterile dressings to cover or re-dress the wound
- Sterile latex-free gloves, optional (these can be used in place of forceps)
- Wound swab (if required)
- Disposal bag.

Note: It is preferable to overestimate your required equipment rather than having to stop the procedure to obtain more.

(See also Wound Care, page 441).

Method for removing wound drains

1. Explain the procedure to the child and parents/carers to facilitate understanding and cooperation.

2. Gather the required equipment and prepare your area for the procedure, i.e. the treatment room or bedside.

3. Wash and dry your hands.

4. If applicable, uncover the wound to obtain access to the drain site. At this point, if the drain is of a suction type, release the vacuum. Sometimes the drain can rest against tissue inside the wound; by releasing the vacuum, any remaining fluid can be drained. Wash and dry your hands.

5. Using aseptic technique (see Aseptic Non-Touch Technique, p. 75), clean the wound if necessary to access sutures or clean away any exudate, which may be a source of infection.

6. Remove any sutures by holding the knot with sterile forceps and gently raising it from skin level; then cut the shortest end of the suture as close to the skin as possible. This prevents any part of the suture which has been exposed externally from passing through the tissue, reducing the risk of infection. This should allow the drain to be released.
   Note: Cut only one end of the suture.

7. Remove the drain slowly by holding the tubing close to the child and pulling gently, but firmly. If there is resistance, which does not yield with firm pulling, stop the procedure and seek advice.

8. Cover the drain site with a sterile dressing. This will minimise infection entering the drain site whilst it heals.

9. Dispose of soiled equipment safely and record the amount of drainage in the appropriate nursing documentation.

10. Regularly check the wound site for any excessive drainage or swelling which could indicate an internal collection of

fluid, i.e. 2- to 4-hourly with routine observations.

11. Further wound management will be as per unit protocol.

Method for shortening a wound drain

1–2. As for removal of wound drain.

3. Wash and dry your hands. Remove wound dressing and expose drain. This is likely to be a tube type of drain, e.g. Penrose or corrugated latex. These drains usually have a sterile safety pin or suture to maintain their position outside the wound.

4. Wash and dry your hands again and clean the wound if necessary.

5. Remove the suture by raising the knot from skin level and cutting the shorter end as close to the skin as possible. When the suture has been removed, grasp the end of the drain and pull gently. It is usually sufficient to shorten the drain by 2–4 cm unless instructed otherwise by the medical staff. If unsure, seek advice. Shortening the drain will ensure that it does not remain in contact with any single structure for any length of time or impede the healing process. It also enables the drain to continue its purpose throughout the depth of the wound. The excess tubing can be cut with sterile scissors.

6. Re-insert a new sterile safety pin just above wound level to prevent the drain slipping into it.

7. Re-dress the wound with an appropriate wound dressing. Copious amounts of drainage may be managed by placing a stoma bag over the drain site. This enables the bag to be emptied and prevents the frequent changing of dressings. This method of collection should be discussed with the child and parents/carers before implementation as they may not feel comfortable with using a stoma bag.

8. Dispose of soiled equipment and record the amount of drainage in the appropriate nurs-

ing documentation. This will aid further management of the drain.

Method for removing a ribbon gauze pack

1–2. As for removal of drain. Confirm the length of ribbon gauze (wick) in situ by either checking the operation notes or consulting the medical staff.

3. Wash and dry your hands. Remove the outer dressing and assess the wound site.

4. Locate the end of the wick and gently ease it upwards out of the cavity. If there is any adherence, the wound and wick can be moistened with saline. Continue to ease the gauze from the cavity until no more is visible.
   Note: Some wounds are managed by shortening the wick gradually over a period of time.

5. Clean the wound as required.

6. Assess the wound bed for signs of healing and the possible need to insert a further wick. If a further wick is required, place an appropriate length in saline or a prescribed solution. (The wick is supplied as a tightly rolled coil in a sterile pack. Lengths are usually indicated on the packaging.)

7. Using two pairs of sterile forceps, one in each hand, grasp the wick with one pair whilst keeping it submerged in the solution, and locate the loose end. Take hold of the end with the other forceps. Gradually unravel the wick and re-roll onto the second forceps, ensuring that it is moistened throughout its length. The moistened wick can then be inserted into the wound from the base up. When the wound has been sufficiently packed, the wick can be cut with sterile scissors.

8. Dress the wound appropriately and dispose of soiled equipment.

9. Complete the nursing documentation and record the length of wick inserted.

10. If the wick has been removed, check the site for excessive leakage.

11. Further wound management will be as per local protocol.

Method for removing a foam pack

1–3. As for removal of ribbon gauze.
4. Grasp the edges of the pack with two pairs of sterile forceps and gently ease it from the wound cavity. Clean the wound if necessary.
5. Assess the wound healing to ascertain whether a further pack is required. If unsure, seek advice. If a pack is required, make up the foam preparation as per the manufacturer's instructions and pour it slowly into the cavity. Allow time for the expansion of the foam and, when it has solidified, cover the wound with an appropriate dressing. It may be necessary to secure the pack in position with tape, but this will depend upon the individual child and the location of the wound.
6. Dispose of soiled equipment and complete the nursing documentation.

COMMUNITY PERSPECTIVE

The removal of wound packs is frequently undertaken in the community, following conditions such as drainage of abscesses.

This procedure can be very frightening for the child and is potentially painful. The CCN must gain the trust of the child and family before undertaking the procedure and organise appropriate pain management (see Pain Management, p. 265). Analgesia should be timed to ensure maximum relief during the procedure. Older children may be able to use Entonox, but as this is self-administered, it is not suitable for the younger child. If the CCN feels that the pain cannot be adequately managed by drugs that can be given in the home, it may be necessary to request admission to hospital as a day case.

The CCN should be prepared to encounter less than adequate facilities for undertaking an aseptic non-touch technique in the home (see Aseptic Non-Touch Technique, p. 75). It may be necessary to take additional equipment (sterile towels, plastic tray, hand-cleansing solutions).

Do and do not

- Do be honest with the child when explaining procedures.
- Do involve and inform the parents/carers.
- Do ensure that the child's safety and privacy are maintained at all times.
- Do involve the play specialist if available.
- Do ensure that adequate analgesia has been given before commencing procedures.
- Do not remove packs or drains without prior instruction.
- Do not assume that older children will cooperate or be brave.

References

Chandratreya A, Giannikas K, Livesley P 1998 To drain or not to drain: literature versus practice. Journal of the Royal College of Surgeons of Edinburgh 43: 404–406

Clancy J, McVicar A 2002 Physiology and anatomy: a homeostatic approach, 2nd edn. Arnold, London

McConnell E A 1999 Clinical do's and don'ts: using a closed wound drainage system. Nursing 29(6): 32

McConnell E A 2001 Clinical do's and don'ts: emptying a closed wound drainage device. Nursing 31(7): 17

Moore P J, Foster L 2000 Clinical cost benefits of two dressings in the management of surgical wounds. British Journal of Nursing 9(17): 1128, 1130–1132

Pulman K 2004 Dressings in the management of open surgical wounds. British Journal of Perioperative Nursing 14(8): 354–357, 359–360

Purushotham A D, McLatchie E, Young D et al 2002 Randomized clinical trial of no wound drains and early discharge in the treatment of women with breast cancer. British Journal of Surgery 89(3): 286–292

Zerbe M, McArdle A, Goldrick B 1996 Exposure risks related to the management of three wound drainage systems. American Journal of Infection Control 24(5): 346–352

Further Reading

Bale S, Jones V (eds) 1997 Wound care in the baby and young child. In: Wound care nursing – a patient centred approach. Baillière Tindall, London, p 70–93

Flanagan M 1997 Wound management. Churchill Livingstone, Edinburgh

Hampton S 1999 In: Miller M, Glover D (eds) Wound management. Theory and practice. NT Books, London

Watret L, White R 2001 Surgical wound management: the role of dressings. Nursing Standard 15(44): 59–69

Practice **27**

Seizures

Louise Simmons

Introduction

Anyone can have an isolated seizure at some point in their life (NSE 2002a). They can happen for a variety of different reasons. Seizures are periods of sudden disturbance of brain function that cause involuntary muscle activity, change in level of consciousness, or altered behavioural and sensory manifestations (Ball & Bindler 1999). Seizures can be frightening and disturbing to observe, both for the professional and the family. A number of dangers can occur during a seizure, i.e. apnoea, airway obstruction, aspiration and injury. The nurse's role is to provide a safe environment for the duration of the seizure and respond appropriately to the situation.

Learning outcomes

By the end of this section you should be able to:

- state the main causes of seizures in children
- describe how to nurse a child during a seizure
- state the possible complications of a seizure

- show awareness of the different anticonvulsant medication that may be administered during a seizure.

Rationale for care of the child having a seizure

At least 20% of children admitted to hospital have a neurological problem, either as the sole or an associated complaint (Waterston et al 1997). Seizures are the most frequently observed neurological dysfunction in children. Although seizures are the main characteristic of epilepsy, a chronic disorder with recurrent and unprovoked seizures (Wong 1997), they can occur with a variety of conditions involving the central nervous system (CNS) (Wong 1997). Approximately 20% of children will experience a seizure in the first 5 years of life, often associated not with epilepsy, but with a febrile illness (Rudolf & Levene 1999). In children who have experienced a seizure associated with a febrile illness, about 15% of cases will have further seizures within the same illness. One in three children is at risk of future febrile seizures with a further third of these at risk of three or more seizures. The risk is even higher if the onset is before the age of 1 year and if there is a positive family history (Lissauer & Clayden 2001). It is therefore important for the paediatric nurse to know how to care for a child during a seizure. Education of parents is also important as to the cause, and how to handle possible future seizures.

Factors to note

Neonatal seizures

The newborn period is the time of life with the highest risk of seizures and epilepsy. The newborn brain is more susceptible to a large number of cerebral and systemic insults. The immature brain is relatively 'excitable' and more likely to seize (Appleton & Gibbs 2004). Neonatal seizures can be difficult to recognise. Many babies in the neonatal period can have abnormal and involuntary movements that must be differentiated from seizures, i.e. jitteriness, startling or spontaneous clonus (Lissauer & Clayden 2001, Appleton & Gibbs 2004).

The features of neonatal seizures are different from those seen in the older infant or child. Most seizure activity in neonates may be subtle, tonic, clonic or myoclonic. The main causes of neonatal seizures are:

- acute infections acquired pre- and postnatally, i.e. toxoplasmosis, meningitis, septicaemia, encephalitis and herpes simplex
- metabolic and electrolyte disturbances, i.e. hypo/hypernatraemia, hypoglycaemia, hypocalcaemia, hypomagnesaemia, which can be due to inborn errors of metabolism or to a single illness, i.e. dehydration due to diarrhoea, vomiting or poor feeding
- birth trauma, i.e. intracranial haemorrhage or anoxic brain damage.

At presentation, all of these possibilities should be considered and various tests – i.e. full septic screen (blood count/culture, urine, lumbar puncture (LP), chest X-ray), computed tomography (CT) scan, magnetic resonance imaging (MRI) scan and electroencephalogram (EEG) – should help confirm/eliminate the various causes.

Many of these causes are treatable and reversible with medications, i.e. antibiotics and electrolyte infusions/medications.

Infants and older children

Convulsions in the infant and older child can still be due to some of the causes seen in neonates.

- Infections, i.e. meningitis, encephalitis and septicaemia can be seen as well as urinary tract infections, otitis media and many viral infections, i.e. colds and coughs.
- Metabolic and electrolyte imbalances can be seen with periods of fasting, i.e. hypoglycaemia or hypernatraemia with dehydration.
- Head trauma can be seen as a result of either accidental (e.g. road traffic accident) or non-accidental injury (e.g. shaken baby syndrome, physical abuse).

Certain neurological conditions, such as febrile seizures, occur exclusively in childhood. It is also important to remember that most of the neuromuscular and neurodegenerative disorders present early in life (Waterston et al 1997).

Febrile convulsions usually occur between 6 months and 3 years but can go up to 6 years of age (Lissauer & Clayden 2001). Febrile seizures are common, occurring in 2–4% of children between 6 months and 5 years, with a peak at 18 months to 3 years (Appleton & Gibbs 2004). They are generalised seizures and occur in children as a result of rapid temperature rise above 39°C (102°F). Up to 75% of all febrile seizures involve a generalised onset, tonic–clonic seizure that lasts less than 15 minutes with no post-ictal neurological deficit or sequelae (Ball & Bindler 1999, Appleton & Gibbs 2004).

The same investigations will be needed on presentation to establish the cause of the seizure. Following the full septic screen, CT scan, MRI scan and EEG as in the neonate, the course of treatment will be determined.

Status epilepticus

Status epilepticus is defined as a continuous seizure lasting more than 30 minutes or a series of repeated seizures between which the child does not fully regain consciousness (Ball & Bindler 1999). It is an emergency situation which is life threatening and in which the child is at risk of permanent brain damage. It is important to support the child's vital functions, i.e. maintain a patent airway, adequate oxygenation and hydration. Monitor vital signs and assess neurologic level. Treatment with intravenous anticonvulsant/sedative drugs will be required. These would start with benzodiazepines such as diazepam, lorazepam, or midazolam, which, if there was no response, could be repeated. Loading doses of phenytoin, or phenobarbital, may be necessary if seizures persist (Ball & Bindler 1999). Clonazepam or thiopental may then be given but these drugs will suppress not only the epileptiform activity but also normal brain function. As this includes the breathing centres, these children will require mechanical ventilation in an intensive care unit.

Epilepsy

Epilepsy is the commonest chronic neurological condition in childhood (SIGN 2003). It means having a tendency to experience recurrent seizures that originate in the brain, which happen when ordinary brain activity is suddenly disrupted. As the brain is responsible for a wide range of functions, seizures associated with epilepsy can take on many forms and affect areas such as memory, sensation, personality, consciousness, mood and movement. Any of these functions may be temporarily disturbed during the course of a seizure (NSE 2002a). The diagnosis of epilepsy has important health, educational and social implications for both the child and family (SIGN 2003). These can include behavioural and emotional problems that are sometimes caused by embarrassment or frustration associated with their epilepsy. Having epilepsy can affect your independence by restricting your access to driving and some people and their families live in fear of the next seizure.

Children diagnosed with epilepsy will be commenced on regular anticonvulsant medication. The type of seizure will determine which medications will be prescribed. Approximately 70–75% of children with epilepsy can be con-

trolled with a single anticonvulsant drug. The current 'recommended' first-line drugs are sodium valproate for generalised seizures and carbamazepine for partial seizures (RCPCH 2003). It often takes time to find the drug most suitable for optimum treatment and dose adjustment is ongoing as the child grows and develops.

Adolescents

Teenagers with epilepsy are frequently caught between paediatric and adult services with neither service being able to understand, or satisfy, their specific needs and concerns (Smith 1998). Adolescents who have epilepsy may find that the onset of puberty and its accompanying hormonal changes can lead to further seizures. This may occur, even though they were previously well controlled on medication. This can be particularly distressing, especially if they had been free of seizures for some time. In addition to the distress of seizures recurring, the adolescent in particular may be extremely sensitive about involuntary loss of control of bladder and bowel which can occur with some seizures.

Types of epileptic seizures

Generalised seizures

These seizures involve the whole of the brain and consciousness is lost. They will often occur with no warning and the child will have no memory of the event (NSE 2002b).

Tonic–clonic

Formerly known as 'grand mal', these are the most commonly recognised seizure. There is a loss of consciousness, muscles contract and the body becomes rigid which is the tonic phase. The clonic phase involves the muscles relaxing and then tightening rhythmically, causing uncontrollable jerks. Respiration is usually irregular and laboured which leads to cyanosis. Saliva may accumulate in the mouth and there may be biting of the tongue. Incontinence may also occur (Lissauer & Clayden 2001).

Myoclonic

Classic features of this type of seizure are brief and abrupt jerking of one or more limbs. If the whole body is involved, the jerkiness is usually bilateral, symmetrical and mostly flexor or extensor jerks. If mild, the head may drop but if more severe, the child may be thrown suddenly forwards or backwards. Myoclonic seizures are frequently associated with learning disability, or abnormal neurological physiology. Infantile spasms are a type of myoclonic seizure with a poor prognosis for the development of an affected infant.

Atonic

Also known as drop attacks, these seizures involve a transient loss of muscle tone, causing a sudden fall to the floor or drop of the head (Lissauer & Clayden 2001).

Absences

Formerly known as 'petit mal', these seizures occur when consciousness is interrupted. They last for only a couple of seconds and often go unnoticed. There is an appearance of staring, blankness and vagueness. Occasionally there is blinking or twitching of the eyelids or face. There may be involuntary movements, e.g. chewing, lip smacking, loss of postural tone, semi-purposeful movements and peculiar sensations. Amnesia is usual throughout the episode and usually lasts for 5–10 seconds (Wong & Whaley 2000).

Partial seizures

These seizures, also known as focal seizures, begin in, or involve, one hemisphere of the brain. Experiences during these seizures will vary, depending on which area of the brain is affected.

Simple partial

Consciousness is not impaired during these seizures. Symptoms include dizziness, numbness, and sensory disturbances to both auditory and visual sensations. The seizure may be confined to a rhythmic twitching of the face, one limb or part of a limb. Pins and needles are often felt in a specific part of the body (Ball & Bindler 1999).

Complex partial

Many symptoms are similar to those of simple partial seizures. They differ in that consciousness is affected so there is limited or no memory of the event. Disturbance of sensation occurs and may affect auditory, olfactory (smell), gustatory (taste) or emotional senses. The child may manifest automatisms (involuntary movements that look purposeful), i.e. lip smacking, mumbling, making chewing movements, fumbling with clothes and generally confused (Delmar 1997).

Secondary generalisation

A partial seizure starts from a focus in one cortex of the brain but the electrical activity then spreads to both hemispheres simultaneously, producing a generalised seizure. If this spread is rapid then there may be an unawareness of the partial seizure onset.

Guidelines

Parental involvement is vital when a child has recurrent seizures. A large part of the nurse's role is to provide support and education. Encourage parents to express their fears and anxieties and answer their questions honestly (Ball & Bindler 1999). This may be to teach about managing their child's fever, as in the case of febrile seizure. In a child who has recurrent seizures, it is likely to be necessary to teach the family how to administer rectal anticonvulsants in an emergency. As with any chronic condition, it is important for the nurse to provide support as well as education in order to help the child and family adjust to the diagnosis and realities of living with a chronic disease.

Equipment

Very little equipment is required to actually care for a child during a seizure. The unpredictable nature of seizures is such that it will most probably have to be gathered as the child is experiencing the seizure. When a child is known to be affected with recurrent seizures, it may be possible to have appropriate equipment available at all times. For example, if the child is known to have problems maintaining adequate oxygenation during a seizure, a resuscitator bag and mask should be kept to hand.

- Pillows/blankets
- Record of seizures chart
- Watch, with second hand, with which the length of seizure can be established.

The following will be needed if the child is unable to maintain adequate oxygenation:

- Oxygen supply: mask and tubing from wall oxygen points if the child is by, or on, their bed. Portable oxygen will be needed if the seizure occurs in the toilet or corridor.
- Suction equipment: as above with the oxygen.
- Resuscitator bag and mask which is age appropriate should be easily accessible if needed.
- Prescription chart: if the patient has just presented in casualty during a seizure, then one must be immediately available.

The following may be needed if the seizure does not stop spontaneously after about 5 minutes:

- Rectal diazepam, paraldehyde or intravenous lorazepam; this will be dependent on the individual hospital/patient protocol or ease of intravenous access
- Filling quill – to enable rectal administration of paraldehyde with olive/sunflower oil
- Non-sterile latex-free gloves
- Lubricating jelly.

Buccal midazolam or lorazepam (administered between gums and lips slowly) may also be administered (again dependent on hospital protocols).

Rectal paraldehyde administration

Rectal paraldehyde may be extemporaneously prepared immediately prior to use, using equal parts paraldehyde and olive or sunflower oil. Arachis oil should be avoided due to the potential of peanut allergy; if it is used, then observe for signs of anaphylaxis, especially if it is the first administration. Avoid contact with undiluted paraldehyde as it reacts with rubber and plastics. This reaction may make it difficult to depress the plunger of the syringe. A plastic syringe can be used if the administration is immediate; if not, a glass syringe should be used. Draw up the diluent prior to the par-

aldehyde (RCPCH 2003). Paraldehyde should be prepared in a well-ventilated room using protective mask and goggles (Merck 1995).

Method

1. If the nurse realises that the seizure is about to occur and the child is standing or sitting, they should be lowered gently to the ground and put on their side if possible. If the infant is sitting, they should also be placed on the ground or in their cot on their side. Do not attempt to restrain them in anyway or try to put anything into their mouth.

2. Call for help. A child should not be left unattended whilst they are having a seizure and a second nurse may be required to fetch equipment/drugs.

3. Note the exact time that the seizure started and continue to observe the passage of time.

4. Remove any objects in the immediate area on which the child may injure themselves. It may be necessary to pad a rigid surface temporarily with a pillow to prevent the child hitting their head or a limb.

5. If possible, ensure privacy – draw curtains, ask onlookers to move away.

6. Observe the child/infant for signs of cyanosis. Be prepared to administer oxygen if they become cyanosed. If they are in repeated spasm for any length of time, it may be necessary to use a resuscitator bag to instil oxygen if they are unable to inspire effectively for themselves.

7. If relatives are present, try to reassure them about what is happening. It can help to reassure them that the child is unaware of what is happening during most types of seizure, even if it looks painful and distressing. Talk calmly and reassuringly to the child during and after the seizure. This will be of comfort at a frightening time.

8. Be aware of how long the seizure has been in progress. Many convulsions are self-limiting and require no emergency intervention (Ball & Bindler 1999). Determine from the child's

prescription sheet when action may need to be taken to administer anticonvulsant drugs. For example, a child is often prescribed rectal diazepam for a seizure lasting longer than 5 minutes. Each child will have different criteria of when to treat the seizures. Children who rarely seize will have quick action but in some cases of degenerative/intractable seizures it may be after 20–30 minutes.

9. If necessary, administer rectal or intravenous anticonvulsant drugs as prescribed, in accordance with local drug policy and procedure, and note their effect.

10. Once the seizure has finished, place the child in the recovery position to prevent a hypotonic tongue from blocking their airway (Campbell & Glasper 1995).

11. If the child has been incontinent they may need a change of clothing. An infant or young child may require a change of nappy.

12. If it was a febrile seizure, take measures to cool the child down. Assess their temperature and identify whether or not they require to be given an antipyretic such as paracetamol or ibuprofen. This may be given rectally if the child is assessed as being insufficiently awake to take it orally, i.e. unable to protect their own airway with a safe swallow, cough and gag reflex. Remove any excess clothing and ensure that the room is not hot and stuffy, but comfortable and well ventilated.

13. Record the seizure and describe it in detail (see Observations and complications, below). Record the precise duration of the seizure and whether or not intervention was required, e.g. oxygen, assistance with breathing or administration of drugs.

Observations and complications

Observation is especially important when caring for a child having a seizure. It can be important both in aiding diagnosis and in helping to achieve effective control. Carefully observe and record all aspects of the seizure. It is important to obtain an eye witness account of the convulsion so that a 'video' image of the episode can be determined (Rudolf & Levene 1999). How did it start? Which part of the body was affected first? Was more than one area of the body affected at one time? What kind of movements occurred? Did the movements change? Was there more than one phase of the seizure? Did it start with spasm and then progress to jerkiness? Did the movements affect more than one part of the body as the seizure progressed? Did the child appear to have any prior warning of any kind? What was the child doing before the seizure occurred? Did they cry out? Can they describe any 'odd' sensations prior to the seizure? Observe the child carefully for signs of cyanosis. Be aware that if the child has had rectal diazepam or IV lorazepam, it may depress their respiratory drive, particularly in the infant.

There are three life-threatening risks of a seizure:

- a complication of a seizure – aspiration, suffocation, injury (including burns), drowning
- status epilepticus (convulsive)
- a related underlying condition – neurodegenerative disorder, severe cerebral palsy (Appleton & Gibbs 2004).

COMMUNITY PERSPECTIVE

One of the most frightening occurrences for parents is to witness their child having a seizure. Much reassurance is required and in some circumstances discussion in their home environment with a CCN may help the parents to adapt to living with a child who has seizures.

The CCN will be able to support the family by allowing time for them to talk about their anxieties and to help educate them about the seizures and any treatment required, as well as monitoring the child's progress. The parents may feel guilt and humiliation and may be

Community Pesspective continues

concerned that the seizures will affect their child's mental capacity and future (Whaley & Wong 1993).

The CCN will be able to:

- Assess how much information the family have understood prior to discharge. Parents may need help to supplement their understanding once the child has been discharged home (Bailey & Caldwell 1997).
- Reinforce the education given in hospital, stressing the importance of drug compliance and the potential complications from sudden drug withdrawal (Kempthorne 1994).
- Ensure parents are competent in administering rectal diazepam/sublingual/buccal midazolam or lorazepam which is now widely used to treat seizures even though it is not licensed for this use (RCPCH 2003).
- Ensure that parents know how long to wait before administering rectal diazepam or sublingual/buccal midazolam/lorazepam
- Ensure parents know when to seek medical help:
  - 10 minutes for the first seizure, or
  - 2 minutes longer than the usual length of seizure, or
  - when a second fit occurs without the child regaining consciousness (British Epilepsy Association 1991).

- Discuss with the family the information that should be given to playgroup, nursery or school staff and any other adults who may take responsibility for caring for the child. The school staff will need to be taught how to administer rectal diazepam (Joint Epilepsy Council 2004) or sublingual/buccal midazolam/lorazepam either by the CCN or the school nurse. It will be necessary for the child to have an individual care plan for use in school, stating the action to be taken if the child has a seizure and the policy for safe storage of medication in school.
- Ensure that parents are aware that their children can undertake sports, although they should not be allowed to swim alone (Joint Epilepsy Council of the UK and Ireland 1995) and restrictions may need to be placed on where they cycle. The wearing of a protective helmet may need to be considered if the child's seizures cause regular falls resulting in injury. Parents may find this difficult to accept as it is an outward sign of their child's seizures.

Most importantly, the family should be encouraged to take a positive attitude and encourage the child to take part in normal activities.

Do and do not

- Do position the child on their side if possible.
- Do observe carefully and thoroughly.
- Do be prepared to provide assistance with breathing.
- Do try to protect the child from injury.
- Do be prepared to administer rectal anticonvulsant drugs if the seizure does not stop spontaneously within 5 minutes.

- Do record all seizure activity.
- Do keep families updated.
- Do speak to the child and give reassurance.
- Do not attempt to restrain the child in any way.
- Do not attempt to put anything into the child's mouth; you may get your finger badly bitten and push their tongue backwards causing a blocked airway.

References

Appleton R, Gibbs J 2004 Epilepsy in childhood and adolescence, 3rd edn. Martin Dunitz, London

Bailey R, Caldwell C 1997 Preparing parents for going home. Paediatric Nursing 9(4): 15–17

Ball J, Bindler R 1999 Pediatric nursing, 2nd edn. Appleton and Lange, Connecticut, CT

British Epilepsy Association 1991 The modern management of epilepsy. Yorkshire Television/Chevron Communications, p G19

Campbell S, Glasper E A (eds) 1995 Whaley and Wong's children's nursing. Mosby, London, ch 31, p 674–679

Delmar 1997 Delmar's textbook of basic pediatric nursing. Delmar, New York

Joint Epilepsy Council of the UK and Ireland 1995 New horizons: a guide for young people with epilepsy. JEC, Leeds, p 16

Joint Epilepsy Council 2004 A guideline on training standards for the administration of rectal diazepam. JEC, Leeds

Kempthorne A 1994 Epilepsy in childhood. Paediatric Nursing 6(4): 30–33

Lissauer T, Clayden G 2001 Illustrated textbook of paediatrics, 2nd edn. Mosby, Edinburgh

Merck 1995 Safety data sheet for paraldehyde GPR ID NO 2944800. Merck, Poole, UK

National Society for Epilepsy (NSE) 2002a Epilepsy: an introduction to epileptic seizures. Chalfont St Peter, Bucks, UK

National Society for Epilepsy (NSE) 2002b Epilepsy: information on seizures and status epilepticus. Chalfont St Peter, Bucks, UK

Royal College of Paediatrics and Child Health (RCPCH) 2003 Medicines for Children. RCPCH, London

Rudolf M, Levene M 1999 Paediatrics and child health. Blackwell Science, Oxford

Scottish Intercollegiate Guidelines Network (SIGN) 2003 Diagnosis and management of epilepsies in children and young people. SIGN, Edinburgh, p 1–7

Smith P E M 1998 The teenager with epilepsy. British Medical Journal 317: 960–961

Waterston T, Helms P, Ward Platt M 1997 Paediatrics: understanding child health. Oxford University Press, Oxford

Whaley L F, Wong D 1993 Essentials of paediatric nursing, 4th edn. Mosby, St Louis, p 973

Wong D 1997 Whaley & Wong's Essentials of pediatric nursing, 5th edn. Mosby, St Louis, MO

Wong D, Whaley L F 2000 Wong and Whaley's clinical manual of pediatric nursing. Mosy, St. Louis, MO

Practice 28

Skin care

Jacqueline Denyer, Rosemary Turnbull

Introduction

The skin is the largest organ of the body and has many functions, the most important being:

- thermoregulation
- protection: from physical and mechanical injury
- waterproofing
- synthesis of vitamin D
- transmission of sensation (Graham-Brown & Bourke 1998).

In the absence of disease it is important to maintain the skin in good condition to minimise infection and dry skin. In many cultures this can be achieved through regular bathing and drying (Denyer & Turnbull 1996).

Often underestimated in their effects on general health and well-being, childhood skin disorders may reduce quality of life through pain and irritation. Although rare, some skin conditions can prove to be life threatening.

Appropriate skin care is essential in those with healthy or diseased skin in order to maintain the functions of the skin as far as possible.

Learning outcomes

By the end of this section you should be able to:

- maintain good skin care in the presence of health and disease

- develop an understanding of children who require additional skin care
- apply topical treatments as prescribed in the correct way
- adapt such treatments to the individual child.

Rationale

Children's nurses are frequently involved in care of children with many skin conditions, including atopic eczema, in general wards when the child is admitted for another condition, in outpatient departments and in the dermatology ward.

The healthy child may suffer from dry skin conditions or infections. The majority of dermatological conditions are exacerbated by the dry hot atmosphere of the hospital. A hospital admission, whether for management of the skin condition or for another reason, provides an ideal opportunity for intensive skin care and for parental education.

Painful and irritated skin has a profound effect on the child's self-image, mood and peer acceptance. Those who will require additional skin care over and above routine cleansing include:

- infants with cradle cap and dry skin
- infants with nappy rash
- children with skin infections
- children with eczema or psoriasis
- the preterm infant whose skin is thin and delicate
- children with serious inherited skin disorders.

Factors to note

- Children can develop a range of skin conditions, many of which are transient, e.g. contact dermatitis, and cause few ill-effects, whilst others can develop into more persistent serious conditions.
- Dry skin is a common problem and its management can be incorporated into the regime of daily hygiene.
- Children enjoy bubble baths but these may have a drying effect and may necessitate restriction. After bathing the skin should be checked for any signs of dryness or irritation and moisturisers applied as necessary.
- Children's skin is often sensitive and an unscented preparation should be chosen.
- Use of coconut and olive oils features in Asian and Afro-Caribbean cultures as a part of daily skin care. Caution must be exercised in using nut oils in view of the increasing awareness of the risk of anaphylaxis in response to such products.
- It is crucial that a detailed history and examination of the skin is made in order to plan, implement and evaluate an individualised treatment plan for the child.
- Where possible, the child and parents should be encouraged to participate in the care. Children may be afraid or fractious and adolescents may rebel against lifelong daily treatments.
- It should be remembered that treatments are often time-consuming and monotonous.
- Preparations can stain all clothing and soft furnishings, and can make carers reluctant to pick up or cuddle the child.

Equipment

- Plastic aprons to protect clothing/uniform
- Gloves, for use when applying medicated creams/ointments or when dealing with children whose skin is infected
- Bath situated in a warm private environment
- Soft towels
- Prescribed bath additive
- Soap substitute
- Prescribed cream/ointment
- Emollient
- Foil bowls and spatula (for decanting creams/ointments not in pump dispensers)
- Selection of toys for distraction
- Clothing
- Nappies if required.

GUIDELINES FOR PERFORMING SKIN CARE

CRADLE CAP/SEBORRHOEIC DERMATITIS

This is characterised by erythema and a yellow scale on the scalp which can spread to eyebrows. Generally affecting infants under 3 months of age, occurring on the scalp (cradle cap), eyebrows, face and limb flexures, it can also favour the nappy area. Unlike atopic eczema, it is not itchy or painful but can look unsightly, causing distress to parents. It will generally clear on its own with mild emollient therapy such as an emollient bath daily and a light emollient cream. It can be complicated by a yeast infection and in this instance an antifungal cream may be indicated. If it does not clear, the infant should be referred to a dermatologist/paediatrician for further assessment.

For cradle cap, olive oil should be applied to the scalp and gently massaged in to loosen the scales and encourage them to separate. The oil can be left in for 30 minutes to overnight, depending on the severity of the cradle cap. A medicated or mild infant shampoo should be used to remove the oil. A soft baby brush can then be used to gently remove the loosened scales. Temptation to remove adherent scales by picking must be resisted as hair loss may result (Gill 2003).

NAPPY RASH

Nappy rash is a relatively common condition of infancy. It can be caused by irritation from faeces and urine or fungal contamination. Infant skin is generally more fragile and therefore more prone to physical and chemical injury/irritation as the dermis is immature due to decreased collagen and elastic fibres as well as immature blood and nerve supply. The normal pH of skin is acidic; moisture in the nappy area increases the pH, making the skin more permeable (Turnbull 2003). Children suffering from gastroenteritis or malabsorption syndromes frequently pass watery stools, which may be acidic and cause damage to the nappy area. These children may require more frequent nappy changes and application of occlusive ointments such as petroleum jelly; this will go some way to reducing contact with irritants. Exposure of the excoriated skin will help minimise nappy rash (Turnbull 2003).

The carer must be educated on prevention of nappy rash by frequent changing and gentle cleansing followed by application of a barrier cream/ointment, such as zinc and castor oil cream or petroleum jelly. The use of fragranced cleansing wipes should be discouraged in the presence of nappy rash as they will only serve to irritate the skin.

When there is no improvement using simple measures, secondary infection such as with *Candida albicans* (thrush) should be suspected and a swab obtained for culture before commencing prescribed treatments (Turnbull 2003). If nappy rash is severe and persists despite all measures, the infant should be referred to a dermatologist/paediatrician for diagnosis.

ECZEMA HERPETICUM

This is caused by the herpes simplex virus (HSV) and many eczematous children have an abnormal response to HSV, which can result in dissemination of the herpes and subsequent toxaemia (Harper 1990).

It is recognised as small clusters of clear fluid-filled vesicles, which can take on a punched-out appearance.

This is a dermatological emergency and all parents should be alerted to this condition and advised to keep the child away from those with cold sores. Healthcare workers with cold sores should not care for the child with eczema and should refrain from work until clear.

IMPETIGO

This is a highly infectious disorder caused by *Staphylococcus aureus* and/or group A streptococci. It is characterised by small blisters that burst easily, releasing a yellow exudate, which in turn forms a pale honey-coloured crust.

The infectious nature of this condition necessitates the child being kept off school or nursery. Sites around the nose and mouth are most commonly affected (Doherty 2001). If the infection is extensive, then systemic antibiotics are indicated and they should be prescribed immediately and not withheld until microbiology results are available.

Topical antibiotics are only of use if the infection is identified early enough and the impetiginised area is localised; however, one must be aware that in some instances such as eczema the possibility of multiresistant strains should be a consideration.

Crusts can be removed by the use of warm saline soaks or a weak solution of potassium permanganate.

Do and do not

- Do isolate the child from others. If in hospital, universal precautions are indicated against infection. At home, the child should have their own towel and avoid using a flannel. Bed linen such as pillowcases should be changed daily to minimise reinfection.
- Do cut the child's fingernails to minimise damage if the skin is scratched. The wearing of mittens/gloves will minimise skin damage.
- Do introduce distraction methods to stop the child scratching or picking at crusts and so spreading the infection.

ATOPIC ECZEMA

Eczema is a chronic inflammatory disorder of the skin. The condition is erratic and varies somewhat in severity. It generally presents in infancy from 3 months of age and there is often a genetic predisposition, i.e. family history of asthma, eczema and allergy. Any area of the body can be affected and education on factors that may exacerbate the condition is crucial in order to give optimum care to the child and promote an adequate quality of life. There is no cure for this condition but several of these factors can assist in the reduction of exacerbations (McHenry 1995).

Factors to note

- Eczema results in intense pruritus (itching) which makes the child irritable and fretful; this in turn results in sleep disturbance and can result in alterations in behaviour.
- The skin becomes red (erythematous) and small blisters (vesicles) occur which, when scratched, result in weeping, bleeding areas of skin.
- There is no cure and the aim is to control the condition and minimise exacerbations.

A basic regime may be enough to maintain control of the skin.

- The ultimate aim of treatments is to replace moisture and reduce inflammation.
- If frequent exacerbations are common, one should establish who does the skin care and how it is carried out. It may be necessary to re-educate the carer and, where appropriate, the child and together negotiate achievable goals.
- One must constantly assess and reassess the child's progress and treatment and alter the treatment accordingly. Attention to the following may serve to improve the child's eczema:
  - Avoid any known aggravating factors.
  - Wear 100% cotton clothing; wool will irritate the skin.
  - Sleep in a well-ventilated room.
  - Use special mattress covers to minimise harbouring of the house dust mite (HDM).
  - Daily vacuuming of the house and mattress, and damp dusting of the room will also reduce HDM.
  - Avoid all hairy/furry animals.
  - Keep finger- and toenails short to minimise damage caused by scratching.
  - Encourage the child to rub on the skin instead of scratching it.
  - Develop distraction techniques and help parents to develop these to minimise anger and frustration.
  - Swimming – where possible, the child should not be excluded. A thin smearing of petroleum jelly or similar will serve to protect the skin. The child must shower thoroughly afterwards, using emollients and soap substitute.
  - To ensure adequate rest and sleep, a prescribed sedative, e.g. antihistamine, should be administered early enough to allow a good 10-hour period before the child is due to rise.

Method

1. Bathing in warm/tepid water at least once daily with added emollient oil and use of a

soap substitute cream will serve to remove surface debris and hydrate the skin.

2. To minimise irritation use a soft towel and pat, not rub, dry.

3. Prescribed topical steroids should be applied twice daily after bathing (unless medical advice differs) to all areas of eczema; there should be enough to show a fine visible film.

4. To avoid dilution of the topical steroid, the prescribed emollient should be applied 30 minutes later and then regularly as necessary throughout the day. Emollients should be applied liberally and in a downward direction to minimise plugging of hair follicles which could result in infection (Atherton 1994). The use of regular emollients serves to soften the skin and therefore reduce pruritus and the need for more potent topical steroids.

If it is not possible to control the child's eczema with this basic regime, it may be necessary to use wet wraps for a short time. These increase steroid absorption as well as cooling the skin and reducing pruritus (Lawton 2002). Wet wraps must be used under the direction of the dermatologist/paediatrician. Wet wraps are lengths of tubefast cut to make a full body suit with normal clothing worn on top. They are relatively time-consuming to apply and should be seen, not as a maintenance treatment, but as a means of regaining control of the child's eczema. The length of time wraps are required will depend on the child's response to treatment; once control is achieved, then the strength of topical steroids should be reduced to achieve maintenance. There are now several brands of tubefast available as well as wet wrap garments; choice generally depends on what is available to carry out the procedure competently. The parent/carer will need additional support during this treatment.

Lichenification is a thickening of the skin as a result of repeated damage through scratching and is visible in knee and elbow flexures. Limbs may respond to application of Ichthopaste/Viscopaste bandages overnight, but the bandages can be left in situ for up to 3 days. They are useful to soften the skin as well as producing a cooling effect.

A low-potency topical steroid can be applied under the bandages if need be; the paste bandage is then covered with Coban elasticated dressing (Robinson 2003).

Note: Occlusive bandages create a warm humid environment which encourages bacterial growth and therefore spread infection; they must not be used in the presence of infection. This also applies to infectious diseases.

Observations and complications

The skin of most children with eczema will be colonised with *Staphylococcus aureus*. Infection should be considered when there is deterioration in the skin. Symptoms may include:

- weeping/wet areas of eczema
- areas of crusting
- enlarged lymph nodes
- pyrexia
- irritability.

Streptococcal infection should be considered if there is family history of sore throats.

Do and do not

- Do educate parents in the management and treatment of the condition and regularly assess and reassess their techniques.
- Do be aware of the side-effects of prolonged or incorrect use of topical steroids. Preparations used in children tend to be mild and should not cause problems. Misuse of stronger steroids can result in thinning of the skin.
- Do monitor growth, as prolonged use of topical steroids, especially moderate and potent types, can inhibit normal growth. Growth should be monitored at each clinic appointment by measuring the child's height and weight and recording the results on a growth chart.
- Do ensure that the school receives education on the child's eczema and conditions that may aggravate the skin, e.g.:
  - avoid sitting in the centre of the room or next to radiators
  - use a soap substitute at all times
  - identify an area where the child can apply emollients.

- Do not bathe in hot water as heat causes vasodilatation and will increase irritation.
- Do not use scented bath oils, creams, laundry powders or fabric softeners as they include fragrance which will irritate the skin.
- Do not dip fingers into pots of cream or ointments as this will increase the risk of contamination and cause infection. The preparation should be decanted onto a saucer each time it is used.
- Do not sit in hot, dry environments.

PSORIASIS

There are various types of psoriasis affecting people in different ways; therefore, treatments are tailored to meet individual needs. Psoriasis can affect any age but is uncommon in children and rarely seen before 3 years of age (Harper 1990).

Factors to note

Psoriasis is a chronic relapsing non-infectious inflammatory disease, the cause of which is not yet understood. There are many factors that can trigger or exacerbate the disease process:

- trauma – lesions appear at the site of injury
- infection – beta haemolytic streptococcal tonsillitis
- stress/emotional upset
- sunlight – the majority will improve but a small percentage will become worse.

Treatments for psoriasis are mainly topical and can only be used when the disease process is active and not as preventive measures.

Method of treatment

- Coal tar preparations: the exact mode of action is unclear but they are known to inhibit DNA synthesis, therefore reducing cell proliferation and inhibiting the psoriatic process.
- Keratolytic agents are creams and ointments that reduce scaling by reducing thick plaques.
- Bathing daily in a prescribed tar-based preparation or emollient bath oil and application of the prescribed keratolytic cream or ointment to affected areas may help to regain control of the disease process.

- The application of emollients regularly throughout the day will promote skin softening and so reduce scaling and flaking of skin.

Care of the scalp

- Cocois or olive oil is massaged into the scalp and left in situ for the prescribed length of time; the hair is then combed out to remove loosened plaques.
- Shampoo using a prescribed tar-based solution.
- Comb again to remove plaques and then allow hair to dry naturally.
- The procedure should be performed separately from the bath to minimise irritation to the skin of the body.

Do and do not

- Do remove the preparation immediately and notify medical staff if irritation during treatment occurs.
- Do inform the parent and child that many preparations are messy and will stain clothing and sometimes skin. It should be stressed that any skin discoloration from treatments will fade.
- Do encourage the wearing of pale clothing to minimise the visibility of shed skin scales.
- Do avoid stressful situations.
- Do inform the child's school and arrange to chat with teachers, which will help reduce teasing; it is also crucial to refer the child to someone who will help them develop coping mechanisms.
- Do not allow the child to see this as a handicap but try to promote positive aspects of body image.
- Do not omit any prescribed treatments or use products prescribed for other people as treatment for psoriasis is individualised.

THE PRETERM INFANT

The skin of the preterm infant is thin and there is absence of subcutaneous fat.

Often, preterm infants receive intensive therapy which involves the use of intravenous cannulae and monitoring with sticky equipment such as cardiac electrodes. Endotracheal tubes are sometimes secured with sticky tapes. Wherever possible, use of such tapes should be avoided and silicone or hydrocolloid dressings used in their place. Where use of adhesive tape is essential, care must be taken on removal to ensure no tearing of the skin results. Petroleum jelly or liquid paraffin may be used to destroy the adhesive properties of the tape prior to removal.

THE CHILD WITH FRAGILE SKIN

Skin fragility may be a feature of prematurity or a genetic defect such as epidermolysis bullosa (EB). EB is a rare genetically determined skin disorder occurring in 1:50 000 live births in the UK. Affected children often require multidisciplinary care at a specialised centre, but day-to-day care is carried out at home with the support of community nurses. Its aim is to:

- maintain skin integrity
- minimise damage.

BATHING

This is a clean, rather than a sterile procedure. Prescribed analgesia must be given and replacement dressings prepared.

Prior to bathing the nurse must consider whether it is an appropriate procedure, or if the child is very sore and bathing is likely to cause added distress. Washing of unaffected areas may be a more suitable alternative (Lin & Carter 1992).

Observation should be made of the site, size and condition of any wounds and the general condition of the skin. Observations should be recorded and photographs taken as necessary in order to monitor progress or deterioration.

Method

1. Line a baby bath with a towelling sling or soft towel to prevent skin damage from the base or sides of the bath by avoiding shearing forces from a hard surface.
2. Add prescribed emollient(s).
3. Use a second person if necessary to assist and minimise trauma.
4. Pat rather than rub the child dry using a soft non-shedding towel to avoid leaving fibres in the wound which may result in over-granulation.
5. Apply prescribed non-adherent dressings to promote a warm moist environment in order to encourage wound healing.

Note: Avoid prolonged bathing which may result in a fall of temperature and result in delayed wound healing.

General care of the child with fragile skin

- Ensure that all who are in contact with the child are aware of the skin fragility and appropriate method of handling.
- Avoid the use of plastic namebands which could rub and cause skin damage.
- Avoid the use of adhesive tapes.
- Use alternative fabrics to secure intravenous cannulae and electrodes, such as silicone dressings or hydrocolloids.
- Choose soft cotton clothing. Turn underclothes inside out to avoid seams rubbing.
- Use glass rather than Tempa DOT thermometers which may stick to the skin and cause tearing.
- Educate theatre and anaesthetic staff prior to any procedures.

COMMUNITY PERSPECTIVE

The health visitor and GP are likely to be the first community healthcare professionals to become aware of skin problems in the younger child. Depending on their level of knowledge of dermatology, health visitors may be confident to manage conditions such as atopic eczema in partnership with the GP. If the eczema is severe, the child should be referred to a consultant dermatologist.

The amount of involvement CCNs have with families of children with eczema will vary according to local policies.

When a child has been admitted to hospital with infected eczema or a severe exacerbation, home visits to check the child's progress and assist the family with the time-consuming treatments have been shown to be beneficial.

Community Perspective continues

Families may find it easier to understand the important aspects of eczema management in their own homes, than in a busy outpatient department. Home visits also enable the CCN to identify factors which may be exacerbating the eczema, e.g. pets or high levels of house dust mite. The CCN will also gain insights into the nature of the condition at its most severe and how exhausted the families may become.

The CCN is in an ideal position to liaise with schools concerning the care of pupils with eczema, thus giving the teachers additional insight into problems that may occur.

Families who give a high input of care to their child with eczema may be entitled to Disability Living Allowance. The CCN may be asked to assist in filling in the application forms.

A multidisciplinary approach to the care of children with eczema has been proved to work well (Masini et al, unpublished work, 1997). Health visitors, CCNs and dermatology nurses, together with their medical colleagues, can develop a service to support the many families who struggle to cope with the demands of a badly affected child.

Useful addresses

Dystrophic Epidermolysis Bullosa Research Association (DEBRA)
DEBRA House
Wellington Business Park
Dukes Ride
Crowthorne
Berkshire RG11 6LS

National Eczema Society
Hill House
Highgate Hill
London N19 5NA
www.eczema.org

Psoriasis Association
Milton House
7 Milton Street
Northampton NN2 7JG

References

Atherton D J 1994 Eczema in childhood: the facts. Oxford University Press, Oxford

Denyer J, Turnbull R 1996 The skin. In: McQuaid L, Huband S, Parker E (eds) Children's nursing. Churchill Livingstone, Edinburgh, ch 17

Doherty C 2001 Infections and infestations. In: Hughes E, Van Onselon J (eds) Dermatology nursing: a practical guide. Churchill Livingstone, Edinburgh, ch 13

Gill S 2003 Infantile seborrhoeic dermatitis and cradle cap. In: Barnes K (ed) Paediatrics: a clinical guide for nurse practitioners. Butterworth-Heinemann, Edinburgh, ch 9, p 10

Graham-Brown R, Bourke J 1998 Mosby's colour atlas and text of dermatology. Mosby, London, ch 1

Harper J 1990 Handbook of paediatric dermatology. Butterworth-Heinemann, London

Lawton S 2002 How to wet wrap. British Journal of Dermatology Nursing 3(1): 8–9

Lin A N, Carter D M (eds) 1992 Epidermolysis bullosa: basic and clinical aspects. Springer-Verlag, New York

McHenry P M 1995 Management of atopic eczema. British Medical Journal 310: 843–847

Robinson J 2003 Atopic eczema. In: Barnes K (ed) Paediatrics: a clinical guide for nurse practitioners. Butterworth-Heinemann, Edinburgh, ch 9, p 3

Turnbull R 2003 Nappy rash. In: Barnes K (ed) Paediatrics: a clinical guide for nurse practitioners. Butterworth-Heinemann, Edinburgh, ch 9, p 11

Further Reading and Viewing

Dystrophic Epidermolysis Bullosa Research Association (DEBRA) Publications, available from: DEBRA House, Wellington Business Park, Dukes Ride, Crowthorne, Berkshire RG11 6LS

National Eczema Society Publications, available from: Hill House, Highgate Hill, London N19 5NA

Nursing Times 1999 Skin care supplement, September 15

Williams R 1991 Guidelines for management of patients with psoriasis. British Medical Journal 303: 829–835

Specimen collection

Christina Maddox, Beryl Pearson

Introduction

Infectious microorganisms/biological agents can refer to the bacteria, viruses, fungi and internal parasites that create a hazard to human health. Most harm through infection but they can also cause allergies or be toxic (ACDP 2003). Specimen collection is undertaken when laboratory investigation is required for the examination of tissue or body fluid, and is an aid to diagnosis.

Specimen collection is a fundamental aspect of children's nursing practice that requires a diverse range of knowledge and skills. Specimens can be taken from a number of areas and the results used for screening, diagnosis, treatment and research. The validity of specimen test results is, however, dependent on using the correct collection technique and safe prac-tice, to avoid contamination and cross-infection. Collecting specimens from children is further complicated by the child's ability to understand what is being asked of them and the parent's willingness and ability to assist. Nurses often have responsibility for both the collection and the safe transportation of samples to the laboratory.

Learning outcomes

By the end of this section you should:

- be aware of the physical and psychosocial implications to the child and family when collecting specimens
- know how to collect appropriate specimens and transport them safely to the laboratory
- be aware of your responsibility and accountability in obtaining specimens, interpreting

and communicating results in conjunction with medical staff and the family
- be aware of the need to record the investigation
- be aware of complications that may arise from specimen collection.

Rationale

Specimen collection is undertaken for the examination of tissue or body fluid. Most samples are sent to the laboratory but some tests are carried out on the ward, for example, blood glucose and urinalysis. Knowledge of correct procedural principles in collecting specimens is essential to effective child and family nursing.

Factors to note

- Always gain consent (NMC 2002) from the parents and the child by explaining the procedure clearly and appropriately (Quick Reference Guide 8 1999) and the reasons for taking the specimen. If specimens are obtained for research purposes, written consent should be obtained. The child and family have a right to refuse without any obligation (Royal College of Paediatrics and Child Health 2000).

- Wherever possible, collect specimens before antimicrobial treatment begins as this may affect the results (Baillie 2001, Royal Liverpool & Broadgreen University Hospitals 2004). However, treatment must not be delayed in serious sepsis.

- The principles of specimen collection are the same, but local protocols may differ. To maintain safe practice the nurse should be familiar with these protocols. Requests for collection of any specimen should be made by a doctor – this is usually on a laboratory request form or sometimes in the medical notes.

- Perform a risk assessment before commencement of any procedure and decide if alternative or additional equipment is necessary. If you are in an unfamiliar environment, for example, the home, it is important to make a risk assessment to ensure safe collection of the specimen (ACDP 2003).

- Pain assessment should be considered before specimen collection and, if required, pain relief should be administered prior to the procedure.

- Hands should be washed according to national protocol, before and after specimen collection. Gloves should be worn when collecting or handling all specimens to avoid cross-contamination of the specimen and the nurse (Infection Control Nurses Association 1997, DoH 2003, Hilton & Baker 2003, Camm 2004).

- Contamination of the specimen must be avoided as this may produce the need for a further sample with implications for the child. It may also cause misleading results and delay in appropriate treatment.

- When collecting the specimen, avoid infecting the child. For example, there is an increased risk of infection if an aseptic technique is not used when collecting a catheter urine specimen or during the collection of cerebrospinal fluid.

- For all specimen samples collected, examine the sample for abnormalities, e.g. colour, content, consistency and odour, and record observations. Record the acquisition of the specimen sample in the nursing documentation.

- All pathological specimens must be treated as potentially infectious and local written laboratory protocols should be followed for the safe handling and transportation of specimens (COSHH 1999, Health and Safety Executive 1999). Specimens for laboratory inspection should be collected in sterile containers with close-fitting lids to avoid contamination and spillage; however, this would only be necessary if examining for infection. For some urine and stool collections, where specimens are being examined for biochemical abnormalities, there would be no need for sterile containers. All specimen containers must be transported in a double-sided, self-sealing polythene bag with one compartment containing the laboratory request form and the other the specimen.

- All specimens must be clearly labelled to identify their source. A laboratory request form with the following information must accompany the specimen. This aids interpretation of results and reduces mistakes.

  - Patient's name, age, ward/department and hospital number
  - Type of specimen
  - How collected, e.g. pad urine, MSU, U-Bag
  - Date and time collected
  - Diagnosis with history and relevant clinical signs and symptoms such as returning from abroad (specify country) with diarrhoea and vomiting, rash, pyrexia, catheters in situ or invasive devices used, or surgical details regarding postoperative wound infection
  - Any antimicrobial drugs given
  - Consultant's name and cost code
  - Name of the doctor who ordered the investigation, as it may be necessary to telephone preliminary results and discuss treatment before the typed report is dispatched
  - Biohazard label, if appropriate.

- When collecting pus specimens, obtain as much material as possible as this increases the chance of isolating microorganisms which may be difficult to grow or are minimal in number, e.g. in tuberculosis.

- Transport medium is used to preserve microorganisms during transportation. Charcoal medium, used for bacteria, neutralises toxic substances such as naturally occurring fatty acids found on the skin. Because many viruses do not survive well outside the body, special viral transport medium is used.

- Specimens sent through the postal system must be packed and labelled according to Post Office guidelines. The specimen must be wrapped in a plastic bag, encased in absorbent material within another plastic bag, placed in a rigid cardboard container and firmly taped. A warning 'Pathological Sample' along with the sender's name and address must be visible on the outside (DoH 1998, Health and Safety Executive 1999).

- In children suspected of suffering from viral haemorrhagic fevers such as Lassa fever, Marburg or Ebola virus, the infection control team must be consulted before any specimens are taken (ACDP 1996).

- Body fluid spillages should be soaked up with paper towels, after which disinfectant or hot soapy water should be used to clean any non-blood spillage (May 2000). For a blood spillage, sodium dichloroisocyanurate (NaDCC) or hypochlorite solution (10 000 ppm) should be sprinkled over and left for a few minutes before cleaning with hot soapy water (May 2000). Local protocols on cleaning bodily fluid spillage may differ (RCN 2004) but universal precautions should always be used and care must be taken, as release of chlorine fumes has occurred when chlorine-releasing agents were mixed with urine (DoH 1990, Health and Safety Executive 2002).

- For advice or further guidance on the collection of any specimen, contact the laboratory.

Equipment

Specific equipment is available in each clinical area for each particular procedure, and should be used. This will vary according to the specimen required but must include:

- disposable gloves – sterile for blood cultures
- a protective tray
- a sterile container for the specimen
- appropriate transport medium, if required
- laboratory specimen form
- a polythene transportation bag
- biohazard label, if required.

Eye swab

This procedure is carried out when infection is suspected. The procedure may be uncomfortable and the child should be prepared appropriately.

- Where possible ask the child to look upwards, then gently pull the lower lid down or gently part the eyelids.
- Use a sterile cotton wool swab and gently roll the swab over the conjunctival sac inside the lower lid. Hold the swab parallel to the cornea to avoid injury if the child moves.
- Place the swab in the transport medium.
- For suspected *Chlamydia* infection:
  - Clean the eye first with sterile normal saline to obtain a clear view of the conjunctiva
  - Use a pernasal wire swab, part the eyelids and gently rub the conjunctival sac of the lower lid to obtain epithelial cells; identification of the organism is by fluorescent monoclonal antibodies
  - Wipe the swab over the marked area on the glass slide and allow to dry
  - Place the glass slide into a slide holder or Petri dish to protect the specimen.

Nose swab

Nasal colonisation with *Staphylococcus aureus* increases the risk of staphylococcal infections at other sites of the body such as postoperative wounds and dialysis access sites. It is also associated with recurrent skin infections and nosocomial infections (Health Protection Agency 2004).

- If the nose is dry, moisten the swab in sterile saline beforehand.
- For viral investigation, moisten the swab in the viral transport medium prior to taking the swab.
- Insert the swab into the anterior nares and direct it up into the tip of the nose and gently rotate. Both nares should be cultured using the same swab to obtain adequate material.
- Plain sterile cotton wool swab. Sample the anterior nares by gently rotating the swab over the mucosal surface.
- Place in transport medium.
- The outside of the nostrils may be rubbed after the procedure to alleviate the unpleasant sensation of swabbing.

Pernasal swab

This investigation is used specifically to diagnose whooping cough (*Bordetella pertussis*). When obtaining this specimen, the nurse must be proficient in the procedure and ensure that suction, oxygen and resuscitation equipment are easily available. The child should be held securely and observed carefully as the procedure may produce paroxysmal coughing and/or vomiting.

- Place the child in a good light to facilitate observation.
- Use a special soft-wired sterile swab to minimise trauma to the nasal tissue.
- Holding the child's head upwards, pass the swab along the floor of the nasal cavity to the posterior wall of the nasopharynx.
- Gently rotate and withdraw the swab and place it in special transport medium or dispatch the swab in its container immediately to the laboratory to ensure maximum enhancement of growth of the organism.

Sputum

Supervised older children, given proper guidance, may be able to provide the specimen themselves. Specimens from younger children and babies may be obtained using a mucus extractor or suction apparatus.

- Encourage the child to cough, especially after sleep, and expectorate into a container. Alternatively, nasopharyngeal/tracheal suction using a sputum trap can be undertaken.
- Physiotherapy may help to facilitate expectoration.
- Ensure that the material obtained is sputum and not saliva, and avoid collecting sputum specimens soon after the child had eaten as food particles may contaminate the specimen.

Throat swab

- Place the child in a position with a good light source. This will ensure maximum visibility of the tonsillar bed.
- Either depress the tongue with a spatula or ask the child to say 'aahh'. The procedure is

likely to cause gagging and the tongue will move to the roof of the mouth and prevent accurate sampling.

- Quickly, but gently, rub the swab over the tonsillar bed or area where there is exudate or a lesion.
- Place the sample into transport medium.

Ear swab

- No antibiotics or other therapeutic agents should have been in the aural region for about 3 hours prior to sampling the area as this may inhibit the growth of organisms.
- If there is purulent discharge, this should be sampled.
- Place a sterile swab into the outer ear and gently rotate to collect the secretions.
- Place the swab in transport medium.
- For deeper ear swabbing, a speculum should be used. This procedure should be undertaken by experienced medical staff as damage to the eardrum may occur.

Wound swab

A wound swab or a sample of wound exudate will help to identify the infection and determine the most effective treatment. Specimen collection from wounds often yields poor results because the swab dries out before it reaches the laboratory. This is a particular problem if the specimen is stored before it is examined. Wherever possible, pus or fluid should be aspirated, but if swabbing is the only practical method, two or three specimens will give more reliable results than a single sample (Gould 2001). Interpretation of results must be in conjunction with clinical signs. In the absence of clinical signs of infection, wound swabs may not provide any useful information (Gilchrist 2000, Hampton 2004).

- Obtain the specimen prior to any dressing or cleaning procedure of the wound. This will maximise the material obtained and prevent killing of the organism by the use of antiseptics.
- Use a sterile swab; gently rotate it on the area to collect exudate from the wound and

place into transport medium. Where there is ample pus, collect as much as possible in a sterile syringe or sterile container and send to the laboratory.

- For detection of *Mycobacterium tuberculosis* a calcium alginate swab can be used. The swab gradually dissolves, maximising the isolation of the organism as its numbers are usually small.

Faeces

- A faecal specimen is more suitable than a rectal swab.

- A specimen can be obtained from a nappy, clean potty or pulp bedpan liner.

- Using a scoop, place faecal material into a container.

- Some investigations require the fresh stool to be taken to the laboratory for analysis immediately (Royal Liverpool & Broadgreen Hospitals 2004). Check with the laboratory prior to specimen collection.

- Where diarrhoea is present, a small piece of non-absorbent material lining the nappy can be used to prevent material soaking into the nappy.

- Examine the sample for consistency, odour or blood and record observations to monitor changes.

- If segments of tapeworm are seen, send them to the laboratory. Tapeworm segments can vary from the size of rice grains to a ribbon shape, 2.5 cm (1 inch) long.

- For the identification of *Enterobius vermicularis* (threadworm/pinworm), material should be obtained first thing in the morning on awakening by using a Sellotape slide. Place the sticky side of a strip of Sellotape over the anal region to obtain the material and stick the Sellotape smoothly onto a glass slide. The eggs of the worm can then be identified under the microscope. Threadworms lay their eggs on the perianal skin at night and therefore they will not be seen in a faecal specimen.

- Where amoebic dysentery is suspected, the specimen of stool must be freshly dispatched to the laboratory. The parasite causing amoebic dysentery exists in a free-living motile form and in the form of non-motile cysts. Both forms are characteristic in their fresh state but difficult to identify when dead.

Urine

Bedside urine testing for the presence of blood, protein, ketones and other analytes is usually undertaken with reagent strips, the results of which are indicative of further laboratory investigation (Cook 1996, Quick Reference Guide 8 1999, Deville et al 2004).

Urine samples should be dispatched to the laboratory as soon as possible, or after no more than 2 hours if kept at room temperature or up to 24 hours if kept at 4°C, to avoid multiplication of organisms and misleading results (Griffiths 1995, Higgins 1995a, Prodigy 2002).

Some laboratories request the specimen to be put into a sterile specimen bottle containing boric acid which inhibits multiplication of most bacteria. However, the growth of some bacteria such as *Enterococcus faecalis* is inhibited by boric acid and therefore it is not always used.

Where laboratory access is limited or rapid testing is required, a commercial dip slide, which consists of a plastic tongue coated with suitable culture medium, can be dipped into the urine immediately after collection, a colour change noted and results obtained in 2 minutes. It tests for leucocyte esterase and nitrites, two indicators of infection. However, these are not 100% accurate and some organisms such as enterococci do not produce nitrites. Enterococci may therefore be missed where there is a real possibility of infection, such as in children with complex renal problems (Griffiths & Woodward 1993). It is also possible that, as the production of nitrites takes at least 4 hours, a young, non-toileting child's urine may be negative to nitrites on urinalysis but positive with later culture (Poole 2002).

Urine collection from disposable nappies for microscopy, culture and biochemical analysis has been described (Ahmed et al 1991, Vernon 1995). According to Poole (2002), this procedure is extremely difficult with modern nappies, due to the level of absorbency, and should be used with caution.

Normal social hygiene such as washing the genitalia with soap and water and drying thoroughly is considered sufficient to minimise contamination from the skin prior to collection of the specimen. Assess the clinical and psychosocial needs of the child as to whether cleaning the genitalia is necessary. The nurse must be sensitive to the cultural issues surrounding touching intimate parts of the body. With sufficient procedural knowledge the child's parents may be able to assist in urine collection.

Midstream specimen

The rationale of a midstream collection is that the first urine, which contains most of the contaminating bacteria from the periurethral area, is omitted, thereby reducing the contamination rate. This is the most reliable non-invasive urine specimen collection method but may not be possible in the very young or uncooperative child. In the female, encourage separation of the labia to prevent perianal contamination whilst passing urine. In the male encourage retraction of the prepuce, if appropriate.

- The first part of the urine stream is passed into the toilet to exclude meatal contamination.
- The middle part of the urine stream is collected into a clean container.
- The remaining urine is passed into the toilet.
- Pour the urine into a sterile container.
- For viral investigation pour the urine into viral transport medium.

Clean-catch, pad or bag specimen

The use of urine pads for collection of urine samples for microbiological analysis was introduced in the mid 1990s and has gained popularity given that the child's comfort is enhanced and that it is possible to extract an appropriate amount of urine without difficulty (Vernon 1995). Given its ease of use, it is possible for parents to collect specimens. However, caution has been raised with regard to the filtering effect of the pad fibres and the high contamination rates of up to 68% (Poole 2002).

Bag samples are equally unhelpful (Al-Orifi et al 2000), whereas clean-catch samples are least likely to need repeating, with several studies reporting low contamination rates for the clean-catch method (MacFarlane et al 1999, Ramage et al 1999, Poole 2002).

1. Select the correct size of sterile urine bag to avoid leakage or contamination with faeces.
2. Remove the protective seal:
   – for the female, place the bag over the vulva, starting from the perineum and working upwards, sticking the bag to the skin
   – for the male, place the bag over the penis.
3. Observe the bag frequently until urine is passed, to avoid leakage.
4. Remove the bag and pour the urine into a sterile container.
5. For viral investigation pour the urine into viral transport medium.
6. Wash the genitalia after the procedure to prevent soreness of the skin (see comments on clinical, psychosocial and cultural issues, above).

Catheter specimen

This is collected from the self-sealing bung of the urinary drainage tubing in a child who is already catheterised. Do not disconnect the closed drainage system as infection may be introduced, nor take the sample from the urinary drainage bag as the specimen may be contaminated.

- Using an aseptic technique, clean the bung with an alcohol swab and allow to dry.
- Using a sterile syringe and needle, insert the needle into the bung at an angle of 45 degrees. This will minimise penetration of the wall of the tubing and subsequent needlestick injury.
- Gently withdraw the urine into the syringe.
- Remove the needle and syringe, wipe the area with the alcohol swab and allow to dry. The rubber bung will self-seal.
- Place the urine in a sterile container.

- Discard the needle and syringe into a sharps container.

Obtaining urine from a Mitrofanoff stoma

The specimen should be obtained by a nurse who is familiar with the Mitrofanoff operation and the specific anatomy of the area on the child.

- The specimen should ideally be taken in conjunction with normal bladder emptying.
- A new sterile catheter of the child's normal catheter size should be used.
- Clean the stoma with soap and water and dry.
- Gently insert the lubricated sterile catheter into the stoma and collect the urine into a sterile container. A water-soluble lubricant should be used.
- Ensure that the bladder is completely empty before withdrawing the catheter.
- Wipe the area dry with a tissue.

Vaginal swab

The taking of this specimen in children should be avoided where possible because of its invasive nature. Also, because of potential legal implications (why the procedure is necessary), it is usually carried out by an appropriately trained health professional or police surgeon.

- In the case of suspected or actual sexual abuse do not clean the area. Identification of semen or sexually transmitted diseases may be required for evidence.
- Expose the vaginal area and part the labia.
- Gently insert a cotton wool swab into the outer entrance of the vagina. Care must be taken not to tear the hymen, if intact.
- Place the swab into transport medium.
- For suspected *Chlamydia* infection:
  – Obtain special transport medium
  – Use a pernasal swab and gently rotate the swab in the vaginal orifice
  – Place in transport medium.

Blood samples

Venepuncture or capillary blood sampling may be performed by a nurse who is trained in the procedure. As there are many haematological (Higgins 1995b, 1997), biochemical (Higgins 1996), immunological and microbiological blood tests, the nurse should check local protocols as to the appropriate laboratory containers required for specific tests and the amount of blood required. Protective clothing such as gloves, aprons and facial protection as appropriate should be used along with an aseptic technique (Jackson 1997, Campbell et al 1999) (see also Control of Infecton, p. 21, Aseptic Non-touch Technique, p. 75, Venepuncture and Cannulation, p. 433).

Blood culture

Isolation of a causative organism is enhanced by careful collection of the blood, using a sterile technique to avoid skin contamination (Higgins 1995c, Campbell et al 1999). Sterile gloves should be used. If possible, avoid palpating the vein after cleansing the skin. The specimen should preferably be taken during pyrexial episodes as the organism may be present in greater numbers.

- Use blood culture bottles according to local policy.
- The skin must be decontaminated with an alcohol-based antiseptic agent and allowed to dry.
- After withdrawing the blood, insert the blood into the container with a new sterile needle as there is a risk of contamination of skin organisms on the needle used to withdraw the blood.
- Place as much blood as possible (up to 3–5 ml) in the bottles.
- Inoculation of the blood into the blood culture bottles should be performed first before inserting blood into other bottles as many of these other bottles are not sterile and accidental contamination may occur.
- In children in whom line sepsis is suspected, blood for culture may be taken from a peripheral vein stab and also from the appropriate intravascular lines to enable identification of colonisation of the line. In cases of suspected bacterial endocarditis, more than one blood culture (three where

possible) should be taken to ensure isolation of organisms which may be low in number.
- Blood culture bottles should be placed into an incubator at 37°C to enhance growth of the organism.

Analysis of antibiotic levels

The relationship between drug dose, drug concentration in biological fluid and the individual child's metabolic process must be understood for interpreting results. The results may be affected by the route of administration, the age of the child and the disease process, such as liver and renal disease. Analysis involves testing levels in blood serum in direct relationship to drug administration.

- For intravenous antibiotic bolus administration, the first blood sample (trough) is taken just before the dose is given. The second sample (peak) is taken 30–60 minutes after the dose is given. The time may vary according to local policy and the drug given.
- Record on the laboratory form the drug, the dose and the mode of administration, the time the drug is given and whether the sample is a peak or trough level.
- Levels of antibiotics given other than intravenously must be discussed locally with the microbiologist because interpretation of the results will differ for drugs given by other routes.
- Blood for antibiotic assay must not be taken through the same catheter which has been used to give the antibiotic at any time. Antibiotics bind to plastic and the drug may release intermittently, giving false results. The same principle applies for some other drugs such as glucose.

Vesicular fluid for electron microscopy

Explain to the child that the procedure is usually pain-free as the needle only penetrates the vesicle not the skin.

Virus particles can be seen under electron microscopy and, combined with the clinical presentation, may aid rapid diagnosis. The vesicular fluid should also be cultured in order to confirm the clinical diagnosis such as varicella-zoster (chickenpox or shingles) or herpes simplex.

- Obtain a glass slide with a marked area for the specimen, a slide holder, sterile syringe and needle, sterile swab and viral transport medium.
- Pierce the top of the vesicle with a sterile needle and, if there is sufficient fluid, draw up the exudate into a syringe. Keep the needle flush to the skin to prevent accidental stabbing if the child moves. Remove the needle and seal the end of the syringe with a sterile cap. Dispose of the needle in a sharps bin.
- If there is minimal fluid, place the marked area of the glass slide over the vesicular fluid to allow the fluid to attach to the slide. Let it dry.
- Place the syringe in a safe container or place the glass slide in a slide holder.
- Dip the sterile swab into the transport medium then rotate it gently over the vesicle fluid on the skin. Place the swab into the transport medium.
- Place a sterile dressing over the vesicle until dry.

Fungal samples of hair, nail and skin

Special containers may be obtained locally from the microbiology department.

- Samples of infected hair should be removed by plucking the hair with forceps or gloves. The root of the hair is infected, not the shaft.
- Samples of the whole thickness of the nail or deep scrapings should be obtained (Smoker 1999).
- The skin should be cleaned with an alcohol swab. Epidermal scales scraped from the active edge of a lesion or the roof of any vesicle should be obtained.

Gastric washings

Swallowed sputum containing tubercle bacilli may be obtained through gastric washings. Children generally do not produce sufficient sputum, therefore gastric washings are obtained for laboratory analysis to aid diagnosis of pulmonary *Mycobacterium tuberculosis*. If alcohol–acid-fast bacilli are seen under the microscope,

further tests are performed to aid the provisional diagnosis. Culture of the organism may take between 6–12 weeks to confirm diagnosis. Three consecutive early-morning specimens should be obtained. There are usually only small numbers of organisms present so as much material as possible should be obtained. As alcohol–acid-fast bacilli are often found in tap water, sterile water must be used.

- Fast the child for at least 6 hours overnight.
- Pass a nasogastric tube (see Enteral Feeding, p. 173).
- Aspirate the stomach contents and place in a sterile container.
- Instil at least 30 ml of sterile water down the tube to obtain as much stomach content as possible.
- Aspirate the contents and place in the same container.
- Remove the tube, if appropriate.

Biopsy material

Specimens such as skin, muscle, kidney, liver, jejunal tissue or brain biopsies are generally obtained by medical staff under either general or local anaesthetic according to the site. A sterile technique is required for all these procedures. All biopsy specimens must be discussed with the relevant laboratory personnel in order that:

- the most appropriate specimen and laboratory tests are undertaken to aid diagnosis; selection of tests may be necessary if the specimen is small
- a fixative such as formalin is not used for microbiological investigation.

Cerebrospinal fluid

Cerebrospinal fluid (CSF) is commonly obtained via a lumbar puncture performed by medical staff (see Lumbar Puncture, p. 233). A sterile technique is required as there is a risk of introducing infection, causing meningitis. Specimens of CSF should be dispatched to the laboratory immediately. Do not store the specimen in a refrigerator as this causes the cells to lyse and deteriorate rapidly, thus giving rise to false results.

COMMUNITY PERSPECTIVE

The types of specimen that can be taken in the home are limited. These may include routine specimens of:

- blood, urine and stools
- swabs from wounds, skin, throat, eyes, etc.

Consideration must be given to the transportation of such specimens to the laboratory. It would not be appropriate for specimens to be carried around in a hot car for several hours, so visits will need to be planned. It is worth considering the use of a cool bag.

Some specimens, e.g. stool and urine samples, can be taken to the GP's surgery, from where they are collected and taken to the local hospital. This may help the family and the CCN by diminishing the need for hospital visits.

References

Advisory Committee on Dangerous Pathogens (ACDP) 1996 Management and control of viral haemorrhagic fevers. HMSO, London

Advisory Committee on Dangerous Pathogens (ACDP) 2003 Infection at work: controlling the risks. A guide for employers and the self employed on identifying, assessing and controlling the risks of infection in the workplace. TSO, London

Ahmed T, Vickers D, Campbell S, Coultard M G, Pedler S 1991 Urine collection from disposable nappies. Lancet 338: 674–676

Al-Orifi F, McGillivray D, Tange S, Kramer M 2000 Urine culture from bag specimens in young children: are the risks too high? Journal of Pediatrics 137(2): 221–226

Baillie L 2001 Developing practical nursing skills. Arnold, London

Camm J 2004 What does it take to ensure effective hand decontamination by nurses? Professional Nurse 19(12): 26–28

Campbell H, Carrington M, Limber C 1999 A practical guide to venepuncture and management of complications. British Journal of Nursing 8(7): 426–431

Cook R 1996 Urinalysis: ensuring accurate urine testing. Continuing Education Article 343. Nursing Standard 10(46): 49–52

COSHH 1999 The control of substances hazardous to health regulations: code of practice. TSO, London

Department of Health 1990 Spills of urine: potential risk of misuse of chlorine-releasing disinfecting agents. Safety Action Bulletin SAB (90)41. DoH, London

Department of Health 1998 Guidance for clinical healthcare workers: protection against infection with blood-borne viruses: Recommendations of the Expert Advisory Group on AIDS and the Advisory Group on Hepatitis. Department of Health, Wetherby, UK

Department of Health 2003 Winning ways: working together to reduce healthcare associated infection in England. Report from the Chief Medical Officer. DoH, London

Deville W, Yzermans J C, van Duijn N P, Bezemec D, van der Windt, Bouter L M 2004. The urine dipstick test to rule out infections. A meta-analysis of the accuracy. BMC Urology 4:4

Gilchrist B 2000 Taking a wound swab. Nursing Times 96(4): 2

Gould D 2001 Clean surgical wounds: prevention of infection. Nursing Standard 15(49): 45–52, 54, 56

Griffiths C 1995 Microbiological examination in urinary tract infection. Nursing Times 91(11): 33–35

Griffiths D M, Woodward M N 1993 Use of dipsticks for routine analysis of urine from children with acute abdominal pain. British Medical Journal 306: 1512–1513

Hampton S 2004 Wound colonization explained. Nurse2Nurse 4(4): 34–36

Health and Safety Executive 1999 Safe Transport of Dangerous Goods Act 1999. TSO, London

Health and Safety Executive 2002 The control of substances hazardous to health regulations (COSHH) 1999: code of practice. TSO, London

Health Protection Agency 2004 Online. Available: www.hpa.org.uk

Higgins C 1995a Microbiological examination of urine in urinary tract infection. Nursing Times 91(11): 33–35

Higgins C 1995b Full blood count (RBC, Hb, PCV, MCV, MCH and reticulocytes). Nursing Times 91(7): 38–40

Higgins C 1995c Microbiological examination of blood for septicaemia. Nursing Times 91(16): 34–35

Higgins C 1996 Laboratory measurement of sodium and potassium. Nursing Times 92(12): 40–42

Higgins C 1997 Erythrocyte sedimentation test as an aid to diagnosis. Nursing Times 93(6): 60–61

Hilton S, Baker F 2003 Transmission of infection. Professional Nurse 18(9): Card insert 2

Infection Control Nurses Association 1997 Guidelines for hand hygiene. ICNA, Edinburgh

Jackson A 1997 Performing peripheral intravenous cannulation. Professional Nurse 13(1): 21–25

MacFarlane P, Houghton C, Hughes C 1999 Pad urine collection for early childhood urinary-tract infection. Lancet 354(9178): 571

May D 2000 Infection control. Nursing Standard 14(28): 51–59

Nursing and Midwifery Council (NMC) 2002 Code of professional conduct. NMC, London

Poole C 2002 Diagnosis and management of urinary tract infection in children. Nursing Standard 16(38): 47–55

Prodigy Guidance 2004 Urinary tract infection – children. Online. Available: www.prodigy.nhs.uk/guidance.asp?gt=uti%20-%20children#Investigations

Quick Reference Guide 8 1999 Urine testing. Nursing Standard 13(50)

Ramage I, Chapman J, Hollman A, Elabassi M, McColl J, Beattie T 1999 Accuracy of clean catch urine collection in infancy. Journal of Pediatrics 135(6): 765–767

Royal College of Nursing 2004 Working well initiative. Good practice in infection control: guidance for nursing staff. RCN, London

Royal College of Paediatrics and Child Health 2000 Guidelines for the ethical conduct of medical research involving children. Archives of Diseases in Childhood 82(2): 177–182

Royal Liverpool & Broadgreen University Hospitals 2004 Joint Pathology Services. Online. Available: www.rlbuht.nhs.uk/jps/mibspcol.htm

Smoker A 1999 Fungal infections. Nursing Standard 13(17): 48–56; 13(19): 43–47

Vernon S 1995 Urine collection from infants: a reliable method. Paediatric Nursing 7(6): 26–27

Practice **30**

Stoma care

Stella Snell

Introduction

The word 'stoma' comes from the Greek word for mouth or opening.

Stoma formation in childhood is generally a temporary measure in the surgical correction of congenital abnormalities. Occasionally a stoma may be permanent. This may be due to trauma, tumour or inflammatory bowel disease. Conditions that may require stoma formation include:

- imperforate anus
- Hirschsprung's disease
- necrotising enterocolitis
- cloacal exstrophy
- ulcerative colitis
- familial polyposis coli
- bladder tumour
- Crohn's disease
- Trauma.

There are three main types of diverting/output stoma; these may be temporary or permanent and act as an outlet for elimination of body waste (Williams 2004).

- Ileostomy: a portion of the ileum is brought out through the abdominal wall and is normally sited in the right iliac fossa.
- Colostomy: a portion of the colon is brought through the abdominal wall and is normally sited in the left iliac fossa. (In children, the transverse colon, descending colon or sigmoid may be used.)
- Urinary diversion:
  - vesicostomy: the neck of the bladder is brought through the abdominal wall low down in the pelvis
  - ureterostomy: one or two of the ureters can be brought out to the abdominal wall, either side by side or at either side of the abdomen
  - ileal conduit: a small segment of the ileum is isolated to act as a reservoir and the ureters implanted into it. This stoma can be sited in the left or right iliac fossa.

There are two main types of continent stoma – a non-refluxing catheterisable channel (Malone et al 1990) – neither of which requires a pouch collection system.

- Antegrade continence enema (ACE): the appendix or portion of ileum is tunnelled out through the abdominal wall, usually in the right iliac fossa, to form a continent catheterisable channel which, when flushed with an enema and saline, irrigates the colon. Faeces are passed via the anus.
- Mitrofanoff: the appendix, a portion of ileum or ureter is used and channelled from the bladder through the abdominal wall. A Mitrofanoff can be sited in the left or right iliac fossa or through the umbilicus, forming a continent catheterisable channel to give access for intermittent bladder drainage.

A stoma nurse, if employed in a hospital where surgery is performed, should be involved in the care of all children requiring stoma surgery (NHS Modernisation Agency 2003). However, this may not be a specialist paediatric stoma nurse. If there is no stoma nurse within the hospital, attempts must be made to refer the child and family to a stoma nurse within the community. Most areas of the UK have stoma nursing support. *The Children's National Service Framework* (DoH 2003) is working towards ensuring that everyone gets the same standard of care, irrespective of where they live. Practice should be evidence based and care should be given by appropriately trained staff.

Learning outcomes

By the end of this section you should be able to:

- identify and describe different types of stoma
- be aware of any dietary implications following stoma formation
- recognise potential problems with stomas
- change a stoma appliance efficiently and effectively
- be aware of how to dispose of used appliances
- help maintain a healthy stoma and peristomal skin integrity
- identify recurring or continuing problems with management of the stoma

- describe how families obtain stoma appliances in the community.

Rationale

Children undergoing stoma surgery and the child and their families will need to be taught how to care for a stoma and be aware of the implications of stoma surgery. Support is needed throughout what can at times be a traumatic experience. The specialist stoma nurse, play therapist and clinical psychologist should all be involved in the care of the child and their family.

Factors to note

Neonates and babies

- After surgery on the small intestine, a large number of babies will have a temporary intolerance to lactose. Ileostomy output is normally loose; however, if lactose intolerance occurs the effluent will be extremely loose/watery, greater in volume and test positive to sugar. This increases the risk of dehydration and failure to thrive. Many will initially be fed by total parenteral nutrition (TPN). Enteral feeding is slowly introduced using a hydrolysed formula, e.g. Pregestimil or Pepti-Junior. These milks are easier to absorb as the shortened gut often lacks some enzymes and bile salts (Shaw & Lawson 2001).

- If an infant is taking a special formula milk, the parents should follow dietetic advice when weaning. It is usual for infants to take a milk-free diet until the ileostomy is closed. Babies with colostomies who take regular formula milks can have a normal weaning diet.

- Sodium depletion can be a common problem for babies and children with ileostomies. The ileum is important in absorption of fluid and electrolytes. Losses can be high, especially in sodium (Shaw & Lawson 2001).

- Dehydration can occur very quickly: if the stools are very loose and an adequate oral intake cannot be taken, especially in the case of gastroenteritis, intravenous therapy will be needed (Shaw & Lawson 2001).

Children with special needs

Siting the position of a stoma in the child who uses a wheelchair needs careful consideration. If any appliances such as callipers or a spinal brace are worn, they should be put on before the siting procedure. The stoma needs to be sited where independence can be maintained.

Children and adolescents

● Privacy should be maintained at all times.

● Older children with ileostomies should be encouraged to take plenty of fluids in hot weather to avoid dehydration.

● Young people and their parents need to be aware of the problems that can be caused by some foods. Examples include popcorn or dried foods which, if eaten in large amounts, can swell in the gastrointestinal tract and cause small bowel obstruction; some foods can produce more odorous stools, e.g. onions, fish, eggs and cheese. Flatus can be increased by beans, greens, onions and fizzy drinks. However, it must be remembered that children need a healthy balanced diet and that nutrient and energy needs are high in relation to their body size compared to adults (Food Standards Agency 2002).

● Children with urinary diversions may benefit from eating foods with a high vitamin C content, which helps to keep urine acid. By doing this and drinking plenty of fluids, especially in hot weather, urine is prevented from becoming concentrated. For those who experience repeated urinary tract infections, drinking cranberry juice may be of benefit (Griffiths 2003).

● Older children may wish to manage their colostomy by means other than a pouch, e.g. colostomy irrigation. This is done by the instillation of warmed water or saline through the stoma via a cone and irrigation equipment. After evacuation of the bowel, a small stoma cap (Fig. 30.1) can then be used instead of a pouch. This system can be used to regulate the colostomy function; however, it is time consuming – up to 1 hour – and may need performing daily (Williams

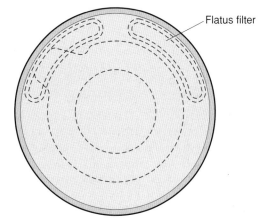

Figure 30.1   Stoma cap

2004). A colostomy plug is again used to gain control over stoma function. This is a soft foam plug, gently inserted into the stoma, often used in association with irrigation (Williams 2004). A stoma nurse must first assess the patient, as not all patients are suitable for these procedures.

● Some children and parents may need extra psychological support in coming to terms with an altered body image. Play therapist and psychologist input can be invaluable and must be considered. All families need support and information to help them cope with the illness (DoH 2003).

Guidelines

The carers of the child should be taught all aspects of stoma care prior to discharge into the community. Support and information should be given to help families plan for getting on with life after leaving hospital (DoH 2003).

TO CHANGE A BAG

Equipment

● Disposable gloves for hospital staff (parents may choose not to wear gloves as they would not normally do so when changing their child's nappy; however, they must be taught correct handwashing procedure to reduce infection)
● Bowl of warm water

- Gauze or dry wipes
- Bag to dispose of used pouch and cleaning materials
- Scissors
- Template – a pattern of the stoma size, usually the adhesive release paper of the previously applied pouch
- Adhesive remover (alcohol free).

Before changing the pouch make sure you have everything to hand. If the stoma is longstanding, the new pouch can be prepared beforehand.

Stoma pouches

There are many different pouches produced by a number of manufacturers. However, there are basically two designs: a one-piece pouch has an adhesive flange with a pouch bonded onto it (Fig. 30.2a), and a two-piece pouch has an adhesive base plate or flange and a separate pouch that attaches to the flange (Fig. 30.2b). Both types can be either closed, for formed stool (Fig. 30.3) or open ended (drainable) for loose stool (see Fig. 30.2) or with a tap for drainage of urine (Fig. 30.4). In the early postoperative period it is advisable to use a transparent drainable pouch. This ensures that the stoma can be observed easily and can be drained rather than changed frequently.

Method

1. Position the child – babies lying down, older children lying or standing.

2. If a drainable or pouch with a tap is worn, empty contents before removing. In the immediate postoperative period the stoma output may require measuring, therefore

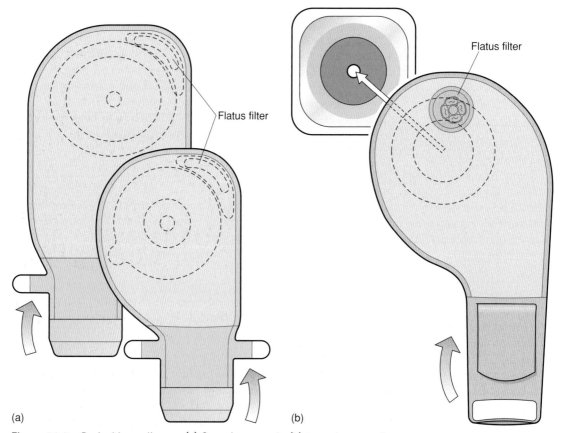

Figure 30.2 Drainable appliances. (a) One-piece pouch; (b) two-piece pouch

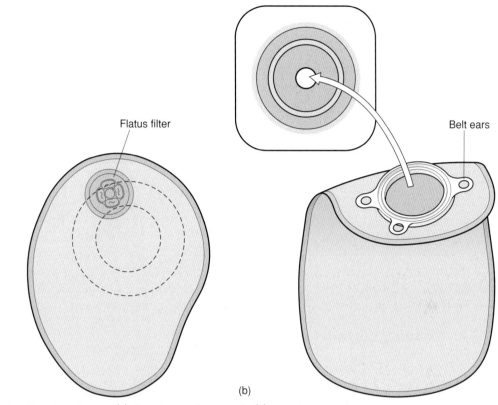

Figure 30.3   Closed appliances. (a) Closed one-piece pouch; (b) two-piece pouch

the pouch will be emptied into a measuring jug, the amount recorded on the appropriate chart and then emptied into a toilet. Before discharge home, children and their carers will need to be taught how to empty the pouch directly into the toilet.

3. Remove the old pouch by carefully peeling it off from top to bottom with one hand whilst supporting the skin with the other. Adhesive remover (non-alcoholic) will make this easier. The used pouch can then be put into a nappy sack or disposal bag.

4. Clean the peristomal skin with warm water and gauze. If some residue of paste or pouch adhesive is left on the skin, remove this first with a dry piece of gauze or adhesive remover. Do not use cotton wool as this can deposit strands that will stick to the stoma and may cause problems with pouch adhesion. Once clean, dry the peristomal skin with dry gauze or a wipe. Prepare the new pouch if not already done. The aperture should be cut to fit snugly around the stoma with no peristomal skin exposed. Put on the new pouch. If a one-piece is being used, fold the adhesive in half, placing the pouch on the underside of the stoma first, then flip the adhesive over the stoma and secure all round. If a two-piece appliance is being used, secure the base plate and then attach the pouch.

5. If a drainable pouch is being used, ensure that the clip/integral closure is secured correctly at the bottom of the pouch. If a tap pouch is used, ensure that the tap is closed.

6. Used pouches should never be put down the toilet (unless they are biodegradable, of which there are some types available). Pouches should be emptied into the toilet, then wrapped in newspaper or placed in a

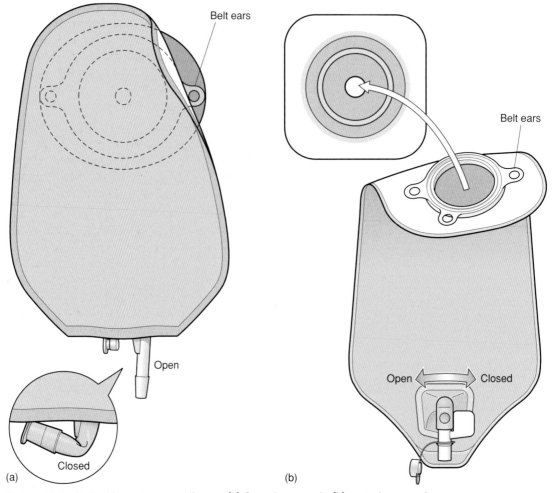

Figure 30.4 Drainable urostomy appliances. (a) One-piece pouch; (b) two-piece pouch

disposal bag designed for this purpose (most ostomy companies provide these free of charge) and then placed in a dustbin or clinical wastebin in hospital. Some local authorities view this as clinical waste and provide a yellow bag collection service (Swan 2001).

Observations and complications

- In the immediate postoperative period the stoma should be observed to determine if there is a good blood supply. To aid easier observation of the stoma, a clear pouch should initially be applied, without a filter;

medical staff will want to know when bowel sounds are returning – any wind passed will inflate the pouch.

- The normal colour of a healthy stoma is pink or red. Any signs of the stoma changing colour to a dusky purple must be reported to medical staff immediately as the blood supply to the stoma could be compromised, risking necrosis (Collett 2002). Observe also for haemorrhage around the stoma and/or into the pouch and excessive oedema.

- When first formed, the stoma will be oedematous due to handling of the bowel (Collett 2002) but over a period of approximately

6 weeks the stoma will shrink in size. It is important to check the size before fitting a new pouch to ensure that no peristomal skin will be exposed. The size of the stoma can be checked by using a template.

- Check for any peristomal skin soreness; this can be caused by stoma effluent being in contact with the skin as a result of incorrect fitting of the pouch or the pouch adhesive not being cut accurately.

- There are specific stoma barrier preparations available to protect the skin around the stoma. They come in creams, pastes, powders, sprays, etc. All have instructions for use and these should be studied carefully. Remember that babies have sensitive skin and non-alcohol-based preparations should be used.

- Surface bleeding can happen if the cleaning routine is too vigorous, the stoma is knocked or the child scratches it. Unless the bleeding is prolonged it should cause no alarm. If the bleeding comes from inside the stoma it should be reported to a doctor.

- It is not uncommon in children for the stoma to prolapse. This is when the bowel intussuscepts (telescopes) out of the skin opening, becoming longer (Burch 2004). This may occur after a period of crying, coughing or strenuous exercise. Generally the stoma will settle back at rest. If it does not and becomes tense or darker in colour, medical advice should be sought.

- If the stoma becomes retracted, problems may arise with pouch leakage. This can be remedied in some cases by using a pouch with a convex flange. If not, the stoma may need refashioning.

- Some children may experience rectal discharge. Usually it is only mucus which continues to be produced in the rectal stump. If the child cannot pass it into the toilet or nappy, or it becomes copious in amount, a gentle rectal washout may be required, which should be carried out by an experienced practitioner.

- Children with stomas can get gastroenteritis like any other child. If a child's stoma output becomes loose or watery they should be encouraged to drink plenty of fluids and an electrolyte replacement drink. Dehydration can occur very quickly, especially in the child with an ileostomy.

- Any complaints of cramp from children with ileostomy should be noted and urinary sodium levels checked; if low, children should be encouraged to take more salt in their diet, or oral supplements can be given.

- Children with urinary diversions can be susceptible to urinary infection due to a shortened urinary tract system (Burch 2004). If the urine smells or is cloudy and the child is unwell, a specimen of urine should be examined. It is important for a child with a urinary stoma to drink plenty of fluids. Drinking cranberry juice may help to prevent urinary tract infections although it is not effective against all organisms. Evidence is still inconclusive as to the effectiveness of cranberry juice as a treatment for urinary tract infection (Griffiths 2003).

ON DISCHARGE

On discharge the family need to be given 1–2 weeks' supply of the type of pouch the child is using. Order numbers along with the manufacturer's name should be written down and given to the parents. This is to ensure that the GP knows which product to prescribe (DoH 2003). Once the prescription is collected the family can obtain the appliances from a local chemist or from a dispensing service which will offer home delivery. One of the benefits of this service is that if a template is sent with the prescription the pouches will be cut to size; they also dispense dry wipes and nappy/disposal sacks free of charge. However, parents must ensure that any medication is on a separate prescription, as these cannot be supplied by home delivery services.

Children up to the age of 16 are exempt from prescription charges; patients aged between 16 and 60 are exempt if they have a permanent stoma. The exemption certificate must be signed by a doctor or stoma care nurse.

The child may also be eligible for disability living allowance for personal care; the hospital social worker will be able to advise on this.

The child should be referred to a stoma care nurse who covers their community area, as well as a children's community nurse and the health visitor (if appropriate), thus ensuring that the team give care in a holistic manner (Black 2000).

COMMUNITY PERSPECTIVE

It is good practice to refer babies and children with newly formed stomas to a CCN before discharge from hospital. The CCN, in conjunction with the stoma nurse, can support the family during the period of adaptation to coping with a stoma and the child's underlying condition, as few areas have access to a paediatric stoma care nurse. The CCN will also liaise and coordinate care between other agencies, such as the health visitor, GP, referring hospital and school nurse, and also help to develop close links with education staff, giving reassurance that, with appropriate staff training, inclusion will proceed smoothly (Rogers 2003). The CCN should ensure that appropriate facilities are in place at the school, e.g. the child has access to an adapted or staff toilet to ensure privacy. The young child or one with dexterity or visual problems will also need the support of an assistant whilst at school. The adolescent may be concerned about changing facilities; again the CCN can support the family in organising this.

Do and do not

- Do refer to a stoma care nurse any child for whom stoma surgery is planned or has taken place.
- Do refer to a children's community nurse prior to discharge.
- Do keep a template of the size of the stoma. This will make preparing new pouches easier. The template will need to be altered as the stoma shrinks postoperatively.

- Do not use cotton wool to clean the stoma. It deposits strands, can hinder pouch application and will be more time consuming.
- Do not cut the pouch adhesive bigger than the stoma as the peristomal skin will become sore.
- Do not cut the pouch adhesive smaller than the stoma as the pouch will leak.
- Do not use general barrier creams on sore peristomal skin; use only preparations specific for this use, otherwise the pouch may leak.

References

Black P 2000 Holistic stoma care. Baillière Tindall, Edinburgh

Breckman B 2005 Stoma care and rehabilitation. Churchill Livingstone, Edinburgh

Burch J 2004 The management and care of people with stoma complications. British Journal of Nursing 13(6): 307–318

Collett K 2002 Practical aspects of stoma management. Nursing Standard 17(8): 45–52, 54–55

Department of Health 2003 The children's national service framework. TSO, London

Food Standards Agency 2002 Feeding your growing child. Food Standards Agency Publications, London

Griffiths P 2003 The role of cranberry juice in the treatment of urinary tract infections. British Journal of Community Nursing 8(12): 557–561

Malone P S, Ransley P G, Kiely E M 1990 Preliminary report: the antegrade continence enema. Lancet 336: 1217–1218

NHS Modernisation Agency 2003 Essence of care. DoH, London

Rogers J 2003 Successful inclusion of a child with a stoma in mainstream schooling. British Journal of Nursing 12(10): 590–599

Shaw V, Lawson M 2001 Clinical paediatric dietetics, 2nd edn. Blackwell Science, Oxford

Swan E 2001 Waste disposal for the ostomate in the community. Nursing Times Plus 97(40): 51–52

Williams J 2004 A stoma for incontinence. In: Norton C, Chelvanayagam S (eds) Bowel continence nursing. Beaconsfield, Oxford, p 165–173

Further Reading

Kean Y 2002 Paediatric stomas and why they are formed. Nurse2Nurse 3(1): 24–26

Metcalf C 2001 Stoma care 1(b): cutting a template. Nursing Times 97(13): 43–44

Rogers J 2004 Paediatric stoma care: advice for carers, 2nd edn. Braun Medical, Sheffield, UK

Support Groups

Contact a Family – *offers advice, information and support for specific conditions and rare disorders*

Family Freephone Helpline: 0808 808 3555
www.cafamily.org.uk

National Advisory Service for Parents of Children with a Stoma (NASPCS)
John Malcolm (Chairman) 51 Anderson Drive, Valley Park View, Darvel, Ayshire KA17 0DE. Tel: 01560 322024
Email: john@stoma.freeserve.co.uk

Practice **31**

Suctioning

Michaela Dixon

Introduction and rationale

Normally, children and babies will keep their airway clear by coughing, sneezing, blowing their noses and by the protective mechanism of the gag reflex. Suction is an invasive procedure, and as such may be traumatic to both the child and their family; it should therefore be used with care after thorough assessment where less invasive treatments are ineffective. The use of careful positioning can also help maintain a patent airway.

Although suction is most often used in intensive care, theatres and emergency departments, it is important for all healthcare workers to understand the principles and techniques, as it forms a vital component of resuscitation and of essential care for both the acutely ill child as well as the child with complex ongoing health needs.

Suction may be performed by the nurse, physiotherapist, doctor or parent/caregiver. For this reason it is important that there are established evidence-based guidelines on an individual unit basis.

Learning outcomes

By the end of this section you should be able to demonstrate that you understand:

- the indications and contraindications for suctioning
- the common techniques used for suctioning
- the problems associated with suctioning.

Factors to note

Infants and toddlers do not always have the necessary ability to clear their airway, due to immaturity of the respiratory system and its functions. Although the respiratory system of a child is mature and fully functional by the age of 8 years, there is a group of children who will have poor respiratory function due to underlying pathology.

Infants are more prone to airway compromise when they have an upper or lower airway infection causing overproduction of mucus and secretions, due to the magnified effect of oedema on their airway when compared to the adult airway (APLS 2001). It can be helpful to give suction prior to a feed in infants.

There are some childhood conditions which can cause overproduction of mucus, or a difficulty in combining swallowing and breathing. Examples include cystic fibrosis, tracheo-oesophageal fistulae prior to surgical repair, some laryngeal disorders and tracheostomy.

After some types of surgery the child may bleed postoperatively, increasing the potential for airway compromise (e.g. after tonsillectomy). These children may require gentle suctioning to remove excessive secretions and prevent airway obstruction.

Some children may not have learnt the coordination skills required to keep their airways clear, whereas others may have lost their previously acquired skills due to illness and/or injury. These children may be unable to cough and clear their airway and so may require suction to prevent airway compromise.

RESUSCITATION

If the child has stopped breathing, firstly assess whether the airway is compromised and, if so, clear it, using suction, if the obstruction is thought to be secretion related. If there is a history of inhalation of foreign object, be very cautious about the use of suction – this may push the obstruction further down into the child's airway, increasing the degree of obstruction present.

Equipment

- Suction catheters:
  - for oro/nasopharyngeal suction: select size according to age of child, size of nostril or Guedel airway, amount and type of secretions, condition of mucosa. If suctioning orally, a larger size of catheter can be used. A smaller-sized Yankauer catheter can be very effective, but should be used with care, due to its more rigid structure. There is no particular formula for calculating suction catheter sizes for oro/nasopharyngeal suction
  - for endotracheal tubes/tracheostomy tubes: the tube size of the suctioning

catheter should be approximately twice the internal diameter of the endotracheal tube. Consequently, for a size 3.5 mm tube, use a size 6 or 7 Fg suction catheter. Using a larger suction catheter would completely occlude the internal diameter of the tube and as a consequence increase the detrimental effects of suction (see below). It is also important to know the length of the endotracheal/tracheostomy tube to ensure that you only suction to an appropriate depth

- Disposable gloves (non-powdered)
- Suction tubing
- Collection device, e.g. disposable bag and container, special suction specimen container
- Wall-piped suction or portable suction machine
- Tap water/clean container
- Sterile normal saline (endotracheal suction only); see discussion below
- Emergency equipment including oxygen and Ambu bag, with appropriately sized face mask, should be available.

All emergency equipment should be checked at the beginning of every shift in accordance with local unit policy.

Indications

If the child is able to clear the secretions independently, do not use suction. Physiotherapy techniques for clearing secretions should be considered, for example percussion and postural drainage (Prasad & Hussey 1995). Discussion with physiotherapists will assist in planning effective care.

- Suction should be considered if the child's respiration is compromised by excessive secretions; this can be assessed visually or through auscultation of the child's chest, using a stethoscope.
- If the child's oxygen saturation is low, i.e. less than 92% in a child without a cyanotic heart lesion, and the respiratory rate and effort high, then breathing may be obstructed and the child may need suction. The child's colour should also be assessed,

in conjunction with heart rate and peripheral perfusion, as these may give an indication of inadequate respiratory function.

Factors to note

- Suction must never be carried out on a child in whom a diagnosis of epiglottitis is suspected. *This is a life-threatening condition* – seek urgent anaesthetic assistance and wait with the child until help has arrived in the department.
- Suction should only be undertaken following careful assessment, not as a matter of routine.
- Any child who requires suction to maintain airway patency should receive humidification to assist in loosening secretions (Prasad & Hussey 1995).
- Laboratory analysis of nasopharyngeal (NPA) or endotracheal secretions will aid in the diagnosis of respiratory infections, e.g. respiratory syncytial virus (RSV +ve) bronchiolitis.

Method

Preparation

1. Assess the need for suction as described above.
2. Explain the procedure fully to the child and family to reduce anxiety levels.
3. Check all equipment is set up correctly and functioning before commencing.
4. Preset suction to appropriate pressure – as a guide the following pressures have been identified:

Neonates: 60–80 mmHg (8–10.6 kPa)
Child: 80–100 mmHg (10.6–13.3 kPa)
Adolescent/ maximum setting of
  adult: 120 mmHg
    (16 kPa)
    (Linton 2000).

When considering nasopharyngeal suctioning, ET suctioning and tracheostomy suctioning, the evidence has shown that there is no difference in the amount of secretions removed using 100 mmHg of suction pressure when compared with secretion removal using a higher suction pressure of 200 mmHg.

There was, however, an increased risk of mucosal trauma when using higher suction pressures and most authors would recommend a maximum pressure of 120 mmHg (16 kPa) (Linton 2000).

5. Place the child in a comfortable, secure position; if necessary, ask for assistance.
6. If the child is receiving oxygen therapy, care must be taken to ensure that the supply is not interrupted to minimise the potential effects of hypoxia.
7. Put on gloves. The glove which is in contact with the suction catheter should be kept clean, and glove and catheter should be changed every time suction is performed. This will depend on local policy – some units will use one suction catheter per suction episode, whereas others will use one for each catheter pass. There is currently limited evidence to support decisions regarding frequency of use.
8. Positioning: If the child is conscious, the best position is lateral, to prevent inhalation of vomit, preferably on a parent's or carer's lap for comfort and reassurance. However, if the child is unconscious the procedure can occur in any position, either lateral or supine.

Technique

There are two main techniques for suctioning, which will be considered separately:

- oro- and nasopharyngeal suction
- suctioning of an artificial airway, e.g. endotracheal tube/tracheostomy suction.

Oro- and nasopharyngeal suction

- Gently insert the suction catheter, not yet applying suction, upwards and backwards into the child's nostril or mouth:
  - If the child has a gag reflex, the child will cough.
  - If the child does not have a gag reflex, measure the catheter from nose or mouth to the suprasternal notch to estimate length (see Fig. 31.1), then insert the catheter as above.
- Gently withdrawing the catheter, apply intermittent suction.

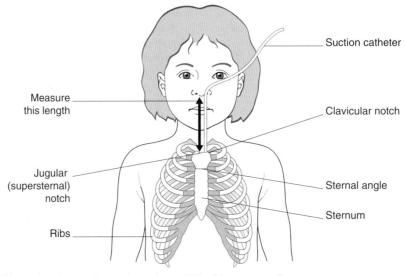

Figure 31.1 Measuring the suction catheter in a child with no gag reflex

Endotracheal suction

It is common practice in many units to instil small amounts of sterile saline, the volume of which is dependent on the size of the child. It is important to note that this is a practice that is not evidence based and about which there is considerable debate. What is important to consider is whether there is adequate humidification as opposed to volumes of sterile saline that should/should not be used when suctioning endotracheal tubes to assist in the removal of secretions. There is considerable debate in the published literature about this practice, with most of the evidence being empirical in nature and inconsistent. Most studies have involved small groups of patients and have examined other variables, e.g. hyperoxygenation prior to suctioning, in addition to the instillation of saline. Akgul and Akyolcu (2002) found a small but not statistically significant detrimental alteration in oxygen saturations and arterial blood gas levels after the instillation of saline for endotracheal tube suction. Other studies have looked at the volume of secretions removed with and without the use of saline and found no statistically significant benefit with the use of saline (Gray et al 1990, Raymond 1995). Other researchers have questioned the amount of saline that is not removed with suctioning and whether this has significant impact on the patient (Blackwood 1999).

It is suggested that, rather than routinely using saline to decrease the viscosity of secretions before suctioning of children with endotracheal tubes in situ, practitioners should concentrate on ensuring adequate airway heat and humidity, paying careful attention to the child's hydration status, and using mucolytic agents/nebulised saline as methods of maintaining the patency of the artificial airway (Blackwood 1999, Griggs 1999, Akgul & Akyolcu 2002).

Closed-system suctioning, designed so that the endotracheal tube does not need disconnection, is advantageous. It has been shown that each time a child is disconnected from the tube, hypoxia occurs. This hypoxia can be alleviated with the integral system (Fiorentini 1992).

It is recommended that the length of the catheter is pre-measured prior to commencing the procedure to avoid the risk of mucosal trauma and to reduce the incidence of right upper lobe collapse in children (Boothroyd et al 1996):

- Gently insert the catheter into the endotracheal tube, with no suction applied.
- Insert the catheter to 0.5 cm beyond the end of the endotracheal tube only; see above regarding selecting appropriate tube size.
- Apply suction and gently withdraw the catheter, interrupting the vacuum briefly every 1–2 seconds to reduce the potential for hypoxia.

Tracheostomy suction

The technique is as for endotracheal suction, but with two important differences:

- Insert the catheter to the tip of the tracheostomy tube, not beyond it (see Tracheostomy Care, p. 399).
- Suctioning a tracheostomy tube should take less time as the tube is shorter in length than an endotracheal tube.

General

- Ensure that the catheter is withdrawn within 10 seconds in the neonate and 15 seconds in a child to reduce hypoxia.
- Flush the suction tubing with tap water to clean it at the end of the procedure or between suction catheter passes if secretions are tenacious.
- Ensure that the child is left in a comfortable position, has recovered from the procedure and their condition is stable (see below).
- Dispose of waste and change equipment as per local procedures.

Observations

- Observe and record the child's colour, oxygen saturation, respiration rate and effort, and heart rate after the procedure to assess the child's response and recovery.
- Inspect the colour, viscosity and amount of secretions.

Summary of possible complications

For further reading, see Ackerman (1998), APLS (2001), Gilbert (1999), Griggs (1999), Johnson (1999), Knox (1993), Page et al (1998) and Turner & Loan (2000).

- Increased intracranial pressure, caused by raised blood pressure (see below).
- Hypoxia: during suction the child receives less oxygen than normal, especially if the procedure is prolonged and the child has pre-existing lung disease.
- Laryngospasm caused by traumatic stimulation of the larynx.
- Mucosal trauma from the same source.
- Microatelectasis, related to trauma and negative pressure.
- Pneumothorax: traumatic suction may perforate the lung.
- Discomfort/pain: described by some children as 'gagging, suffocating'.
- Overstimulation of secretions, often from too frequent suction.
- Sepsis, due to poor infection control techniques and a child who may be more susceptible to infection.
- Hypo/hypertension: caused by indirect vagal stimulation through hypoxaemia, as well as direct stimulation of the vagal nerve by the suction catheter.
- Tachycardia/bradycardia, due to direct and indirect vagal stimulation, and hypoxaemia.

COMMUNITY PERSPECTIVE

Some babies and children will be discharged home with ongoing care needs including the need for suction. There are an increasing number of children who require long-term home ventilation, have artificial airways (tracheostomies) in situ for airway protection, or who have complex medical conditions and are unable to maintain a patent airway independently. For many of these children, their parents/caregivers have primary responsibility for their day-to-day care, with support from a children's community nursing (CCN) team. It is vital that parents are, first of all,

Community Perspective continues

comfortable with the responsibility involved and, second, have received full training, prior to the child's discharge from the acute setting.

A partnership involving the child, their family and all health professionals involved is important to facilitate a smooth transition from hospital to home care. Consideration should be given to the following prior to discharge:

- Provision of both home and portable equipment in the event of mains failure
- Availability and supply of disposables, e.g. suction catheters and gloves
- Regular servicing of equipment and availability of loan equipment
- Resources available in the event of equipment failure.

Most families are likely to need ongoing support from the CCN team, although the intensity of the input required will obviously vary according to the individual family. For some children, particularly those with complex needs, an 'open door' access agreement with the appropriate hospital will be necessary.

Do and do not

- Do check the emergency equipment at the beginning of every shift as per local policy.
- Do wear gloves when carrying out this procedure.
- Do note the infant/child's colour and other vital signs and document these in the nursing records.
- Do not undertake suctioning as a matter of routine.

References

Ackerman M H 1998 Installation of normal saline before suctioning in patients with pulmonary infections: a prospective randomized controlled trial. American Journal of Critical Care 7(4): 261–266

Advanced Paediatric Life Support Group (APLS) 2001 Advanced paediatric life support: the practical approach, 3rd edn. BMJ Publishing Group, London

Akgul S, Akyolcu N 2002 Effects of normal saline on endotracheal suctioning. Journal of Clinical Nursing 11: 826–830

Blackwood B 1999 Normal saline instillation with endotracheal suctioning: primum non nocere (first do no harm). Journal of Advanced Nursing 29(4): 928–934

Boothroyd A E, Murthey B V, Darbyshire A, Petros A J 1996 Endotracheal suctioning causes right upper lobe collapse in intubated children. Acta Paediatrica 85: 1422–1425

Fiorentini A 1992 Potential hazards of tracheobronchial suctioning. Intensive and Critical Care Nursing 8: 217–226

Gilbert M 1999 Assessing the need for endotracheal suction. Paediatric Nursing 11(1): 14–17

Gray J E, MacIntyre N R, Kronenberg W G 1990 The effects of bolus normal-saline instillation in conjunction with endotracheal suctioning. Respiratory Care 35(8): 785–790

Griggs A 1999 Tracheostomy: suctioning and humidification. Emergency Nurse 6(9): 33–40

Johnson L 1999 Factors known to raise intracranial pressure and the associated implications for nursing management. Nursing in Critical Care 3: 117–120

Knox A M 1993 Performing endotracheal suction on children: a literature review and implications for nursing practice. Intensive and Critical Care Nursing 9: 48–54

Linton M 2000 Endotracheal tube suctioning. In: Sinha S K, Donn S M (eds) Manual of neonatal respiratory care. Futura, New York

Page N, Giehl M, Luke S 1998 Intubation complications in the critically ill child. AACN Clinical Issues 9(1): 25–35

Prasad S A, Hussey J 1995 Paediatric respiratory care. A guide for physiotherapists and health professionals. Chapman and Hall, London

Raymond S J 1995 Normal saline instillation before suctioning: helpful or harmful? A review of the literature. American Journal of Critical Care 4: 267–271

Turner B, Loan L 2000 Tracheobronchial trauma associated with airway management in neonates. AACN Clinical Issues 11(2): 283–299

Practice 32

Temperature control

Toby A. Mohammed

Introduction

Despite wide fluctuations in environmental temperature, through homeostatic mechanisms the human body can maintain the internal temperature at 37°C ± 1°C (Tortora & Grabowski 2005). This internal temperature is referred to as the core temperature or set point. The difference between the core temperature and that of the body surface can be as much as 0.5°C in normal circumstances (Casey 2000).

The production of heat and the promotion of heat loss are maintained by a delicate balance of physiological mechanisms. Heat loss is increased by vasodilatation and sweating, while heat production and conservation are stimulated by shivering and vasoconstriction (Casey 2000). The balance between heat production and heat loss is controlled by a group of specialised neurones located in the anterior portion of the hypothalamus.

If the blood temperature rises, these neurones fire nerve impulses more rapidly; if the temperature decreases, the opposite occurs (Tortora & Grabowski 2005). These impulses are sent to other portions of the hypothalamus, which stimulate either a temperature increase or decrease. Thus these cells serve as an internal thermostat. An increase in body temperature is one of the most common symptoms of illness in children and may be caused either by an infection or by a head injury in which the temperature control centre of the hypothalamus has been affected.

Learning outcomes

By the end of this section you should be able to:

● identify the child at risk of pyrexia
● initiate appropriate action to reduce or maintain a child's body temperature
● understand the use of antipyretic medication and environmental interventions to reduce temperature in the fevered child
● appreciate the problems of maintaining temperature in the term and preterm neonate (see Incubator Care, p. 205).

Rationale

The primary aim of reducing an ill child's temperature is to promote comfort by relieving the discomfort caused by the fever.

Factors to note

Research has indicated that fever has a therapeutic purpose (Holtzclaw 2003). Fever is caused by the raising of the set point as a result of the initial infection. The raising of the set point is thought to be stimulated by the action of protein-like substances, produced by phagocytic white blood cells, on the cells of the hypothalamus. This action causes a release of prostaglandins, which resets the set point or core temperature at a higher level. The resetting of the core temperature may induce shivering and vasoconstriction to enable the body to reach the new temperature even if the body temperature is recorded at a higher than normal level. This will occur until the new set point has been reached (Porth 1994, Tortora & Grabowski 2005).

The rise in body temperature decreases the level of free serum iron, required for bacterial/viral growth, as well as damaging the cell membranes of the microorganisms (O'Connor 2002).

Under normal conditions, body temperature fluctuates throughout the day. The temperature of a child is higher in the late afternoon and early evening.

As children have a higher metabolic rate, they tend to have higher body temperatures.

An increase in temperature caused by bacterial, or viral, infection renders the child more prone to febrile seizure (see Seizures, p. 347). This occurs in approximately 4% of children (Campbell & Glasper 1995, Johnson 1996).

Reducing the temperature of a child may not affect the course of the child's illness, but may aid in the reduction of parental/carer anxiety (Adams 1999).

In the infant, overheating has been identified as a risk factor for sudden infant death syndrome (Lynch 2004).

Infants and young children are highly susceptible to alterations and fluctuations in temperature. Their body temperature is altered not only by the environmental temperature, but also by crying, playing and emotional upset. Body proportions of infants and young children are different from those of the older child or adult, with the head of the infant or young child being larger in proportion to the rest of the body. Consequently, a greater amount of heat can be lost via the head (Wong 1997) (see Incubator Care, p. 205).

Equipment that may be required for aiding comfort for the child with a fever

- Thermometer
- Cotton sheets/blankets
- Cool fan
- Medicine cup/spoon for antipyretic medication.

Guidelines

The main reason for treating a fever is to relieve discomfort; however, it is widely recognised that clinical practitioners continue to believe that diminishing a child's temperature will alter the outcome of febrile illness (Holtzclaw 2003). In fact Casey (2000) recommends that elevations less than 38°C, in otherwise healthy children, probably should not be treated and left to run their course.

However, within clinical practice measures are routinely taken to reduce the temperature, including pharmacological and environmental intervention. It must be remembered for the reasons aforementioned that this practice does not alter the course of the illness, but relieves discomfort.

The most effective intervention is the use of antipyretic medication (O'Connor 2002).

Pharmacological intervention

- The most effective way of reducing a child's temperature is to utilise an antipyretic medication to lower the set point (O'Connor 2002), although the use of such medication in children is controversial. Paracetamol is the main drug of choice; however, more recently ibuprofen is being used for older children. Both of these medicines act by inhibiting the synthesis of the prostaglandins secreted by the hypothalamus (Casey 2000), as described previously. Casey (2000) implies that temperatures below 38°C require little intervention and may indeed reduce the length of the illness.

- There is a misconception amongst nurses and medical staff regarding the route of administration of paracetamol, with most thinking that rectal administration is a quicker way of reducing temperature (Chandler 2000, O'Connor 2002). The Royal College of Paediatrics and Child Health (1997) identified that rectal paracetamol was absorbed at a much slower rate than oral doses, with absorption being 90–120 minutes compared to 60 minutes, respectively.

- The antipyretic of choice will be given at the prescribed amount.

Environmental intervention

The use of environmental measures to reduce a child's temperature has been much debated within the literature (Kinmonth et al 1992, Harrison 1998, Blumenthal 2000). Although rarely used on its own, sponging the child with warm water, following administration of antipyretic medication, may give more relief and comfort (Kinmonth et al 1992, O'Connor 2002). However, Blumenthal (2000) suggested that there is little therapeutic difference between the use of antipyretics and warm sponging compared to antipyretics alone.

Environmental measures that can be taken following administration of an antipyretic to aid the comfort of the child include:

- reducing the amount of clothing
- using loose-fitting cotton clothing
- reducing the amount of bedding; use sheets and blankets rather than quilts
- reducing the room temperature by opening windows, using a cool fan (directed away from the child)
- encouraging cool oral fluids
- warm (rather than tepid) sponging of the child's body surface (Harrison 1998).

Avoiding chilling is imperative as this will cause the child to shiver and subsequently raise the set point.

Observations and complications

- Check the child's temperature (see Assessment, p. 83) after an antipyretic has been given to assess its effect. This will normally be done around 30 minutes to 1 hour after the dose. There is no need for continued frequent monitoring; however, a return to regular monitoring, e.g. 4-hourly, would help in the continued evaluation and assessment of the effect of the intervention.
- The child should be observed to ensure that they are gaining some comfort from the antipyretic, i.e. becoming more settled, reduced flushing.
- The child should be observed for seizure activity.

COMMUNITY PERSPECTIVE

Temperature taking by the CCN is usually only required for children who:
- have malignant disease
- are prone to febrile seizures
- are particularly vulnerable to infection.

Routine temperature taking can heighten the parents' anxiety.

Do and do not

- Do ensure that the child's temperature is monitored regularly (see Assessment, p. 83).
- Do ensure that the parents are provided with information related to febrile seizures. This helps relieve anxiety.
- Do ensure that parents are provided with both verbal and written information on discharge.
- Do not use environmental measures to reduce the temperature in the febrile child before the use of antipyretics. They may induce shivering, which will cause a further rise in the temperature.
- Do not use cool moist compresses on the skin before the use of antipyretics.
- Do not use aspirin for fever in children under 12 years of age because of its identified correlation with Reye's syndrome (McGovern et al 2001).

References

Adams S 1999 What to do with febrile children. Professional Care of Mother and Child 9(1): 2–3

Blumenthal I 2000 Fever and the practice nurse: measurement and treatment. Community Practitioner 73(3): 519–521

Campbell S, Glasper E A (eds) 1995 Whaley and Wong's children's nursing. Mosby, London

Casey G 2000 Fever management in children. Nursing Standard 14(40): 36–42

Chandler T 2000 Paracetamol doses: practice variation. Paediatric Nursing 12(4): 7–8

Harrison M 1998 Childhood fever: is practice scientific? Journal of Child Health 2(3): 112–117

Holtzclaw B J 2003 Use of thermoregulatory principles in patient care: fever management. Cinahl Information Systems, Glendale, CA

Johnson W 1996 Childhood fevers: advising parents on management. Community Nurse 2(2): 20, 22–23

Kinmonth A, Fulton Y, Campbell M J 1992 Management of the feverish child at home. British Medical Journal 305(6862): 1134–1136

Lynch E 2004 A bed of their own. Nursing Standard 18(48): 18–19

McGovern M C, Glasgow J F T, Stuart M C 2001 Reye's syndrome and aspirin: lest we forget. British Medical Journal 322(7302): 1591–1592

O'Connor S 2002 Antipyretics in the paediatric A&E setting: a review. Paediatric Nursing 14(3): 33–35

Porth M 1994 Pathophysiology – concepts of altered health states, 4th edn. Lippincott, Philadelphia, PA

Royal College of Paediatrics and Child Health (RCPCH) 1997 Prevention and control of pain in children: a manual for health care professionals. BMJ Publishing Group, London

Tortora G J, Grabowski S R 2005 Principles of anatomy and physiology, 11th edn. HarperCollins, New York

Wong D 1997 Whaley and Wong's essentials of pediatric nursing, 5th edn. Mosby, St Louis, MO

Practice **33**

Tracheostomy care

Jane Hutchins, Melanie Wilson

Introduction

A tracheostomy is an artificial opening into the trachea via the neck (Fig. 33.1), providing a channel for effective respiration and for the removal of tracheobronchial secretions when circumstances make breathing impossible via the mouth and nose.

Indications for tracheostomy include:

- **congenital abnormalities:** laryngeal papilloma, laryngeal haemangioma, laryngeal webbing, vocal cord paralysis, choanal atresia, subglottic stenosis, tracheo-oesophageal anomalies and micrognathia (underdevelopment of the mandible as in Pierre–Robin syndrome and Treacher–Collins syndrome)
- **trauma:** subglottic stenosis, children requiring long-term ventilation, children with facial or neck tumours, emergency situations, e.g. road traffic accidents
- **infections:** acute epiglottitis, laryngotracheobronchitis and polyneuritis (e.g. Guillain–Barré syndrome)
- **a foreign body** may totally occlude the upper airway resulting in the need for an emergency tracheostomy.

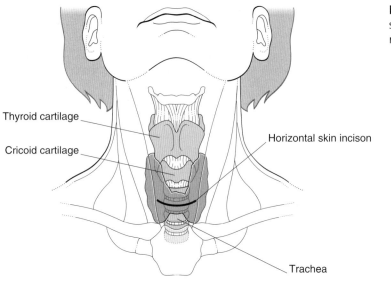

Thyroid cartilage

Cricoid cartilage

Horizontal skin incison

Trachea

Figure 33.1 Tracheostomy showing the landmarks of the neck and the incision site

It is therefore essential that paediatric nurses are aware of the signs and symptoms of airway obstruction:

- **Stridor** – a high-pitched sound produced by narrowing within the more rigid confines of the larynx or trachea. In laryngeal obstruction the stridor is inspiratory; in tracheal lesions it is usually both inspiratory and expiratory (Bull 2002).
- **Stertor** – the noise produced by obstruction in the throat, i.e. above the larynx; it is usu-ally a low-pitched choking type of noise (Bull 2002).
- **Use of accessory muscles** of respiration resulting in intercostal and sternal recession (Fig. 33.2).
- **Pallor**, sweating and restlessness.
- **Nasal flaring.**
- **Tachycardia** (limits vary according to age).
- **Cyanosis** – the lips will show a subtle dusky coloration.
- **Exhaustion** – a late stage. The child makes less effort to breathe, stridor and recession

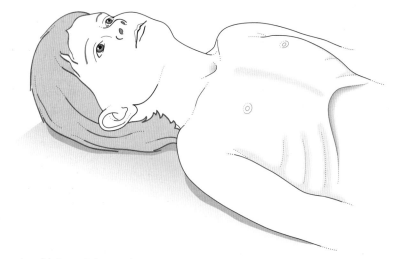

Figure 33.2   Sternal and intercostal recession

become less pronounced and apnoea is not far off (Bull 2002).

Learning outcomes

By the end of this section you should:

- be able to identify the conditions which more commonly necessitate the formation of a tracheostomy
- understand the rationale behind the various procedures required to maintain a patent airway in a child with a tracheostomy
- be able to list the various pieces of equipment required to perform certain necessary procedures
- understand the rationale of when these different procedures are required
- be able to list the skills that staff and the child's carers need to acquire to care for a child with a tracheostomy
- be able to list the equipment required at home prior to the child's discharge.

Rationale for tracheostomy care

Children requiring tracheostomies may initially be in intensive care units. Some children may require long-term tracheostomies and will be cared for in general children's wards or at home. The main aim when caring for a child with a tracheostomy is to maintain patency of the tube, so ensuring a clear airway at all times. Tracheal suction must be applied to achieve this. The frequency of suction varies from child to child, and is dependent upon the age of the child and the viscosity and amount of secretions. The child may need extra humidity to help keep the secretions thin and easily removable (Clarke 1995). This is because the normal mechanisms of warming and humidifying air as it is breathed (i.e. passage through the nose) are bypassed while a tracheostomy is in place (Harkin & Russell 2001). If necessary, humidity is administered, e.g. via an East Blower Humidifier connected to a tracheostomy mask or headbox. Regardless of the method of humidification used, the equipment must be set up according to the manufacturer's instructions.

Guidelines

Nurses must provide knowledge, information, support and resources, and facilitate the skills development of the family in order for the family to be fully capable to act as the agents of care for the child with a tracheostomy (Kang 2002). These include suction, irrigation, cleaning the stoma site, changing the tapes and changing the tracheostomy tube. Theoretical knowledge includes what to do if there are changes in secretions, signs of infection or aspiration, signs of a mucus plug or blocked tracheostomy tube, and cardiopulmonary resuscitation (CPR). In addition, nursing staff should understand and be competent in the anatomy of children's airways; predisposing factors which may lead to the formation of a tracheostomy; operative procedures; preparation of bedside equipment; immediate postoperative care (including the treatment of potential complications); care of a child following decannulation; care of an East Blower Humidifier; discharge planning; education of parents and relatives and allowance entitlements. They should also have an awareness of current research (Allan 1987).

Equipment required at the child's bedside

The following are required at the bedside of all children with a tracheostomy, both in hospital and at home, so that accidental displacement of the tracheostomy tube can be dealt with immediately and tracheal suction and irrigation can be performed when necessary.

- Oxygen point and tracheostomy mask (not required at home unless the child is oxygen dependent, where an oxygen cylinder would be used)
- Suction apparatus with tubing and a box of suction catheters of appropriate size; one catheter attached to the suction tubing
- Several 5 ml ampoules of 0.9% saline
- 2 ml syringes, several of which have 0.5 ml of 0.9% saline already drawn up (to save time in an emergency)
- Sachets of sterile 0.9% saline
- Sterile gallipot

- Latex-free disposable gloves (non-sterile, non-powdered)
- Bowl of water (to rinse the suction tubing)
- Disposal bag for hazardous waste in a solid bin (infection control guidelines)
- Spare tracheostomy tube (same size as the child has in situ)
- Spare tracheostomy tube (one size smaller)
- Equipment for cleaning of the stoma, e.g. cotton applicators
- KY jelly (as per local policy)
- Tracheostomy tape
- Scissors.

Factors to note

- Gloves are worn to prevent the spread of infection should the child have infected secretions. Some health authorities may insist that parents wear gloves while suctioning, therefore local policy should be followed.
- Non-powdered gloves are used to prevent the introduction of powder into the trachea.
- Ideally, latex-free gloves should be worn to reduce the incidence of latex allergy.
- Unsterile, non-powdered gloves are used because tracheostomy care does not need to be carried out using a sterile procedure. A clean technique, i.e. thorough handwashing and not touching the part of the suction catheter that goes inside the tracheostomy, is sufficient.
- The bowl of water and the syringes filled with 0.5 ml of 0.9% saline should be renewed after 24 hours, to prevent the growth of *Pseudomonas*.
- Irrigation of the tracheostomy tube prior to suction may be used to remove thick tenacious secretions, to aid with the inability to pass a suction catheter or to help a child experiencing breathing difficulties. However, this is a potentially hazardous procedure and must be undertaken with care (Clarke 1995). This is supported by the American Thoracic Society who submitted an official statement in July 1999 about the care of children with tracheostomies. In the review of all aspects of tracheostomy care in children, the guidelines state that **isotonic sodium chloride should not be instilled routinely** (Ridling et al 2003).
- Evidence consistently shows that such instillation is detrimental in adults, most often resulting in decreased oxygen saturation. The effects of its use in children, however, have not been well studied (Ridling et al 2003). In many paediatric intensive care units and ENT wards, instillation of such solution is still part of routine practice; however, many nurses continue to question its use. Therefore, hospital policy should be followed.
- Tracheal dilators may cause trauma to the trachea. As a result of this these are rarely used in practice. However, some hospitals may still have them in the tray at the child's bedside for emergency purposes; therefore local policy should be followed.
- Due to the recent issues regarding bovine spongiform encephalopathy (BSE) and the re-sterilising of equipment, the Sheffield Children's NHS Trust now supplies each child with three silver tracheostomy tubes of their own. They must only be used for the same patient and thrown away after decannulation.
- Advances in laryngeal reconstruction have reduced the need for long-term tracheostomies, which in turn has meant that silver tubes are rarely used now. Children are being decannulated earlier due to reconstructive surgery. Depending on the extent of the surgery, they may keep their tracheostomy for a few weeks longer until the trachea has healed sufficiently. Usually children are decannulated in theatre whilst having reconstruction and then they are ventilated on the intensive care unit for 5 days to allow the trachea to heal.
- The ward resuscitation trolley should contain an appropriately sized Ambu bag for use in an emergency. The 15 mm connector fits directly onto the tracheostomy tube. Ambu bags are now given to parents in the community.
- If the child has a silver tracheostomy tube, a blue endotracheal connector will be needed to connect the Ambu bag to the tube.

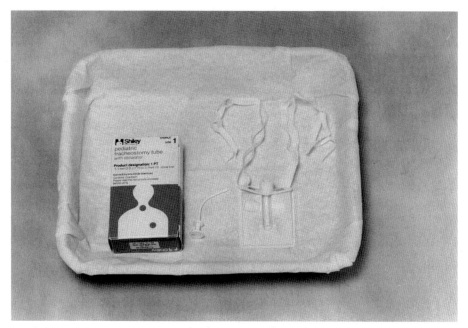

Figure 33.3 Shiley tracheostomy tubes: box (left); introducer (centre); spare tracheal tube with tapes attached (right)

Examples of tracheostomy tubes

Shiley tracheostomy tubes

These are plastic tubes with an introducer (Fig. 33.3). Sizes are 3.0, 3.5, 4.0 and 4.5 in the neonatal design and 3.0, 3.5, 4.0, 4.5, 5.0 and 5.5 in the paediatric design. Neonatal tubes have a different design of flange from the paediatric tubes; the angle of the curve also differs although the internal diameter is the same. This make of tube tends to be used most frequently in children and in newly formed tracheostomies. This type of tube needs to be changed approximately every 3–4 weeks unless it becomes blocked. You may find that parents are keen to change them weekly in order to gain more practice and confidence. These types of tube are for single use only.

Sheffield tracheostomy tube

This is a silver tube with an introducer, two inner tubes (one being a spare), a speaking tube and a blocker (Fig. 33.4). The inner tube can safely be removed and cleaned without disturbing the outer tube. The consultant may choose a silver tube for children who require long-term airway management without ventilation.

There are other types of tubes available and their use will vary according to surgeon preference as selection is based upon the child's presenting upper airway anatomy, physiological requirements, treatment, e.g. long-term ventilation, and body size (Abraham 2003).

TRACHEOSTOMY SUCTION

Rationale

Suctioning of the tracheostomy tube prevents the build up of secretions, which may narrow the lumen of the tube and make it difficult for the child to breathe. Suctioning of the tube should be undertaken with care as, performed incorrectly, it can lead to damage of the air passages or to infection.

Factors to note

- Suction catheters – it is important to use the correct size of suction catheter (NHS QIS 2003). A catheter that is too small will not aspirate the secretions efficiently, and a catheter that is too large will block off too much of the airway during suction. Generally, the sizing of the catheter is twice the

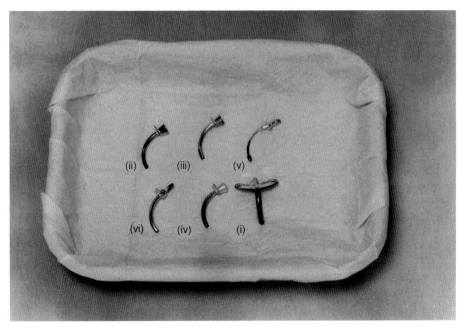

Figure 33.4   Sheffield tracheostomy tubes: (i) tracheostomy tube; (ii) and (iii) inner tubes; (iv) speaking tube; (v) introducer; (vi) blocker

diameter of the tracheostomy tube, e.g. a 3.5 neonatal or paediatric tube would require a size 7 Fg catheter.

- Suction – it is important to apply only enough suction to remove secretions. Suction that is too vigorous can damage the tracheal mucosa. Suction that is too gentle is inefficient at removing secretions and may mean that the procedure has to be repeated. Research has shown that suctioning at a negative pressure of 100 mmHg is effective in most clinical situations, whilst causing minimal tracheal damage (NHS QIS 2003). Some models of portable suction machines require a higher pressure to remove minimal secretions. The manufacturer's guidelines should be referred to before using such machines.

Equipment

- Suction equipment (either wall or portable)
- Appropriate size of suction catheters
- A box of disposable gloves (non-sterile, non-powdered)
- Disposal bag for hazardous waste in a solid bin
- Bowl filled with tap water
- A pre-measured guide to measure the length of suction catheter, e.g. a piece of suction catheter that has been previously cut to the length required.

Method

1. To prevent trauma during the procedure, check that the suction equipment is set to 100 mmHg and that there is a suction catheter of the correct size attached to the suction tubing.

2. In order to gain the child's/parents' cooperation, allow the child to perform their own suction if this is usual. If not, explain the procedure.

3. To reduce the risk of infection, wash hands thoroughly.

4. To minimise the risk of cross-infection, put on gloves and withdraw the suction catheter from the sleeve. Do not touch the part of the catheter that will be introduced into the tracheostomy.

5. To prevent damage to the tracheal mucosa, which can lead to trauma and respiratory infection, turn the suction equipment on, do not apply suction, check the length of suction catheter to be used against the pre-measured guide and gently introduce the catheter to this length. The length of the suction catheter should be equal to the length of the tracheostomy tube + 0.5 cm (*no further*).

6. To minimise irritation of the mucous membranes, apply suction as the catheter is gently withdrawn. Catheters have previously been rotated on removal in the belief that this will pick up more secretions and prevent adherence to the tracheal wall. Although this was practice when single-eyed catheters were used, Day (2000) states: 'It is not necessary to rotate the catheter in the fingers as withdrawal takes place if the preferred multiple eyelet catheters are being used'. Do not apply suction for more than 15 seconds at a time, as prolonged suction can damage mucous membranes and also cause the child to become bradycardic. The child cannot breathe effectively when the suction catheter is partially occluding the tracheostomy tube.

7. Repeat the procedure if necessary, using both a fresh suction catheter and glove.

8. To prevent a build-up of secretions in the suction tube, discard the catheter and glove and rinse the tubing. Apply a fresh suction catheter to the tubing to ensure that suction can be rapidly applied when necessary.

9. Ensure that the child is comfortable and able to continue with the activity they were involved with prior to suction (Kleiber & Krutzfield 1988).

Observations

If the secretions are particularly copious, which often occurs routinely when a child first wakes up after sleeping, unusually tenacious (thick), green in colour, bloodstained or have changed in any way, record this information in the nursing documentation and liaise with medical staff. This ensures that any evidence of infection or other problems are detected as early as possible. If tenacious secretions persist for longer than 1 hour, humidified air will be required for a few days until the secretions return to their usual consistency. Bloodstained secretions on a well child may suggest the catheter has been introduced too far into the tracheostomy tube when suctioning and has caused a minimal amount of trauma.

CLEANING THE TRACHEOSTOMY STOMA SITE

This is a socially clean technique, usually performed once or twice a day. Tracheostomy stoma care aims to keep the area clean and dry, reducing the risk of skin irritation and infection (St George's Healthcare NHS Trust 2000). It also allows you the chance to check for any redness or chaffing of the flange against the skin which, depending on the consultant's advice, may require treatment.

Equipment

- Gallipot
- Cotton buds
- Cool boiled water, a sachet of 0.9% saline or Saliwipes (impregnated sterile swabs with 0.9% sodium chloride) as per local policy
- Non-sterile latex-free gloves as per local policy.

Method

1. Wash your hands.
2. Explain the procedure to the child and parent.
3. Empty the normal saline or cooled boiled water into the gallipot/open Saliwipe pack.
4. Put on non-sterile latex-free gloves as per local policy.
5. Dip the end of the cotton bud into the solution or using Saliwipe, wipe in one direction underneath the flange of the tracheostomy tube.
6. Dispose of that cotton bud or using a clean Saliwipe, repeat the procedure as many times as necessary, i.e. until the area is clean.

7. Finally, dry under the flange with a cotton bud.
8. Dispose of all used equipment appropriately.

Observations

Observe, record and report to medical staff:

- any offensive smell which may indicate an infection
- any bleeding which may indicate an excessive growth of new skin around the stoma (granulation) (Fig. 33.5).

CLEANING A SILVER TRACHEOSTOMY INNER TUBE

This is a socially clean procedure and needs to be performed 3- to 4-hourly or more or less frequently as the child's condition dictates. The aim of this procedure is to maintain a clear airway at all times; frequency therefore depends upon the consistency and amount of secretions produced.

Equipment

- Two gallipots, one labelled 'clean' and one labelled 'dirty'
- Disposable latex-free gloves
- Pipe cleaners
- Sodium bicarbonate.

Method

1. To prevent cross-infection, keep gallipots in their bags and label one 'clean' and the other 'dirty'. Also write the date and time that the bag was opened. These should be replaced every 24 hours.
2. To protect yourself and to prevent cross-infection, wash your hands and put on a pair of gloves prior to starting this procedure.
3. To prevent cross-infection, keep the gloves on and remove the dirty inner tube from the tracheostomy tube and place in the 'dirty' gallipot.
4. Take the 'clean' gallipot and the 'dirty' gallipot containing the inner tube to the sink.
5. To ensure that the inner tube is free from secretions, place some sodium bicarbonate and water into the 'dirty' gallipot and clean the inner tube by passing pipe cleaners through it until all the secretions have been removed. Finally rinse the inner tube with tap water to remove any pipe cleaner fibres.
6. Place the clean tube in the 'clean' gallipot. Take the equipment back to the child's bedside and replace the clean tube into the child's tracheostomy.

Observations

Record in the nursing documentation any increased amount of secretions, or tenacious

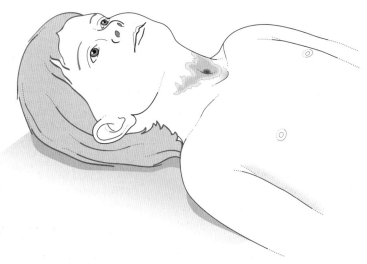

Figure 33.5 Excoriated skin with granulation

secretions, and inform medical staff if the tracheostomy tube requires changing more frequently than is usual for each individual child.

Factors to note

- Some silver tubes have a spare inner tube, e.g. Sheffield tubes. In this case, the clean tube should be kept in the 'clean' gallipot and, once the dirty tube has been removed, the clean tube can be immediately placed into the child's tracheostomy site. The dirty tube can then be taken away for cleaning as described earlier.
- Do not place silver tubes in Milton as this turns them black and the caustic nature of Milton will cause trauma to the trachea.
- Shiley (plastic) tubes are meant for once-only use. They should not be cleaned and replaced.

CHANGING THE TRACHEOSTOMY TUBE TAPE

This is a socially clean procedure (i.e. thorough handwashing) which is vital to prevent the tube becoming dislodged or removed altogether (Docherty & Bench 2002). This procedure is performed at least once a day, more frequently if the tapes become wet (McGee 1990).

Equipment

- Two equal lengths of tracheostomy tape
- Pair of clean scissors
- Blanket to wrap child in
- Neck roll (e.g. rolled-up towel).

Method

1. To minimise anxiety and gain cooperation, explain the procedure to the child and parent.
2. Wash your hands.
3. It may be easier to see the tracheostomy if the child's head is extended slightly. To do this, place a rolled-up pillowcase or towel under the child's shoulders.
4. If the child is young or a baby, it may be useful to wrap them up in a blanket to keep their arms secure.
5. Thread a piece of tape through the flange on each side of the tracheostomy tube.

6. To ensure that the tracheostomy tube does not fall out, *always* secure the new tapes by tying a reef knot (right over left and under, left over right and under) on one side of the neck before cutting the old tapes. Alternate the sides daily to prevent soreness. On young babies *never* fasten the tapes behind, as this may become confused with the ties on a bib.
7. To ensure that the tapes are not too tight (which leads to sores) or too loose (which may allow the tube to fall out) check the tightness of the new tapes by inserting the tip of your little finger under the new tapes.
8. Carefully remove the old tapes.
9. Remove the neck roll and ensure that the child is comfortable and able to continue with the activity that they were involved with prior to changing the tapes.

Observations

Observe and report immediately to medical staff any redness or excoriation around the child's neck.

Factors to note

- If the tracheostomy is new, the child's neck may be swollen, making it difficult to insert the clean tapes. This is made easier by wrapping a small amount of Sellotape around the end of the tracheostomy tape, like the ends of a shoelace.
- *Never* remove the old tapes before securing the new ones as the tracheostomy tube may fall out.
- The use of Velcro tapes on active children who are nursed on the wards is not recommended. This is due to lack of research regarding the security and safety of their use. However, you may find that children who are nursed in intensive care, or on home long-term ventilation and who are immobile will have Velcro tapes. These are then changed for linen tapes when they reach the ward.

CHANGING A TRACHEOSTOMY TUBE

This is a socially clean procedure. Normally, the first change of a tracheostomy tube is undertaken by the consultant ENT staff, senior registrars or competent nursing staff. It is recommended that two people perform this procedure when possible, one to support the child. In an emergency situation, i.e. when the child is experiencing respiratory distress and irrigation and suction have failed to clear the tube, this procedure may be performed without the presence of medical ENT staff; however, following the tube change ENT medical staff must be informed. It is recommended that a tube change should be avoided in newly formed tracheostomies for at least 4–5 days to allow swelling to subside and the removal of the black stay sutures. If a new tube change needs to be performed as an emergency within the first 5 days, you can pull on these sutures to allow for traction on the opening in order to insert the tube (Bull 2002).

The position of the child during a tube change is determined by their age, ability to cooperate and their comfort. The older child may have their tube changed sitting with their neck extended, whereas the infant may require to be swaddled in a blanket.

Equipment

- KY jelly (as per local policy)
- Sterile dressing towel
- Sterile tracheostomy tube (appropriate size)
- Sterile tracheostomy tube one size smaller
- Scissors
- Hand towel (used as a roll to extend the child's neck)
- Suction apparatus with the appropriate size of suction catheter connected
- Oxygen via a tracheostomy mask
- Non-sterile latex-free gloves (as per local policy).

Method

1. To promote a safe procedure, prepare the correct equipment.
2. To minimise anxiety and gain cooperation, explain the procedure to the child and parent.
3. Wash your hands.
4. For tracheostomy tubes with inners, prior to starting the procedure ensure that the inner tube fits correctly inside the main tube, thus avoiding the need for a second tube change.
5. To prevent trauma to the trachea, insert the introducer into the main tracheostomy tube and apply a small amount of KY jelly to the tip and place on the sterile towel.
6. In order that the new tracheostomy tube can be secured immediately, insert the new tapes into the flanges of the new tracheostomy tube prior to performing the tube change (Fig. 33.6).

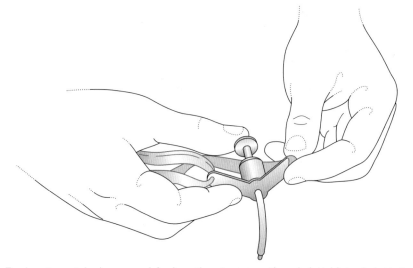

Figure 33.6 Tracheostomy tube is prepared for insertion: tapes are threaded and introducer is inserted

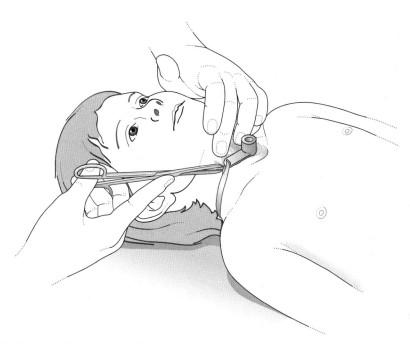

Figure 33.7   Existing tracheostomy tape is cut

7. To promote easy insertion of the tube, place a rolled towel under the child's head and ensure that the neck is extended and the child held securely.

8. Cut the old tapes, remove the old tube and immediately insert the new tube (Figs 33.7–33.11). *Immediately* remove the introducer as the airway is occluded whilst this is in situ. The child may cough following this

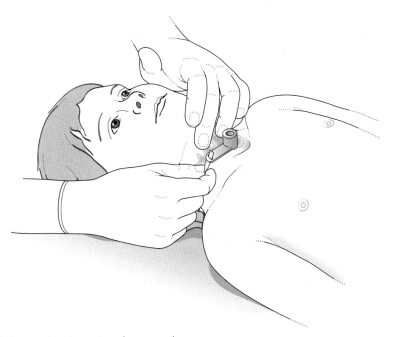

Figure 33.8   Existing tracheostomy tape is removed

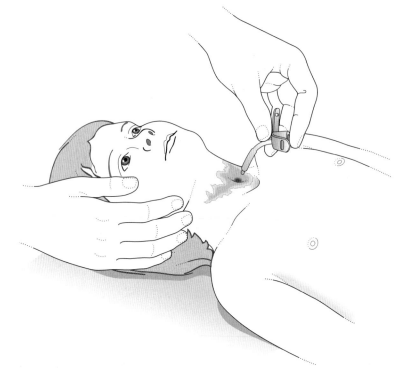

Figure 33.9   Tracheostomy tube is removed

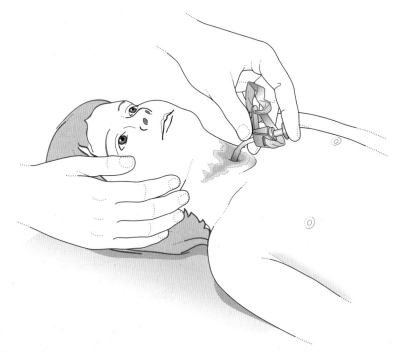

Figure 33.10   New tracheostomy tube is reinserted and introducer removed

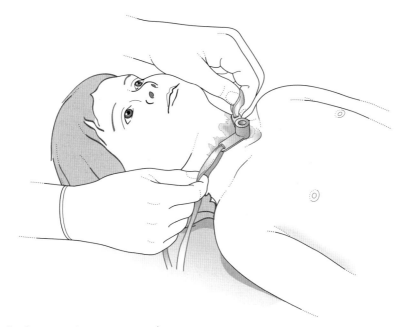

Figure 33.11   Tracheostomy tapes are secured

procedure, so perform suction immediately and secure the tapes. If you are changing the tube in an emergency, after insertion, tie the tapes loosely before performing suction, then re-tie the tapes appropriately when the child's condition has improved.

9. Dispose of the dirty tracheostomy tube appropriately – plastic tubes are disposable; silver tubes are re-sterilised.

Observations

Observe and report to medical staff any inflammation or excessive granulation around the stoma site.

Factors to note

- If the tracheostomy tube is changed in an emergency situation (i.e. the tube has totally blocked), the child will need oxygen therapy and suction until their condition stabilises.
- If the new tube is difficult to insert, i.e. the tracheostomy is newly formed, try a smaller size. Ensure that the appropriate ENT surgeon is informed immediately of the problem.

- To ensure the safety and well-being of the child, a qualified nurse who is experienced in looking after the tracheostomy tube must accompany the child on any escorts from the ward. Typical escorts may be to X-ray, theatre, the playroom or school-room, etc.
- When the child is away from the bedside, either on an escort or in the playroom, they *must* have the following equipment with them at all times:
  - portable suction machine with tubing and catheters of the appropriate size
  - portable oxygen (only if the child is oxygen dependent)
  - several 5 ml ampoules of 0.9% saline and a 2 ml syringe
  - spare tracheostomy tube of the size in use
  - spare tracheostomy tube a size smaller
  - scissors.
- If parents have received teaching on how to care for their child's tracheostomy and nursing staff are happy with their level of competence (it is vital that they have performed a tube change before), they may be allowed to take their child away from the ward unsupervised for short periods of time.

Tips for day-to-day life

● When bottle-feeding an infant, do not prop the bottle up or feed the child while they are lying down as liquid can enter the lungs via the tracheostomy tube. Hold the infant in a nearly upright position during feeding.

● Always prepare a shallow bath. Take care to prevent bath water from getting into the tracheostomy tube because it goes directly into the lungs. For extra safety you may attach a 'Swedish nose' onto the tracheostomy which will cover the end of the tube yet still allow active respiration.

● Do not use talcum powder on a child with a tracheostomy. The upper airway has been bypassed and this means that they lose the normal filtering mechanism of the nose and normal defences such as coughing (Griggs 1998). If talcum powder entered the tracheostomy it could cause the secretions to become thick and dry up, forming a plug, which could easily block the tracheostomy tube.

● Take care when placing children in car seats or bouncy chairs. You must make sure that they do not occlude the tracheostomy with their chin. If this is the case, the use of a thin neck roll placed over their shoulders should correct their position.

● If the child requires an inhaler, use an Aerochamber device, usually available from pharmacy. They work in exactly the same way as a volumatic device but connect neatly onto the tracheostomy tube.

● Likewise, if the child requires a nebuliser, use a standard nebuliser kit and replace the mask/mouthpiece with a tracheostomy mask (never connect the reservoir directly onto the tracheostomy tube as the vapour is unable to escape and will result in serious damage to the child's lungs).

COMMUNITY PERSPECTIVE

Safety dictates that parents/carers caring for children with a tracheostomy will have been fully trained in the necessary care and management and assessed as competent in that care prior to planned discharge from hospital.

The family and/or child will need to be able to take full responsibility for routine tracheostomy care.

The specific details of tracheostomy care will depend on the child's individual needs, the type of tracheostomy device and the types of ancillary equipment being used. The CCN must be familiar with these variables before accepting a child for home care.

All children discharged home with a tracheostomy must have both a mains and a portable suction machine. A maintenance schedule must be agreed and cleaning instructions given.

Responsibility for the supply of essential equipment such as tracheostomy tubes and suction catheters should be agreed before discharge.

Direct humidification, e.g. via an East Blower, should only be supported in the home at the direction of the referring paediatrician and then only if home conditions are appropriate and safe. Warm air delivered by a humidifier to a tracheostomy mask can be dangerous in the home environment as the child can suffer burns or scalds, or condensation can enter the tracheostomy tube. The hot humidifier containing boiling water is a danger to the child and others. The close supervision that is required if this equipment is to be used in the home may be impossible.

A sick child with a tracheostomy is likely to be extremely dependent and this can affect the freedom and mobility of the whole family. Discharge planning should include a bid being made for continuing care monies so that respite care can be provided in the home.

It is sensible to notify electrical and telephone companies in writing so that the home can be given priority for restoration of power in the event of a failure.

- Should the child require oxygen therapy, there are several ways to achieve this. The use of oxygen via a Swedish nose is acceptable for a maximum of 2 litres. Any dose higher than this would be required through humidification.

References

Abraham S 2003 Babies with tracheostomies: the challenge of providing specialised clinical care. ASHA Leader 8(5): 4–5, 26

Allan D 1987 Making sense of tracheostomy. Nursing Times 83(45): 34–38

Bull P D 2002 Diseases of the ear, nose and throat, 9th edn. Blackwell Science, Oxford

Clarke L 1995 A critical event in tracheostomy care. British Journal of Nursing 4(12): 676, 678–681

Day T 2000 Tracheal suctioning: when, why and how. Cited in Docherty B, Bench S 2002 Tracheostomy management for patients in general ward settings. Professional Nurse 18(2): 100–104

Docherty B, Bench S 2002 Tracheostomy management for patients in general ward settings. Professional Nurse 18(2): 100–104

Griggs A 1998 Tracheostomy: suctioning and humidification. Nursing Standard 13(2): 49–53, 55–56

Harkin H, Russell C 2001 Tracheostomy patient care. Nursing Times 97: 25, 34–36

Kang J M 2002 Using a self-learning module to teach nurses about caring for hospitalised children with tracheostomies. Journal for Nurses in Staff Development 18(1): 28–35

Kleiber C, Krutzfield N 1988 Acute histologic changes in the tracheobronchial tree associated with different suction catheter insertion techniques. Heart and Lung 17: 10–14

McGee L 1990 Case study: maintaining skin integrity during the use of tracheostomy ties. Osteotomy Wound Management 30: 37–40

NHS QIS 2003 Caring for the patient with a tracheostomy. Best Practice Statement. NHS Quality Improvement Scotland, Edinburgh

Ridling D A, Martin L D, Bratton S L 2003 Endotracheal suctioning with or without instillation of isotonic sodium chloride solution in critically ill children. American Journal of Critical Care 12(3): 212–219

St George's Healthcare NHS Trust 2000 Guidelines for the care of patients with tracheostomy tubes. St George's Healthcare NHS Trust, London

Further Reading

Carron J D, Derkay C S, Strope G L et al 2000 Paediatric tracheostomies: changing indications and outcomes. Laryngoscope 110: 1099–1103

Dougherty J M, Parrish J M, Hock-Long L 1995 Part 1: developing a competency-based curriculum for tracheostomy and ventilator care. Pediatric Nursing 21(6): 581–584

Serra A 2000 Tracheostomy care. Nursing Standard 14(42): 45–55

Wellitz P B, Dettenmeier P A 1994 Test your knowledge of tracheostomy tubes. American Journal of Nursing 94(2): 46–50

Tracheostomy Websites

A Guide to Tracheostomy Care for the Child, University of Kentucky Hospital
www.mc.uky.edu/PatientEd/ukbook.htm

Aaron's Tracheostomy Page
www.tracheostomy.com

The American Thoracic Society www.thoracic.org

Breathing Easier, University of Chicago Children's Hospital
www.ucch.org/ucch/healthpages/pulmcrit/breath/noframe/index.html

Care Card, Children's Mercy Hospital, Kansas, Missouri
www.childrens-mercy.org/CareCard

Paediatric Tracheostomy, University of California, Davis Medical Center
http://wellness.ucdavis.edu/childhealth/specialneeds/paediatric tracheostomy

Stiftung NOAH Tracheostomy Care Guide
www.stiftung-noah.de/en/index.aspx?bhcp=1

Tracheostomy, University of Michigan Health System
www.med.umich.edu/1libr/pa/pa_tracheos_hhg.htm

Support Group

ACT – Action For Children With Tracheostomies
72 Oakridge
Thornhill
Cardiff CF14 9BQ
Tel/Fax: 029 2075 5932
email: claire@claire-act.fsnet.co.uk

Practice 34

Traction

Brian Silverwood

Introduction

Traction is a pulling force. In orthopaedics, traction therapy is used as a conservative intervention. It is used to reduce and maintain alignment of fractures, immobilise inflamed or injured joints, relieve pain, correct mild deformities and reduce muscle spasm.

Learning outcomes

By the end of this section you should:

- understand why traction is used
- be able to identify the different types of traction
- recognise the methods of applying traction
- be able to care for a child on traction
- recognise the common complications that may occur as a result of the use of traction.

Rationale

Traction, in all its many guises, is extensively used in orthopaedic practice, including paediatrics. Like many aspects of orthopaedic ther-apy, it does not remain constant and therefore requires a high degree of nursing input.

Factors to note

Effects of hospitalisation on the family

Traction is often indicated following trauma such as a road traffic accident. The parents often feel shocked, guilty or angry about the trauma and find the application of traction very stressful at an already difficult time. An emergency admission, however routine for nursing staff, or a planned admission, is a time of great stress for both the parents and child. It is essential that explanations of all that is happening and why are given to the child and parents. When appropriate, the child and parents should be encouraged to participate in care of the traction when they feel able to do so. It is important that they feel confident and happy with this and do not undertake it out of a sense of duty. Traction equipment can be daunting to a nurse unfamiliar in its use and may be very frightening to a parent. Traction is often used for prolonged periods of time.

This can be disruptive to family life. Parents should feel welcomed onto the ward and be able to stay with their child if they wish, though this may be difficult if there are siblings at home.

Equipment

Traction equipment and terminology can be confusing and anxiety provoking to nurses who do not fully understand the components and how each attaches to the other. The type and method of traction used is indicated by the type and position of the fracture, the age of the child and the desired outcome. Other factors such as trauma, surgeon's preference and availability of equipment will also be considered.

Nurses caring for patients on traction need a working knowledge of each of the various types of traction along with its rationale, correct set up and maintenance. Folick et al (1994) recognise that there are many variations in practice, all of which fulfil the same purpose. What is essential is that a uniform approach is used once the traction is established. There are many types of traction and the names may vary from centre to centre. There may also be variations and alterations to accommodate individual needs.

Types of traction

Traction is either fixed or balanced:

- Fixed traction is achieved by exerting a pulling force on the point splinted between two fixed points.
- Balanced traction exerts a pulling force on the part held between two mobile points, and works by using the patient's weight against the applied load.

Both skin and skeletal traction are used in paediatrics.

Skin traction

This is the first choice of treatment and involves applying adhesive strips of material to either side of the affected limb. The limb is then bandaged, taking care to leave the knee free. The skin traction kits include cords to allow a pull to be exerted on the strips, which is transmitted from the material and skin to the underlying tissues and bone. Only a moderate amount of pull can be exerted using weights and the bed end is then elevated.

Skeletal traction

This is used at the surgeon's preference if the alignment of the fracture is difficult to achieve and maintain and internal fixation is not possible. This involves the insertion of a sterile pin through an area of strong bone such as the femoral condyles, tibial tuberosity or calcaneum. This is performed under general anaesthetic using aseptic conditions. A metal stirrup is then attached to the pin ends and cord fastened to it. Weights are then attached to the stirrup and hang over a pulley; they are then left free hanging over the elevated bed end. Skeletal traction is also used following trauma, such as when the integrity of the skin is damaged and the application of skin traction would be difficult. Skeletal traction allows for easier access to wounds, dressings or any other injuries. It is now rarely used in paediatric practice due to advances in orthopaedic surgical techniques in the management of complicated long bone fractures.

The following types of traction are most commonly used in paediatrics:

- Simple leg traction or Buck's extensions: used for pre- and postoperative positioning and immobilisation, rest for inflammatory disorders such as irritable hip syndrome – this is either fixed or balanced, and is usually skin traction.
- Gallows or Bryant's traction: used in infants usually under 1 year of age for femoral fractures and preoperative positioning prior to hip surgery – this traction is always bilateral and is fixed (Fig. 34.1).
- Thomas splint traction: used for femoral fractures – this can be either skin or skeletal, fixed or balanced. Now often used for femoral fractures as splintage to allow swelling to subside prior to internal fixation of the fracture using the nancy nailing system (Fig. 34.2).
- Slings and springs traction: often used for children with Perthes disease or other hip conditions. Enables the child to have bed rest

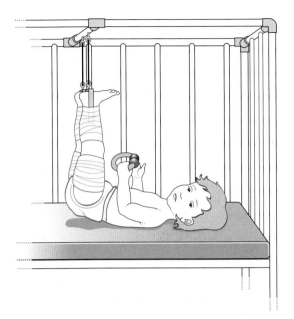

Figure 34.1 Gallows traction. This is fixed traction

and the physiotherapist to teach and perform specific exercises of the hip and lower limbs.

The following forms of traction are now rarely used in paediatrics:

- Burns frame, Japanese frame or hoop traction: used in infants to correct congenital dislocation of the hip – fixed skin traction.
- Dunlop traction: used for contractures of the elbow and immobilisation of supracondylar fractures of the elbow – this can be skin or skeletal and is balanced (Fig. 34.3).
- 90–90 traction: used for displaced femoral fractures – balanced (Fig. 34.4).
- Pelvic traction: used for low back pain – fixed or balanced.
- Halter neck traction: used for torticollis, cervical injuries or disease processes – balanced (Fig. 34.5).
- Halo traction: used for cervical injuries – this is skeletal and fixed.
- Hamilton–Russell or modified Hamilton–Russell traction: used for immobilisation of fractured femur, postoperatively following hip surgery and for treatment of hip dislocation. It combines balanced traction with suspension – skin or skeletal (Fig. 34.6).

Guidelines

Developmental issues
Traction is used for all age groups from the newborn in gallows traction, to the adolescent

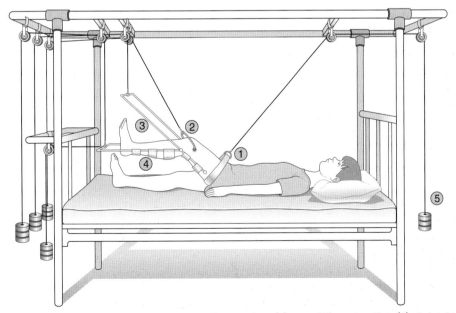

Figure 34.2 Thomas splint. The figure shows complex traction: (1) use of Thomas splint; (2) skeletal traction; (3) skin traction (below the knee); (4) Pearson knee piece; (5) counterbalance traction. This is balanced traction

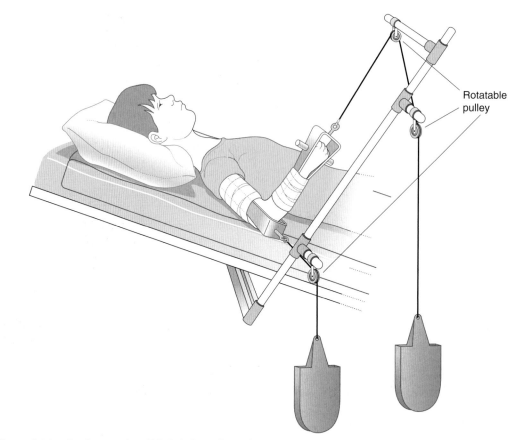

Rotatable pulley

Figure 34.3 Dunlop traction. This is balanced traction

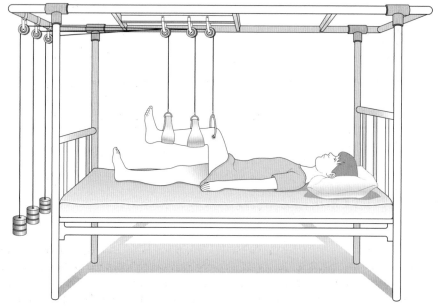

Figure 34.4 90–90 traction. This is balanced traction

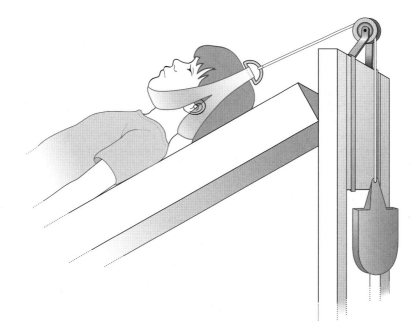

Figure 34.5 Halter neck traction. This is balanced traction

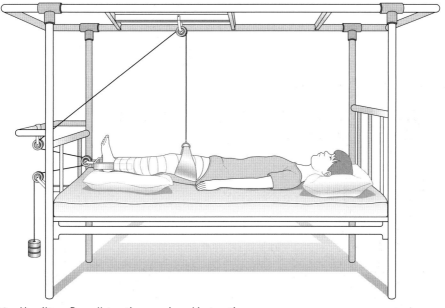

Figure 34.6 Hamilton–Russell traction – using skin traction

on Thomas splint traction. It is an immobilis-ing device and therefore restricts independ-ence and the freedom to move. Consideration should be given to the environment and where these children are to be nursed.

Infants and young children should have their developmental needs met whilst in hos-pital. An open ward and the company of other children may provide a stimulating environ-ment, but equal consideration must be given to parents who wish to be resident and will require a degree of privacy.

Young children often regress in their development, for example a child who is toilet trained may start to wet the bed. This can be upsetting for both the child and parent, but it is common and only temporary, so reassurance and support must be given.

Adolescents sometimes wish to be with their peer group, as they are often in for prolonged periods. However, some find it difficult to adjust to the loss of control over their environment and will prefer to be on their own.

All children and parents need to know what is expected of them, they need explanation of procedures and routine and they should be given choices (Houston 1996).

The multidisciplinary team

Children requiring traction have input from many members of the team during their stay in hospital.

Physiotherapists

Their role can be vital to the overall outcome of the traction. Their aim is to prevent complications of joint stiffness, muscle wasting and deformities by using exercises, which are taught and supervised. Early intervention is required to prevent complications arising and should be within 24 hours of the application of traction.

Occupational therapists

If splints or slings are required as a result of complications such as foot drop or toe/finger deformities, the occupational therapist will assess the child's needs and organise the necessary equipment.

Play specialists

A child experiencing regressive behaviour may benefit from play therapy. Play specialists provide activities not only to prevent boredom but also to support staff in carrying out painful procedures with the use of distraction therapy. Physiotherapy and exercise can often be disguised as play and can be quite imaginative and developmentally stimulating (see Play, p. 457).

Ward-based schoolteacher

Traction is often a prolonged therapy and may cause long absences from school. *Services for Children and Young People* (DoH 1996) states: 'Your child has a right to receive suitable education while in hospital for a long time.' Liaison often takes place with the child's school to ensure continuity of education needs, and home education can be arranged if necessary.

Dietitian

The role of the dietitian is important as children on traction frequently have reduced appetite as a result of immobility and are subsequently more prone to constipation.

Parental participation

Once the traction has been established and is no longer daunting to the parents, they can often participate in their child's care. This is usually with the activities of daily living, but particular activities relating to the care of the traction, such as care of splints and greasing Thomas splint rings, can also be undertaken. Supervision of exercises as taught by the physiotherapists can be done by the parent and child together, though parents must be willing participants and must not feel that they have to undertake these roles.

When administering care, the nurse should be constantly thinking of ways to help the child care for themselves or assisting the nurse with the daily care of the traction system, for example, helping to change the bandages.

Equipment

For all skin traction
- Commercial skin traction kits, either adhesive or non-adhesive foam backed
- Bandages and securing tape
- Traction cord
- Traction beams and frames.

Other equipment that may be used for all traction
- Wooden blocks (for fixed traction, used to keep the heel off the bed)
- Weights and pulleys (for balanced traction)
- Balkan beams on four-poster frame

- Splints, e.g. Thomas splint
- Slings, e.g. foot and knee or halter neck
- Padding – gauze or cotton wool
- Monkey poles
- Polymer gel pads to prevent sore heels.

Equipment used specifically for skeletal traction

- Skeletal pins, e.g. Steinmann or Denham
- Stirrups, e.g. Bohler
- Knee piece, e.g. Pearson.

Application of skin traction

A full nursing assessment needs to have been completed prior to the application of traction to obtain baseline information upon which all plans of care are based (see Assessment, p. 83).

1. Prepare the child and parent for the procedure with careful explanation of the plan of care.

2. Ensure that the child has had adequate analgesia prior to the procedure. Application of traction can be stressful and sedation may be required in addition to analgesia. Entonox (50% nitrous oxide and 50% oxygen) provides excellent pain relief for procedural pain (Pickup & Pagdin 2000). If manipulation of the fracture is required, a general anaesthetic will be given.

3. Maintain privacy.

4. Clean the skin prior to the application of traction.

5. Leave the ankle free. This allows for movement of the joint and prevents stiffness.

6. Bony prominences, especially of the malleoli and head of fibula, should be left free from pressure. Padding may be applied to these areas.

7. Strapping must be firm but not tight or constricting (Pritchard & David 1990) and must be applied wrinkle-free to prevent sores developing.

8. Two people are required to apply traction safely, one to do the application and one to support the affected limb.

9. If weights are to be used, pulleys and cord cut to the appropriate length will be required. The medical staff should indicate the amount of weight to be used. Too much can result in the child being pulled down the bed, and not enough will be ineffectual in providing any form of traction. When using weights, the bed end should be slightly elevated to provide some counter balance.

Nursing care of the child in traction

Having applied the traction, the nursing care is then based on the care of the immobilised child, with additional factors implied by the traction.

Pain and discomfort

Once traction has been applied the child is usually more comfortable. Pain needs to be assessed and analgesia given. One of the most common causes of discomfort is muscle spasm; this is resolved with antispasmodics but does settle after a short time on traction.

Positioning

Traction often demands the patient to be nursed in an unnatural position, such as lying flat, head down (e.g. gallows traction). This often affects the usual activities of daily living in the early stages but children quickly adapt.

Skin care

The skin on the injured limb needs to be checked at least daily. It is important to look for signs of allergic reaction to traction kits and adhesive tapes. Following trauma, damaged skin must be monitored and dressings applied as directed and necessary. Skin care also extends to washing and pressure area care as the child is immobile. Frequent change in position if possible, or relief of pressure on bony prominences such as sacrum, elbows and heels, is extremely important. Often the child will naturally move position and the use of a high-specification mattress, along with the use of a pressure-reducing device such as polymer gel pads, will reduce the risk of pressure sore development (Silverwood 2004).

When skeletal traction is in use, care of the pin sites is essential. The aim is to prevent infection which, if undetected or untreated, can develop into osteomyelitis. There may be variations in the care of pin sites; usually the dressings applied in theatre are left intact for the first 48 hours, then a regime of daily cleaning with normal saline is established. The sites are then left exposed. Observe for redness and swelling or presence of any exudate and report any changes to the medical staff.

Elimination

Changes in the child's usual bowel and bladder activities are common. Constipation frequently occurs owing to decreased gastrointestinal motility. A high-fibre diet and increased fluid intake can help. Bowel movements should be monitored. Urinary tract infections can also be an initial problem owing to awkward positioning and fear of using bedpans. Bed wetting due to regression in younger children is common.

Eating and drinking

This can be difficult because of the position of the patient, and reduced appetite can be expected. Frequent small meals should be encouraged and these can be in the form of milky drinks, or milk shakes, to promote high calcium intake. Fluid balance should be recorded.

Small children on gallows traction should always have their meal times supervised to prevent the dangers of choking.

Observations and complications

Trauma and constriction of a limb due to traction can cause disturbance to the circulatory system, the muscles and the nerve supply.

Neurovascular observations including colour, movement, sensation, pulse and pain should be recorded half hourly for the first 4 hours and then hourly for the first 24 hours following the injury and at least 12 hours following application of the traction. The orthopaedic team must be contacted immediately should any alterations in neurovascular observations occur.

The circulatory system

Circulatory problems are indicated by the change in colour of the injured limb, usually to a pale or blue colour, temperature change from warm to cool and the absence of a distal limb pulse.

The muscles

Damage to muscles can occur after injury or surgery to a limb. Muscle damage is known as acute compartment syndrome or Volkmann's ischaemic contracture. Early detection of damage to the muscle is critical as muscle, once infarcted, can never recover.

The signs and symptoms are:

- **Pain** – often disproportionate to the injury
- **Pallor** – a mottled, bluish or pale colour
- **Paraesthesia** – tingling or altered sensation
- **Paralysis** – inability to move the limb
- **Pulselessness** – absence of a distal pulse (Danby & Edwards 2001).

These are known as the five Ps. Not all symptoms are present at the same time. As with changes in the circulatory system, any change must be reported immediately.

Observation and monitoring of the above are undertaken for at least 24–48 hours at a frequency of half- to 1-hourly intervals according to the child's condition.

Joints

Joint stiffness can result from bad positioning and inactivity. Passive and active exercise taught by the physiotherapist can prevent this. Excessive traction force or overdistraction (more than 2.5 cm (1 inch) of buttock off the mattress), especially in gallows traction, must be avoided as this can cause damage to infants' hips.

Nerves

Nerve damage is indicated by numbness, pins and needles or altered sensation. Prolonged nerve damage can cause foot drop.

Osteomyelitis

Infection of the bone is a potential but serious hazard of skeletal traction. Observation for signs of infection around pin sites and regular cleansing are necessary.

COMMUNITY PERSPECTIVE

In some areas, orthopaedic surgeons are in favour of children with femoral fractures or congenital hip dislocation being nursed at home on traction for part of the treatment (Clayton 1997, Orr et al 1994). A child nursed on gallows traction or with a Thomas splint can be considered for home traction.

Prior to discharge

The child should be well established on traction and fractures should be stable.

Pain should be well controlled with oral analgesia.

Parents/carers must understand the principles of the traction, be familiar with the equipment and be able to recognise any problems.

The suitability of the home to accommodate the equipment must be assessed by the CCN. This includes measuring the doorways to ensure that frames will go through and that there is sufficient room to negotiate round corners. A ground floor room will be most suitable as the child will feel more included in family life. It has to be accepted that some homes will be unsuitable for this type of home care and the family's hopes should not be raised unrealistically.

Parents need to be aware of whom to call in an emergency. If the CCN is able to provide 24-hour cover, this is not a problem. If this facility is not available, it may be necessary to involve ward staff (Clayton 1997) or have a re-admission policy organised which would need to include the ambulance service. The family should have access to a telephone.

Liaison with the ambulance service will be necessary prior to discharge to prevent problems.

Parents should be aware of the dates of their outpatient appointments and transport should be arranged.

Equipment to be supplied by the hospital

- Traction frame either specially adapted (Clayton 1997) or a hospital bed
- Weights and pulleys
- Supply of traction extension kits, cord, bandages and securing tape
- Tincture benzoin compound
- Pressure-relieving device may be necessary (see Pressure Area Care, p. 321)
- Bedpan and urinal if required
- Incontinence aids if appropriate
- Hairwashing aids.

Following discharge

Initially, there should be daily visits by the CCN to check traction and pressure areas and ensure that the family are coping.

Strategies for relieving boredom can be suggested to the family. Work can be sent from school for the school-aged child. A home tutor may be arranged via the school education department.

All children will benefit from the involvement of a community play specialist if available.

Before the child returns to hospital for removal of the traction, the family will need information and reassurance concerning the child's mobility following the removal. They may also require information concerning physiotherapy.

Children can be cared for with home traction most successfully, but there will need to be commitment from both family and professionals.

Do and do not

- Do check the condition of equipment before assembly.
- Do size the patient correctly for traction to ensure comfort and maximum therapeutic outcome.
- Do ensure that traction pull is maintained at all times.
- Do check visible skin daily for signs of irritation or blistering.
- Do ensure that traction cords run in a straight line to aid smooth running in the pulleys.

- Do not allow traction cord to become knotted and frayed.
- Do not allow weights to rest on the floor – they must be free hanging.

- Do not bandage over the knee when the leg is in traction – the knee should be visible.

References

Clayton M 1997 Traction at home: the Doncaster approach. Paediatric Nursing 9(2): 21–23

Danby D J, Edwards D J 2001 Essential orthopaedics and trauma, 3rd edn. Churchill Livingstone, London

Department of Health 1996 Services for children and young people. HMSO, London

Folick M A, Carina-Garcia G, Birmingham J J 1994 Traction: assessment and management. Mosby, London

Houston M S 1996 Care of the school-aged child in 90/90 traction. Orthopaedic Nursing 15(2): 57–64

Orr D J, Simpson H D, John P J, Bell D W 1994 Home traction in the management of femoral fractures in children. Journal of the Royal College of Surgeons of Edinburgh 39(5): 329–331

Pickup S, Pagdin J 2000 Procedural pain: Entonox can help. Paediatric Nursing 12(10): 33–36

Pritchard A P, David J A 1990 The Royal Marsden manual of clinical procedures, 2nd edn. Harper and Row, London

Silverwood B 2004 Prevention of sore heels – evidence and outcomes. Paediatric Nursing 16(4): 14–18

Further Reading

Apley A P, Solomon L 2001 Concise system of orthopaedics and fractures, 2nd edn. Arnold, London

Benson M K D, Fixsen J A, MacNicol M F, Parsch K (eds) 2002 Children's orthopaedics and fractures, 2nd edn. Churchill Livingstone, London, p 464–477

Lee-Smith J, Santy J, Davis P, Jester R, Kneale J 2001 Pin site management. Toward a consensus: part 1. Journal of Orthopaedic Nursing 5(1): 37–42

Nicol D 1995 Understanding the principles of traction. Nursing Standard 9(46): 25–28

RCN 2003 Pinsite Care Project. Focus for research in orthopaedics group. RCN, London. Online. Available: www.man.ac.uk/rcn/ukwide/frogpinsite.htm

Spansella P D, Stevens H M 1996 Handbook of paediatric orthopaedics. Little, Brown, Boston, MA

Practice **35**

Urine testing and urinary catheterisation

Margaret Henderson, Karen Leitch

Introduction

Development of the urinary and renal system starts around the third week of fetal development and continues until the fetus reaches a gestational age of 34 weeks (Tortora & Grabowski 2003). At 34 weeks' gestation the urinary system is fully formed and the kidneys have their composite number of one million nephrons per kidney; however, these nephrons are immature and continue developing until around 12–18 months (Terrill 2002, Tortora & Grabowski 2003). The glomerulus of the fetal kidney will filter approximately 0.5 ml/min of filtrate prior to 34 weeks' gestation, increasing thereafter in a linear fashion with age to approximately 120 ml/min achieved during adolescence (Terrill 2002). In a healthy child, the volume and acidity of the urine and the concentration of solutes will vary according to the child's own metabolism. During pathological conditions, the composition of urine can change dramatically. An analysis of the chemical composition, the volume and the physical properties of the urine can tell us much about the metabolism of the child and the internal body environment (Poole 2002, Tortora & Grabowski 2003).

Learning outcomes

By the end of this section and following further reading and practice you should be able to:

- identify the normal constituents of urine
- correctly use urine-testing equipment
- recognise abnormal constituents in urine
- prepare a child and parents for urethral catheterisation
- select the appropriate size and type of urethral catheter
- safely insert a urethral catheter, minimising trauma and distress
- perform appropriate catheter care
- understand the need for suprapubic aspiration of urine
- provide comfort and support to child and parents during suprapubic aspiration
- understand the use of bladder irrigation
- recognise the need for bladder irrigation
- safely execute bladder irrigation.

Rationale

The examination of urine is the oldest clinical laboratory test. Performed either in the laboratory, or at ward level, urinalysis is one of the commonest clinical tests ordered and it can determine whether a child is dehydrated and/or infected, or has a renal or metabolic disorder (Liao & Churchill 2001, Poole 2002).

Factors to note

- Daily urinary output will vary with oral fluid intake, environmental temperature and the child's activity (Marshall 1995).

- Urine volume can also be influenced by blood pressure, diet, temperature and general health (Tortora & Grabowski 2003).

- Urinalysis is frequently performed both within the hospital and in the community.

- Urine is normally transparent and amber in colour with a variable odour.

- Urinary pH may range from as low as 4.5 to as high as 8.0, depending on the acid–base balance (Rigby 2004). Accurate measurement can be obtained only from freshly voided specimens.

- Specific gravity measures the ability of the kidney to concentrate or dilute the urine. High values indicate underhydration (Liao & Churchill 2001). The normal range is 1.001–1.025 (Cook 1996).

- Traces of protein (>200 mg/day), normally albumin and globulin, can be present, but are not detectable using strip reagent tests. This is normal and is insignificant (Marshall 1995, Cook 1996). Additionally, transient proteinuria may be seen in as many as 75% of febrile patients with little clinical significance (Liao & Churchill 2001).

- Minute traces of ketones and urobilinogen are normal in the urine; however, these are undetectable using strip reagent tests (Cook 1996). The diagnostic use of urobilinogen in urine is limited (Liao & Churchill 2001).

- A positive nitrite test indicates the presence of a significant number of bacteria in the urine (Poole 1999). The test is most sensitive when urine has been incubated in the bladder for approximately 4 hours. Bayer multistix are commonly used.

- A positive leucocyte esterase test results from the presence of significant leucocytes in the urine, common in people with a urinary tract infection (UTI) (Poole 1999); however, this does not necessarily indicate a UTI. The term pyuria refers to the presence of abnormal numbers of leucocytes (Liao & Churchill 2001).

- A urine sample can be obtained from an infant, or child, in a number of ways including midstream specimen for children who are toilet trained and have urethral sphincter control. For those who are not toilet trained, a specimen can be obtained by clean-catch urine or obtaining the specimen using a sterile bag or absorbent pad (Ramage et al 1999, Farrell et al 2002, Poole 2002).

– midstream specimens are the method of choice in cooperative children who are toilet trained. This method ensures that the bacteria of the periurethral area do not contaminate the specimen by omitting to collect the first urine (Poole 2002)

– clean-catch technique has been identified as being an efficient method for collecting a sterile urine specimen (Ramage et al 1999). However, the method can be time consuming and technically difficult

– bag specimens are obtained from attaching an adhesive sterile bag to the infant. Although an easy technique, there is a greater risk of bacterial contamination (Al-Orifi et al 2002)

– urine collection pads, launched in 1994, have been introduced widely within the NHS. This method is cheap and technically easy to use in infants; however, concern has been raised regarding the filtering effect of the pad fibres and reported high contamination rates (Farrell et al 2002, Poole 2002)

– suprapubic aspiration may be performed in emergency situations and will be addressed later in this section.

● The method used for urine sampling may be determined by the type of test that is being undertaken and may be considered as sterile or non-sterile, e.g. a specimen for bacteriological analysis will mean that there should be minimal contamination and would be regarded as a sterile specimen, whereas one required for biochemical analysis would not require a sterile specimen. In practice, however, bacteriological and biochemical tests are frequently done concurrently and therefore a sterile specimen would be obtained.

URINE TESTING

Urinalysis with reagent strips is a common routine examination seen both in the community and in hospital. It plays an important role in the diagnosis and screening of several diseases (Armstrong 2004). Urinalysis can also be used to monitor the progress of disease and in monitoring the efficacy of treatment. The reagent strips contain impregnated reagent areas and can test for one or more constituents when the reagent area comes into contact with the urine. Urinalysis with reagent strips is a cheap, reliable and simple non-invasive method of detecting and monitoring disease (Armstrong 2004).

The following practice guide refers to the testing of urine, using reagent strips, within the hospital or community setting.

Factors to note

● Urine examination can yield valuable information on the early signs of disease (Poole 2002, Armstrong 2004).
● Careful and accurate use of reagent strips for urine testing can prove to be cost-effective as this may help to reduce the number of sterile specimens that are analysed within the laboratory (Armstrong 2004). Reagent strips are also used within the laboratory setting. The use of an automated urine chemistry analyser has been shown to improve accuracy of urine testing (Rowell 1998).
● If urine is not to be tested within 1 hour of being obtained, the specimen can be stored in a refrigerator until such time as it can be tested, when the specimen should be allowed to return to room temperature (Cook 1996).

Equipment

● Reagent strips
● Manufacturer's instruction for use
● Manufacturer's colour chart
● Urine container
● Stopwatch/watch with second hand
● Recording chart
● Non-sterile latex-free gloves
● Automated analyse (if available).

Method

1. Explain to both the child and parent the reason for the test and how the specimen is to be collected.

2. Obtain a sample of urine in a suitable container, which should be clean, dry and free from contaminants (Poole 2002).
3. Check the expiry date on the bottle of test strips; ensure that the test strips are not damp.
4. Read the instructions carefully.
5. Wearing non-sterile gloves, dip the reagent strip into the fresh urine specimen, ensuring that all reagent areas are covered. Remove immediately and tap the edge of the strip on the side of the urine container to remove excess urine.
6. Closely observe the reagent strip areas and compare with the manufacturer's colour charts at the stated times. If using an automated analyser, follow the manufacturer's instructions.
7. Record the findings on an appropriate recording chart and report any abnormalities.
8. Replace the cap on the container tightly and store as per manufacturer's instructions.

Observations and complications

- Preferably use a fresh urine sample.
- Urine which has been stored in the refrigerator should be returned to room temperature before testing.
- Check that the reagent strips are dry and have not exceeded their expiry dates.
- Ensure accurate timing by using a stopwatch or a watch with a second hand. Inaccurate timing will give false results.
- Check the reagent area with the manufacturer's colour chart at the appropriate time.
- Always replace the lid of the bottle immediately after use, ensuring that it is tightly closed.

Do and do not

- Do ensure that the reagent areas are fully covered with urine.
- Do ensure accurate timing prior to comparing with the colour chart.
- Do record results on the appropriate chart.
- Do send a specimen of urine to the bacteriology laboratory for analysis should blood or protein be detected. This may indicate infection.
- Do send a specimen of urine to the bacteriology laboratory if the specimen is foul smelling, cloudy, dark red/brown in colour. This may indicate infection.
- Do not use damp reagent strips.
- Do not cut the strips as this may alter their effectiveness.
- Do not check more than one urine specimen at a time.

URETHRAL CATHETERISATION

Urethral catheterisation is the insertion of a drainage device into the urinary bladder, using an aseptic technique, to drain the bladder of urine (NHS QIS 2004). Catheterisation can be intermittent or continuous, when the catheter is referred to as being indwelling (Pomfret 2000, Robinson 2001). Intermittent catheterisation is commonly used where the child has a neurogenic bladder.

The following practice guide is focused on the catheterisation of the acutely ill child or the child requiring investigation. Adaptations to the practice may be made for intermittent catheterisation of the chronically ill child or the child with long-term urinary problems, as indicated below.

Factors to note

- Urethral catheterisation may be performed for many reasons including the relief of urinary retention, following surgery to rest or help heal the bladder or urethra, to dilate a urethral stricture, and for diagnostic testing such as voiding cystogram or urodynamics. In rare circumstances it may be performed to obtain a specimen of urine (Campbell & Glasper 1995, Gray 1996, Robinson 2001, Sanders 2001).
- Intermittent catheterisation may be performed on children. This may be necessary for children with neurogenic bladder as a result of myelomeningocele. This is performed at home by the parents and/or the child and is a clean procedure rather than aseptic. Where nursing staff perform the procedure, whether in the community or hospital

setting, then the procedure should be aseptic to reduce the risk of infection (NHS QIS 2004).

- For intermittent catheterisation, the genital area may be cleansed with soap and water and thoroughly dried.

- Relaxation exercises may be taught to the child.

- The use of anaesthetic lubricant is indicated in both boys and girls (MacKenzie & Webb 1995, Gray 1996).

- It is now thought to be safer to use single-use catheters (single non-ballooned) for intermittent catheterisation (Addison 2001).

- Urinary catheters manufactured within the UK must conform to British Standard BS1695; thus they are tested to ensure a high level of safety (Willis 1995a). European Community guidelines for medical equipment are also adhered to.

- The choice of catheter is important and based not only on the child's urethral size but also on the reasons for use and whether or not the catheter is to be indwelling (EPIC 2001, Robinson 2001, 2004). Accurate assessment of the patient along with evidence-based decision making, record keeping (time and date of insertion, type of catheter and any complications). Type and size of catheter are increasingly important aspects of care (Buckley 1999, EPIC 2001, NHS QIS 2004). MDA (2001) clearly advocates that a device should only be used for the purpose for which it is intended. This calls into question the use of polyvinyl chloride (PVC) nasogastric tubes in neonates identified by Gray (1996). Smith (2003) identifies this practice as persisting, primarily as a result of suitable catheters not being available for their use. Smith urges that practitioners raise this with the manufacturers.

- Consideration needs to be given to latex allergy when selecting a urethral catheter. Urethral catheters are made from silicone, PVC and latex, and therefore appropriate catheters are available for children with latex allergy.

- Suprapubic catheterisation is becoming more common and at times preferable to urethral catheterisation. This may be used following bladder and ureteric surgery if there is a urethral problem (e.g. stricture), or if a child/family chooses this option for long-term urinary management (Sanders 2001, NHS QIS 2004).

Equipment

- Sterile dressing pack
- Two pairs of sterile latex-free gloves
- Appropriate size of catheter
- Cleansing solution, e.g. sterile sodium chloride
- Lidocaine gel
- Appropriate size of syringe for lidocaine gel (if required)
- Sterile water (for catheter balloon)
- Appropriate size of syringe for sterile water
- Urinary drainage bag.

Method

1. A careful explanation of the procedure and reasons for it being needed should be given to the child and parent.
2. The parent may be asked to comfort and support the child during the procedure.
3. The child may be sedated prior to catheter insertion. Sedation is prescribed by the medical staff.
4. Asepsis is important to prevent infection (EPIC 2001).
5. Select an appropriate catheter size (see Table 35.1).
6. Prepare sterile equipment.
7. Wearing sterile gloves, cleanse the urethral meatus with the cleansing solution (NHS QIS 2004).
8a. *For girls:* gently separate the labia and cleanse the meatus thoroughly, cleansing the full length of the labia from the front to back (Rushing 2004).
8b. *For boys:* gently retract the foreskin and cleanse the entire surface of the glans penis. Replace the foreskin once dry (Simpson 2002).
9. Gently pat the genitalia dry with a clean sterile swab.

Table 35.1 Selecting an appropriate size-for-age urethral catheter (Gray 1996)

Age of child	Size of catheter	Rationale
Infants (0–1 year)	6–8 French Foley catheter	Small French Foley catheters are preferred for long-term drainage or where urinary debris is present. Catheters are manufactured using inert material, which reduces urethral discomfort
13 months to 12 years	6–8 French Foley catheter with 3 ml retention balloon	Preferred to feeding tube for prolonged drainage. Standard balloon sizes preferred over larger sizes, which increase bladder neck irritation and bladder spasm
13–18 years	8–14 French Foley catheter with 5 ml retention balloon	Smaller sizes promote comfort and adequate drainage

10. Insert 2–3 ml (up to 10 ml for older children) of lidocaine local anaesthetic gel into the urethra, using the nozzle provided (Gray 1996).
11. Allow 3–5 minutes for the gel to have full effect.
12. Change gloves to ensure the utmost protection against infection.
13. Cover the catheter with more lubricant and gently insert it into the urethra until urine is obtained. Allow the urine to flow into a sterile container. Obtain a specimen, if required, for bacteriology.
14. Insufflate the catheter balloon (if used) with the appropriate amount of water as instructed by the manufacturer. Overfilling the catheter balloon may cause the balloon to rupture or cause bladder irritation (Robinson 2004).
15. For the neonate, if the catheter is to be indwelling and does not have a balloon, it should be secured to the infant with surgical tape in such a fashion as to prevent undue tension.
16. Attach the urine drainage bag.
17. Reassure the child and parent.

Observations and complications

- An assistant to help with catheterisation is essential. Parents should **not** be used for this role.
- Assemble all equipment prior to going to the child and parent.

- Ensure that the anaesthetic gel has taken effect prior to inserting the catheter.
- Insert the catheter gently, using aseptic technique.
- Do not use excessive force to insert the catheter. Contact medical staff if any difficulty with insertion is experienced.
- Obtain a specimen of urine for bacteriology prior to attaching the drainage bag.
- Ensure that urine is flowing freely before insufflating the catheter balloon (if applicable) or securing the catheter (Belfield 1998).
- Ensure that there are no kinks in tubing and that the drainage bag is properly positioned (see Catheter care, below).

Do and do not

- Do ensure that the catheter is secured in position.
- Do ensure that anaesthetic lubricant gel is used in both girls and boys.
- Do ensure that sterile gloves are changed prior to insertion of the catheter.
- Do record the type/size of catheter and the amount of water in the balloon in the child's nursing documentation (Buckley 1999).
- Do ensure that a trusted chaperone is present to support a child who has been, or is suspected of having been, sexually abused.

- Do not use excessive amounts of lubricant jelly as this may lead to infection (Willis 1995a).
- Do not use excessive force when advancing the catheter.
- Do not continue with the procedure if the child is extremely distressed.

CATHETER CARE

Following urethral catheterisation, the care of the catheter is of the utmost importance. The primary aim of catheter care is to reduce infection, which accounts for some 30% of hospital-acquired infection in adult patients (Winn 1996). Although indwelling urethral catheters are uncommon in children, it is important to ensure that the risk of infection is reduced, as they are often used in children who are acutely unwell and at their most vulnerable and susceptible.

Catheter-associated infection is a concern with indwelling catheters for prolonged periods, e.g. acquired UTI. The risk of infection with routine catheterisation is 1–2% per procedure; the risk with indwelling catheters is 5% risk per day, accumulating (Tambyah & Maki 2002). Short-term catheterisation is intermittent and up to 14 days; long term is >14 days (Getliffe 1995).

Factors to note

- There are two main routes of bacterial infection in the catheterised child:

  - periurethral: bacteria travelling between the urethral wall and the outside of the catheter
  - intraluminal: bacteria travelling up the inside of the catheter lumen (Willis 1995b).

- Maintaining urethral meatus hygiene is of utmost importance in preventing periurethral infection. Maintaining meatal hygiene with soap and water is now thought to be sufficient (EPIC 2001). The use of antiseptic solutions is not recommended.

- As important as the insertion of the indwelling catheter, is the removal. This is partly due to the fact that whilst the catheter is in situ, the bladder is shrunk (empty) and the insufflated balloon comes into contact with the bladder wall and can cause irritation and haematuria. A high-capacity balloon sits higher in the bladder and can rest on the trigone, at times causing spasm, irritation, haematuria and erosion of the bladder wall. It is essential to ensure that the balloon is fully deflated prior to removal and to remove with extreme care as the balloon can become creased and cause trauma to the urethra (Semjonow et al 1995, Robinson 2000, MDA 2001).

- Urinary pH has been recognised as being a contributory factor in catheter encrustation (Sanders 2001, Rigby 2004). An increase in urinary pH is thought to be the result of bacterial infection, which causes an increase in bacterial colonisation of the catheter surface and subsequent encrustation (Getliffe 2002).

- Increasing fluid intake to prevent catheter blockage, by reducing or preventing infection, is not indicated; however, maintaining a balanced diet will help to prevent susceptibility to infection (Getliffe 1995, Wilson 1996, Pomfret 2000).

Equipment

- Catheter bag holder
- Alcohol wipes (for cleansing drainage port of catheter bag)
- Urine container
- Latex-free gloves and apron.

Method

1. Catheter care commences with the selection and insertion of the urethral catheter (see Urethral catheterisation, above).
2. Ensuring a closed system is important in reducing infection (NHS QIS 2004). However, all systems have points of entry for infection, normally at connection sites (Pomfret 2000).
3. Selection of drainage equipment is dictated by the reasons for catheterisation. Some drainage bags are designed for hourly or more frequent urinary volume measurement. Some are drainable, with others being totally closed.

4. Always ensure that the catheter drainage bag is kept below the level of the bladder. This ensures good drainage and prevents backflow of urine. Some bags may be fitted with a non-reflux valve; however, it is good practice to position the bag below bladder level to ensure that there is minimal chance of backflow.

5. Use an appropriate catheter bag hanger for suspending the bag. This should prevent contact of the bag with the floor (EPIC 2001).

6. When emptying the catheter bag, wear gloves and apron. Clean the drainage tap with an alcohol wipe before and after emptying, and empty the urine into a clean container.

7. Urine drainage bags should be emptied frequently enough to maintain urine flow and prevent reflux (EPIC 2001). Drainage bags should not become more than two-thirds full before emptying (NHS QIS 2004).

8. Cleanse the urethral meatus with soap and water (Pomfret 2000). This can be performed during the child's normal bath-time routine (EPIC 2001).

9. Cleansing the urethra twice daily, morning and evening, is considered sufficient (Willis 1995b).

10a. *For girls:* cleanse the labia majora, then the labia minora followed by the urethral meatus and down the catheter for approximately 3 cm. Dry the area.

10b. *For boys:* cleanse around the glans penis by retracting the foreskin, then cleanse from the urethral meatus down the catheter for approximately 3 cm. Dry and replace the foreskin over the glans penis. In young boys it is not desirable to retract the foreskin, as this may cause discomfort.

11. Always ensure that hands are washed before and after care.

Observations and complications

● Ensure that the catheter is secured with tape to the child's upper inner thigh. This will help prevent undue traction on the catheter.

● Use a catheter bag holder to ensure that the bag does not come into contact with the floor.

● Ensure that hands are washed before and after emptying the catheter bag. Gloves should also be worn.

Do and do not

● Do involve parents.
● Do tape the catheter to the thigh to prevent undue traction.
● Do ensure that the urethral meatus is clear of debris.
● Do ensure that gloves are worn when cleaning the urethral meatus.
● Do keep the urine drainage bag below the level of the bladder.
● Do clean the drainage outlet before and after emptying.
● Do not allow the drainage bag to rest on the floor.
● Do not use a variety of different cleansing agents for cleansing the meatus.

BLADDER IRRIGATION

Children with an indwelling urethral catheter may require bladder irrigation to relieve catheter blockage, the most common cause of which is encrustation of the catheter surface caused by mineral constituents of the urine (Winn 1996, Robinson 2004). In boys following hypospadias repair, where a urethral catheter has been inserted to aid urinary drainage and/or act as a stent, blockage of the catheter may occur, necessitating bladder irrigation (Ellsworth et al 1999).

Factors to note

● Catheter blockage can be caused by bladder spasm, twisting of the tube or constipation (Simpson 2001). Each of these should be considered if a child's urinary catheter drainage diminishes.
● Urine infection is known to increase the incidence of catheter blockage (Pomfret 2000).
● Urine infection produces an alkaline urine which encourages encrustations (Simpson 2001).

- Citric acid solutions may be used to dissolve crystals that have formed as a result of alkaline urine. Mandelic acid solution will help reduce microorganisms which produce urease creating alkaline conditions. Sodium chloride (0.9%) can be used to flush out blood, pus and mucus (NHS QIS 2004).
- Bladder washout does not prevent catheter-associated infection. Using antibiotic solutions for bladder instillations is not effective in treating catheter-associated infection.

Equipment

- Sterile dressing pack
- Sterile latex-free gloves
- Sterile solution for irrigation
- Syringe (catheter-tipped if required)
- Drainage bag (if required)
- Sterile bowl for collecting returned fluid.

Method

1. Where possible, a closed system should be used, e.g. Urotainer system. However, it must be noted that performing a bladder irrigation will entail the opening of the closed system with the potential for introducing infection. Always follow the manufacturer's instructions when using these bladder irrigation solutions.
2. Explain to the child and parent the need for the bladder irrigation and what will happen.
3. This is an aseptic procedure and sterile equipment should be used.
4. Select an appropriate volume of bladder irrigation solution. The volume used will be dependent on the child's bladder capacity. Different volumes of solution in 'closed containers' are now available.
5. Wearing sterile gloves, clean the connection between the catheter and drainage bag (if used) with antiseptic solution, approximately 2.5 cm (1 inch) above and below the connection.
6. Disconnect the drainage bag from the catheter and attach the syringe/solution container.

7. Push the fluid into the catheter following the manufacturer's instructions. This will flush out the inside of the catheter.
8. Disconnect the syringe from the catheter and allow the fluid to drain into a sterile receptacle.
9. Repeat the procedure until the returned fluid flows freely.
10. Clean the insertion end of the catheter and attach a new drainage bag (if required).
11. Record the total amount of fluid used and returned.

Observations and complications

- Prepare equipment prior to collecting the child.
- Ensure that the solution has been warmed to room temperature prior to insertion.
- Ensure accurate recording of all fluid instilled and drained.
- Observe the returned fluid for clarity, blood or any particles.

Do and do not

- Do ensure that the bladder irrigation fluid is at room temperature prior to insertion.
- Do use a closed system if available.
- Do record the volume of fluid instilled and returned.
- Do observe the returned fluid for clarity, blood and particles.
- Do not use excessive force to instil fluid.
- Do not apply negative pressure, using the syringe, to drain the bladder.

SUPRAPUBIC ASPIRATION

Suprapubic aspiration of urine is performed by experienced medical staff to obtain a sterile specimen of urine for urinary investigation in infants and children less than 2 years old. This technique is used when the specimen is required urgently, dictated by the child's condition, normally when the child is unable to produce a specimen by clean-catch technique. Suprapubic aspiration should be performed when the urinary bladder is known to contain urine, normally if the child has not passed urine for 1 hour or the bladder is palpable above the symphysis pubis and is considered the best way to minimise bacterial contamination (Campbell & Glasper 1995, Jakobson & Esbjorner 1999).

Factors to note

- Suprapubic aspiration of urine is usually performed in young children who are not toilet trained, normally less than 2 years of age and who are very unwell, a specimen of urine being required to rule out urinary tract infection (Carter & Dearmun 1995).
- It is important that the child's bladder contains urine; therefore this procedure should only be performed if the child has not passed urine for at least 1 hour.
- Although invasive, this method of specimen collection is the technique of choice in the sick febrile infant. The use of ultrasound assistance improves success rates in obtaining a urine sample (Ramage et al 1999).

Equipment

- Sterile dressing pack
- 70% alcohol
- Sterile latex-free gloves
- 5–10 ml syringe
- Size 20, 21 and 22 gauge needles
- Airstrip dressing
- Sterile urine container.

Method

1. Explain to the parent the need for the bladder aspiration.

2. The parent may wish to comfort the child during the procedure. This should be encouraged; however, the parents should not be coerced as they may find the aspiration distressing.
3. This is an aseptic procedure; therefore a sterile technique should be used.
4. The child should be in a supine position with legs in the frog-leg position and securely restrained to prevent undue movement.
5. The area above the child's symphysis pubis should be cleaned with 70% alcohol and allowed to dry.
6. A member of the medical staff will insert the needle into the bladder approximately 1 cm above the pubic bone at a 90 degree angle.
7. Urine is then aspirated from the bladder.
8. The needle is then withdrawn. Pressure should be applied to the insertion site for 1–2 minutes. A dry dressing, e.g. Airstrip, should be applied.
9. The urine should be put into an appropriate sterile urine container and sent for bacterial or biochemical analysis.

Observations and complications

- Ensure that the child is firmly held in the supine position during the procedure.
- Ensure that pressure is applied to the needle insertion site once the needle is removed. This helps to stem bleeding and leakage of urine.
- Advise parents that some fresh blood may be present in the urine for a short period following the procedure.
- Observe the child for signs of increasing abdominal pain, as bowel perforation during the procedure is possible.

COMMUNITY PERSPECTIVE

There will be situations where parents are taught to test their child's urine, e.g. to monitor protein levels in Henoch–Schönlein purpura and nephrotic syndrome, and glucose in diabetes. The families will be in direct contact with the hospital and are likely to have been taught the techniques prior to discharge. The role of the CCN will be to ensure that the parents are confident and to occasionally check techniques.

The CCN may be involved in teaching parents or children the technique of intermittent self-catheterisation, and in some cases will be asked to support Learning Support Assistants in schools who care for children with catheters. This may be undertaken by the continence advisor.

Do and do not

- Do ensure that the child is held firmly.
- Do observe the insertion site for signs of bleeding.
- Do observe nappies for haematuria.
- Do not perform the procedure if the child has voided urine within the previous hour.
- Do not coerce parents or carers into holding the child firmly.

References

Addison R 2001 Intermittent self catheterisation. Nursing Times 67(20): 67–69

Al-Orifi F, McGillivray D, Tange S, Kramer M 2002 Urine culture from bag specimens in young children: are the risks too high? Journal of Pediatrics 137(2): 221–226

Armstrong K 2004 Urinalysis. Practice Nurse 27(4): 25–30

Belfield P 1998 Urinary catheters. British Medical Journal 296(6625): 836–837

Buckley R 1999 Keep it legal. Nursing Times 95(6): 75–77

Campbell S, Glasper E A (eds) 1995 Whaley and Wong's children's nursing. Mosby, London, ch 8

Carter B, Dearmun A K 1995 Child health care nursing – concepts theory and practice. Blackwell Science, Oxford, UK

Cook R 1996 Urinalysis: ensuring accurate urine testing. Nursing Standard 10(46): 49–52

Ellsworth P, Cendron M, Ritland D, McCullough M 1999 Hypospadias repair in the 90's. AORN Journal 69(1): 148–150, 152–153, 155–156

EPIC 2001 Guidelines for preventing infections associated with the insertion and maintenance of short term indwelling urethral catheters in acute care. Journal of Hospital Infection 47(Suppl): S239–246

Farrell M, Devine K, Lancaster G, Judd B 2002 A method comparison study to assess the reliability of urine collection pads as a means of obtaining urine specimens from non-toilet trained children for microbiological examination. Journal of Advanced Nursing 37(4): 387–393

Getliffe K 1995 Care of urinary catheters. Nursing Standard 10(1): 25–29

Getliffe K 2002 Managing recurrent urinary catheter encrustation. British Journal of Community Nursing 7(11): 574–580

Gray M 1996 Atraumatic urethral catheterisation of children. Pediatric Nursing 22(4): 306–310

Jakobson B, Esbjorner E 1999 Minimum incidence and diagnostic rate of first urinary tract infection. Pediatrics 104(2): 222–227

Liao J, Churchill B 2001 Paediatric urine testing. Paediatric Clinics of North America 48(6): 1425–1434

MacKenzie J, Webb C 1995 Gynopia in nursing practice: the case of urethral catheterisation. Journal of Clinical Nursing 4: 221–226

Marshall W J 1995 Illustrated textbook of clinical chemistry, 3rd edn. Lippincott Gower, London

MDA 2001 Problems removing urinary catheters. SN2001(02). Medical Devices Agency, London

NHS QIS 2004 Urinary catheterisation and catheter care. Best practice statement. NHS Quality Improvement Scotland, Edinburgh

Pomfret L 2000 Catheter care in the community. Nursing Standard 14(27): 46–51

Poole C 1999 The use of urinary dipstix in children with high risk renal tracts. British Journal of Nursing 8(8): 512–516

Poole C 2002 Diagnosis and management of urinary tract infection in children. Nursing Standard 16(38): 47–55

Pullen R L 2004 Inserting an indwelling urinary catheter in a male patient. Nursing 34(7): 24

Ramage I J, Chapman J P, Hollman A S 1999 Accuracy of clean-catch urine collection in infancy. Journal of Pediatrics 135(6): 765–767

Rigby D 2004 pH testing in catheter maintenance: the clinical debate. British Journal of Community Nursing 9(5): 189–194

Robinson J 2000 Removing catheters. Journal of Community Nursing 14(12): 8

Robinson J 2001 Urethral catheter selection. Nursing Standard 15(25): 39–42

Robinson J 2004 A practical approach to catheter-associated problems. Nursing Standard 18(31): 38–42

Rowell D M 1998 Evaluation of a urine chemistry analyser. Professional Nurse 13(8): 533–534

Rushing J 2004 Inserting an indwelling urinary catheter in a female patient. Nursing 34(8): 22

Sanders C 2001 Suprapubic catheterisation risk management. Paediatric Nursing 13(10): 14–18

Semjonow A, Roth S, Hertle L 1995 Reducing trauma whilst removing long-term indwelling balloon catheters. British Journal of Urology 75(2): 241

Simpson L 2001 Indwelling urethral catheters. Nursing Standard 15(46): 47–54, 56

Simpson L 2002 Patient information: 4. Intermittent self-catheterisation. Nursing Standard 16(29): Essential Skills Booklet

Smith L 2003 Which catheter? Criteria for selection of urinary catheters for children. Paediatric Nursing 15(3): 14–18

Tambyah P A, Maki D G 2002 Catheter-associated urinary tract infection is rarely symptomatic: a prospective study of 1497 catheterized patients. Archives of Internal Medicine 160(5): 673–677

Terrill B 2002 Renal nursing: a guide to practice. Radcliffe Medical Press, Oxon, UK

Tortora G J, Grabowski S R 2003 Principles of anatomy and physiology, 10th edn. Wiley, New York

White M, Oliver H 1997 Developing guidelines on catheterisation in schools. Professional Nurse 12(12): 855–858

Willis J 1995a Intermittent catheters. Professional Nurse 10(8): 523–528

Willis J 1995b Catheters. Urinary tract infections. Nursing Times 91(35): 48–49

Wilson M 1996 Control of infection in catheterisation. Nurse Prescriber/Community Nurse 2(2): 31–32

Winn C 1996 Basing catheter care on research principles. Nursing Standard 10(18): 38–40

Further Reading

Greaves J, Buckmaster A 2001 Abolishing the bag: quality assurance project on urine collection. Journal of Paediatrics and Child Health 37(5); 437–440

Lowthian P 1998 The dangers of long-term catheter drainage. British Journal of Nursing 7(7): 366–397

Practice **36**

Venepuncture and cannulation

Maureen Lilley

Introduction

Children may require blood sampling or the insertion of an intravenous cannula for many reasons, including the monitoring of the progress of a condition, the administration of medicine or the administration of fluids, blood or nutrition.

In the majority of circumstances the children's nurse will be assisting medical staff in this procedure by providing support to the child during the procedure.

However, more recently, some nurses have been extending their scope of professional practice to include venepuncture and intravenous cannulation.

Learning outcomes

By the end of this section you should be able to:

- demonstrate an awareness of the differences between arteries and veins
- identify the common sites for venepuncture and intravenous cannulation
- support the child during the procedure
- choose the appropriate size of intravenous cannula/needle for the individual child
- safely perform venepuncture/intravenous cannulation if extending the scope of practice under supervision and as per local policy
- apply the necessary precautions to prevent dislodgement of the needle/cannula
- safely dispose of equipment used during the procedure.

Rationale

Obtaining access to the blood vessel of a child is a relatively common occurrence within paediatric practice. However, it should be borne in mind that obtaining a blood sample or insertion of an intravenous cannula is a traumatic and distressing event for the child and parents. The children's nurse plays an important role during this procedure, not only in the provision of support and comfort to the child and/or parents but also in providing expert assistance to the healthcare professional obtaining the blood sample or inserting the intravenous cannula. Firm support of the child will help to reduce the distress that they may be experiencing.

Children's nurses, in a variety of settings, are extending their scope of professional practice to include such areas as venepuncture and intravenous cannulation.

Guidance from the Nursing and Midwifery Council (NMC) emphasises knowledge and skills as prerequisites for taking the responsibility for practice (Davies 1998, NMC 2002).

Factors to note

- Intravenous access may be more difficult to obtain in young children owing to the size of their veins and the possibility of the veins being covered with subcutaneous fat, as well as their level of cooperation (Willock et al 2004).

- Both arteries and veins are composed of three layers or tunics and have a hollow core called the lumen (Tortora & Grabowski 2003).

- Arteries contain blood at higher pressure than within veins, with the blood moving within the artery in a pulsatile manner caused by the longitudinal arrangement of smooth muscle. Arterial blood is brighter in colour than venous blood.

- When an artery is punctured, the blood will leave in a pulsatile fashion. Greater quantities of blood can be lost from an artery; however, constriction of the walls of the artery helps to delay the escape of blood (Tortora & Grabowski 2003).

- Veins have less elastic tissue and smooth muscle than arteries; however, they contain more white fibrous tissue.

- Veins are distensible and adapt to changes in volume and pressure. Gentle squeezing of the area above a vein will cause the blood to pool within the vein and the vein to become palpable.

- Veins tend to be more superficial than arteries.

- The pressure of the blood within the vein is low and when the vein is punctured the blood will tend to flow out of the vein evenly.

- The venous anatomy differs in each individual child; hence a thorough examination of all possible sites will help relieve distress by identifying the best site. Possible sites for intravenous cannulation and venepuncture are displayed in Figure 36.1. Care must be taken to avoid adjacent structures, e.g. arteries, nerves.

- Accidental puncture of an artery may cause painful spasm and will result in prolonged bleeding.

- If the nerve is touched severe pain may result.

- Venepuncture and intravenous cannulation are painful procedures. The use of local

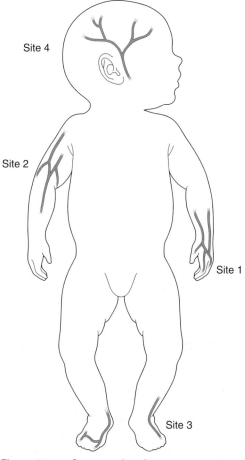

Figure 36.1 Common sites for venepuncture

topical anaesthetic cream has been proven to reduce the pain of these procedures. EMLA (eutectic mixture of local anaesthetic) cream is one such cream that is universally used in children (Riendeau 1999). In children less than 6 months of age, the use of EMLA cream is contraindicated as the risk of methaemoglobinaemia is thought to be increased (Brisman et al 1998) and therefore EMLA cream is only licensed in the UK for children aged 1 year and over. Tetracaine gel (Ametop) is another local anaesthetic and can be used in children/infants over 1 month old (Hewitt 1998, Jain & Rutter 2000). Local topical anaesthetics should be applied as prescribed by medical practitioners.

- Methaemoglobinaemia is a condition wherein the haemoglobin of the blood has been altered to a form that cannot transport oxygen (Wong 2003).

- EMLA cream should be applied 1 hour prior to the needle puncture; Ametop can be applied 30 minutes prior to procedure. A thick layer of cream/gel should be applied over the site and should be covered with an occlusive or semi-permeable dressing, e.g. Tegaderm (Hewitt 1998, Willock et al 2004).

- It is important to have a thorough examination of all sites to ensure that the best site is chosen. Distal sites should be used to preserve the proximal sites in case the initial attempts are unsuccessful (Wong 2003).

- Some hospitals/trusts employ phlebotomy technicians to perform venepuncture and cannulation. Healthcare assistants may also be trained to perform these tasks.

- Registered nurses should be fully conversant with the NMC *Code of Conduct* (2002) if considering extending their scope of practice within this area.

VENEPUNCTURE

Venepuncture is the term used for the procedure of entering a vein with a needle, normally for the purposes of obtaining a blood sample for laboratory analysis.

Equipment

- Correct size of needle/butterfly needle
- Tourniquet
- Gauze swabs or equivalent for spillage whilst sampling
- Syringe(s)
- Appropriate blood sampling bottles (correctly labelled)
- Swabs soaked in 70% alcohol (e.g. Mediswab)
- Non-sterile, latex-free gloves
- Cotton wool balls/gauze swabs
- Spot plasters.

METHOD

1. Explain the procedure to the child and parents prior to the venepuncture.
2. Always examine all potential sites to ensure that the best vein is obtained. Ensure that this is explained to the child. Common sites used for venepuncture are the back of the hand and the antecubital fossa; however, the feet and scalp may be used (see Fig. 36.1, site numbers 1–4).
3. Once sites have been identified, apply local topical anaesthetic, as prescribed, to the two most suitable sites for venepuncture and cover with a dressing.
4. Firmly hold the child's limb and provide tourniquet by gently squeezing the limb. Parents can support and hold the child, to reassure them, but should not be used to provide tourniquet. Apply tourniquet if no-one is available to assist.
5. Wipe off the local topical anaesthetic.
6. Warming child's limb will help the vein to dilate.
7. Palpate the vein to ascertain its calibre and direction. (Palpation – evaluate the vein by gently placing finger tips over the protruding vein.)
8. Wash hands prior to commencing the procedure.
9. The area should be cleaned with an alcohol-impregnated swab, e.g. Mediswab, and allowed to dry.

10. Wearing non-sterile, latex-free gloves, insert the needle into the vein approximately 0.5–1 cm at a 30 degree angle.
11. Because of the size and calibre of a child's veins, a flow-back of blood may not always be seen.
12. Withdraw the appropriate amount of blood and instil into appropriate blood bottles. Paediatric vacuum systems are available for obtaining blood samples and should be used wherever possible.
13. Once all samples have been obtained, release the tourniquet, place a cotton wool ball or gauze swab over the insertion site and withdraw the needle. Then apply pressure over the site for approximately 2–3 minutes.
14. Once bleeding has stopped, a dry dressing, e.g. Airstrip dressing, may be applied if the child does not have an allergy to this type of dressing.
15. Reassure the child and parents during the procedure and afterwards.
16. Dispose of waste and sharps as per local policy.
17. Most areas now give the child a bravery award following venepuncture. This may be a sticker, a badge or a certificate.

INTRAVENOUS CANNULATION

Peripheral intravenous cannulation is required when a child is to receive intravenous fluid therapy or intravenous medication. An intravenous cannula consists of a plastic catheter, which is inserted with the aid of a stylet or needle placed in the lumen of the catheter with the sharp point protruding from the end.

Equipment

- Correct size of intravenous cannula
- Tourniquet
- Gauze swabs or soft paper for spillages whilst cannulating
- T piece or equivalent, primed with heparin sodium (Hepsal) or 0.9% sodium chloride
- Tape to secure cannula: this should be Transpore or a sterile dressing for intravenous use, e.g. IV 3000

- Bandage
- Splint for limb/cover for cannula site (if sited in scalp)
- Swabs soaked in 70% alcohol (e.g. Mediswab)
- Latex-free gloves
- Hepsal to flush inserted cannula
- Intravenous administration set if fluids required
- Fluids or drugs as per drug prescription sheet
- Appropriate drug prescription sheet (as per hospital policy)
- Syringes if blood sampling
- Appropriate blood-sampling bottles correctly labelled.

Method

1. Examine potential cannulation sites thoroughly. Apply local topical anaesthetic as prescribed.
2. If the scalp vein is chosen, consent should be obtained from the parents for the shaving of the section of head. The parents may wish to keep the sample of hair.
3. Select the appropriate size of intravenous cannula.
4. Cut tape to desired length.
5. Gently hold/support the child in a supine position if possible. Parents can assist in supporting their child and providing reassurance during the cannulation, if they feel able to do so.
6. Wipe off topical anaesthetic and clean site with an alcohol-impregnated swab. Allow to dry.
7. Apply tourniquet to aid identification of the best vein for cannulation, particularly if no-one is available to assist.
8. Insert the cannula at a 15–30 degree angle, advance the catheter and withdraw the stylet needle. A flash-back of blood should be seen before advancing the catheter.
9. Securely tape the cannula in place (see Fig. 36.2).
10. Flush the cannula as per local policy to maintain patency.
11. Immobilise the limb using a suitable splint, which immobilises the joint close to the

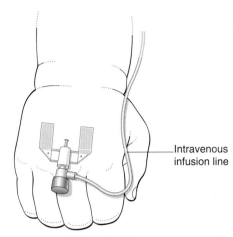

Figure 36.2   Taping of an intravenous cannula to secure its position

Intravenous infusion line

site of insertion, hence preventing excessive movement (see Fig. 36.3).

12. Protect a scalp cannula using a gallipot (see Fig. 36.4).

13. Attach an intravenous fluid administration set to the cannula if it is to be used for intravenous therapy.

14. Apply a sterile SmartSite (needle-free system) if the cannula is to be used for intravenous medication.

15. Dispose of waste and sharps as per local policy.

Observations and complications

● Ensure that blood flows freely and that there is no swelling at the insertion site.

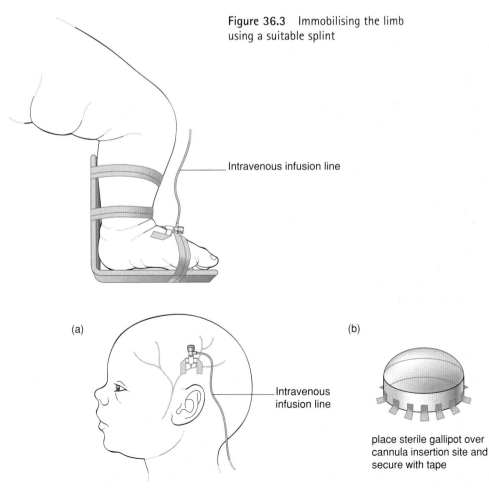

Figure 36.3   Immobilising the limb using a suitable splint

Intravenous infusion line

(a)

(b)

Intravenous infusion line

place sterile gallipot over cannula insertion site and secure with tape

Figure 36.4   (a, b) Protecting the scalp cannula

- Blood spurting into the syringe may indicate puncture of an artery. If this occurs, remove the needle and apply firm pressure for 5 minutes.
- Extreme pain may indicate nerve involvement.
- If either of the two aforementioned complications arises, immediately remove the needle, allow the child to rest and then try again.
- Failure to ensure a free flow of blood may result in haemolysis and an inaccurate biochemical result.
- Using a needle that is too small may lead to haemolysis.
- Intravenous cannulae should be secured with tape or dressings; however, approximately 1–2 cm above and below the insertion site should be clearly visible to allow for close observation.
- Splints should be used on limbs with an intravenous cannula sited, the aim being to immobilise the limb and prevent the cannula from becoming dislodged. These again should be secured in place by surgical tape and bandaged. Approximately 1–2 cm above and below the insertion site should be clearly visible to allow for close observation.
- Poor application of pressure following removal of the needle may result in bruising and swelling around the site.

Care of in situ intravenous cannula

On a daily basis:

- check patency of cannula by flushing as per local policy
- check cannula is secured and remains in position
- check site for redness, swelling, inflammation and pain as per local policy
- record all checks in patient documentation.

The cannula should be changed on a weekly basis.

COMMUNITY PERSPECTIVE

CCNs trained in the techniques of venepuncture and cannulation may be able to save families visits to hospital by undertaking these procedures in the home. This can save families many hours as outpatients and therefore the procedure becomes less of an issue for the child. However, in practice, the necessity for the procedure may arise so infrequently that the CCN may need to consider whether they are having sufficient practice to retain the necessary skills.

Some areas may use Ametop, which is a quicker and cheaper alternative to EMLA and can be used on full-term babies from the age of 1 month. The CCN may carry sharps bins, although children having care requiring regular use of sharps may keep these in the home. Local collection for disposal can be arranged.

Do and do not

- Do involve parents in the support of their child.
- Do ascertain the child's previous experience of venepuncture/cannulation.
- Do ensure that all possible sites for use are thoroughly examined.
- Do palpate the vessel to identify its position.
- Do ensure that local topical anaesthetic (EMLA or Ametop) is used, if the child wishes, to help prevent pain.
- Do ensure that the child has had an explanation of the procedure.
- Do use the play therapist/leader if available to help with explanation and assist with distraction.
- Do ensure that the child is firmly yet gently supported. An experienced assistant will help ensure a successful procedure.
- Do apply tape or dressing to secure intravenous cannulae. The dressings should keep the site dry and prevent contamination.

Dressings with a high water permeability should be used (Wong 2003).

- Do not coerce parents into being present. Some parents may not wish to be present or may feel anxious and scared, which will heighten the child's anxiety.
- Do not ask the parents to restrain their child. They should be providing support and reassurance. However some parents may wish to help restrain their child.
- Do not tell the child that it will not hurt.
- Do not use EMLA cream on children less than 1 year old.
- Do not use fragile, inflamed or fibrosed veins.

- Do not use sites that may interfere with a child's normal activity, e.g. do not use the right hand of a right-handed child; avoid the feet of an active toddler if possible.
- Do not use wooden tongue depressors as splints.
- Do not use non-sterile tape to cover the insertion site of an intravenous cannula as this may contaminate the site. (This does not usually happen in practice where either Transpore or zinc oxide tape is used most commonly.)
- Do not use adult vacuum systems for venepuncture as these are often not suitable and may cause the vein to collapse.

References

Brisman M, Ljung B M, Otterbom I et al 1998 Methaemoglobin formation after use of EMLA in term neonates. Acta Paediatrica 87(11): 1191–1194

Davies S 1998 The role of nurses in intravenous cannulation. Nursing Standard 12(7): 43–46

Hewitt T 1998 Prolonged contact with topical anaesthetic cream: a case report. Paediatric Nursing 10(2): 22–23

Jain A, Rutter N 2000 Does topical amethocaine gel reduce the pain of venepuncture in newborn infants? Child: Care Health and Development 83(3): 207–210

Nursing and Midwifery Council (NMC) 2002 Code of practice. NMC, London

Riendeau L 1999 Evaluation of analgesic efficacy of EMLA cream. Regional Anesthesia and Pain Medicine 249(20): 165–169

Tortora G J, Grabowski S R 2003 Principles of anatomy and physiology, 10th edn. Wiley, New York

Willock J, Richardson J, Brazier A, Powell C, Mitchell E 2004 Peripheral venepuncture in infants and children. Nursing Standard 18(27): 43–50

Wong D L 2003 Nursing care of infants and children, 7th edn. Mosby, St Louis

Further Reading

Crosby C, Mares A 2001 Skin antisepsis: past, present and future. Journal of Vascular Access Devices 6(1): 26–31

Fisher J, Harrison D 2000 Managing pain in critically ill children. In: Williams C, Asquith J (eds) Paediatric intensive care nursing. Churchill Livingstone, Edinburgh

Frey A M 2001 Infusion therapy in clinical practice, 2nd edn. W B Saunders, Philadelphia, PA

Halimaa S L 2003 Pain management in nursing procedures on premature babies. Journal of Advanced Nursing 42(6): 587–597

Heilskov M A 1998 A randomised trial of heparin and saline for maintaining intravenous locks in neonates. Journal of the Society of Pediatric Nursing 3(3): 111–116

Kolk A M, van Hoof R, Fiedeldij Dop M J 2000 Preparing children for venepuncture. Child: Care Health and Development 26(3): 251–260

Rohm K D, Schollhorn T A, Gwosdek M J et al 2004 Do we necessarily need local anaesthetics for venous cannulation? European Journal of Anaesthesiology 21(3): 214–216

Practice **37**

Wound care

Vikki Garrick

Introduction

A wound can be defined as 'a cut or break in continuity of any tissue caused by injury or operation' (Weller 2000) and, as with adults, wounds in children can occur for a variety of reasons. In general, wounds can be classified in two categories: acute and chronic.

Acute wounds include injuries caused by trauma, e.g. road traffic accidents, scalds, bites, lacerations, burns and those caused by surgical intervention. Chronic wounds in the child population have very different wound aetiologies from their adult counterparts. Much of the current literature covers common chronic wound types in the adult population, e.g. diabetic foot ulcers, pressure ulcers and venous leg ulcers. With the exception of pressure ulcers, these wounds are almost never seen in the paediatric population. Chronic wounds in children include congenital abnormalities, e.g. ulcerated haemangiomas; underlying medical conditions, e.g. epidermolysis bullosa (EB); pressure ulcers and lesions caused by acute medical conditions, e.g. meningococcal septicaemia.

Although children have the same physiological response to injury as adults, they can regenerate the cells required for the wound-healing process more rapidly, resulting in faster wound closure (Tendra Academy 2004).

The nurse's role in paediatric wound care, therefore, begins with an understanding of the wound healing process. This understanding is paramount in making an accurate assessment of any wound as the subsequent treatment plan will be heavily dependent on the outcome of that assessment. The nurse, in collaboration with the multidisciplinary team, must be able to choose the appropriate wound management strategies for the child and their family. A fundamental part of this process is recognising the need for individualised, family-centred care.

Learning outcomes

By the end of this section you should be able to:

- understand the physiological processes involved in healing

- describe the factors that can delay wound healing
- describe each phase of wound healing and the associated wound tissue type
- understand the need for holistic wound assessment
- use a paediatric wound assessment chart
- understand the theory behind applied wound management
- consider wound healing within the context of other childhood disorders
- understand how wound dressings work and what role they play in applied wound management
- recognise the role of the multidisciplinary team in the assessment and management of paediatric wounds
- understand the importance of family-centred care in the management of paediatric wounds.

Rationale

Children's nurses learn to develop holistic nursing skills and this is no different in the field of wound management. The goals for holistic wound management in children are to control pain, reduce emotional discomfort and minimise the risk of scarring (Bale & Jones 1997). Many factors can delay and complicate healing: poor tissue perfusion and oxygenation, poor nutritional status, infection, underlying medical conditions and extremes of age (Bryant 1992). The principal objectives of wound care are, first, to restore the function of injured tissue and second, to do no damage during that process of restoration (Box 37.1).

What is healing?

Wounds heal in two different ways: by primary or by secondary intention. Healing by primary intention indicates a process in which the wound edges are closed as soon as possible using sutures, staples or glue. As there is no tissue loss, healing is rapid and usually occurs within 24 hours. When wounds are closed in this way, granulation tissue is not visible and scar formation is minimal (Collier 1996). Surgical wounds without complications heal in this way. Healing by secondary intention occurs when there is tissue loss into the dermis and deeper layers of the skin. The wound edges are not opposed and tissue gradually regenerates from the bottom of the wound to fill the defect. This type of wound requires skilful and holistic assessment (Russell 2002a).

Healing occurs more rapidly in children than in adults for the following reasons:

- formation of granulation tissue is faster
- production of collagen and elastin is faster
- quantity of fibroblasts in the wound is greater (Tendra Academy 2004).

Phases of wound healing

An understanding of the physiological process of wound healing is vital in making an accurate assessment of any wound; subsequent treatment will depend on the outcome of the assessment. There are three phases of wound healing:

- the inflammatory phase
- the proliferative phase
- the maturative phase.

Box 37.1 Aims of wound care

- Create the optimum environment for the natural healing processes to take place
- Promote moist wound healing
- Protect from trauma and cooling
- Remove devitalised tissue and excess exudate

- Prevent infection
- Promote dignity, comfort and well-being
- Restore the function of injured tissue
- Maintain the function of the skin
- Cost effective

Based on data from Dealey (1994), Bale & Jones (1997) and Casey (1999).

Inflammatory phase

When tissue is injured, blood vessels are also injured and the clotting process is started. Damaged cells release histamine causing vasodilatation and increased permeability of the blood vessels, delivering neutrophils and monocytes to the area (Collier 1996). This inflammatory response, therefore, results in all of the signs and symptoms of inflammation:

- pain
- heat
- swelling
- erythema (redness)
- exudate production.

This is a normal and natural response and does not indicate infection. The fluid produced by the inflammatory response contains factors which actively promote healing. Its greatest importance is that it contains antibodies, leucocytes and macrophages. These collectively keep bacterial invasion and infection under control. Providing there is no infection or further injury or invasion, the inflammation gradually subsides and the exudate drains back into the circulation.

The main function of this phase is to keep the wound bed free from bacteria or other contaminants so that the optimal environment for tissue regeneration can be achieved (Collier 2003).

Proliferative phase

The main cells involved in this phase are macrophages and fibroblasts. Macrophages influence the healing process in several ways: they clear the wound of devitalised and unwanted material, release enzymes which break down necrotic tissue and are responsible for producing the cells which regulate new tissue formation (Kingsley 2002).

Fibroblasts are responsible for the production of the delicate collagen matrix laid down in the wound at this time. The matrix acts as a frame on which new capillary loops 'grow' into the wound bed. This process is known as angiogenesis. The formation of the capillary loops in the wound bed gives it a red appearance; this is known as granulation tissue. The new capillary loops are numerous and very fragile and therefore are easily damaged (Kingsley 2002).

Maturative phase

Once the wound bed is filled with granulation tissue, re-epithelialisation begins. Epithelial cells divide and begin to migrate over newly granulating tissue. A moist wound healing environment has been shown to accelerate the rate of epithelialisation and dermal repair (Winter 1962, Field & Kerstein 1994, Miller 2000, Bryan 2004). Collagen fibres, which have been randomly laid down during the proliferative phase, are also reorganised. The scar appears large but as the collagen fibres reorganise into tighter positions, the scar is reduced. Owing to the disappearance of vascular granulation tissue during this stage, there is progressive decrease in the vascularity of the scar, thus changing its appearance from dusky red to white over a period of time (Miller 2000, Bryan 2004).

Factors affecting healing

Conditions or factors that may compromise wound healing should be considered when undertaking wound assessment.

Nutrition

All children require a diet which contains appropriate nutrients and vitamins. The value of nutrition in the healing process is paramount – nutrition provides the raw materials required for tissue regeneration (Bryant 1992).

Encouragement must be given to the child to maintain an adequate oral intake and some creative thinking may be required to accomplish this. Encouraging small amounts regularly may be preferable to having three large meals daily. Simple snacks such as yoghurts, cheese, chicken and fruit can be offered at regular intervals throughout the day.

- Children who are deficient in nutrients as a result of illness, or disease, are susceptible to impaired healing:
  - vitamin C deficiency inhibits formation of collagen fibres and capillary development
  - protein deficiency reduces the supply of amino acids for tissue repair
  - zinc deficiency impairs epithelialisation.
- Children with special needs may have difficulty eating, drinking and swallowing;

skilled assistance is therefore needed to ensure adequate intake of nutrition.

- The assistance of the dietitian is also useful to ensure nutritional requirements are being met (Shepherd 2003).

Disease or pathology

- Diabetes mellitus: hyperglycaemia impairs phagocytosis, which is the engulfing and destruction of bacteria, foreign bodies and necrotic tissue by phagocytes. It also inhibits collagen synthesis and impairs circulation and capillary growth.
- Anaemia: healing is likely to be impaired through the reduction in oxygen transportation (Casey 2000).
- Compromised immunological status, such as in children with a malignancy, HIV/AIDS or an immunodeficiency disorder: healing in these conditions is delayed because of reduced efficiency of the immune system. Secondary to this is a decreased resistance to infection, which in turn will delay healing.
- Impaired circulation, as seen in some children with cardiac disorders, reduces the supply of nutrients to the wound area, and inhibits the inflammatory response and removal of debris from the wound.

Medication

- Cytotoxic drugs and radiotherapy interfere with cell proliferation during the process of healing.
- Radiation inhibits fibroblastic activity and capillary formation; it may also cause necrosis.
- Prolonged steroid therapy delays healing during the inflammatory and proliferative phases (Bale & Jones 1997). It impairs phagocytosis, inhibits fibroblast proliferation, depresses formation of granulation tissue and inhibits wound contraction.

Other causes

- Pain and stress can affect the immune system and thus interfere with wound healing.
- Foreign bodies inhibit wound closure and prolong the inflammatory response.
- Infection prolongs the inflammatory response and increases tissue destruction.

- Mechanical friction damages or destroys granulation tissue.

Wound assessment

Collins et al (2002) define assessment as 'information obtained via observation, questioning, physical examination and clinical investigation in order to establish a baseline'. This is a concise definition which encourages holistic assessment of the child and family and not just assessment of the wound. The importance of holistic assessment and early identification of any factors which could delay the natural healing response is essential for a successful patient outcome (Bale 2000).

It is helpful to consider the following factors when assessing a wound:

- Cause of the wound – remove where possible (e.g. pressure)
- Site of the wound – this will have an impact on product choice
- Clinical condition of the patient – this will impact on healing rates
- Size of the wound.

After assessing these factors, the nurse must then assess the wound itself. As this process is so subjective, a standardised approach to wound assessment is advisable (Russell 2002b). The theory of 'applied wound management' has been developed to facilitate a logical and systematic approach to wound management (Gray 2004).

This tool uses a simple set of observations to decide the status of the wound and, when used in conjunction with clinical judgement, aids the nurse in developing a treatment plan for the wound.

Applied wound management splits the process of wound assessment into three steps (see Fig. 37.1):

1. the wound healing continuum
2. the wound infection continuum
3. the wound exudate continuum.

The wound healing continuum

This is a colour-coded guide to wound tissue type which defines the aim of the appropriate

THE WOUND HEALING CONTINUUM

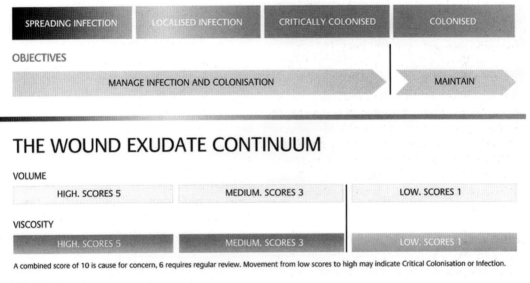

| BLACK | BLACK/YELLOW | YELLOW | YELLOW/RED | RED | RED/PINK | PINK |

OBJECTIVES

DEBRIDEMENT   PREVENT STATIC WOUNDS AND SPEED HEALING

THE WOUND INFECTION CONTINUUM

| SPREADING INFECTION | LOCALISED INFECTION | CRITICALLY COLONISED | COLONISED |

OBJECTIVES

MANAGE INFECTION AND COLONISATION   MAINTAIN

THE WOUND EXUDATE CONTINUUM

VOLUME

| HIGH. SCORES 5 | MEDIUM. SCORES 3 | LOW. SCORES 1 |

VISCOSITY

| HIGH. SCORES 5 | MEDIUM. SCORES 3 | LOW. SCORES 1 |

A combined score of 10 is cause for concern, 6 requires regular review. Movement from low scores to high may indicate Critical Colonisation or Infection.

OBJECTIVES

MANAGE EXUDATE TO PREVENT MACERATION OF SURROUNDING SKIN AND TO MAINTAIN MOIST HEALING ENVIRONMENT

Figure 37.1   The applied wound management chart

wound management for that tissue type (e.g. debridement, protection).

The wound infection continuum
This is a colour-coded guide to wound tissue type which helps to identify the bacterial burden on the wound and possible treatment strategies to help reduce that burden.

The wound exudate continuum
This categorises levels of wound exudate by volume and viscosity and identifies treatment aims accordingly.

This is a useful tool in helping the nurse prioritise the various aspects of the wound itself and is also an aid for product selection. By using clinical judgement and the applied wound management tool to identify the tissue type, bacterial burden and level of exudate, the nurse has enough information on the wound to make an informed choice when selecting a wound management product.

An effective wound assessment should therefore consider the components identified above and document all findings accurately in the wound assessment chart or nursing notes. An example of a wound assessment chart is presented in Figure 37.2.

Guidelines when undertaking wound care

Local policies and guidelines may be in place to help the nurse when undertaking wound care. An example of Best Practice Guidelines is presented in Box 37.2.

Ongoing wound assessment is essential to a positive wound care outcome for the child and their family. The children's nurse, in consultation with other members of the multidisciplinary team, must make an informed decision on what approach is the most appropriate for a particular child and their family. It is essential for the nurse to have the required information regarding the child and the wound prior to undertaking any wound care practice.

Wound cleansing

The purpose of wound cleansing is to remove dressing debris or wound debris (necrotic tissue, sloughy tissue), both of which can act as a focus for infection (Bale & Jones 1997). It follows, therefore, that routine wound cleansing is not advised and may indeed be detrimental to the wound healing process. This procedure should only be performed when there is an indication that it will either benefit the healing process or prevent infection (Blunt 2001). Modern interactive dressings such as hydrocolloids and hydrogels can be used to soften and hydrate necrotic tissue before cleansing. This makes the process less traumatic when removing dead tissue. The use of this type of product has implications for practice and suggests daily changes of dressing and cleaning of wounds should be discouraged where possible to allow the product to work to its fullest potential.

Irrigation

Cleansing by irrigation with warmed solutions (tap water, sterile water, normal saline) will prevent the shedding of fibres into the wound bed and is less traumatic for the child. This technique is now being advocated (Bale & Jones 1997). However, one of the difficulties of this method is in assessing the amount of pressure to be used when irrigating; it should be enough to dislodge debris without causing damage to the underlying tissues.

Cleansing by bathing and showering

Bathing and showering are appropriate methods for wound cleansing, particularly for children. The use of bathing and showering in paediatrics is much less frightening and traumatic than other methods of wound cleansing and it can also be a playful experience. Many children prefer to remove their own dressings by soaking them off in the bath or shower. In surgical wounds, once skin edges have sealed, bathing or showering is not likely to present any further risk (Briggs 1997). In hospitals the issue of cross-infection must be considered; therefore careful measures for disinfection of the bath must be taken between children using it.

Wound dressings

Children are a challenging group where wound dressings are concerned. Box 37.3 illustrates the specific requirements of wound management products for the paediatric population. There are many and varied dressings available for the paediatric nurse to choose from; Table 37.1 contains examples of and information on some products suitable for use on children.

Equipment

- Trolley or appropriate clean surface
- Sterile dressing pack containing plastic tray, non-woven swabs, pair of gloves, sterile towel
- Sterile latex-free gloves if not contained in dressing pack
- Plastic disposable apron
- Large disposable plastic bag for soiled disposables
- Appropriate dressing materials.

Method

Preparation of the child

1. Assess the child for the need for analgesia, which should be given half an hour prior to the dressing change.
2. Explain the procedure to the child in an age-appropriate manner and to the main

caregivers. Ensure understanding and identify their role throughout the dressing change.

3. Use play and involve the play specialist if appropriate.

4. Allow enough time between information giving and performing the practice – too much time may cause the child to become anxious, too little may not allow the play specialist time to prepare the child adequately.

5. Introduce the use of distraction, where appropriate.

6. Ensure that all the potential equipment required is on the dressing trolley.

7. Positioning of the child will depend on the site or location of the wound. Choose a

Paediatric Wound Assessment Chart

(a)

Name: . . . .

Unit No: . . . . DoB: . . . . Consultant: . . . .

Date of initial assessment: . . . .

Does drug therapy at present include any of the following:

	YES	NO
Steroids	☐	☐
Chemotherapy	☐	☐
Insulin	☐	☐
Antibiotics	☐	☐
Inotropes	☐	☐

Draw site of wounds:

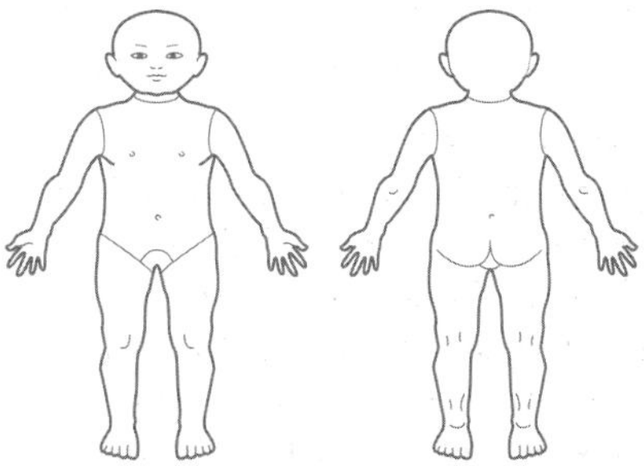

Front   Back

Cause of wound: . . . .

Now include wound care in nursing care plan

Initial wound assessment:

| NB | There may be more than one type of tissue in wound |

✓

Pink ☐
Red ☐
Yellow ☐
Black ☐
Dark red and raised ☐

Describe:
· Wound appearance . . . .
· Wound size . . . .
· Type of exudate (if any) . . . .
· Condition of surrounding skin . . . .

If wound is a PRESSURE SORE please plan to use a pressure relieving surface and document in care plan

---

Nutritional status: If poor contact Dietitian

Dietitian contacted: YES ☐   NO ☐

☐ Good   ☐ Satisfactory   ☐ Poor

Figure 37.2   (a, b): Paediatric wound assessment chart

(b)

Paediatric Wound Assessment Chart

Name . . . . Hosp No. . . . . DoB. . . . . Consultant . . . .

	Date	Date	Date
Analgesia used	YES☐ NO☐	YES☐ NO☐	YES☐ NO☐
Wound appearance and size (cm)			
Colour of wound bed:	Pink ☐ Red ☐ Yellow ☐ Black ☐ Dark red ☐	Pink ☐ Red ☐ Yellow ☐ Black ☐ Dark red ☐	Pink ☐ Red ☐ Yellow ☐ Black ☐ Dark red ☐
Exudate and type			
Odour			
Swab taken NB After wound cleansing			
Photograph (✓)			
Document treatment carried out			
Document dressing applied			
Reviewed by:	Dietitian / Tissue viability nurse / Medical staff	Dietitian / Tissue viability nurse / Medical staff	Dietitian / Tissue viability nurse / Medical staff
	Next dressing change / Signature and designation	Next dressing change / Signature and designation	Next dressing change / Signature and designation

Document wound care in care plan after each dressing change

Figure 37.2   Cont'd

position that is most comfortable and reassuring for the child, ensuring that the wound is easily accessible. Infants or small children can lie or sit on an adult's lap, if the wound site permits. Ensure that the child is in a safe position throughout.

8. If wound cleansing is required, a bath or shower is a less traumatic method for the child and is an effective way to soak off dressings (Bale & Jones 1997).

9. Ensure that the child is kept warm and dressing time is kept to a minimum, thus decreasing heat loss and discomfort for the child.

10. Ensure that a young child has their favourite cuddly toy, or comforter, with them throughout.

Wound care practice

1. Ensure adequate time is available to undertake the wound dressing.

2. Explain all the steps of the practice, in advance of them occurring, and throughout, to the child and parent.

3. Perform the dressing using a non-touch technique. Ensure thorough handwashing.

4. If appropriate, allow the child, in as far as is possible, to remove the dressing gently, avoiding damage to new granulation or epithelial tissue (this may be undertaken in the shower or bath).

5. If further cleansing is required after the bath or shower, irrigate using a syringe with a warmed solution (tap water, normal saline).

6. Assess the wound and surrounding skin.

Box 37.2   Best Practice Guidelines for caring for patients with wounds

Statement

Wound assessment and treatment should be based on a basic understanding of tissue repair and factors affecting the healing process.

The named nurse is personally accountable for their practice and, in exercising professional accountability, may therefore enhance their skills by caring for a patient with a wound as per trust hospital guidelines.

The named nurse should recognise when they are unable to deal with a wound due to lack of experience/knowledge and should contact the Tissue Viability Nurse for advice.

Aim

- Wound management will be approached holistically and tailored to the needs of the child and family
- Wound assessment will be carried out prior to application of any wound management products
- Wound management products used will be appropriate for the stage of healing
- Accurate documentation will be undertaken at each dressing change
- The nurse will work in partnership with medical staff, seeking their cooperation when necessary to ensure patient needs are met in a safe and effective manner

Guidelines

- Nursing staff caring for patients with wounds should have a basic understanding of the stages of wound healing
- Nursing staff caring for patients with wounds should be aware of factors affecting healing
- Wound assessment should take place prior to application of any wound management product
- Progress will be documented on the wound assessment chart at each dressing change

Dressing procedure

- Ensure the patient has had adequate analgesia prior to the procedure
- Assemble all equipment required prior to the procedure to ensure wound exposure time is kept to a minimum
- Apply the principles of aseptic technique to reduce the risk of infection
- Clean the wound only if necessary using warmed normal saline or tap water and a 20 ml syringe
- *Do not* dry the wound
- Select an appropriate dressing product using the wound assessment flow chart and wound formulary
- Document assessment and treatment on the wound assessment chart and in the care plan
- Plan and document the wound review date
- If the wound is complex or slow to heal, contact the Tissue Viability Nurse
- Contact other relevant members of the multidisciplinary team if required (e.g. medical staff, community nursing team, pharmacy)
- If dressing products are required for wound care at home, contact the Community Nursing Team and provide the patient with a 7-day supply of products

Box 37.3   Dressing requirements for children

- Comfortable
- Conformable
- Non-adherent
- Pain-free on application
- Pain-free on removal
- Easy to apply
- Hypoallergenic
- Waterproof
- Non-restrictive
- Non-bulky
- Manufactured in small sizes
- Skin-friendly adhesives
- Able to withstand children's activities: crawling, climbing, running, cycling
- Reasonable wear time

Table 37.1 Examples of and information on dressings suitable for use on children

Category of product	Example of product	Mode of action	Indications for use	Contraindications for use	Special considerations	Frequency of dressing change
Non-adherent	Mepitel (Mölnlycke) NA Ultra (Johnson & Johnson) Tegapore (3M) Telfa clear (Tyco Healthcare)	Protects fragile tissue Non-adherent over wound surface area	Clean granular wounds Epithelialising tissue Wounds with low-moderate exudate	Necrotic tissue Suitable for most wound types as long as correct secondary dressing chosen to absorb exudate	Requires secondary dressing Can be used with topical applications, e.g. silver sulfadiazine (Flamazine)	May be left in place for up to 7 days NB: If wound heavily exudating, not advisable to leave dressing for 7 days; 3–5 days more realistic in paediatric arena
Hydrocolloid	DuoDERM, Granuflex (ConvaTec) Hydrocoll (Hartmann)	Mixture of sodium carboxymethy-lcellulose, pectin and adhesive polymers Occlusive therefore fulfils many of ideal dressing criteria Forms a gel which bathes the wound as it absorbs fluid	Superficial grazes, minor skin abrasions (extra thin versions only) Rehydrating dry, crusty wounds, e.g. pressure sores Necrotic tissue	Wounds with large amounts of exudate Clinically infected wounds	Products come in an extra-thin variety and small sizes, particularly appropriate for paediatric population Waterproof therefore child can bath/shower with dressing in situ No secondary dressing required	May be left in place for up to 7 days Dressing needs to be changed when gel 'bubbles' in centre of dressing

Hydrofibre	Aquacel, Aquacel Ag (ConvaTec)	Hydrocolloid fibres Converts to gel when in contact with exudate Locks bacteria in dressing facilitating reduction of bacterial burden at wound surface area Aquacel Ag is combined with silver to increase bactericidal effect	Wounds with moderate–high exudate levels Heavily colonised wounds	Dry wounds or those with low exudate levels	Needs a secondary dressing Foam dressings appropriate	May be left in place for up to 5 days NB: If wound heavily exudating, not advisable to leave dressing for 5 days; 3–5 days more realistic in paediatric arena
Film dressings	Tegaderm (3M) IV 3000 (Smith & Nephew)	Semi-permeable therefore allows passage of varying amounts of moisture from the wound surface Covers and provides protective layer over shallow, non-exuding wounds	Used to secure IV cannulae (IV 3000) and for the application of topical local anaesthetics, e.g. EMLA cream As a secondary dressing with hydrogels as they maintain moisture at the wound surface	Wounds with high levels of exudate which gathers under the film	Potential for adhesive trauma on removal from skin Ensure correct technique used for removal Can be difficult to apply as dressing can stick to itself if backing removed incorrectly	May be left in place for up to 7 days If used as secondary dressing with hydrogel, 3–5 days more realistic in paediatric arena

Continued

Table 37.1 Examples of and information on dressings suitable for use on children—cont'd

Category of product	Example of product	Mode of action	Indications for use	Contraindications for use	Special considerations	Frequency of dressing change
	Cavilon non-sting barrier film (3M)	Non-sting protective transparent barrier film 'Coats' skin to act as protective barrier from adhesive tapes, urine, faeces Is not removed by washing	Protects fragile and excoriated skin Used as treatment for severe nappy rash Good for prevention of excoriation under nasogastric tubes	Sensitivity to film contents	Non-sting property means pain-free application Comes in foam applicator or pump spray	Re-apply every 48–72 hours
Alginate	Sorbsan (Unomedical) Kaltostat (ConvaTec)	Manufactured from seaweed Combination of mannuronic and glucuronic acid Also contain varying concentrations of calcium Turns to gel when in contact with exudate	Wounds with moderate–high exudate levels Donor sites/ haemangiomas (Kaltostat is also a haemostat) Heavily colonised wounds	Dry wounds or those with low exudate levels	Needs a secondary dressing which will cope with exudate levels; foam dressings appropriate Can be difficult to remove from cavities Have potential to adhere if exudate level not sufficient to make dressing gel	May be left in place for up to 5 days NB: If wound heavily exudating, not advisable to leave dressing for 5 days; 3–5 days more realistic in paediatric arena
Hydrogel	Intrasite gel, Intrasite conformable (Smith & Nephew) ActiFormCool (Activa Healthcare)	Carboxymethyl-cellulose gel. Draws exudate into gel while donating fluid to the wound Promotes a moist healing environment	Dry, crusting wounds Superficial grazes	Wounds with large amounts of exudate Maceration to surrounding skin	Needs a secondary dressing; film dressings most appropriate Be careful not to use a secondary dressing which will absorb the gel (e.g. gauze swabs)	May be left in place for up to 5 days NB: Not always appropriate to leave dressing for this long; 3 days more realistic in paediatric arena

Foam dressings	Lyofoam (SSL) Tielle (Johnson & Johnson) Allevyn (Smith & Nephew)	Absorb exudate into dressing, thus controlling level of moisture at the wound surface Insulates wound surface Depending on product chosen, can also protect epithelialising tissue, e.g. Tielle Lite	Depends on type of foam used. Will absorb varying degrees of exudate Wounds with moderate–high exudate levels, e.g. Tielle, Tielle Plus, Allevyn Flat wounds and shallow cavities Foam conforms to shape of cavity Wounds with low exudate levels, e.g. Tielle Lite, Allevyn Thin	Necrotic tissue Suitable for most wound types as long as correct type of foam chosen after exudate assessment	Some foams require a secondary dressing If using adherent foam dressing, remove carefully as adhesive can damage sensitive skin Some adherent foam dressings can be removed painlessly using water	May be left in place for up to 5 days NB: If wound heavily exudating, not advisable to leave dressing for 5 days; 3 days more realistic in paediatric arena
Silver dressings	Actisorb Silver 220 (Johnson & Johnson) Aquacel Ag (ConvaTec) Arglaes Silver (Unomedical) Urgotul SSD (Parema)	Reduces bacterial burden in wound through mechanism of silver on tissue	Wounds which are critically colonised or locally infected Product chosen will depend on exudate level of wound	Necrotic tissue Sensitivity to silver	Some silver products require a secondary dressing	May be left in place for up to 7 days NB: If wound heavily exudating, not advisable to leave dressing for 7 days; 3–5 days more realistic in paediatric arena

7. The choice of dressing for the contact layer, which is the primary dressing, will depend on the type of tissue categorised and the level of exudate (Harding & Jones 1996).
8. The choice of secondary dressing will often depend on the contact layer (Harding & Jones 1996).
9. Assess pain at the wound site.
10. Secure the dressing using an appropriate method. For neonates, Surgifix is a good alternative to adherent dressings or adhesive tapes.

11. For children who have special needs, it may be difficult to carry out aseptic non-touch technique at dressing changes. With this group of children, it is even more important that their dressing is secured; to avoid the use of tape that can be easily removed may require some creative thinking.
12. Document the assessment and management by completing the wound assessment and treatment chart, and record information in the child's nursing notes.

COMMUNITY PERSPECTIVE

The principles when undertaking wound care in the community are the same as in hospital; however, the CCN may need to be adaptable to maintain safe practice in the home (see Aseptic Non-Touch Technique, p. 751).

Analgesia, if required, may be given prior to the CCN's visit, allowing time for the drug to work; alternatively, Entonox may be self-administered by the child during the procedure.

Do and do not

- Do involve the child and family.
- Do ensure that the multidisciplinary team are involved.
- Do individualise the child's wound care.
- Do assess the wound systematically, using where possible an assessment tool, and categorise the tissue status and exudate level.
- Do record wound assessment and wound care on the wound assessment chart and in the nursing notes
- Do minimise wound care problems by introducing evidence-based care.

- Do consider the factors that may influence wound healing.
- Do use play and distraction when undertaking wound care practice.
- Do assess the child for the need for analgesia.
- Do complete the dressing change as quickly as is practical.
- Do encourage bathing or showering as a wound cleansing option.
- Do not use cotton wool balls.
- Do not routinely cleanse the wound.
- Do not use force to remove a dressing.
- Do not use alcoholic solution of povidone–iodine (Betadine) on wounds.

References

Bale S 2000 Ch. 4, cited in Bale S, Harding K, Leaper D (eds) An introduction to wounds. EMAP Healthcare, London

Bale S, Jones V 1997 Wound care nursing – a patient centred approach. Baillière Tindall, London

Blunt J 2001 Wound cleansing: ritualistic or research-based practice? Nursing Standard 16(1): 33–36

Briggs M 1997 Principles of closed surgical wound care. Journal of Wound Care 6(6): 288–292

Bryan J 2004 Moist wound healing: a concept that changed our practice. Journal of Wound Care 13(6): 227–228

Bryant R 1992 Acute and chronic wounds: nursing management. Mosby Year Book, London

Casey G 1999 Wound management in children. Paediatric Nursing 11(5): 39–44

Casey G 2000 Modern wound dressings. Nursing Standard 15(5): 47–57

Collier M 1996 The principles of optimum wound management. Nursing Standard 10(43): 47–52

Collier M 2003 Wound bed preparation: theory to practice. Nursing Standard 17(36): 45–52

Collins F, Hampton S, White R 2002 A–Z dictionary of wound care. Quay Books, Mark Allen Publishing, Surrey, UK

Dealey C 1994 The care of wounds. Blackwell Science, Cambridge, UK

Field C, Kerstein M 1994 Overview of wound healing in a moist environment. American Journal of Surgery 167(Suppl 1a): 25–30

Gray D 2004 Applied wound management: a new conceptual framework in wound management. Applied Wound Management Supplement. Wounds-UK, Aberdeen, UK

Harding K, Jones V 1996 Wound management: good practice guidelines. Macmillan Magazines, London

Kingsley A 2002 Wound healing and potential therapeutic options. Professional Nurse 17(9): 539–544

Miller M 2000 Moist wound healing. Essential wound healing. EMAP Healthcare, London

Russell L 2002a Ch. 1, cited in White R, Harding K 2002 Trends in wound care. British Journal of Nursing Monograph. Quay Books, Mark Allen Publishing, Surrey, UK

Russell L 2002b Ch. 10, cited in White R, Harding K 2002 Trends in wound care. British Journal of Nursing Monograph. Quay Books, Mark Allen Publishing, Surrey, UK

Shepherd A 2003 Nutrition for optimum wound healing. Nursing Standard 18(6): 55–58

Tendra Academy 2004 Best practice statement: issues in paediatric wound care. Minimising trauma and pain. Mölnlycke Health Care, Dunstable, Bedfordshire, UK

Weller B F 2000 Nurses dictionary, 23rd edn. Baillière Tindall, London

Winter G D 1962 Formation of the scab and the rate of epithelialization of superficial wounds in the young domestic pig. Nature 193: 293–294

Further reading

Casey G 2002 Wound repair: advanced dressing materials. Nursing Standard 17(4): 49–53

Dowsett C 2002 The role of the nurse in wound bed preparation. Nursing Standard 16(44): 69–76

Hampton S 2004 Wound colonisation explained. Nurse2Nurse 4(4): 34

Miller M, Glover D 1999 Wound management: theory and practice. EMAP Healthcare, London

Morgan D 2000 Formulary of wound management products: a guide for healthcare staff, 8th edn. Euromed Communications, Haslemere, Surrey, UK

Stephen-Haynes J, Gibson E 2003 Anatomy and physiology: wound healing and wound assessment. Wound Care Society Educational Booklet 1(2), Huntingdon, UK

Watret L, White R 2001 Surgical wound management: the role of dressings. Nursing Standard 15(44): 59–69

Willock J, Maylor M 2004 Pressure ulcers in infants and children. Nursing Standard 24(18): 56–62

World Union of Wound Healing Societies 2004 Principles of best practice: minimising pain at wound dressing-related procedures. A consensus document. MEP, London

Appendix 1

Play

Joyce Stebbings

INTRODUCTION

Play forms an integral part of the care of the sick child. Most practical procedures involving the child will at some stage include some aspect of play. Play facilitates communication between the child and their carers, thereby providing a sense of control, trust and understanding. 'Hospitalisation, medical procedures and surgery are a source of anxiety for children/young people and their families' (Lansdown 1996). There are a variety of different types of play applicable to children according to their age and stage of development. These will be described, citing examples from practice of children who have successfully used play to help them understand and cope with their illness. Play programmes designed for the hospitalised child, taking into account the child's individual needs, age, cognitive understanding and illness, can provide a positive introduction to the ward environment, thus aiding the nurse in the holistic care of the child. The core of this text is designed to explore the importance of play in the life of the sick child. It is hoped that those who use this book will find this section a useful addition. Figures A1.1 and A1.2 show a visual interpreta-

tion of a child's experiences and what play in hospital represents.

'Through play, a child will make sense of the world' (OMEP 1966, cited in Morris 1989). When children are provided with an environment where play occurs naturally, they are able to express feelings, indulge in fantasy and work through difficult situations if appropriate. This last aspect is one where the intervention of skilled and trained adults may be needed. Hospital play specialists (HPS) are people who have undergone an appropriate training and have the in-depth knowledge and skills to work with children when they are sick, to help them cope with their illness through play. As play is a pleasurable activity, its normality helps to promote confidence in an unfamiliar environment, thus aiding the recovery process. As Pam Malcolm, Hospital Play Specialist once said: 'No child is too sick to play. For some children, even a simple hand massage is a gentle way of letting them know that you are there.'

The use of play was initially introduced into paediatric wards in 1963, when Consultant Paediatrician, Dr Morris, noted how withdrawn and unnatural children appeared to be when admitted to hospital (Morris 1989). He believed

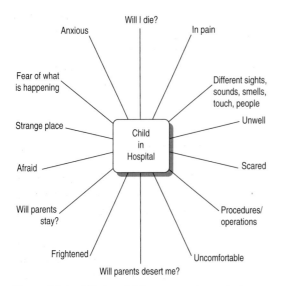

Figure A1.1 What a child may experience during their stay in hospital

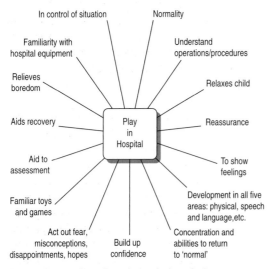

Figure A1.2 Benefits of play in hospital

play session with an older child, both are forms of play. The involvement and cooperation of the child with the adult has healing potential for the child. Some people may think that they have forgotten how to play, or have never experienced play themselves. To those of you in this situation, just relax and do what comes naturally; let the children take the lead, copy them, laugh with them, get down to their level physically as well as spiritually. The child's uncomplicated mind will easily show us how to enjoy play, but sometimes our expectations and inhibitions get in the way. Once the child's trust has been obtained, the ability to play becomes one of the greatest assets of a children's nurse.

PREPARATION

Play in hospital aims to inform children about the unusual situation in which they find themselves and thereby allay fears and increase confidence. It will also provide a much-needed link with home and normality. Using play preoperatively, or prior to other frightening procedures (venepuncture, radiotherapy, nasogastric feeding), goes a long way in helping children to express their real feelings. 'Harris (1981) suggests that preparation for hospitalization not only facilitates the reduction of anxiety but the benefits include an improved response to treatment' (Broadhurst 2003).

Before preparing a child for a procedure or operation, various factors have to be taken into consideration. These are the age of the child or adolescent, cognitive development, emotional maturity, previous experiences, cultural differences, coping strategies and parental anxiety. Where possible, a trusting relationship should be formed before any preparation begins. It is also important that whoever is leading the session is fully aware of the implications of the operation or procedure for the child. During preparation, the use of real hospital equipment is vital. The use of syringes, masks, anaesthetic cream, clear plasters, stethoscopes, etc. will allow children to familiarise themselves with equipment that may be used during their own procedure or operation. Picture books, photographs and videos may help a child by

that just because a child was in hospital, opportunities for play should not be taken away. Save the Children Fund set up play schemes with the aim of reducing stress and anxiety and encouraging normal play.

Play is an activity that we are all involved in, often without realising it. From waving to a baby in a cot, which involves eye contact and communication, to a more involved imaginative clarifying images and thoughts. Wolfer (1979) showed that by providing the child with accurate information about procedures in a safe, non-threatening environment, the child was able to cope more effectively in a potentially stressful situation (see examples in Box A1.1).

During preparation sessions the child must be given physical and emotional space to express feelings and fears. The session should not be rushed as this may add to the child's feeling of loss of control. The whole hospital experience tends to remove control from the child. If the child can be given space to think through and explore the forthcoming procedure through play, they can be given back some control over the situation, and this will help boost their confidence. In some cases it may be appropriate to include sessions for the parent/carer and siblings, as the child being treated may pick up their feelings towards the procedure: '...we have found it important to prepare the parent as well as the child, parental anxiety being mirrored in the child ... siblings are also prepared for any future admission they may have' (Maglacas 1986).

It is really important that you do not miss out those children with additional needs. It is easy to think that just because their understanding or communication is different from what is usually seen they will not see the potential procedure as frightening. In these cases adapting aids is necessary. Consulting other colleagues for ideas on doing this may be the solution. As stated in the article *Play Preparation for Children with Special Needs*, 'professional standards and the requirement for equitable care demands that play preparation is available to every child, whatever his or her level of development' (Crawford & Raven 2002).

Note: The child should *always* be warned if the procedure is going to hurt as this will help build up a trusting relationship.

Preparation guidelines

1. Always be honest with the child.
2. Give information that is child friendly, using words and phrases that the child and family will understand, ensuring that it is consistent and allows time for questions. Always use the correct names of equipment to avoid confusion.
3. Timing: Young children who have limited or no understanding of time cannot manage their anxiety about a future event if told far in advance. Where possible discuss with parent/carer.
4. Avoid using phrases such as 'We will give you medicine to put you to sleep.' This can be confused with when a pet dies and is 'put to sleep'. 'Can I take your temperature?' may evoke anxiety as to where you are taking it: 'Will I get it back?'
5. Most children benefit from individual preparation.
6. Stress sometimes results in the child being unable to fully absorb what is being said. Be aware of non-verbal indications that the child may no longer be listening. Remember to acknowledge feelings and give reassurance and further explanations when needed.
7. Use breathing techniques: During venepuncture, some children will be helped by getting them to breathe in; then, as the needle is inserted, they can be asked to breathe out.

Box A1.1   Examples of ways in which play can allay fear in children

1. A 5-year-old with leukaemia, who was 18 months into his treatment, had a cannula inserted to administer antibiotics. During the procedure he displayed his anger by reacting violently. It was not until 2 days later, through a play session with the HPS, that the child realised it was only a piece of tubing in his arm and not a needle. He then became much more relaxed about the situation and cooperated well during follow-up procedures.
2. 'Jack', a doll with a Hickman line attached, allows children to work through their own personal medical experience.

This may help them feel that they have more control over the situation.

8. In some situations where the child is upset and screaming, it is possible to scream with them, thereby showing that this expression of pain and fear is understandable. This must be used with caution, as it can be most upsetting for other children and their parents.

9. It is important that everyone dealing with the child is as relaxed as possible, as this will give confidence to both child and family.

10. Children often regress whilst in hospital and may require repetitive explanations and information about their procedures.

11. Some parents may be anxious that telling their child about a procedure will cause more anxiety. It is worth explaining that a child who is not given accurate information may fantasise and fear something worse.

12. Be aware of the implications for children, especially when procedures are performed on vulnerable body parts such as the eyes, genital or anal areas. They may have anxieties about this.

13. All children and families are different, with a variety of previous experiences. The preparation must be tailored to fit the particular situation.

14. If siblings are present, then find out from parents what their understanding of the procedure is so that, if necessary, time can be spent with them.

Emergency admissions and procedures often do not allow for effective preparation; it is worth ensuring that a preparation book (a book with a series of descriptive photographs about procedures) is always available.

TYPES OF PLAY

Play in hospital can be based around the work of Sylva (1993) who describes two main categories of play: normative and therapeutic.

The purpose of normative play is to establish norms and rules. This sort of play, which children use most often, engages others, including friends and siblings and uses the toys around the child. Normative play helps to bring familiarity to an unfamiliar situation such as an experience in hospital. Normative play is undertaken voluntarily and is pleasurable. Very rarely does it have any goals and the child is in control. In a safe, relaxed and inviting environment children can feel able to carry out their play.

Therapeutic play is structured by adults and followed through by the child. Its purpose is to help the child to achieve 'emotional and physical well-being' by means of various activities, in order to achieve therapeutic ends. Through play, a child is given the opportunity to overcome fears and anxieties by bringing unconscious feelings to the surface. This play also incorporates desensitisation. A child who developed a needle phobia was able, with great pleasure, to work through his feelings of anxiety by handling and familiarising himself with the properties of a syringe, firstly without a needle, and then progressed to using a needle and injecting into an orange. The mother was also present during this session and felt comfortable handling the syringe and working through her own anxieties relating to her son's treatment.

Puppets allow children to talk about their illness through the third person and are very simple and quick to create; for example, draw a face on your finger and bring the child into conversation. A 3-year-old with cancer was able to express her feelings of anger with ease when encouraged to do so with a finger puppet. She talked to the puppet about the horrible taste of the medicine in her mouth and about how cold it felt when it went into her tummy.

Another 4-year-old with arthritis expressed her anger at her consultant by using 'play-mobile' people. She positioned the characters in such a way that the one she had decided was to become the consultant was in a bed and she was the nurse inflicting pain on him; she squealed with delight when he cried. The most favourite activity postoperatively is 'gunging' the imaginary doctor or nurse with cornflour mixture.

After an uncomfortable procedure has been carried out, silent play or simple discussion using any of the above examples can allow the child to be angry about the invasion of their body in a secure and non-threatening environment.

Needle play

This type of play is used to help children who have fears with any procedure that involves needles of any kind. This is done on a one-to-one basis with the child using real needles in a controlled manner. It leads to a better understanding of the procedure and provides an opportunity for feelings to be discussed. A needle plan can be drawn up depicting how the child wants to sit or whether to have cream or not, etc. This gives the child a feeling of control where they previously felt they had none. As the child psychologist Richard Lansdown wrote in his pamphlet *Helping Children Cope with Needles* (1987), 'the overall aim is to help all children cope by reducing the sensation of pain to one of pressure'. He went on to say that it would be ideal to 'enable all children to keep still (most important for medical and nursing staff) and to come away from the experience without anxiety about the next time'. A qualified play specialist or staff who have attended a 'needle play' workshop should carry out this type of play. In extreme cases a referral to a child psychologist may be necessary.

Messy play

Messy play is an activity that allows children to be as messy as they wish, 'giving considerable pleasure and satisfaction to the sick child. The finished work is admired, bringing self-esteem and a good self image, helping the child to gain confidence and to cope with situations' (Play Focus 2002). This is very beneficial in the clinical environment of the hospital. It is a great kick against the system and an outlet for expression of emotion, be it frustration, anger, despair, loneliness or isolation. Play dough, cornflour and water, and syringe painting all provide therapeutic opportunities for expressive play. A young sibling showed great pleasure in thumping the play dough very hard when her sister was readmitted to the children's ward on her birthday, which was seen as a reflection of her inner feelings.

Use of paintings and drawings may also allow children to express how they are feeling about a situation.

Distraction

Distraction therapy during an unfamiliar procedure helps to limit the anxiety and stress that a child may feel. You must also be aware that not all children like to be distracted and should be given the opportunity to watch if they so choose. This is something which can be discussed prior to the procedure taking place.

Bubbles

Encourage the child to blow the bubbles high and low. Look at colours and shapes within them.

Sticky bubbles

These bubbles can be made into a game of trying to catch them on your finger or how many you can cover the doctor in.

Counting

Use number games; count up and down.

Puppets

Encourage the child to talk about procedures, using the puppet.

Imagination

Talk with the child about their favourite activity or hobby.

Breathing

Encourage the child to control their breathing. Breathe in and hold for a few moments.

Relaxation tapes

Play the tape during a procedure. Gently talk the child through the forthcoming procedure.

Shouting

Allow the child to shout. Shout with the child, if appropriate.

Squeezing

In stressful situations, give the child a ball to squeeze.

Design a distraction box full of bubbles, sticky bubbles, musical toys and interactive books. The items used for distraction must not be readily available for normal play as this will reduce the attention span of the child. Leave the box in the treatment room for easy accessibility.

VISUALISATION

Visualisation exercises can be easily learned and can assist in the care offered to the anxious child (Ott 1996). Visualisation exercises are helpful when undertaken by those familiar with the procedure. They should be used with caution and not by inexperienced practitioners. There are possibilities for such exercises to be done pre- or postoperatively. Such exercises are a useful form of support, which may be used to help children through other stressful times in their life (Ott 1996).

SIBLINGS

Siblings often experience feelings of abandonment, guilt, loss and uncertainty. Introducing play that includes the sibling will go a long way to encourage harmony within the family during an unfamiliar experience of hospitalisation. 'Those who are well informed, and who assume a helping role, seem more able to accommodate the changes in the family and to perceive the experience in positive terms' (Whitaker 2002).

PRAISE AND REWARDS

It is really important to give praise to the children when they have done well. It makes them feel good about themselves. This can be done with a reward of a certificate or a sticker. It is a good idea to call them star patient awards as

bravery implies that one child is braver than the other.

PLAY AND THE WAY FORWARD

Play specialists are now employed on most children's wards across the country. The introduction of a team member who works regular hours and is responsible for creating a safe, fun and non-threatening environment gives the child some normality in an abnormal situation. The ability to create an environment where play occurs naturally is the best gift offered to sick children and their families.

The recently published *National Service Framework for Children, Young People and Maternity Services* (DoH 2004) states that child-centred hospital services should be services that 'consider the "whole child", not simply the illness being treated' and 'are concerned with the overall experiences for the child and family'. It goes on to explain the essential need for play as 'evidence shows that play hastens recovery as well as reducing the need for intervention to be delivered under anaesthesia. The use of play techniques should be encouraged across the multi-disciplinary team with play specialists taking a lead in modelling techniques that other staff can adopt', and that a play service should be able to 'offer a wide variety of play interventions to support the child at each stage of his/her journey through the hospital system'.

The ability to understand the importance and value of play will add a vital component to the skills of the children's nurse, not only on the ward but also en route to theatre, in the anaesthetic room and in all other areas where children are nursed.

References

Broadhurst J 2003 Making changes. NAHPS Journal 33: 10–16

Crawford C, Raven K 2002 Play preparation for children with special needs. Paediatric Nursing 14(8): 27

Department of Health 2004 National Service Framework for children, young people and maternity services. DoH, London

Harris P 1981 Children in hospital (Parts 1 and 2). Nursing Times October 7th and 14th, cited in Broadhurst J 2003 Making changes. NAHPS Journal 33: 10–16

Lansdown R 1987 Helping children cope with needles – a guide for parents and staff, cited in Broadhurst J 2003 Making changes. NAHPS Journal 33: 10–16

Lansdown R 1996 Children in hospital. Oxford University Press, London

Maglacas S 1986 Learning about hospital. Nursing Times January 15th, cited in Broadhurst J 2003 Making changes. NAHPS Journal 33: 10–16

Malcolm P Lifeline playtime in intensive care. An information pamphlet for parents and staff. Great Ormond Street Children's Hospital, London

Morris D 1989 Hospital – a deprived environment for children. A case for hospital play schemes. Save the Children Fund, London

Organisation Mondiale pour l'Education Prescolaire (OMEP) 1966 Play in hospital. Report by the World Organisation for Early Childhood Education, London

Ott M 1996 Imagine the possibilities: guided imagery with toddlers and preschoolers. Pediatric Nursing 22(1): 34–38

Play Focus 2002 Messy play for children in hospital. National Association of Hospital Play Staff, Beaconsfield, Bucks, UK

Sylva K 1993 Play in hospital – when and why it's effective. Current Paediatrics 3: 247–249

Whitaker J 2002 Making connections: play and siblings. NAHPS Journal (Summer)

Wolfer J 1979 Psychological preparation for surgical patients: the effects on children's and parents' stress responses and adjustment. Paediatrics 56: 2

Further Reading

Amylase R 1994 The excellence of play. Open University Press, Buckingham, UK

Cohen D 1993 The development of play. Routledge, London

Collier J 1993 Painful procedures: preparation and coping strategies for children. Maternal and Child Health 9: 282–283

Cook P 1999 Supporting sick children and their families. Baillière Tindall, Edinburgh

Copley B, Forryan B 1997 Therapeutic work with children and young people. Cassell, London

Craft M 1993 Siblings of hospitalized children: assessment and intervention. Journal of Paediatric Nursing 8(5): 289–297

Davenport G 1991 An introduction to child development. HarperCollins, London

Edwards M, Davis H 1997 Counselling children with chronic medical conditions. British Psychological Society Books, Blackwell Science, Oxford, UK

Hogg C, Rodin J 1990 Quality management for children: play in hospital. Play in Hospital Liaison Committee, London

Hughes F 1991 Children, play and development. Allyn and Bacon, Boston, MA

Lansdown R 1990 More than sympathy. Tavistock, London

Lansdown R, Walker M 1991 Your child's development from birth through adolescence. Alfred Knopi, New York

Lowson S 1998 Innovations in paediatric ambulatory care. Palgrave Macmillan, London, p 72–89

Miller S A 1987 Adolescents: promoting self esteem in the hospitalized adolescent. Comprehensive Paediatric Nursing 3: 187

Muller D, Harris P, Wattley L 1999 Nursing children – psychology research and practice. Lippincott Nursing Series, Philadelphia, PA

National Association of Hospital Play Staff 2002 Guidelines for professional practice. NAHPS, Beaconsfield, Bucks, UK

Rodin J 1983 Will this hurt? Preparing children for hospital and medical procedures. Royal College of Nursing, London

Sadler C 1990 Child's play. Nursing Times 86(11): 16–17

Savins C 2002 Therapeutic work with children in pain. Paediatric Nursing 14(5): 14–16

Shuttleworth A 2003 Children first: a health website for children. Nursing Times 99(44): 18–19

Smalley A 1999 Needle phobia. Paediatric Nursing 11(2): 17

Sparshott M 1997 Pain, distress and the newborn baby. Blackwell Science, Oxford, UK

Weller B 1980 Helping sick children play. Baillière Tindall, London

Wolfendale S 2000 Special needs in early years: snapshots of practice. Routledge Falmer, London, ch 4

Appendix 2

Complementary therapies

Julia Fearon

INTRODUCTION

Interest in complementary medicine continues to increase amongst the UK general population (Ernst & White 2000, Harris & Rees 2000, Thomas et al 2001). Although the literature relating specifically to children is scarce and primarily from overseas, it would appear that children and families are utilising complementary medicine, especially for chronic illness such as musculoskeletal disorders, skin, oncological and respiratory disease (Armishaw & Grant 1999, Ernst 1999, Simpson & Roman 2001, Davis & Darden 2003). Many of these conditions are those in which orthodox medicine has limited success in offering sustained relief or for which orthodox treatments have unpleasant side-effects. It would appear also that children and families value complementary medicine for the psychological support it can provide (Kemper 2001, Buckle 2003, Fearon 2003). There is a wide variety of books available on different therapies, targeted at both the lay person and the healthcare professional, as well as a range of courses available from certificate to higher degree level. With this interest and uptake comes the need for careful consideration when introducing the different therapies into nursing care.

This appendix will give a broad overview and definition of some of the more commonly used therapies; identify where and why they may be offered, particularly in relation to some of the procedures discussed in the main text; suggest aims for integrating complementary therapies; consider the question of consent; and provide some cautionary notes about specific therapies. At the end is a list of useful addresses and contacts where further informa-tion can be accessed by the reader. The thera-pies included are aromatherapy, therapeutic massage, reflexology, therapeutic touch, cran-iosacral therapy, visualisation and guided imagery, hypnotherapy and homeopathy.

Defining complementary therapy is notori-ously difficult (Harris & Rees 2000), not least because of the huge number and diversity of treatments and techniques which can be included under the complementary banner. The British Medical Association (1993) identi-fied well over 100. The terms complementary and alternative therapies are often used syn-onymously and many texts will refer to com-plementary and alternative medicine (CAM). The House of Lords (2000) defined CAM as 'a diverse group of health-related therapies and disciplines which are not considered to be part of mainstream medical care'.

It is suggested that children's nurses should utilise the term 'complementary therapies' as it implies that the therapy is an 'adjunct to' main-stream care rather than alternative, which implies being used 'instead of' mainstream care.

Complementary medicine is not new. Some of the principal therapies used today have their roots in ancient times, for example aro-matic plant material is known to have been used over 5000 years ago (Price & Price 1999). Despite the relative antiquity of some thera-pies, it should not be assumed that they are automatically endowed with credibility. How-ever, in the face of increasing patient demand for therapies (Luff & Thomas 2000), orthodox health care is now seeing greater integration of complementary therapies (Prince of Wales's Foundation for Integrated Health 2003). Com-plementary therapies can offer the nurse an enhanced set of tools for practice (Frisch 2001), but nurses must be rigorous in their under-standing of each chosen therapy in order to ensure safe integration of therapies and not fragment existing care (Avis 2003). Nurses should also consider carefully if administra-tion of a complementary therapy is appropri-ate to their nursing role or better delivered by a complementary therapy practitioner. How-ever, there may be complementary therapy techniques which can legitimately be incorpo-rated into nursing practice (Richardson 2001), for example, simple head massage during a hair wash.

Nurses who undertake courses in comple-mentary therapy should not be disheartened by challenges to their therapy, but should con-tinue to develop their knowledge base and reflective skills. They should be rigorous and analytical of the quality of their work and also the literature they may use to argue the bene-fits of their chosen therapies. They should develop their communication and negotiation skills, in order to build a team around them of like-minded people for mutual support, whilst putting forward sound strategies for policy development and subsequent integration and implementation of the therapies. Likewise, they should value their role in furthering the dialogue within the healthcare arena to ensure that the interests and well-being of patients, practitioners and organisations are appropri-ately served. The Royal College of Nursing Complementary Therapies in Nursing Forum is a useful means of networking with other practitioners around the country.

Once implemented, the benefits of therapies should be evaluated and nurses in practice are in the best position to do this. A mechanism for evaluation and also for supervision and sup-port for practitioners by specialists in the field of complementary medicine should be estab-lished (Tavares 2003).

SUGGESTED AIMS OF COMPLEMENTARY THERAPIES IN CHILD CARE

- To improve the quality of a child's experience, communications and continuity of care.
- To enhance the quality of a child's life, in terms of symptom management for acute, chronic and terminal conditions.
- To reduce anxiety and fear that may exacer-bate the child's experience.
- To enhance the relationships between child and nurse, child and parent(s), nurse and family.
- To encourage fun and distraction.

- To improve motivation, alertness and healing potential.
- To provide different approaches to care to empower and enable children to work towards realising their potential.
- To provide an opportunity for nurses to observe and enhance their understanding of child development and behaviours and for the children to learn and understand more of themselves.

Complementary therapies have an important part to play in the care and well-being of children. When offering a therapy, one should be cognisant of the individuality of children and the place each child holds in their family. Every child has their own story to tell and each visit or therapy session may bring different issues. Therefore, the therapist should be alert to the responses, verbal and non-verbal, of children and their families and be skilled in the art of reflective practice.

CONSENT

The question of informed consent is especially pertinent since the publication of the Report of the Public Inquiry into Children's Heart Surgery at Bristol Royal Infirmary (2001). Informed consent for a child to receive a complementary therapy must be obtained in the same way as for any other healthcare intervention. Proof of informed consent is important not just for the child and family's sake but also serves to protect the practitioner in the event of any complaint arising following treatment.

A BRIEF EXPLANATION OF THE THERAPIES

Aromatherapy

Aromatherapy is the use of concentrated, aromatic plant extracts (essential oils) for their therapeutic effects. Essential oils can be extracted from a variety of sources, e.g. flowers, herbs, trees, fruit and roots. René Gattefosse coined the term aromatherapy in the 1930s, but oils and herbs have been used for thousands of years for medicinal purposes

(Ernst 2001, Rankin-Box 2001). The oils are used to treat the whole person. They can be applied in a variety of ways including massage, inhalation, compresses, creams, lotions, baths. They are very concentrated and must be diluted in a carrier oil or cream/lotion before being administered to the skin.

Essential oils affect an individual on a psychological, physiological and cellular level. When applied via massage, the scent of the oil activates the olfactory sense which triggers the limbic area of the brain – that which is concerned with memory and emotion (Ernst 2001). The oil is also absorbed into the bloodstream via the skin. The therapeutic properties of essential oils are thought to relate to responses to the chemical constituents (Price & Price 1999). There are possible harmful effects associated with some constituents and the use of oils that contain them may therefore be contraindicated in certain conditions, such as pregnancy or epilepsy.

Buckle (2003) identified how aromatherapy may offer positive benefits for children:

- Where a child has a learning disability:
  - to promote parent/child bonding
  - to encourage tactile development
  - to improve sleep patterns
  - to promote endorphin production and improve pain relief
  - to empower parents by giving them control over one area of their child's care.
- For children generally, aromatherapy has been shown to:
  - reduce anxiety
  - relieve constipation (Shireffs 2001)
  - help relieve chronic pain and undoubtedly has a supportive and qualitative role to play in the field of children's palliative care.

There is also evidence that some essential oils have antibacterial action (Caelli et al 2001).

Some essential oils are toxic under certain conditions whilst others may cause skin sensitivities. It is important, therefore, that whoever uses the oils has a sound knowledge base and is accountable for their use. They are not the panacea for all ills and should be used with caution by appropriately qualified practitioners. It is important that the recipient likes the smell, because, by virtue of its links with the limbic system, it may evoke memories or emotional reactions or put in place memories for the future – either positive or negative. This is an important consideration in such areas as haematology/oncology where smells may be negatively associated with, for example, chemotherapy and may cause problems for the child and carers if they come into contact with the same smell at a later stage.

The dilutions need to be very much higher for children and even more so in newborn and preterm infants (Tisserand & Balacs 1995) who have fewer layers of epidermis than an older child or adult. Price and Price-Parr (1996) suggest 1 drop of essential oil per 12 kg of body weight to a maximum of 15 drops per 50 ml of base carrier, and a maximum of 8 drops for use in the bath, vaporiser, compress, etc. for a child weighing over 50 kg. The choice of oils is more limited in the younger age group because of the possibility of adverse reactions to some of the constituents of particular oils. This also has implications for the mode of administration. In-depth knowledge of oil derivation, constituents and actions is essential. Likewise, it is necessary to have a good knowledge of anatomy and physiology in order to understand the implications of application, e.g. the structure and development of infant skin, excretory capabilities of the immature kidney, the dynamics of dysfunctional systems and musculoskeletal splinting of an injured or unstable area.

Carrier oils are also of considerable importance, not least because of their varied therapeutic qualities and also their varying dermal uptake (Price & Price 1999). It would appear from anecdotal evidence that some hospitals will only allow the use of arachis (groundnut) oil as a carrier oil. If there is a risk of nut allergy it would seem sensible to use a non-nut derivative such as grapeseed (*Vitis vinifera*) oil instead.

Therapeutic massage

Holey and Cook (2003) describe therapeutic massage as 'the manipulation of the soft tissue of the body by a trained therapist as a component of a holistic intervention'. As a therapeutic intervention, massage can improve health and well-being, especially through a reduction in pain and anxiety (Brownlee & Dattilo 2002). Massage is probably one of the oldest therapies known to man, but it is only in the last 150 years that it has become more formalised into the methodologies we know today. Massage offers a means of communicating through caring touch that is very different from the 'clinical' touch associated with much of nursing (Estabrooks 1992). Touch can also be influential in the development of tactile sensitivity and motor development (Eliot 1999) although as Cullen and Barlow (2002) highlight, touch has not been extensively explored as a vehicle of communication.

Research has demonstrated the benefits of massage for babies and children (Barlow & Cullen 2002) and massage has been shown to improve the outcome for neonates in terms of weight gain, length of stay in hospital and subsequent development (Vickers et al 2000). It has also been shown to reduce cortisol levels (Acolet et al 1993); however, it is important that therapists recognise that preterm infants may be hypersensitive to touch and handling. Nerve pathways and pain modulation in the neonate need to be considered (Melzack & Wall 1994). It may be inappropriate for some neonates to receive massage. Similarly, nurses should be aware that children affected by autism may have heightened (or reduced) sensory responses in any of the five main senses, including touch (Cullen & Barlow 2002) and should consider if it is more or less appropriate to instigate massage for these children.

Permission from a child may be acquired through non-verbal means and it is important to identify this (Russell 1993). For example, babies who have had a difficult delivery or received numerous heel pricks may reject or become distressed by specific contact, which may appear as a threat. Babies should always be approached with respect and openness and if a baby demonstrates, by means of facial expressions or other body language, that the contact is too close, that must be respected. It may be appropriate to make contact via another part of the body.

Careful assessment of need is required, together with awareness of body language (Horgan & Choonara 1996). A child who has a disordered perception of touch, as in abuse, is someone on whom massage must be used with extreme caution, if at all.

Reflexology/reflex zone therapy

Gentle pressure is applied to specific areas or zones of the hands and feet which are believed to correspond with different parts of the body (Ernst 2001). It is suggested that stimulating these zones through specific touch can promote health and well-being (Griffiths 2001). It is said to have been used very successfully in inducing a state of relaxation in an anxious person, in lowering blood pressure (Griffiths 2001), in relieving chronic constipation and encopresis (Bishop 2003) and in other functional disorders such as headache (Ernst 2001).

When working with children, there is a general rule of thumb that they cannot tolerate the same length or depth of treatment as an adult (Bayly 1982). It is important to note that the therapy is not without its contraindications and a practitioner should be cognisant of these.

Therapeutic touch (TT)

This is defined as 'an energy field interaction between two or more people, aimed at re-balancing or re-patterning the energy field to promote relaxation and pain relief and activate self-healing' (Sayre-Adams & Wright 2001).

TT is a therapy based on principles of quantum physics and the notion that we interact with our environment in an 'energetic' way. The view was promoted by Martha Rogers who suggested that human beings may be seen as dynamic energy fields, whole entities, not to be viewed in terms of their parts (Sayre-Adams & Wright 2001). Dr Dolores Krieger, formerly Professor of Nursing in New York University, studied and researched the particular method of 'laying on of hands' and coined the term 'therapeutic touch'. The therapist incorporates non-contact touch with a high degree of 'centredness' to promote balance and well-being. 'Intention' is at the core of the TT process and has been termed a 'healing meditation' (Sayre-Adams & Wright 2001). Ernst (2001) includes therapeutic touch within the spiritual healing modalities and identifies several research studies that yielded positive results and it has been a recognised part of nurse education in the USA for a number of years.

Bach flower remedies

During the early part of the 20th century, Dr Edward Bach, physician and bacteriologist, identified 38 flower remedies, one for each of the most common negative moods or states of mind. Bach flower remedies derive from non-poisonous wild flowers and act as a form of supportive therapy used to establish equilibrium and harmony through the personality, addressing such behaviours as fear, envy, jealousy, guilt, self-recrimination, rigidity of attitude, intolerance, impatience, procrastination, self-pity, and so on (Chancellor 1990).

In order to store the essences, the remedies are preserved in brandy. They should be taken in non-carbonated spring water – although they can be taken neat. Dilution particularly applies to children who would probably find the effect of alcohol on the tongue too strong and unpleasant. Parents must be aware of the alcohol content of the remedies, but since only two to four drops are used at a time it should not be a problem for most parents to accept. Rescue remedy – a combination of five remedies – which offsets the effects of shock and severe anxiety and distress, calming the individual by 'quietening' the autonomic nervous system in response to shock, is probably one of the most useful of all the remedies.

Craniosacral therapy

The technique is a form of therapeutic manipulation developed by J E Upledger in the 1970s based upon concepts derived by W G Sutherland in the 1930s (Ernst 2001). Sutherland believed that restricted movement at the sutures of the skull negatively affects rhythmic impulses of the cerebrospinal fluid as it flows from the cranium to the sacrum. Gentle manipulation of the sutures of the skull and/or of the sacrum is believed to normalise movement restrictions of the skull sutures and therefore normalise cerebrospinal circulation. This in turn can improve the function of the nervous system and relieve a wide variety of symptoms (Upledger 2000). Ernst (2001) describes no well-documented benefits of craniosacral therapy, but conversely identifies several direct and indirect risks of the technique.

Visualisation and guided imagery

Visualisation and guided imagery can be used as coping strategies for reducing anxiety and stress (Payne 2000) and as a means of handling a difficult situation more easily (Ryman 2001), such as prior to venepuncture. It is a form of relaxed, focused concentration and is a natural and powerful coping mechanism. It can be easily learned and used as an adjunct to the care of toddlers and preschool children, as well as older children, who are experiencing anxiety and pain (Bullock & Shaddy 1993, Ott 1996).

There are important steps that should be taken in preparation for the visualisation, which involves the therapist being very relaxed, 'centred' and focused on the child and their needs; the parents should be informed of goals and permission for the visualisation obtained; the therapist should have an open and honest relationship with the child about the visualisation, listen to any expressed concerns and then help the child to refocus their anxiety on the goals and images.

However, this is not a treatment to be used with those who are experiencing emotional instability. It can be harmful to those who are suffering from mental health disorders (Payne 2000), e.g. freely dissociating or acutely psychotic (Ott 1996). However, it can be used to teach the child and parents relaxation techniques and to enable the child to cooperate with treatment, for example immunisations, venepuncture, bone marrow aspirations, biopsies or radiotherapy (Decker & Cline-Elsen 1992). It can improve self-esteem by enabling children to see themselves as having coped positively with a difficult situation.

Hypnotherapy

This is the conscious use of an altered level of consciousness or state of deep relaxation through suggestion to enhance the sense of health and well-being (Rankin-Box 2001). It can be a valuable tool for pain management, reducing anxiety and phobias, and has many potential benefits in child care (Ernst 2001). Whether it can be used effectively in the clinical setting depends largely on the clients' willingness to manage their own health care (Rankin-Box 2001).

Homeopathy

Homeopathic preparations are made by diluting substances from natural sources many, many times in a water and alcohol base. Each successive solution is shaken very vigorously, a process known as succussion (Atherton 2001). Orthodox scientists state that the resulting liquid is nothing more than water, but homeopaths believe the energetic imprint or 'memory' of the original source remains in the substance. The homeopath works on the assumption that you treat like with like. Hence a symptom of vomiting will be treated with an extreme dilution of an emetic. Homeopathy is thought to be extremely safe which is probably why it is one of the more commonly used complementary therapies in children (Ernst 1999, Lee & Kemper 2000, Simpson & Roman 2001). However, nurses should be aware that, in around 20% of cases treated with homeopathy, an aggravation of symptoms will be seen and that some homeopaths will advocate rejection of orthodox treatments such as immunisation (Lee & Kemper 2000, Ernst 2001).

THE 'CLINICAL' ENVIRONMENT

Some therapies can, in part, be taught either to the child or to the parent/carer and so encourage sharing, a sense of responsibility towards the child's own health, empowerment and positive coping mechanisms (Ott 1996). Consideration should be given to the environment in which therapies can be offered in terms of quiet, freedom from outside distraction where possible, privacy, lighting, warmth and so on.

They can be offered in a variety of settings:

- at home – by parents, dually qualified children's community nurses, play specialists, physiotherapists, occupational therapists, etc.
- in hospital wards
- in hospital departments, such as accident and emergency, or outpatient clinics
- general practice surgeries
- hospices
- schools and nurseries.

CONCLUSION

The appropriate integration of complementary therapies into mainstream healthcare settings has the potential to offer much to children and families. For example, helping to provide psychological support for children and families (Buckle 2003, Fearon 2003) and teaching children coping strategies which can stand them in good stead for the future (Burgess 2001, Kemper 2001, Brue & Oakland 2002). To apply them effectively requires sound education and skills acquisition through accredited organisations, together with access to supervision by experienced practitioners. The personal development that accompanies this learning can flourish with encouragement, experience and reflection. The healthcare arena is challenging to the complementary practitioner, but it offers an ideal setting for collaboration, evaluation and advanced patient care.

References

Acolet D, Modi N, Giannakouplopoulos X et al 1993 Changes in plasma cortisol and catecholamine concentrations in response to massage in preterm infants. Archives of Disease in Childhood 68: 29–31

Armishaw J, Grant C C 1999 Use of complementary treatment by those hospitalised with acute illness. Archives of Disease in Childhood 81(2): 131–137

Atherton K 2001 Homeopathy. In: Rankin-Box D (ed) The nurses' handbook of complementary therapies, 2nd edn. Churchill Livingstone, Edinburgh

Avis A 2003 Complementary therapies in nursing, midwifery and health visiting practice: RCN guidance on integrating complementary therapies into clinical care. Royal College of Nursing, London

Barlow J, Cullen L 2002 Increasing touch between parents and children with disabilities: preliminary results from a new programme. Journal of Family Heath Care 12(1): 7–9

Bayly D 1982 Reflexology today – the stimulation of the body's healing forces through foot massage. Thorsons, London

Bishop E 2003 Reflexology in the management of encopresis and chronic constipation. Paediatric nursing 15(3): 20–21

British Medical Association 1993 Complementary medicine: new approaches to good practice. British Medical Association, London

Brownlee S, Dattilo J 2002 Therapeutic massage as a therapeutic recreation facilitation technique. Therapeutic Recreation Journal 36(4): 369–382

Brue A W, Oakland T D 2002 Alternative treatments for attention deficit disorder/hyperactivity: does evidence support their use? Alternative Therapies in Health and Medicine 8(1): 68–74

Buckle S 2003 Aromatherapy and massage: the evidence. Paediatric Nursing 15(6): 24–27

Bullock E A, Shaddy R E 1993 Relaxation and imagery techniques without sedation during right ventricular endomyocardial biopsy in pediatric heart transplant patients. Journal of Heart and Lung Transplantation 39: 215–217

Burgess C 2001 Complementary therapies: guided imagery and infant massage. Paediatric Nursing 13(6): 37–41

Caelli M, Porteous J, Carson C F, Hellier R, Riley T V 2001 Tea tree oil as an alternative topical decolonisation agent for methilicillin-resistant Staphylococcus aureus. International Journal of Aromatherapy 11(2): 97–99

Chancellor P M 1990 Illustrated handbook of the Bach flower remedies. C W Daniel, Saffron Walden, Essex, UK

Cullen L, Barlow J 2002 Kiss, cuddle and squeeze: the experiences and meaning of touch among parents of children with autism attending a touch therapy programme. Journal of Child Health Care 6(3): 171–181

Davis M, Darden P M 2003 Use of complementary and alternative medicine by children in the United States. Archives of Pediatric and Adolescent Medicine 157(4): 393–397

Decker T W, Cline-Elsen J 1992 Relaxation therapy as an adjunct in radiation oncology. Journal of Clinical Psychology 48: 388–393

Eliot L 1999 What is going on in there? Penguin, London

Ernst E 1999 Prevalence of complementary/alternative medicine for children: a systematic review. European Journal of Pediatrics 158(1): 7–11

Ernst E 2001 The desktop guide to complementary and alternative medicine: an evidence based approach. Mosby, Edinburgh

Ernst E, White A 2000 The BBC survey of complementary medicine use in the UK. Complementary Therapies in Medicine 8(1): 32–36

Estabrooks C A 1992 Toward a theory of touch: the touching process and acquiring a touching style. Journal of Advanced Nursing 17: 448–456

Fearon J 2003 Complementary therapies: knowledge and attitudes of health professionals. Paediatric Nursing 15(6): 31–35

Frisch N 2001 Nursing as a context for alternative/complementary modalities. Online Journal of Issues in Nursing, www.nursingworld.org

Griffiths P 2001 Reflexology. In: Rankin-Box D (ed) The nurses' handbook of complementary therapies, 2nd edn. Churchill Livingstone, Edinburgh, p 133–140

Harris P, Rees R 2000 The prevalence of complementary and alternative medicine use amongst the general population: a systematic review of the literature. Complementary Therapies in Medicine 8(2): 88–96

Holey E, Cook E 2003 Evidence based therapeutic massage: a practical guide for therapists, 2nd edn. Churchill Livingstone, Edinburgh

Horgan M, Choonara I 1996 Measuring pain in neonates: an objective score. Paediatric Nursing 8(10): 24–27

House of Lords 2000 Complementary and alternative medicine. Select Committee on Science and Technology, 6th Report. TSO, London

Kemper K 2001 Complementary and alternative medicine for children: does it work? Archives of Disease in Childhood 84(1): 6–10

Lee A C, Kemper K 2000 Homeopathy and naturopathy: practice characteristics and pediatric care. Archives of Pediatrics and Adolescent Medicine 154(1): 75–80

Luff D, Thomas K 2000 Sustaining complementary therapy provision in primary care: lessons from existing services. Complementary Therapies in Medicine 8(3): 173–179

Melzack R, Wall P 1994 Textbook of pain. Churchill Livingstone, Edinburgh

Ott M J 1996 Imagine the possibilities! Guided imaging with toddlers and preschoolers. Pediatric Nursing 22(1): 34–38

Payne R 2000 Relaxation techniques, 2nd edn. Churchill Livingstone, Edinburgh

Price S, Price L 1999 Aromatherapy for health professionals, 2nd edn. Churchill Livingstone, Edinburgh

Price S, Price-Parr P 1996 Aromatherapy for babies and children. Thorsons, London

Prince of Wales's Foundation for Integrated Health 2003 Setting the agenda for the future. Prince of Wales Foundation for Integrated Health, London

Rankin-Box D (ed) 2001 The nurses' handbook of complementary therapies, 2nd edn. Churchill Livingstone, Edinburgh

Report of the Public Inquiry into Children's Heart Surgery at the Bristol Royal Infirmary 1984–1995 Learning from Bristol (the Kennedy Report) 2001 Cmnd 5207(1). TSO, London

Richardson J 2001 Integrating complementary therapies into health care education: a cautious approach. Journal of Clinical Nursing 10(6): 793–798

Russell J 1993 Touch and infant massage. Paediatric Nursing 5(3): 8–11

Ryman L 2001 Relaxation and visualisation In: Rankin-Box D (ed) The nurses' handbook of complementary therapies, 2nd edn. Churchill Livingstone, Edinburgh, p 141–149

Sayre-Adams J, Wright S 2001 Therapeutic touch: theory and practice. Churchill Livingstone, Edinburgh

Shireffs C 2001 Aromatherapy and massage for joint pain and constipation in a patient with Guillain–Barré. Complementary Therapies in Nursing and Midwifery 7(2): 78–83

Simpson N, Roman K 2001 Complementary medicine use in children: extent and reasons. A population based survey. British Journal of General Practice 51(472): 914–916

Tavares M 2003 National guidelines for the use of complementary therapies in supportive and palliative care. The Prince of Wales's Foundation for Integrated Health, London

Thomas K J, Nicholl J P, Coleman P 2001 Use and expenditure on complementary medicine in England: a population based survey. Complementary Therapies in Medicine 9(1): 2–11

Tisserand R, Balacs T 1995 Essential oil safety – a guide for health care professionals. Churchill Livingstone, Edinburgh

Upledger J E 2000 Craniosacral Wirth therapy. In: Novery D W (ed) The complete reference to complementary and alternative medicine. Mosby, St Louis, MO

Vickers A, Ohlsson A, Lacy J B, Horsly A 2000 Massage for promoting growth and development of preterm and/or low birth-weight infants. Cochrane Database of Systematic Reviews (2)CD000390

Further Reading

Mantle F 2004 Complementary and alternative medicine for child and adolescent care. Butterworth-Heinemann, Edinburgh

Useful addresses

Association of Reflexologists
27 Old Gloucester Street
London WC1 3XX

Tel: 0870 567 3320
E-mail: info@aor.org.uk

British Holistic Medical Association (BHMA)
59 Lansdowne Place
Hove
East Sussex BN3 1FL
Tel: 01273 725951
E-mail: bhma@bhma.org

British Hypnotherapy Association
67 Upper Berkeley Street
London W1H 7GH
Tel: 020 7723 4443

Complementary Medicine
Peninsula Medical School
Universities of Exeter and Plymouth
25 Victoria Park Road
Exeter EX2 4NT
Tel: 01392 424872

Craniosacral Therapy Education Trust
78 York Street
London W1H 1DP
Tel/Fax: 07000 785778

Accredited courses for registered nurses, midwives and pharmacists

Institute for Complementary Medicine (ICM)
PO Box 194
London SE16 1QZ
Tel: 020 7237 5165
E-mail: info@icmedicine.co.uk

International Federation of Professional Aromatherapists (IFPA)
82 Ashby Road
Hinckley LE10 1SN
Tel: 01455 637987
E-mail: admin@IFPAroma.org.uk

Natural Medicines Society (NMS)
PO Box 205
Hampton
Middlesex TW12 3WP
Tel: 0870 240 4784
E-mail: enquiries@the-nms.org.uk

Prince of Wales's Foundation for Integrated Health
12 Chillingworth Road
London N7 8QL
Tel: 020 7619 6140
E-mail: info@fihealth.org.uk

Research Council for Complementary Medicine (RCCM)
27a Devonshire Street
London W1G 6PN
Tel: 020 7935 7499
E-mail: info@rccm.org.uk

Society of Homeopaths
4a Artizan Road
Northampton NN1 4HU
Tel: 01604 62262
E-mail: info@homeopathy-soh.org

Index